121

Drugs and Human Behavior

Denise De Micheli
André Luiz Monezi Andrade
Richard Alecsander Reichert
Eroy Aparecida da Silva
Bruno de Oliveira Pinheiro
Fernanda Machado Lopes
Editors

Drugs and Human Behavior

Biopsychosocial Aspects of Psychotropic Substances Use

Springer

Editors
Denise De Micheli
Department of Psychobiology
Universidade Federal de São Paulo
São Paulo, Brazil

André Luiz Monezi Andrade
Department of Psychology
Pontifícia Universidade Católica de Campinas
Campinas, São Paulo, Brazil

Richard Alecsander Reichert
Department of Psychology
Universidade do Vale do Itajaí
Itajaí, Santa Catarina, Brazil

Eroy Aparecida da Silva
Department of Psychobiology
Universidade Federal de São Paulo
São Paulo, Brazil

Bruno de Oliveira Pinheiro
Department of Education
Universidade Federal de São Paulo
Guarulhos, São Paulo, Brazil

Fernanda Machado Lopes
Department of Psychology
Universidade Federal de Santa Catarina
Florianópolis, Santa Catarina, Brazil

The translation was done with the help of artificial intelligence (machine translation by the service DeepL.com). A subsequent human revision was done primarily in terms of content.

ISBN 978-3-030-62854-3 ISBN 978-3-030-62855-0 (eBook)
https://doi.org/10.1007/978-3-030-62855-0

This Springer imprint is published by the registered company Springer Nature Switzerland AG
The registered company address is: Gewerbestrasse 11, 6330 Cham, Switzerland

To Alba Zaluar (in memoriam), who made us look critically to the complexity of the social and human phenomena through contesting simplistic reductionism and emphasizing the importance of formulating public policies based on evidence in favor of a more equal, democratic, and fair world. We are very grateful for her contributions to science and, especially, to this book's writing.

Contents

Contributors

Marcelo Mayora Alves Universidade Federal do Pampa (Unipampa), Santana do Livramento, RS, Brazil

André Luiz Monezi Andrade Pontifícia Universidade Católica de Campinas, Campinas, SP, Brazil

Ilana Andretta Universidade do Vale do Rio dos Sinos, São Leopoldo, RS, Brazil

Karina Borgonovi Silva Barbi Pontifícia Universidade Católica de Campinas, Campinas, SP, Brazil

Beatriz Cortese Barbugli Pontifícia Universidade Católica de Campinas, Campinas, SP, Brazil

André Bedendo Universidade Federal de São Paulo, São Paulo, SP, Brazil

Julia Bernardo Universidade Federal de São Paulo, Guarulhos, SP, Brazil

Flávia Zacouteguy Boos Universidade Federal de São Paulo, São Paulo, SP, Brazil

Silvia Brasiliano Universidade de São Paulo, São Paulo, SP, Brazil

André Amaral Bravin Universidade Federal de Jataí, Jataí, GO, Brazil

Eric C. Brown University of Miami, Miami, FL, USA

Fernanda Calixto Paradigma Centre, Sciences and Behavioral Technology, São Paulo, SP, Brazil

Universidade Federal de São Carlos, São Carlos, SP, Brazil

Fabio Carezzato Universidade de São Paulo, São Paulo, SP, Brazil

Veronica Vidotto Caricati Pontifícia Universidade Católica de Campinas, Campinas, SP, Brazil

João Carlos Caselli Messias Pontifícia Universidade Católica de Campinas, Campinas, SP, Brazil

Janaina Luisi Turisco Caverni Universidade Federal de São Paulo, São Paulo, SP, Brazil

Camila Chagas Universidade Federal de São Paulo, São Paulo, SP, Brazil

Roberto Moraes Cruz Universidade Federal de Santa Catarina, Florianópolis, SC, Brazil

Fernanda Rasch Czermainski Universidade Estácio de Sá, Rio de Janeiro, Brazil

Weridiane Lehmkuhl da Luz Universidade Federal de Santa Catarina, Florianópolis, SC, Brazil

Dianne da Rocha Prado Universidade Federal do ABC, São Bernardo do Campo, SP, Brazil

Andressa Melina Becker da Silva Universidade de Sorocaba, Sorocaba, SP, Brazil

Eroy Aparecida da Silva Universidade Federal de São Paulo, São Paulo, SP, Brazil

Rubens Espejo da Silva Universidade Paulista, São Paulo, SP, Brazil

Daniel da Silva e Silva National Institute on Alcohol Abuse and Alcoholism, Rockville, MD, USA

Rogério da Silva Ferreira CAPS AD III Antônio Carlos Mussum, Rio de Janeiro, RJ, Brazil

Caroline Matilde da Silva Ribeiro Pontifícia Universidade Católica de Campinas, Campinas, SP, Brazil

Pollyanna Santos da Silveira Universidade Católica de Petrópolis, Petrópolis, RJ, Brazil

Fabrício de Araújo Moreira Universidade Federal de Minas Gerais, Belo Horizonte, MG, Brazil

Vívian Vargas de Barros Universidade Federal de São Paulo, São Paulo, SP, Brazil

Luana Martins de Carvalho University of Illinois at Chicago, Chicago, IL, USA

João Mendes de Lima Júnior Universidade Federal do Recôncavo da Bahia, Santo Antônio de Jesus, BA, Brazil

Denise De Micheli Universidade Federal de São Paulo, São Paulo, SP, Brazil

Tassiane Cristine Santos de Paula Universidade Federal de São Paulo, São Paulo, SP, Brazil

Lucas Guimarães Cardoso de Sá Universidade Federal do Maranhão, São Luis, MA, Brazil

Ygor Diego Delgado Alves Universidade Federal de São Paulo, São Paulo, SP, Brazil

Júlio Cézar Gonçalves do Pinho Universidade do Vale do Itajaí, Itajaí, SC, Brazil

Liz Paola Domingues Universidade Federal de São Paulo, São Paulo, SP, Brazil

Hudelson dos Passos Faculdade Guilherme Guimbala, Joinville, SC, Brazil

Vitor Leite Ferreira Universidade Federal de Juiz de Fora, Juiz de Fora, MG, Brazil

Cleusa Pinheiro Ferri Universidade Federal de São Paulo, São Paulo, SP, Brazil

Neliana Buzi Figlie Universidade Federal de São Paulo, São Paulo, SP, Brazil

Antonio Nery Filho Universidade Federal da Bahia, Salvador, BA, Brazil

Gabrielle Fernandes Fronza Pontifícia Universidade Católica de Campinas, Campinas, SP, Brazil

Cainã Gomes Instituto de Psicologia Baseada em Evidências, São Paulo, SP, Brazil

Pedro Paulo Gomes Pereira Universidade Federal de São Paulo, São Paulo, SP, Brazil

Liliana Andolpho Magalhães Guimarães Universidade Católica Dom Bosco, Campo GrandeMSBrazil

Marília Zaluar Passos Guimarães Instituto de Ciências Biomédicas, Universidade Federal do Rio de Janeiro, Rio de Janeiro, RJ, Brazil

Luisa Fernanda Habigzang Pontifícia Universidade Católica do Rio Grande do Sul, Porto Alegre, Rio Grande do Sul, Brazil

Patricia Brunfentrinker Hochgraf Universidade de São Paulo, São Paulo, SP, Brazil

Ian Carlos Hübner Sociedade Educacional de Santa Catarina – Unisociesc, Joinville, SC, Brazil

Dan Josua Instituto de Psicologia Baseada em Evidências, São Paulo, SP, Brazil

Jamir João Sardá Junior Universidade do Vale do Itajaí, Itajaí, SC, Brazil

Luís Pereira Justo Universidade Federal de São Paulo, São Paulo, SP, Brazil

Maria Lorena Lefebvre Universidad Nacional de Tucumán, San Miguel de Tucumán, Tucumán, Argentina

Jan Luiz Leonardi Instituto de Psicologia Baseada em Evidências, São Paulo, SP, Brazil

Renata Thurler Lessa Pontifícia Universidade Católica de Campinas, Campinas, SP, Brazil

Helena Maria Medeiros Lima Universidade de São Paulo, São Paulo, SP, Brazil

Fernanda Beatriz Hodar Lobato Pontifícia Universidade Católica de Campinas, Campinas, SP, Brazil

Fernanda Machado Lopes Universidade Federal de Santa Catarina, Florianópolis, SC, Brazil

Gelsimar Machado Universidade Federal do Espírito Santo, Vitória, ES, Brazil

Mayra Pires Alves Machado Universidade Federal de São Paulo, São Paulo, SP, Brazil

Gabriella Di Girolamo Martins Pontifícia Universidade Católica de Campinas, Campinas, SP, Brazil

Leonardo Fernandes Martins Universidade Salgado de Oliveira, Niterói, RJ, Brazil

Anderson Nazareno Matos Conselho Regional de Psicologia de Minas Gerais, Divinópolis, MG, Brazil

Fúlvio Rieli Mendes Universidade Federal do ABC, São Bernardo do Campo, SP, Brazil

Sheila Giardini Murta Universidade de Brasília, Brasília, DF, Brazil

Gilda Ângela Neves Instituto de Ciências Biomédicas, Universidade Federal do Rio de Janeiro, Rio de Janeiro, RJ, Brazil

Ana Regina Noto Universidade Federal de São Paulo, São Paulo, SP, Brazil

Emérita Sátiro Opaleye Universidade Federal de São Paulo, São Paulo, SP, Brazil

Richard Alecsander Reichert Universidade do Vale do Itajaí, Itajaí, SC, Brazil

Joana Bender Remus Universidade Federal de Santa Catarina, Florianópolis, SC, Brazil

Liana Romera Universidade Federal do Espírito Santo, Vitória, ES, Brazil

Telmo Mota Ronzani Universidade Federal de Juiz de Fora, Juiz de Fora, MG, Brazil

Adriana Scatena Universidade Federal de São Paulo, São Paulo, SP, Brazil

Daniela Ribeiro Schneider Universidade Federal de Santa Catarina, Florianópolis, SC, Brazil

Jaluza Aimèe Schneider Pontifícia Universidade Católica do Rio Grande do Sul, Porto Alegre, Rio Grande do Sul, Brazil

Drielle Feitosa Silva Universidade Federal de Jataí, Jataí, GO, Brazil

Sarah Raphaella Fonseca Silva CAPS AD III Antônio Carlos Mussum, Rio de Janeiro, RJ, Brazil

Marcelo Sodelli Pontifícia Universidade Católica de São Paulo, São Paulo, SP, Brazil

Priscilla dos Santos Peixoto Borelli Tavares CAPS AD III Antônio Carlos Mussum, Rio de Janeiro, RJ, Brazil

Charlene Fernanda Thurow Universidade Federal de Santa Catarina, Florianópolis, SC, Brazil

Camila Vasconcelos Universidade Federal da Bahia, Salvador, BA, Brazil

Victor Distefano Wiltenburg Universidade Federal do ABC, São Bernardo do Campo, SP, Brazil

Adriana Mokwa Zanini Instituto Porto Alegre da Igreja Metodista, Porto Alegre, RS, Brazil

Part I
Introductory Aspects and Main Concepts

Chapter 1
Humanity and the Use of Substances: A Historical Overview

Helena Maria Medeiros Lima

Introduction

The history of the use of substances by mankind brings a specific cut: the chronology of discovery, uses and man-object-drug relationships, and the paradigms involved. If, for example, in Greece the drug itself was considered just another object in the world, indifferent per se, and its adjectivation as beneficial or malefic depended only on the quantity ingested, we reach the Middle Ages with the demonization of the drug object and the concomitant elevation of the substances to the category of "malefic objects." If the pagan use advocated freedom and recreational, medicinal and relaxing uses, with shamans protagonists of various possibilities of treatment and healing with the use of substances, after the advent of Christianity and the symbiotic alliance Church-State any unauthorized uses by the Church were considered heretical and condemned non-medical, curious, shamans, and consults to gallows, bonfires or decapitation (Castro 2002, 2008).

The records of the ancestral use of substances are accessible to us in contemporaneity by different means: fossils, hieroglyphs, painting—which, until the advent of photography, was, along with sculpture and ceramics, the means of documentation of medical and humanitarian facts (Couto 2013)—with the invaluable contribution of fields of knowledge such as Paleo and Ethnobotany, Anthropology, Medicine, Psychology, Law, History, Literature, as well as Religions.

The systematic consumption of a large set of substances capable of altering the behavior, consciousness, and mood of human beings is proven to be millennial. However, its elevation to the category of social problem is historically recent, just under a century ago (Labate 2008). One of the greatest authors in the history of drug use in humanity is Antonio Escohotado, who in his work *General History of Drugs*

H. M. M. Lima (✉)
Universidade de São Paulo, São Paulo, SP, Brazil
e-mail: helenali@usp.br

D. De Micheli et al. (eds.), *Drugs and Human Behavior*,
https://doi.org/10.1007/978-3-030-62855-0_1

(Escohotado 2000) did a thorough socio-anthropological-biomedical survey on drugs published to date and expanded the studies to include socio-political and legal analysis.

It is considered important to study the way in which the use of substances takes on varied features in different times and cultures, in the context of which individual needs are formed (MacRae 2010). There is a *naturalization* of the prohibitive character when it comes to drugs. The historical amnesia that feeds the prohibitionist rhetoric of converting "drugs" into absolute evil no longer considers that many of them played a central role in the configuration of the world we know today: sugar, tea, coffee, tobacco, alcohol (Simões 2008). Not to mention the non-problematic use of drugs like opium, cocaine, hemp, psilocybin (Escohotado 2004). The construction of prohibitionist policy is directly linked to politics, religion, and economic relations in each society, as will be seen here, having been initiated with the literal "witch hunt."

It is worth mentioning that not every drug user is or will become "addicted," with dependence being a statistical minority in relation to the total number of users in the world (Nery 2019b). The attribution of the beneficial/malefic character of the substance is essentially determined by the social and historical context. There is a double moral when talking about drugs; from the adulteration of compounds to the "cause–effect" link among violence, criminality, and drug use that configures a scenario of terror and simplification: *drug use sustains criminality*, a phrase that needs to be constantly deconstructed. The diversity of uses and consumptions mirrors our own cultural diversity; all cultures start from the enormous diversity of practices, representations, symbols and arts of Brazil and the world. Drugs are and are in different cultures and times, so they cannot be understood outside of them (Labate 2008).

The relationship between the use of substances and different existential aspects such as suicide, death (euthanasia), festivities, sources of energy, escape/ cushioning, science and magic, art and religion, makes the work of historicization infinite, depending on the aspect addressed. Here will be presented a timeline, from the tenth century BC to the present day, considering the paleontological, anthropological, and historical records recognized by science.

Timelines as a Way of Reading History

The not very extensive specific bibliography on the subject brings two forms of record: the chronological, by times and ages, and the thematic record, by type of drug over time. Here a reading of the timeline will be presented, with the records ordered chronologically and following the classification of the periods according to General History. The articulation with History brings inevitable priorities, considering the already mentioned naturalization of prohibitionism, the emphasis on human relations in the different forms of substance use and the silenced role of the shamans (Castro 2008). These, throughout history, range from protagonists to charlatans, from community leaders to outcasts, and even today—particularly in the peripheries of Brazil's large cities and in most of the 54 countries on the African continent—are references in terms of attention, treatment, and existential support for a broad mass of people (Lima 2018).

Definitions and practices related to substances are historical and cultural products, which refer to particular modes of understanding, experimentation, and engagement in the world (Simões 2008); sociocultural scenarios involve the whole concept in the field of substance use: Moral and cultural factors have a determining action in the constitution of the regulating or structuring patterns of consumption of all types of substances (Labate 2008); the subject must be approached from a multidisciplinary perspective, since its understanding involves the consideration of several aspects, such as pharmacological, psychological, and sociocultural, without disregarding the risks and biochemical complexities of the use of substances—but it is necessary to open more space for reflection beyond Biology. The increase in the pharmaceutical industry and the various strategies for improving adherence to treatments for acute and chronic diseases highlights the sophistication of research in Chemistry, Biochemistry, and Human Physiology, but it is also increasingly difficult to maintain patients under treatment when only the intake of tablets is considered as a focus (Lima 2012, 2018).

Contemporary tele-tecno-media (Fernández 2009) brings imperatives of success aimed at productivity, materiality, and the accumulation of goods as synonyms of success and, not by chance, the painful counterpart in suffering. What are the names of suffering in the face of drug use? How is it necessary to evaluate and think about the responsibility of the subject and the social field in such complex issues? (Dunker 2015; Ribeiro 2019; Rosa 2016).

How is this systematization carried out and in what way does the triumphalist official discourse of success in the face of the seizure of tons of drugs confront realities like the so-called Cracolândia in São Paulo—Brazil? Does the enunciation of the drug user as a "bandit" start from which social sectors and how does this nomination contribute to the maintenance of the problems in which drugs, violence, social ties, and punishment are directly articulated?

The World Health Organization brings the suicide epidemic as the highest in history (World Health Organization 2019). In this journey, drugs considered legal such as alcohol, caffeine, yerba mate and tobacco, great allies of both professionals in the market and *homeless*, population on the street, live side by side with amphetamines, barbiturates, hypnotics (legally sold under prescription), *crack,* cocaine, marijuana, MMDA,[1] and other drugs considered illegal in a society where the slogan is consumption.

Political control and determination over the harm and benefits of individual drug use and social impact have been increasingly distanced from biochemical or molecular factors: the economic empire, taxes, billions in money circulating through legalization or illegality of certain substances are preponderant factors when one thinks of the global dimension of the phenomenon. Prescribed or licit drugs, such as

[1] 3-methoxy-4,5-methylenedioxyamphetamine; 5-methoxy-MDA.

anxiolytics, hypnotics, alcohol, and tobacco, which are known to cause more dependency and are responsible for more social problems, do not have the same stigma as certain drugs considered illicit, such as marijuana and cocaine, despite the studies and results that point in opposite directions (Araújo 2012; Lima 2012; Seibel 2010).

From shamans (Castro 1986, 2008; Narby and Huxley 2004) to tobacco chewers to the present day[2]ices, from the records of the first seeds and rituals to contemporary pills, from Prehistory to raves, facts about the different relationships established between people and drug objects will be presented here. Relationships of pleasure, delight, abstraction, inspiration, party, studies, research—and the counterpart, sufferings, stigmas, evils, according to human possibilities and stories (Nery 2017).

The assumption sustained here is that *people* establish relationships with drugs, as well as establish policies and norms about what is allowed and what is prohibited at any given time, in any given place, the punishments and labels (Nery 2019a).

Puritanism as explanatory system, although quite widespread, do not contribute to a scientific and methodical debate. Despite the growing recognition of the relevance of approaches, studies and research that emphasize the cultural aspects of drug use, there is still a tendency to give greater legitimacy to studies on the subject developed in the health sciences, such as medicine, pharmacology, biology, biomedicine (Labate 2008). Social approaches tend to be taken more into consideration when they are carried out in the field of crime, trafficking, urban violence or poverty, and are devalued when they directly address the issue of drug use and cultural uses, as well as the complete social demoralization of shamans (Castro 2008; MacRae 2010; Narby and Huxley 2004).

Thinking about drugs is also thinking about human suffering. Suffering is reflected as a significant aspect of the human condition, not with the perspective of reducing or naturalizing it, but of being attentive to it, understanding ways of assigning meaning, reframing, intensifying, and prioritizing care. Besides relating this issue also to drug use as an attempt to alleviate some level of suffering and the reflections that permeate from the debates of bioethics, harm reduction, and subject autonomy, it is necessary to broaden the debates beyond prejudices, moral impositions, and pseudo-scientific misrepresentations (Nery 2019a).

The drug concept is quite complex. The very etymology of the term drug is considered one of the most controversial (Vargas 2008): among the various hypotheses raised, from the Latin *drogia*, the Arabic *durâwa,* and the Celtic *druko,* for example, the Dutch hypothesis brings the term drug as a word derived from the Dutch *droghe vate,* which means "barrels of dry things" and whose use would be registered since the fourteenth century. This hypothesis allows us to situate the emergence of the word in the last centuries of the Middle Ages, in the "aftermath" of the Crusades,

[2] *Ice*: is a methamphetamine developed in the Far East, used as a liquid, with a drop in the tip of the cigarette; its potency ensures an effect that lasts for several hours with an administration, or for a day or more using larger doses, providing hyperexcitation that the Japanese, Chinese and Indonesians (major consumers) balance with large quantities of alcohol and pharmaceutical sedatives (Escohotado 2004).

when the societies of courtship and the "civilizing" process entered into development in the Western world (Castro 1977; Labate 2008).

In this chapter, *drugs are* considered—psychoactive or not—substances which, instead of being "overcome" by the body (and absorbed as a simple nutrient), are capable of "overcoming" it, causing—in insignificantly small doses compared to those of other foods—major organic, psychic or both types of alterations (Escohotado 2004).

According to Nery (2017), we are unique and in this existential particularity we have tastes, experiences, schools, affinities, and disaffections. The difference in our choices marks and characterizes us. When the subject chooses a drug, that choice has to do with his life story. Whether by boredom or suppressed desire, our stories determine our choices. Instead of considering the user as an object, without will, without capacity, without any possibility of discernment, here the user is considered as a human being: with possibilities, choices, and limits (Lima 2012).

The time travel of this chapter brings information that does not always circulate when talking about drugs: The effective use promoted by the shamans in several continents; the fact that there has been, since prehistoric times, the adulteration of substances and this is a public concern; to know that the use of injectable drugs has already been public and a symbol of status, which can be inferred from finding gold cases and syringes, referred to as precaution and increased safety margins for users; to remember that the non-problematic use of countless substances has proven to be more the rule than the exception; that accidental dependencies and fatal overdoses occurred in much smaller numbers than imagined by contemporary media discourses; that the transformation of the drug from *object* to *subject in* the imaginary and in prohibitive policies (subsidizing the "War on Drugs" paradigm or Prohibitionism), far from being "natural," is a construct based on several factors and not related to a real, biochemical, inexorable danger of the *drug object*. To know that dependence is a condition in which some people arrive according to their needs, their relationship with the world, their condition of life and, finally, that the initial movement towards drug use is always the subject, the human being (Nery 2018).

Reiterating the inorganic character of the drug object and emphasizing the role of the human being in the use, labeling, evaluation, and stigmatization of this object is one of the objectives of this chapter.

Drugs: Concepts and Prejudices

It is important for this journey through time to remember that the Greek word for drug is *pharmakon*, while *pharmakós*, changing only the final letter and the accent—means *scapegoat*. According to Escohotado (2004), far from being a coincidence, this manifests to what extent in our early days medicine, religion, and magic are inseparable. The oldest fusion of these three dimensions, shamanism, an institution originally spread throughout the planet, whose meaning is to minister techniques of ecstasy, meaning ecstasy a trance that eliminates the barriers between vigil and dream, the sky and the subsoil, life and death; taking a drug, or giving it to another, the shaman throws a bridge between the common and the extraordinary, which serves both for magical divination and religious ceremonies, for therapies and cures (Castro 1986, 2008; Escohotado 2004; Lima 2018; Narby and Huxley 2004).

The purely physiological effect of the drug is considered to matter little, since it is a question of understanding the interpretation that the individual gives of his experience, his state and the motivation that drives him to repeat drug use (MacRae 2010; Castro 2008). Instead of just asking about *when* humanity began to use drugs, one can add to the question of *why* this use took place—and so we approach religious and therapeutic/healing activities, especially the figure of the shamans and the non-casual silence of these leaders and their practices throughout history (Araújo 2012; Castro 1977, 1986, 2008).

Before Civilizations: The Prehistoric Drug Registries

In the Andean civilization, a plant that appears represented in ceramics since the tenth century BC is the so-called St. Peter: a cactus that usually contains mescaline, although some species contain DMT (dimethyltryptamine)—alkaloid with a fast and intense effect (Escohotado 2004). St. Peter is the "doorman" of Christian heaven—giving this name to a pagan drug, used for religious gathering and divination purposes, shows the shamanic gaze over herbs and plants (Narby and Huxley 2004).

The first Mesopotamian reference to hemp was only made in the ninth century BC, in the Assyrian domain, with the use being mentioned as incense; the open brazier was already frequent among the Scythians, who threw large pieces of hashish on heated stones and closed the enclosure to prevent the smoke from coming out, a technique similar to that used by the Egyptians for their *kiphy,* another ceremonial incense loaded with hemp resin.

When one thinks of the period before writing and civilization, in front of the paleontological registers it is important to highlight the wide diffusion and constancy of the use of the most diverse substances to provoke alterations in the psychic and behavioral functions of human beings (MacRae 2010). According to Escohotado (2004), the poppy plantations in southern Spain, Greece, northwestern Africa, Egypt, and Mesopotamia are probably the oldest on the planet. The opium extracted from there has up to three times more morphine than in the Far East.

Since prehistory, members of different human cultures have known how to use plants and some substances of animal origin to cause changes in consciousness for a variety of purposes. In archeological sites from 8000 B.C. onwards, there is firmer evidence that psychoactive plants were already part of man's life (Araújo 2012), who used stimulating plants in funerary and visionary rituals in religious cults; consumed drinks with opium and cultivated poppy to produce it; drew hallucinogenic lotus flowers in pots; and made ropes and fabrics with *Cannabis sativa* fibers. According to Flandrin and Montanari (1998), the oldest known recipe is a beer production recipe (with barley malt as the main ingredient) and is credited to Sumerians around 8000 BC. A drawing of the Sumerians dated 4000 B.C., with two men and their straws around a pitcher, is interpreted as a record of prehistoric beer consumption.

The first written reference to the poppy (known as 'slumber') appears in Sumerian plates of 3000 B.C., by means of a word that also means "to enjoy"; Egyptian hieroglyphs already mention medicinal uses of opium, with reference to the juice extracted from the poppy's head, opium, recommended as an analgesic and soothing agent, in rectal and oral ointments and, according to Ebers' papyrus, "to prevent babies from shouting loudly." Egyptian opium or "Thebes" symbolizes the highest quality in the entire Mediterranean basin, mentioned even by Homer in the Odyssey as "something that makes you forget any suffering" (Escohotado 2004).

According to paleobotanical scholars, remains of hemp fiber dated 4000 B.C. show that the fiber was already used for therapeutic purposes.

In America dozens of hallucinogenic plants are known: records from 7000 b.C., in colonies, the Paleobotanists have already found corresponding seeds (spores and hyphae) of hallucinogenic mushrooms, especially *Amanita muscaria.* From the tenth century B.C. there are stone mushrooms among the monuments of the Izapa culture in present day Guatemala, which continued to be carved by different parts of Central America for more than a 1000 years; it is also in the tenth century B.C. that activities of the Chavin culture, whose headquarters was present day Peru, date back to certain stone carvings holding a hallucinogenic cactus (Araújo 2012).

The coca bush originates from the Andes and, since the third century B.C., there are sculptures of faces with swollen jaws by chewing their leaves; guarana and mate (containing caffeine) and cocoa (containing theobromine) are also American; in India and Indonesia similar effects are obtained thanks to betel, a drug little known in the West. In China, tea and ephedra, a concentrated stimulant, have been used for 4 or 5 millennia. From Africa, *kola nut* (a coffee stimulant) and *kat* (a bush consumed in Yemen, Somalia, and Ethiopia) originate.

From the fourth century b.C. there is a ceramic deer-shaped pipe—which has a *peyote* button between its teeth. Texts from Mesopotamia and Syria, dating from 3000 and 2000 b.C. bring descriptions of banquets where alcoholic beverages were considered indispensable. It is considered that practically all civilizations invented some beverage fermented with the raw material they had within their reach, the oldest being a kind of Chinese wine, dated 7000 b.C., with herbs and spit-up rice (Narby and Huxley 2004).

Most Shamanic religions, which predominated before the Christian era, had cults involving the use of psychoactive substances. In the oldest sacred books that exist, the *Rig Veda* (base of Hinduism), the same word was used to designate god and drug: sum. The drink was consumed as a fundamental part of the cult; with time, the ecstasy caused by the psychoactive lost importance in the ritual, which began to use plants without psychoactive effect. The original plant was considered to be *Amanita* muscaria, the red "hat" mushroom and white spheres. The hallucinogenic power of this mushroom was cultivated by the tribes of Siberia—some rituals involved the indirect consumption of the drug, drinking the urine of the shaman who had consumed it (Araújo 2012; Narby and Huxley 2004).

Also in the *Rig Veda*—with hymns radically opposed to any alcoholic beverage—they speak of *ebriety* as the one that "lifts the chariot from the winds." Ebriety is sometimes a religious experience—others only hedonistic—that the ancient man practices with various psychoactive substances (Escohotado 2004). Within sacramental ebriety, *possession* and *travel* are distinguished:

1. Ebriety of possession is that which induces to raptures of body frenzy in which the critical conscience disappears, in the use of alcohol, tobacco, belladonna, and similar drugs; accompanied by music and violent dances, these raptures are all the more reparative the less they resemble lucidity and memory; is the ebriety that reigns in Africa, and from this center has possibly passed to the Mediterranean and the great Indonesian arch of islands; in historical times, arrived in America with the slave trade, under names like voodoo, candomblé or *mandinga*;
2. Briefness of travel is based on drugs that potentiate the senses without erasing the memory: its use can be accompanied by music and dance, but above all it arouses a conscious, introspective psychic incursion before or after. This is ebriety proper shamanic, having been initiated in Central Asia, expanding to America, the Pacific and Europe.

In Western Europe, in the seventh century BC, the Celts of today's Marseilles region traded ropes and hemp tow with the entire Mediterranean; archeological finds (data obtained and analyzed by Paleobotanists) in the area include several pipes and the druids' fame as medicine connoisseurs indicate that this culture probably knew its use as a conscientious altered (Escohotado 2004; MacRae 2010).

The use of alcoholic beverages, therefore, goes back to this prehistoric period and its use as a medicine was already mentioned in the cuneiform writing tablets of Mesopotamia in 2200 BC. About 15% of the almost 800 ancient Egyptian medicines included beers or wines in their composition; there are also numerous references to wine in the Old Testament.

Greek Civilization

The Greeks inaugurate an intermediate type of society, in which population density is compatible with respect for individual freedom. In this scenario, the Hypocratic school presents disease and cure as a result of natural processes; by separating magic and religion from medicine, the Hypocratic denies the validity of any cure based on the symbolic transference of evil from someone to another—it therefore breaks with the institution of the *scapegoat*. The new medicine uses the appropriate *pharmakon* or drug for the cure of the problem, instead of the *pharmakós* (scapegoat). Drugs are *substances that act by cooling, heating, drying, contracting, relaxing, making you sleep*. The essential and differential of each one is the proportion between active dose and deadly dose—*because it is the quantity that distinguishes the medicine from the poison* (Escohotado 2004). Thus, the drugs were seen as basically neutral, their effects, positive or negative, being dependent on the dosage and the way of use (MacRae 2010). No substance was good or bad in itself, and the way to use it was to say whether its effects were benign or malignant. The essential notion is that *the danger is not in the drug, but in the way it is used*, not only in the pharmaceutical context, but also in the social, religious, and political environment (Araújo 2012; Lima 2018).

For the Greeks, the medicinal, religious, and social use of drugs had more or less the same condition, with the exception of wine. Besides wine, the Greeks used for ceremonial and playful purposes beers, hemp, belladonna, mandrake, in smoking or incense, and an extract of hashish with wine and myrrh for specific stimuli. However, the most popular drug was opium, the first mention of this drug in Herodotus' time; Hippocrates baptized it as *opós mekonos,* "sleeping juice," "capable of calming any pain."

Theriaka or *triaga* was the name of the antidotes, since in Antiquity poisoning was an obsession. It was a Greek remedy made of opium, used as vitamins in the contemporary world—to prevent diseases. Together with pure poisons like hemlock and aconite, in homeopathic doses, opium composes all the antidote potions (Araújo 2012; Escohotado 2004). From the first reference to opium to even the elaboration of the triages, *there is not a single reference of someone harmed by its use*. Every possible danger to a drug was concentrated in wine, for the Greeks. Important debates in philosophical schools were dedicated to the nature of wine: if it had been granted to drive humans crazy or for their good—wine was forbidden to women and men under 30 (Escohotado 2000).

Elleusis

The Mysteries of Elleusis was, for about 2000 years, the spiritual symbol of Greek culture. Initiation took place in the temple of the Greek city of Elleusis, annually, until the year 400. In the autumn, at night, and the pilgrims (*epoptés*) received a potion, the *kykéon*, composed of flour and peppermint, in addition to taking an oath for their lives to keep the details of the experience absolutely secret (MacRae 2010; Escohotado 2004). The average attendance was 2000–3000 people each fall and initiation was forbidden to murderers. This ritual was known as one of the greatest mysteries of the classical era. The promise was never to talk about what was going on inside.

Several researchers consider that it had some psychoactive principle, possibly the *ergote*, a fungus that is found in the wheat of the region until today, and that would explain the profound effect of the experience. In the 1960s an ethnobotanist, a chemist and a specialist in classical Greece presented an answer to the "Mysteries of Elleusis." Comparing what was known about the time and the ritual with the variety of cereals in the region and the knowledge about drugs developed until that decade, they concluded that the cult involved the consumption of *ergot* or *ergote*, a fungus that produces hallucinogenic substances from which LSD developed in 1938. Ergot is a common pest of wheat and other cereal species, including some common in this region of Eleusis; the toxins of this fungus are water soluble, and capable of producing powerful hallucinations without causing unwanted side effects. According to these scholars, the ergot dissolved in the flour with water that the participants drank at the beginning of the cult would then be a secret ingredient and the cause of the mystical experience that the Greeks enjoyed together (Araújo 2012; Escohotado 2000). The Elleusian religion, based on a single act of great intensity, oriented towards producing an ecstatic experience of death and resurrection, is considered as an ingenious adaptation of ancient shamanic rites to the new Greek culture, as a bridge between the so-called natural cults, proper to villages, and the civil (purely formal) cults that were beginning to consolidate in cities.

Romans and Christianity

The Greeks' view of the psychoactive has been fully assimilated by Roman civilization. It is the wine that will give rise to personal and collective conflicts, as Plato suggests, in Rome the use of wine was forbidden to women and those under 30. Men of that age could drink, and those over 50, until they got drunk "to deal with the difficulties and boredom of old age" (Escohotado 2000).

The only general precept on the subject, in force from republican times until the decadence of the Empire, the *lex Cornelia*, says textually: *Drugs are an indifferent word, where both what is used to kill, and what is used to cure, and the filters of love, but this law only reproves what is used to kill someone* (our griffon).

The *sobria ebrietas* (sober ebriety), seen as a form of self-knowledge, led to relaxation with dignity (MacRae 2010). The *pharmakon* of the Hypocratic school was maintained and developed by Roman doctors; the *theriaka*, with opium, became very popular in the Roman Empire, being widely used by emperors, such as Marcus Aurelius—who began the mornings with a portion of opium "big as an Egyptian bean and diluted in tepid wine" (Araújo 2012.

Opium was consumed in large quantities throughout the Empire, being its sale taxed and its price fixed by the government, to avoid speculation and capital flight. Opium from Mesopotamia and Egypt was considered of better quality, and in the year 312 there were 793 drug stores in Rome, which gave the government 15% of the total taxes collected in the city. According to Araújo (2012), there are no records of health problems caused by the use of the substance among the Romans, in which opium was used in agonic therapy and as a euthanasia. It was during this period that the demand for the drug exceeded supply, and its adulteration was frequent (Escohotado 2000). Adding to the substances similar elements in appearance (to increase quantity and profit) is a concern and a habit since it is understood the use of any substance by humanity. The "baptism" of drugs can be extremely harmful when, for example, glass powder is added to cocaine powder, pool cleaning liquid in merla, mix.

This consumption does not create problems of public or private order. Opium consumers do not exist either as clinical cases or as outcasts in society. The custom of using this drug is no different from any other custom, such as dawn, exercise, going out or staying at home—and for this reason there is no Latin expression equivalent to "opiomaniac."

Hemp was smoked at social gatherings, but the plants most consumed for their medicinal and psychoactive effects were the poppy and the vine. However, Rome's great contribution to the history of drugs is considered her alliance with Christianity, which in the fourth century became the official religion of the Empire.

Christianity and Witch Hunt

Like the shamanic religions, whose disciples ingested psychoactive drugs to find or talk to God, Christians have in wine a constant in their rituals. The role of alcohol in Christianity was more symbolic than practical: while the ancient religions used drugs to produce drunkenness, which was their own mystical experience, Christians relied on the Eucharist itself as the source of this state of mind. Religious ecstasy was no longer provided by an external agent, but by the exercise of faith, of autosuggestion (Araújo 2012).

The tendency to transfer the importance of drugs to rituals and their priests included religions whose tradition required drinking hallucinogenic plants. The ritual became more important, to the detriment of the delirium caused by drugs. Christianity not only abandoned but prohibited the use of substances with these effects; its doctrine preached suffering and mortification of the pleasures *of the flesh* as a form of approaching God.

The need for Christianity to establish itself as the dominant religion in Europe and its surroundings was another reason for prohibiting and persecuting the use of herbs for medicinal and, above all, hallucinatory purposes. They used the biblical argument *"You shall not let sorcery survive"* to persecute shamanic leaders who provided healing and trance through plants (Escohotado 2004; Narby and Huxley 2004). In 392, when Christianity became the official religion of the Roman Empire, the Church took effective steps to extinguish the competition represented by other religions. Between 424 and 589 several Roman laws and Christian decrees emerged that inaugurate the official persecution of all kinds of shamans, leaders of other religions and herbalists. The penalties varied from execution to the sale of the accused as slaves. Possession of any plant or book for herbal use was sufficient evidence of crime; many centuries before marijuana was called "devil's herb," all medicinal plants had already been demonized by the Church. The penalties extended to those who consulted with these people for any purpose; Catholic bishops also incited the burning of temples of other religions and entire libraries, such as that of Byzantium and the Basilica of Julian. In 391 Bishop Theophilus incited the burning of the Library of Alexandria, with 120,000 volumes, an incalculable loss to humanity (Escohotado 2004). Fire was used as an instrument of purification for many centuries.

The Christianization of the Roman Empire led to the collapse of ancient pagan notions about drug neutrality, sober ebriety, self-medication, and the boundary between morality and law. The priests of the new state religion began to persecute worshippers seen as rivals, trying to obliterate any trace of their old beliefs and practices, including their vast pharmacopeia (MacRae 2010). Drugs began to be stigmatized for their association with magical and religious cults, as well as for therapeutic uses to alleviate suffering—since pain and the mortification of the flesh were conceived by Christians who were in power as a form of approach to God.

The pursuit of pharmacological knowledge was such that in the tenth century (when Church and Empire had already become a unit) the use of drugs for therapeutic purposes became synonymous with heresy. All the rites of the Mediterranean came to be considered *treaties with satanic powers* (Araújo 2012; Escohotado 2000). The search for healing was limited to the use of resources of purely symbolic efficacy, such as "mummy dust," "unicorn horn dust," in addition to ecclesiastical indulgences, holy oils, candles, and holy water.

Criminalization and Stigma of Substance Use

Christianity has brought suffering, martyrdom, and pain as values of closeness to God. The Christian faith proclaims a considerable measure of affliction, because pain is grateful to God; what is not to alleviate momentary pathologies is unworthy flight; all ebriety implies guilty weaknesses. The goal of a *timely* death is condemnable. Pagan knowledge, especially concerning drugs, is considered contaminated by witchcraft; St. Augustine declares that "scientific eagerness is, in itself, insane curiosity" (MacRae 2010). An edict of King Hilderico warns that the use of diabolical plants is a betrayal of the Christian faith; Charlemagne calls opium "the work of Satan." The criminalization of the use of substances is beginning according to the apostle Paul, it *is necessary to eliminate all stimulus to "relaxed behavior."* Sects such as the Tacians, Marcionites, and Aquarius, in which drinking constitutes a mortal sin, are rigorously abstemious (Araújo 2012).

In a few centuries Europe has gone back a millennium. Natural disasters and feudalism caused many villages to be abandoned, no real trade, collapse in incipient industry, impossible communications; the prolongation of this state of affairs suggests the search for *causes* for "so much disaster". They begin to put the cause of the problems on the witches—and at that time shamanistic traditions have resurfaced in isolated nuclei and in the poorest counties, where fewer nobles and clerics pass through. The expression "witch hunt" began in this scenario—at the same time, in the Islamic world a greater tolerance to the use of substances persisted—except the restriction to the use of alcohol.

The crusade against witches shows that persecution can multiply to infinity. When Europe had about 3 million inhabitants, the Catholic and Protestant inquisitors burned 500,000 people alive between the fifteenth and seventeenth centuries, confiscating the possessions of so many millions more. Few humanists disagreed with the inquisition. This war can be seen as an attempt at control launched by the rural nobility and the clergy at the height of the urban bourgeoisie and national monarchies, a great change that is heralded in the West, demolishing the logic of the inexorable destiny determined by birth.

Meanwhile, in Islam..

Islam dictates precepts about food, schedules, and drugs; however, there are no *sacred drugs* (such as the wine of mass), nor any *sacrilegious drugs*. In relation to alcohol, drunkenness is deplored because *it makes the person ridiculous and fallacious*. Opium is used as a euthanasic, having a dominant place in the pharmacopoeia. The triaga magna is resumed, and several books on medicinal botany and pharmacy appear. It is the Arabic translators, the schools of Toledo and Sicily, who return to the West the part of pagan knowledge that was able to escape the incendiary fervor (already mentioned) of the first Christians.

The rapid expansion of Islam spreads the opium from Gibraltar to Malaysia, taking Turkish and Iranian plantations as producer nuclei (Escohotado 2000). By the ninth century, consumers were already in the habit of eating and smoking opium, in addition to consuming it in grape syrups mixed with hashish. The Arab culture uses opium as a general euphoriant, recommended for transit from the second to the third age.

According to Escohotado (2004), in the eleventh century Hassan Ibn Al-Sabbah founded the order of *haschischins*. Model for European orders of cavalry, as Templars, their members received abundant amounts of opium before leaving for combat: hence the word "assassin." The *haschischins* were not murderers, they were warriors, less cruel and arbitrary than their enemy. As for hemp, it is not mentioned in the Koran, being called *bangah* in the eleventh century Arabia (Seibel 2010). It is advised in pharmacopeia for several specific uses, although also as a playful drug, associated with opium and alcohol. By the end of the thirteenth century, the Arabic language comprises more than a hundred terms to say "hashish." Al-Zarkasi charges the drug one hundred and twenty damages.

Coffee was discovered in Arabia after the tenth century, considered "Arab pride," next to liquid opium. Considered of great utility to avoid fatigue and only from 1551 was allowed the opening of public coffees. In principle, the undesirable is alcoholic drunkenness, which "leads to lying," but this does not presuppose giving up the gifts of ebriety in general, since *being sober is proper to animals*. In a second moment, any form of ebriety is to blame, because *the induced relaxation is not a sign of culture, but a forbidden pleasure*. From the fourteenth century on, Islamic power declines and is taken over by fundamentalist and intolerant movements, with book burning, persecution and punishment of alcohol and hashish users.

Middle Ages and Modern Ages: Money and Power on the Agenda

One of the most significant contributions of the Arab world has been his efficiency in medicine—the Arab doctor as a generous supplier of psychoactive drugs. Already in the late eleventh century some *Solanaceae sp* such as opium and hemp were used by doctors of kings, nobles, and prelates to treat various complaints (Escohotado 2004; MacRae 2010).

In the twelfth century we found the first "soporiferous sponges," anesthetics composed of opium, *meimendro* and mandrake, ground and macerated in water—*when you want to saw or cut a man, soak a rag in it and apply it to his nostrils for a while*, recommended Miguel Escoto, from the school of Salerno. During this period, there was a relationship between drug use, lust, and witchcraft, and it was believed that sorcerers used drugs to maintain sexual relations with the devil.

Several recipes for different types of ointments used to produce a sensation of flight or sexual delight are included in the Inquisition's records from the thirteenth to eighteenth centuries—which punished with torture and death the use of any drug other than alcohol. One of the main components of the ointments were plants of the *Solanaceae* families, which cause visions (Araújo 2012).

Other authorized and widely used expedients of Catholic and Protestant inquisitors were testimonies paid or provided by criminals in exchange for freedom. The penalty was to be burned in a public square, which offered the people the security that evil was being defeated. By the end of the fifteenth century the witches were able to live together in relative peace, providing the peasants with their medicines and their hallucinogenic or aphrodisiac delusions. Later, in 1484, Pope Innocent VIII decided that witches are dangerous and the 'witch hunt' gains momentum.

While witches were persecuted and burned, others were able to study and apply knowledge about medicinal and psychoactive plants without accusations of connection with the devil: the alchemists. Still in the twelfth century, the School of Salerno—a milestone in teaching and medicine in Middle Ages Europe—recommended the use of opium as an anesthetic and sedative, and the main remedy was *Antidotarium nicolai*, whose recipe mixed poppy with mandrake root and Belgian. These three ingredients were among the most common in witches' recipes.

The alchemists were, together with the first doctors, protected by the Inquisition and by their connections with the University and the kings. They were a certain kind of magicians who mixed knowledge in botany, medicine, and chemistry in search of the philosopher's stone (which would transform any metal into gold) and the elixir of youth (which would guarantee eternal life). In the fourteenth century the *Manual of Inquisitors* made it explicit that witches should be closely watched, for *when they do not obtain the discoveries they desire, they soon turn to the devil.*

In the Americas, part of the popular work was the production of the so-called *coca bread,* consumed by the nobility in great quantity. The conquest of Inca America brought, at first, a democratization of consumption and with that the Spaniards made fortunes; after the conflict between the inquisitors (who saw the use of the plant as an idolatrous practice) and the landowners (defending their profit), the resolution was to clearly allocate a tithe on all trade on the plant, whose export exceeded 1300 tons of the leaf.

While America proved to be an abundant source of raw materials, in Europe it followed ambivalence through the use of drugs. In this context, alchemists were important to the development of modern medicine and pharmacy by preserving the use of opium and other psychoactive substances during the Middle Ages and allowing the popularization of these substances later.

The Renaissance and the resumption of closer contact with Eastern cultures allowed a gradual resumption of non-criminalized drug use. For a long time, however, those who had a more in-depth knowledge of the subject continued to be viewed with suspicion. The reestablishment of opium as a therapeutic panacea of the West began, although with the restriction: anyone could be prosecuted, tortured, and burned alive for suspicion, and it was then necessary to create unpopular, university class therapeutic crafts to resist the inquisitors.

Paracelsus, an alchemist famous for creating laudanum (dye or opium solution), whose application resisted for two centuries and influenced a whole generation of drugs from the nineteenth century. He was a great advocate of the use of opium and used substances from the classical pharmacopeia and the arsenal of medieval alchemy and witchcraft in his medical practice. Your lesson? The same happens with drugs as with weapons: such objects remain undetermined until they are used for good or evil (Vargas 2008). Paracelsus argued that illnesses were not the result of the imbalance of moods or bodily fluids and should not be treated through diet, bleeding, and purging; according to him, illnesses possessed entities—*ens*—that should be treated through the use of chemical substances. He also postulated that all substances in nature could exert positive (and constitute *essentia*) or negative (*poison)* influences, the difference between *essentia* and *poison* being basically a matter of dose—*Dosis sola facit venenum* (Araújo 2012; Escohotado 2004).

The discovery of America, as we have already mentioned, in addition to contact with indigenous cultures, served to expand the European pharmacopoeia, despite the vigorous persecution of them by the conquistadors. Cocoa, yerba mate, and tobacco were thus introduced into Europe. In all the narratives of Europeans, the astonishment at the tobacco habits of natives from all parts of America appears. In addition to smoking, they smelled of powdered plant, made drinks and ointments.

The Arab influence had a huge impact on European development in the following centuries. Partly because Europe lost much of its importance on the world stage since the barbaric invasions and the fall of the Roman Empire, while the peoples of the East, especially after Islamic expansion, had occupied an increasingly hegemonic economic, political, and social position in the Old World; partly also because the resurgence of Europe as an important pole on the world stage only came at the cost of breaking with certain traditions long rooted in European soil. This break-up, augmented by the incorporation of the experiences and traditions of others, was named *Renaissance*.

The appreciation of exotic spices was amplified in the centuries after the end of the Crusades, called “the madness of spices” (Vargas 2008). Their use has come to be recognized as a means of social distinction, plus symbolic value: dream values, the values attributed to the East, a mysterious and distant land on which the West projected desires and utopias. If, on one hand, the "taste of paradise" was the privilege of the wealthy, the cosmological-photographic drift in search of paradise was not their prerogative.

Returning to tobacco, the Europeans brought to America the prejudice and obsession they lived with the witches: the Indians used the plant for pleasure, as medicines, to reduce hunger or to celebrate and talk with their gods. These Europeans claimed that "it was the devil's doing. They associate shamans with the devil, but tobacco did not unexpectedly trigger a 'witch hunt' in America as it did in Europe. The settlers were interested in finding gold and silver, and took some tobacco seeds to Europe in the 1550s. From then on, the spread of tobacco was unprecedented: the French ambassador to Portugal, Jean Nicot, presented Catherine de Medici with a seedling of the plant and, after some medicinal tests, spread the news that it cured cancer (Araújo 2012; Escohotado 2004). In 1571, Nicolás Monardes described tobacco ("nicotiana herb") as a cure for practically all diseases known at the time. The Pope of that time had tobacco planted in the Vatican, and priests and bishops from Europe helped spread the plant to the rest of the continent; but when they began to smell snuff and smoke during Mass, Catholics turned against the drug. Pope Innocent VIII threatened to excommunicate anyone using tobacco near the churches. In the Arab world, it is estimated that the Ottoman emperor Murad IV had 25,000 smokers executed over 14 years. In Persia the death penalty against smokers was also adopted, and it was executed by throwing melted lead down the throats of the condemned. In China, between 1640 and 1644, the penalty for smokers was beheading.

The wide and rapid spread of tobacco created a powerful market that motivated the first drug policies in the modern era. One of the first anti-smokers, King James I of England, decreed in 1604 a 4000% tax on the value of tobacco imported into the country; in addition to tax policies, in the seventeenth century Japan, the Ottoman Empire, Sweden, Denmark, Russia, China, and the Mongol Empire banned tobacco consumption. As users multiplied, despite high taxes and punishments, and fortunes were made with the sale and collection of taxes, the laws cooled down and by the end of the seventeenth century economic interests took precedence over moral and religious ones.

During the eighteenth century, it was of rationalism and enlightenment, there was a cooling down of the persecution of religious heterodoxies and a return of the drugs of paganism to daylight. It no longer seemed evident that pain pleased and brought man closer to God and the medical and playful use of substances regained its legitimacy. A large production and trade of cheap opium-based drugs began used to treat a range of symptoms ranging from insomnia to uterine contractions and stomach disorders. Ludans were used by kings, plebs, soldiers, prelates, and artists. In this eighteenth century, opium became the main export commodity of the European powers to the Chinese market, generating economic problems for that empire—which, in an attempt to prevent the product from entering the country, started two wars with England, losing both and being forced to pay heavy compensation to the British.

Regarding alcohol, the first mention of the use of refrigeration appears in a twelfth century treaty called *Aqua vitae,* resulting from distillation, and *Aqua ardens*, resulting from bidestillation, 96° alcohol. The liqueurs were popularized, offering a fast and deep drunkenness, obtained with less liquid and with more options to choose aromas and flavors compared to wines. A more commercially stable product, the production and sale achieved great commercial margins. Since the fifteenth century distillers were expanding their European market by taking alcohol to China. Faced with the alluvium of alcohol promoted by distilled beverages, several measures were taken in Europe. The most ambitious was a foundation aimed at promoting sobriety, presided over by German nobles and bishops; others, like in China, condemned the user; Francis I, from France, had the ear of a recidivist alcoholic cut off. It is worth mentioning that the Arabs, despite their reputation for rigor, had never applied punishments of this nature to the user.

The double moral and hypocrisy in relation to drugs are on the scene: members of the clergy themselves produce mass liquors of great popular acceptance, while they are responsible for formulating and applying punishments to alcohol users. The clergy also receive large sums of money as tithes on coca plantations, liquor exports, and at the same time act as informers to users and consumers (Araújo 2012). On the scene, the transformations of social ties (Rosa 2016) that will culminate in blaming users as criminals. In 1613, the tithe on coca trade in Latin America is the most important part of the revenues for the bishops of Cuzco and Lima. The ambiguity is made explicit: *chewing the leaf would become an "unauthorized social activity,"* even with an evident increase in productivity by the stimulating character of coca.

Still in the seventeenth century, the caffeine-rich yerba mate begins to enter the market and receives contradictory definitions: mentioned as a means to talk to God, it was also labeled "diabolical herb," "whose leaves were deadly poison." In 1620, the Company of Jesus intended to export mate to Europe, to compete with Mexican cocoa, coffee and tea from the Orient. It is estimated that in Asunción, Paraguay, 14,000 arrobas were consumed each year by the then 500 Spanish residents (Escohotado 2004). One plant that sprouts in the southern tributaries of the Amazon is *Paulinia cupana*, known as Guarana. It has a higher caffeine concentration than mate and coffee. As it grows in the middle of the jungle, having, therefore, difficult access for the colonizers, this drug did not motivate neither literature nor polemic during the first centuries. Currently, it is one of the main Brazilian exports. The Middle Ages and the Renaissance are times, according to Escohotado (2004), when the consumption of alcoholic beverages reaches previously unknown levels. In the Modern Age, the return to thinking about euphoria and euthanasia is considered as goods, since now the absolute value is the individual and his or her auspices of freedom.

New World, Old Problems

According to Narby and Huxley (2004), at the beginning of European expeditions to America shamans were respected and the culture of indigenous pharmacopeia was valued. Instead of colonizing and imposing European medicine and pharmacology, pharmacists and doctors moved from Europe to Peru and other places to learn from native herbalists. Doctor Francisco Hernández, in 1580, published 17 volumes of the *Natural History of the Indies,* mentioning more than 3000 plants (Castro 1977; Escohotado 2000).

The Aztec culture maintained botanical gardens with pharmacological deposits and archives; herbalists and drug addicts were constant in public markets, and the poor population could obtain free diagnoses and drugs. However, it was very difficult to differentiate Indians from wizards, healers, and malicious deceivers.

Peyote, ololiuhqui (lysergic acid amide), and tobacco were the most common herbs, and the author Juan de Cárdenas defends drug neutrality: the same drug, in the same doses, can be *for good or for bad* (Castro 2002). A long period of persecution began, and in 1629 the inquisitor Ruiz de Alarcón launched a crusade against the natives of Morelos y Guerrero, with the burning of seeds, destruction of plantations, lawsuits, and convictions. Around 1700 inquisitorial trials are held in America against sorcerers and herbalists; they present original indigenous concepts as a *secret organization opposed to Christianity and the government.*

In Central America, the first drug that caught the attention was the *Theonanácatl* ("wonderful mushroom"), a name that covers several species of psilocybin mushrooms. The first chroniclers appeared the *Theonanacatl* with none other than Lucifer. The mentioned ololiuhqui is the mixture of the seeds of two climbing plants and, according to Bernardino de Sahagún, *serves the natives to commune with the Devil.* This same anathema received the *peyote*, a cactus containing mescaline, whose use was quickly considered a *pagan ritual and superstition.* Carlos Castanheda, a social anthropologist who has become an apprentice shaman in Mexico, described his experience with psychoactive drugs in the book "The Devil's Herb" (Paula 2014).

In the Caribbean Islands, the Amerindians discovered in Santo Domingo by Columbus used *yopo* or *yakoana*, cohoba powder, in the territories that currently belong to Venezuela and Colombia. The drug is extracted from a plant *Anadenanthera peregrina*, whose active ingredient is DMT (dimethyltryptamine), alkaloid with a fast and intense effect.

Cocoa, whose cultivation seems to originate in Mexico—where the Aztec emperors consumed it ceremonially, with cutlery and gourds made of gold—contains a substance called *theobromine*, an alkaloid that belongs to the coffee family. The Greek naturalist Linneu named it *theobroma*, literally, *divine food.*

The tendency of human beings to symbolic uses of substances pervades the history of civilizations: in each context, a mode of use, a desired effect, an effect obtained. The notion of self-control, for centuries, is stronger than any idea of 'superpowers' of drug objects. Accountability for attitudes (Rosa 2016) is a theme of clinic, politics, religion: what are the social ties involved in blaming users as being *without character, bad, violent?*

The change in the world scenario with the Opium Wars ratifies the double moral rooted in the theme "drugs": production, trade, money, and power involved on the one hand and, on the other, politics and the legal regime. To what extent does the political system determine the type of drug use and subsequent adjectivation of producers and users?

XIX and XX Centuries: Isolated Active Principles

In the nineteenth century chemists, pharmacists, doctors, literati, philosophers, and artists have an interest in all kinds of psychoactive. The needs of some seem to converge to the possibilities opened by others and, ultimately, the goal is to submit the mood to the will, having the emotion and perception as instruments. Nietzsche defined ebriety as *nature's play with man*. Combined with commerce, the advances in chemistry resurrect the idea of *perfect drugs*—Panakeiai or panaceas—incarnated as modern and superior versions of the old *trigas*. In the middle of the nineteenth century, there are about 70,000 secret formula remedies in Europe and America, with free access.

With the technological increase, scientists began to isolate the active principles of several plants, producing drugs such as morphine (1806), codeine (1832), atropine (1833), caffeine (1841), cocaine (1860), heroine (1883), mescaline (1896), and barbiturates (1903). Being purer and easier to handle, their dosages could be calculated more accurately. Ether, chloroform, and nitrous oxide (dentists' gas), potent anesthetics, were also developed. Hectares of crops now fit into a single case, and the uncertainties derived from unequal concentrations in different plants are eliminated—purity would allow accurate dosing, increasing safety margins for the consumer.

There is a paradigm shift: drugs cease to be more or less magical vegetables, linked to rites and sacraments; their active principles are free from the mythical emphasis by Pharmacology and Medicine.

In the context of wars, industrial revolution (overwork, insomnia, exhaustion) and the spread of the most diverse diseases, there was great demand for medicines. In the era of industrialization and urbanization, the formation of large proletarian masses exploited, piled up, alienated from the productions of which they were part, concomitantly with revolutions and political restorations and the technological transformation of the world, the context facilitated an enthusiastic look at drugs as an influence on the spirit.

Not by chance, the first great drug of the nineteenth century was morphine (one of the alkaloids of opium), used in the American Civil War and in the Franco-Prussian of 1879, its ability to soothe or suppress pain. The first monograph on cases of morphine links "vice" to "weakness of character." As an epidemiological profile, 25% were women; 65% were therapists, health professionals or family members; 10% were clergy, bohemians and some sex professionals. Almost all kept their use discreetly, although in some of the most elegant European salons it was fashionable to sting publicly, and offer cases signed by famous goldsmiths with gold or platinum syringes (Escohotado 2004). The daily use of morphine could *be daily, without shortening life or reducing work capacity*, concluded the study.

Diacetilmorphine, or heroin, due to its energetic virtues (*heroisch*) appeared on the market and was sold together with the aspirin by a small dye factory owned by F. Bayer. It was launched with great publicity in 1898, on a free sale basis even after opium and morphine were controlled. A curious reference appears in his prospectus: *morphinomaniacs treated with this substance immediately lost all interest in morphine.* Both morphine and heroin are advocated by Western missionaries to rehabilitate opium-dependent people in the Far East. To this day, morphine is known in China as "Christ's Opium." Between 1911 and 1914, England exports 40 tons of morphine to these territories, and Germany, 10 tons of heroin (as a power, is equivalent to 10,000 tons of Indian opium). The health plan that Westerners recommended to the Emperor was based on the "anti-opic pill," whose main ingredient was heroin. The foundations were laid for the harm reduction strategy: half a century later, the plan will be to cure the habituation of heroin with methadone.

Cocaine was isolated in 1859 and soon traded on a large scale, with more intense advertising than morphine and heroin. Sigmund Freud undertakes a global investigation, with extensive review of all existing literature and proposals for use. Parke-Davis and Merck laboratories have subsidized his studies. His experiments—which earned him a place of reference at one time—had their results distorted, promoting a defamation that still appears as an argument against Psychoanalysis. The compilation of her studies was carried out a posteriori by Anna Freud (Freud 1975; Lima 2017).

Around 1890 there are hundreds of drinks with coca or pure cocaine extracts. The most famous will be the *French Wine of Coca, Ideal Tonic*, marketed as *Coca Cola* by an apothecary in Georgia in 1885. In 1886 the embryo of the Dry Law began, and the inventor J. S. Pemberton suppressed the alcohol and added-cola nut (which contains caffeine), launching Coca Cola in the market as *sovereign remedy.* Pemberton sold his share to another pharmacist, A. Grigs Candler, who added the gasified pressure tap to the product.

Prohibitionism

In 1800, Napoleon Bonaparte forbids the use of hashish throughout Egypt in order to *avoid violent delusions and excesses of any kind.* The psychiatrist J. Moreau de Tours, considering that hemp is a mode of knowledge of the mind and can be the object of scientific investigation, brings together a group—called *Haschischins Club*—with Baudelaire, Delacroix, Verlaine, Rimbaud, Victor Hugo, and Balzac. As one of the results, a publication by Baudelaire with articles related to its sessions: *Artificial Parks.*

The British government, through the *Indian Hemp Drugs Commission*, published seven volumes in 1894 which concluded: *Considering the issue in general, it should be added that in India the rule is the moderate use of hashish and marijuana, and that excessive use is exceptional.*

After all, what would be the "truth" about the effects of psychoactive substances? Would they promote inspiration? Destruction? Would there be a "standardized effect," common to all users?

Official prohibitions and authorizations regarding drug prescription, use, production and marketing involve millions in cash. The dispute for the territories of action—medicine/health, police/repression, researchers/know-how involves political and social alliances that do not always bring as a result the well-being of humanity. The first major prohibitionist movements in the USA began with the *Harrison Act in* 1914, which aimed to control the production and use of substances; in 1919, the *Volstead Act* (Dry Law), which took effect between 1920 and 1932, prohibiting the consumption of alcoholic beverages. Thousands of doctors were sent to prison for prescribing opiates to their patients.

Synthetic drugs, identical molecules or very similar to natural remedies, have transformed laboratories into large pharmaceutical industries. For example, ephedrine was the active ingredient used in Chinese medicine for millennia in the treatment of asthma and bronchitis; in 1890, it was isolated in a laboratory. The application for patents, the use in people close to and, the free supply were standards of the time. Let us consider that the ethical norms for research with human beings—Bioethics—appeared only after the Second World War. The use of amphetamines in the post-War period; the use of LSD in research on human psychism and the treatment of alcoholism; the emergence of ecstasy and MDMA (methylenedioximethamphetamine); the release of alcohol and tobacco as legal drugs and of many opiates only as "controlled" drugs. This whole scenario is an amplification of what is legitimate as a *human experience*. A drug is produced, released, consumed, and without detailed analysis of its contexts, it is criminalized, becomes clandestine, loses its purity and receives frightening adulteration, and the guilty/punished is the user. But this did not come from one day to another.

In the twentieth century, U.S. foreign policy began to emphasize the issue of controlling the production and international trade of various psychoactive substances, focusing on opiates and expanding into *cannabis*.

International agreements, promulgated under strong US pressure, address the drug issue from a markedly binary, dualistic perspective, with pharmacological approaches and excluding social or cultural factors (MacRae 2010). The drugs to be reached by the legal provisions do not receive a scientific definition, and the term "psychotropic substances" is attributed to anyone who is included in a series of four different lists, the so-called List I being composed of substances that admittedly do not create dependency or tolerance—and yet receive the heaviest restrictions, without any space for studies or research (Seibel 2010).

Both in international treaties and in the legislation and national policies resulting from them (Torcato 2016), the profound heterogeneity of the modes of consumption, the reasons, beliefs, values, rites, lifestyles, and worldviews that sustain it is ignored. Treating this use in a separate way to the study of the evolution of society, its conflicts, imbalances, and power relations, closes the question as "fight against drugs," making it impossible to adopt effective measures to deal with the most harmful consequences, and excludes the whole political, social, and economic set that sustains and maintains the relationship between marginality and the use of psychoactive drugs.

Reflecting from..

Historical issues such as the "witch hunt," the silencing of shamans, the disqualification and demoralization of the work of experts in herbs and plants, the sensationalism in the face of different drugs, the billions that the pharmaceutical industry invoices annually are subsidizing the *pathologization* of all and any use of psychoactive substance that, in a certain time and space, is called illicit use.

The concept of *social imaginary* is elucidative as to the relationship that culture establishes with subjective formation. The social imaginary is a device that helps the necessary interdisciplinary dialogue in the field of drugs. According to Rosa (2016), this set of meanings, norms, and logics that determine the concrete place occupied by individuals in society. Are drug users delinquent? Or would social exclusion subsidize the problems of psychoactive abuse? How can drug addiction be explained among middle-class urban youth, considering only biomedical factors?

In any case, drug users are closer to being strangers, those who, by Freud's (1919) considerations, carry the possibility of bringing out what should remain hidden. They must always be circumscribed in a space of visibility/invisibility, so that they do not denounce with their presence, because they are denied the possibility of narrative, the hole, the gap, that exists in every act of governing and regulating civilizations (Rosa 2016). The *strangers* (users) are those whom capitalism should erase, make silent, by producing the illusion that they are mortified, in the most complete des-subjectivation. Erasure and mortification on life, which results in survival. The world is divided between "the world of drugs" and "ours," haughty, clean, correct, impeccable, and unassailable. When we approach the history of drug use, its periods of permission, its contexts of use in which it was possible to quantify and qualify the few abuses and problems, we see that the relationships in which there is demonization of the drug object are permeated by economic interests of the market, international power, and very little sensitive to anthropological, cultural, and social issues. Public health issues today are much more related to licit drugs such as alcohol, tobacco, anxiolytics, and antidepressants (misuse, abuse, direct relationship with cancer, accidents, violence, fatal overdoses) than to illicit drugs (WHO 2019).

In 1998, the UN General Assembly called on all member countries to campaign for "a drug-free world and 10 years after the result of 'stabilizing consumption' was questioned. At the end of the twentieth century, the system of control of some psychoactive drugs that had developed since the Shanghai International Conference (1909) began to be severely questioned. Drugs began to be controlled, supposedly, because they caused harm—but a 100 years later they became increasingly dangerous because of control, clandestinely. The UN does not review the need for control or question the complex causes of prohibitions of certain substances to the detriment of others.

Understanding the drug issue requires this dive into human history. To understand critically what is reported, what is presented as "scientific," what is sold as "natural" and what is impregnated in our culture as "good" and "evil."

In the 1980s, with the introduction of the Harm Reduction Strategy, there was a revision of concepts and emphasis on combating trafficking rather than repression of users. These changes reflect a closer alignment of drug policies in Europe and further away from the USA.

In Harm Reduction, the pagan idea that drugs can only be used and objects of pleasure, relief from suffering, elevation of mood, sociability, happiness is recovered, as well as the priority to the understanding that the user *is us*. We are all, in public, users of caffeine, cocoa, aspirin, anxiolytics, antidepressants; by punitive imposition, we do not admit the use of marijuana, cocaine, heroin. The double standard exists even among us, scholars, educators, researchers, and public health professionals—we cannot admit the use of substances considered illicit under penalty of exile, exclusion, and stigmatization. In other words, we still have a long way to go. Man's relationship with drugs needs to be revisited and contextualized. A first step is taken here: to know a little about history.

References

Araújo, T. (2012). *Almanaque das drogas*. São Paulo, Brazil: Leya.

Castro, E. V. (1977). *Indivíduo e sociedade no Alto Xingu: os Yawalaptí* (Master's thesis) Museu Nacional/Universidade Federal do Rio de Janeiro, Rio de Janeiro, Brasil.

Castro, E. V. (1986). *Araweté: os deuses canibais*. Rio de Janeiro, Brazil: Zahar/ANPOCS.

Castro, E. V. (2002). *A inconstância da alma selvagem e outros ensaios de antropologia*. São Paulo, Brazil: Cosac Naify.

Castro, E. V. (2008). Xamanismo transversal: Lévi-Strauss e a cosmopolítica amazônica. In R. C. Queiroz & R. F. Nobre (Eds.), *Lévi-Strauss: leituras brasileiras*. Belo Horizonte, Brazil: Editora UFMG.

Couto, D., Jr. (2013). *As flechas de Apolo: aspectos culturais da medicina ocidental, desde a Guerra de Troia até a Primeira Conflagração Mundial*. Rio de Janeiro, Brazil: Rubio.

Dunker, C. I. L. (2015). *Mal-estar, sofrimento e sintoma: uma psicopatologia do Brasil entre muros*. São Paulo, Brazil: Boitempo Editorial.

Escohotado, A. (2000). *Historia general de las drogas*. Madrid, Spain: Espasa.

Escohotado, A. (2004). *História Elementar das Drogas*. Lisboa, Portugal: Antígona.

Fernández, A. (2009). *La atencionalidad atrapada*. Buenos Aires, Argentina: Buena Vista Ed.

Flandrin, J., & Montanari, M. (1998). *História da Alimentação*. São Paulo, Brazil: Estação Liberdade.

Freud, S. (1919). *Das Umheimlich. O Infamiliar*. São Paulo, Brazil: Autêntica Ed.

Freud, S. (1975). *Escritos sobre la cocaína*. Barcelona, Spain: Editorial Anagrama.

Labate, B. C. (2008). *Drogas e cultura: novas perspectivas*. Salvador, Brazil: EDUFBA.

Lima, H. M. M. (2012). *Adesão ao tratamento de AIDS por pacientes com AIDS, tuberculose e usuários de drogas*. Curitiba, Brazil: CRV.

Lima, H. M. M. (2017). *Freud Pré-1900* (Monografia de especialização). Departamento de Psicanálise do Instituto Sedes Sapientiae, São Paulo, SP, Brasil.

Lima, H. M. M. (2018). Diagnóstico Situacional da Opção B+ e Sífilis congênita nos países da Comunidade de Países de Língua Portuguesa – CPLP. Retrieved from www.cplp.org/id-4879.aspx

MacRae, E. (2010). Antropologia: aspectos sociais, culturais e ritualísticos. In S. Seibel (Ed.), *Dependência de Drogas*. São Paulo, Brazil: Atheneu.

Narby, J., & Huxley, F. (2004). *Shamans throught time—500 years on the path to knowledge*. New York, NY: Penguin.

Nery, A. F. (2017). *Conversando com Nery. As drogas escolhem os humanos*? [Video file]. Retrieved from https://www.youtube.com/watch?v=sbTmJSED8qk

Nery, A. F. (2018). *Conversando com Nery. Dependência química, uso e abuso: como fazer a diferença?* [Video file]. Retrieved from https://www.youtube.com/watch?v=P0RABJnvhwA

Nery, A. F. (2019a). *Drogas: fique por dentro. #177*. Retrieved from https://drogasfiquepordentro.com/2019/05/18/drogas-fique-por-dentro-177-20-04-19/amp/

Nery, A. F. (2019b). *Conversando com Nery. Usar drogas não é (necessariamente) uma doença alienante: o que é, então?* [Video file]. Retrieved from https://www.youtube.com/watch?v=uC76-sK3UBA

Paula, C. F. C. (2014). *Sobre saberes e verdades: as discursividades científica e feiticeira no livro-enunciado de Carlos Castaneda* (Masters's thesis), Universidade Federal de Goiás, Catalão, Brasil. Retrieved from http://repositorio.bc.ufg.br/tede/handle/tede/3816

Ribeiro, A. L. (2019). *Usuário de drogas em situação de rua numa perspectiva interseccional de raça, classe e gênero: análise bioética da (não) responsividade do sistema de saúde* (Doctoral dissertation), Universidade de Brasília, Brasília, Brasil. Retrieved from https://repositorio.unb.br/handle/10482/35161

Rosa, M. D. (2016). *A clínica psicanalítica em face da dimensão sociopolítica do sofrimento*. São Paulo, Brazil: Escuta/FAPESP.

Seibel, S. (2010). *Dependência de drogas*. São Paulo, Brazil: Atheneu.

Simões, J. A. (2008). Prefácio. In B. C. Labate (Ed.), *Drogas e cultura: novas perspectivas*. Salvador, Brazil: EDUFBA.

Torcato, C. E. M. (2016). *História das Drogas e sua proibição no Brasil: da Colônia à República* (Doctoral dissertation), Faculdade de Filosofia, Letras e Ciências Humanas da Universidade de São Paulo, São Paulo, Brasil. Retrieved from https://www.teses.usp.br/teses/disponiveis/8/8138/tde-05102016-165617/publico/2016_CarlosEduardoMartinsTorcato_VCorr.pdf

Vargas, E. V. (2008). Fármacos e outros objetos sócio-técnicos: notas para uma genealogia das drogas. In B. C. Labate (Ed.), *Drogas e cultura: novas perspectivas*. Salvador, Brazil: EDUFBA.

World Health Organization (WHO). (2019). *Mental Health Newsletter*. Retrieved from https://mailchi.mp/who/who-mental-health-newsletter-december-2019?e=ac9c2b8605

Chapter 2
Drug Use and Substance Use Disorders in Brazil and the World: Epidemiological Data

Liz Paola Domingues, André Bedendo, Emérita Sátiro Opaleye, and Ana Regina Noto

Introduction

What Is Epidemiology?

Epidemiology is one of the scientific ways of studying health and disease conditions, considering these phenomena at the population level. Thus, it can be understood as the study of what affects the population, usually to identify the correlated factors that influence the occurrence and distribution of such phenomena in the territories, as well as new occurrences and longitudinal monitoring of already known problems (Jekel et al. 2006).

Alcohol, tobacco, and other drugs use are considered a public health problem, given the social, economic, and health implications that they cause on society (UNODC 2019; WHO 2014, 2015a, b) and, for this reason, several countries conduct periodic surveys to obtain information on substance consumption patterns in their population. Although the procedure of these surveys is of national responsibility, many countries report their data to the United Nations (UN), which is responsible for analyzing and disseminating periodic reports on the epidemiology of drug use worldwide.

Some information is essential to report epidemiological data, such as the population studied, the phenomenon observed, the incidence of the event, the place, and the period in which the observations were made. Regarding substance use, it is also relevant to note the frequency and patterns of use. The most verified frequency in epidemiological surveys is lifetime use, i.e. use of the substance at least once in life; past-year use, regarding the use of the substance at least once in the last 12 months; and recent use or past-month use, considering the use of the substance at least once

L. P. Domingues (✉) · A. Bedendo · E. S. Opaleye · A. R. Noto
Universidade Federal de São Paulo, São Paulo, SP, Brazil
e-mail: liz.paola@unifesp.br

D. De Micheli et al. (eds.), *Drugs and Human Behavior*,
https://doi.org/10.1007/978-3-030-62855-0_2

in the previous 30 days (Carlini et al. 2006; Bastos et al. 2017). Equally essential is to explore the consumption patterns since they relate to different social and health consequences. There is no risk-free substance intake, just as not all drug use is necessarily harmful. Therefore, one should consider the low-risk consumption pattern or just substance use. The latest editions of the International Disease Catalogue (ICD-11) consider that uses that bring negative consequences should be regarded as Mental and behavioral disorders due to psychoactive substance use, while the Diagnostic and Statistical Manual of Mental Disorders (DSM-5) consider that any use that brings negative consequences should be regarded as a dependence syndrome or substance use disorder, and may be classified as mild, moderate or severe according to the number of criteria met (Araújo and Lotufo 2014; Oliveira et al. 2017).

Challenges of Epidemiological Drug Research

A particular challenge when researching stigmatized subjects like substance use is a tendency for some participants in omitting their behavior. This makes research subject to biases in addition to those already known in epidemiological studies, as well as requiring multidisciplinary understanding and careful procedures that increase confidence in data while ensuring specific ethical care for the participants.

With the advancement of reliable laboratory techniques for the detection of substances in biological material, it could be said simplistically that this would be the ideal way to obtain drug exposure in a given population. However, this approach makes the investigative processes more costly and often not feasible, it requires elaborate infrastructure and staff with expertise for sample collection and analysis, in addition to ethical issues to be raised. There are also environmental surveys, such as the one recently conducted in Brasília that showed a greater presence of cocaine metabolites from sewage samples during the 2014 World Cup event compared to previous samples (Sodré et al. 2017). This type of study sheds light on consumption geographically over time but answers little about who, how, and how much was consumed.

The most common way of collecting substance use data is based on self-report questionnaires. There are limitations, but on a large scale, this is the most cost-effective technique. Self-report questionnaires are preferred for sensitive topics since they enhance anonymity and are more convenient to participants. On the other hand, they are not useful for surveying a large amount of information with high complexity, besides requiring at least literate survey subjects. For these cases, in-depth interviews are more beneficial, which also increases the adherence of participants and response rate, minimizes errors, and improves the quality of the information collected. However, compared to self-report questionnaires, the interviews require well-trained technical staff to collect data systematically, thus increasing survey costs, and execution time (Miller et al. 2010).

Despite the challenges, it is a consensus that systematic surveys to monitoring consumption, knowing users' characteristics, and related risk behaviors are essential for an effective approach to the issue. Equally important is to develop research in order to evaluate the broad possibilities of preventive measures and treatment as the most successful and more cost-effective. Updated information enables the development of public policies that meet the real interests and needs of the population to allocate public resources better. The following sections describe findings derived from the main epidemiological studies conducted in the world and Brazil.

Current Scenario on Drug Use

Historical Overview

The consumption of psychotropic drugs accompanies the history of humanity, inserting itself into the daily lives of different people around the world over time, affecting and being affected by local cultures. Therefore, it is to be expected that the predominantly used drugs, substance use patterns, and the consequences related to their use are different from one region to another, which is essential to be taken into account at the time of public policies and interventions.

Many countries conduct periodic surveys to monitoring the drug use in their territory, while the UN is concerned with monitoring results at a global level. The latest global data report on alcohol use was published in 2018; smoking reports, with the most recent edition published in 2019; and the reports on other drugs, with the last edition also dated 2019.

Epidemiological studies evaluating alcohol and other drugs used in Brazil have been conducted since the 1980s. The studies addressed different populations, including elementary and high school students (EHS), university students, household population, street children and adolescents, crack-cocaine users, and motor vehicle drivers. Despite a large gap between them, some of these surveys were repeated at different times, allowing a certain level of comparison between them. Among these, six epidemiological surveys with EHS students and three with household population stand out.

Alcohol

It is known that the consumption of alcoholic beverages is present in several populations around the world, often associated with socialization, which emphasizes its social relevance. However, although socially accepted, the consumption of alcoholic beverages is considered a public health issue, since its use is a risk factor for several social and health problems (WHO 2014, 2018a, b).

In the last world report on alcohol, it can be observed that the worldwide percentage of people who consume alcoholic beverages has decreased at about 5% since the 2000s. However, although there is a relative decrease, the absolute number of drinkers in the world has increased, reflecting the growth in the world population. In practice, in 2016 there were 336,000 more drinkers in the world compared to the 2000s. In 2016, 44.5% of the world population over 15 years of age had never consumed alcoholic beverages, and 43% reported consumption during the previous year, of which 62.4% were men. The prevalence of alcohol use disorders is 10.3% of the world population, of which 5.3% is related to dependence. Again, men represent the highest prevalence among individuals with alcohol use disorders, representing 8.6% of the world population. Europe has the highest prevalence of alcohol use disorders, with 18.1% of its population, while the Eastern Mediterranean region has the lowest prevalence, with a total of 1.5% of its population. The prevalence of alcohol use disorders is higher in areas with larger economies (WHO 2018a, b).

The pattern of alcohol use is also explored by the world reports, looking at Heavy Episodic Drinking, defined as 60 g of pure alcohol on a single occasion, at least once a month (WHO 2018a, b). This pattern of consumption deserves to be highlighted, since the ingestion of large quantities of alcohol leads to intoxication levels related to several negative consequences, such as intoxication, accidents, and violence (WHO 2014). Among the excerpt of the population that consumed alcohol in 2016, 39.5% reported the practice of Heavy Episodic Drinking (WHO 2018a, b), a decrease from the 44.4% that reported this pattern of consumption in the 2000s (WHO 2014).

Regardless of the population evaluated, alcohol is the most used drug in Brazil, according to the III National Survey on Drug Use by the Brazilian Population—III LNUD (Bastos et al. 2017). This most recent national study evaluated 16,273 participants aging from 12 to 65, from 351 cities. This study showed that 66.4% of the Brazilian population (almost 102 million people) consumed alcohol at least once in their lives. Regarding the prevalence of dependence, it is estimated that approximately 2.3 million Brazilians have criteria for dependence. This is equivalent to 3.5% of individuals who consumed alcohol in the 12 months before the survey, a prevalence notably higher among men (4.6%) than women (2.1%). These estimates were lower than those available in the previous 2005 survey of the 108 largest cities in the country, which indicated that 74.6% of the respondents consumed alcohol during their lifetime, and 12.3% met the criteria for dependence (Carlini et al. 2006). Even so, when considering only the 108 largest cities in the country in the most recent study, a lower prevalence of alcohol use is still noticeable, suggesting a reduction in consumption.

Figure 2.1 presents different patterns of alcohol use among several populations. College students showed the highest alcohol use prevalence for every pattern. However, data also highlight the use among street children and adolescents. The numbers reflect the cultural aspects associated with the use of alcohol during college life. In contrast, for the street population, the highest use is related to the individual and social vulnerabilities associated with street status. Binge drinking (consumption of 4 or more doses or 5 or more doses on the same occasion among

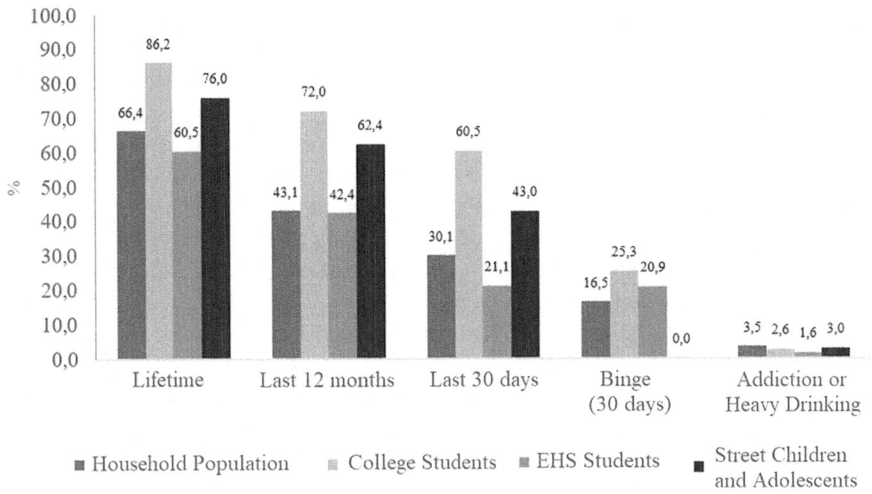

Fig. 2.1 Patterns of alcohol use among different populations. Sources: Andrade et al. (2010), Bastos et al. (2017), Carlini et al. (2012), Noto et al. (2004). (1) Among EHS students and street children and adolescents, data on heavy use were considered (20 or more times in the last 30 days). (2) Dependency criteria according to DSM-IV. (3) Data for college students assessed as being at high risk for addiction according to the Alcohol, Smoking and Substance Involvement Screening Test (ASSIST). (4) The data on binge among EHS students comes from a subsample of the national survey that considered only high school students aged between 14 and 18 years old ($n = 17{,}297$) (Sanchez et al. 2013). (5) Binge data not available among street children and adolescents. Legend: *EHS* elementary and high school

women and men, respectively) was also more prevalent among university students, underlining university students as a risk group for alcohol-related problems. In turn, the highest prevalence of dependence was observed among the household population.

It is also interesting to note that, according to III LNUD, the highest prevalence of alcohol consumption is observed among men, participants between 25 and 34 years of age, and people with higher education levels in all the patterns of use previously mentioned (except for dependence, whose highest prevalence was among Brazilians with no level of education or with lower education levels). These data suggest that although consumption is frequent among people with higher levels of education, the impact of dependence tends to affect people with lower levels of education.

Tobacco

Smoking is considered a major global public health issue. Tobacco use is related to more than 6 million deaths per year, even when its consumption is performed as adverted by the manufacturers (WHO 2015a, b). It is the second most consumed substance in the world, with 19.2% smokers in 2017. On the other hand, there was a reduction in the number of smokers from 1.46 billion in 2007 to 1.07 billion in 2017. Brazil has been recognized for adopting successful public policies resulting in successful outcomes (Levy et al. 2012). Similar to alcohol use, men represent 76.8% of smokers worldwide, while 92% of individuals who quit between 2007 and 2017 were women. Like alcohol, tobacco consumption is also higher in more economically developed regions (WHO 2019a, b).

In the last 15 years, there has been a rise in electronic devices for nicotine consumption, such as electronic cigarettes and vaporizers. Still, the consequences of such devices for the health of users and their impacts on public health are not yet well described. These devices deliver nicotine, leading the World Health Organization (WHO) to advise that these substances should be subjected to the same regulations and policies as tobacco (WHO 2019a, b).

In Brazil, tobacco is the second most consumed drug. The most recent household survey estimated that one-third of participants (33.5%) have already smoked industrialized cigarettes in their lives, which is equivalent to more than 51 million Brazilians (Bastos et al. 2017). Regarding past-year or past-month use, the same study estimated quite similar prevalence, respectively, 15.4% and 13.6%, which is expected for a highly addictive substance.

Figure 2.2a shows a summary of tobacco use patterns among different populations. The figure highlights the higher prevalence in all measures among children and adolescents in a street situation, which emphasizes the vulnerability associated with such condition. Data from the fifth and sixth surveys among EHS students showed a reduction in tobacco use across all use patterns (Carlini et al. 2012; Galduróz et al. 2004). Despite lower comparability due to methodological variations, III LNUD data also indicate reductions in tobacco use prevalence compared with the previous study (Carlini et al. 2006) (Fig. 2.2b). These data reflect remarkable advances in Brazilian tobacco control public policies that have helped reduce tobacco use and the prevalence of tobacco dependence in the country.

Other Drugs

Contrary to alcohol and tobacco data, the prevalence of other drugs use has increased globally in recent years beyond population growth, from 4.8% in 2009 to 5.5% in 2017. There are currently about 271 million drug users in the world, of which 13% have a substance use disorder (UNODC 2019).

Marijuana

Marijuana is the third most used drug in the world, with 188 million users (3.8% of the world population). Marijuana consumption increased by 30% between 1998 and 2017. However, from 2009 onwards, the growth in the number of users remained stable, following the population growth. Marijuana is also the third most consumed substance among young people, with 4.7% of users among the population aging between 15 and 16 years old. This substance is used by 89.6% of young people reporting any other drug use, except for alcohol or tobacco (UNODC 2019).

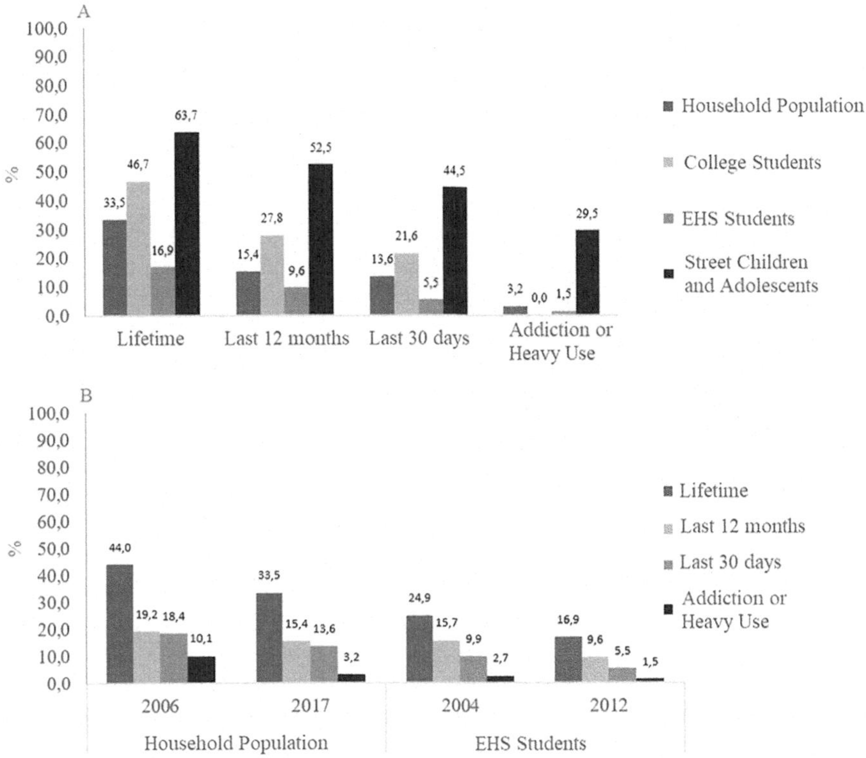

Fig. 2.2 (**a**) Patterns of tobacco use among different populations; Sources: Andrade et al. (2010), Bastos et al. (2017), Carlini et al. (2012), Galduróz et al. (2004), Noto et al. (2004). (1) In the household study, it refers to the use of industrialized cigarettes; (2) Among EHS Students and street children and adolescents, data on heavy use were considered (20 or more times in the last 30 days); (3) Dependency criteria according to DSM-IV; (4) Dependency or heavy use data not available among college students. (**b**) Comparison of tobacco use between the last two national studies between household population and EHS students. (1) EHS students considered data on heavy use. Legend: *EHS* elementary and high school

Among the illicit substances, marijuana is the most consumed by the Brazilian adult population (university and household populations). The III LNUD estimated that 7.7% of Brazilians (almost 12 million people) have already used marijuana in their lives. This prevalence reduces substantially when considering past-year use (2.5%), past-month use (1.5%), and dependence (0.29%) (Bastos et al. 2017). If we consider only the 108 Brazilian municipalities also accessed in the II household survey, it was observed that the prevalence of marijuana use was higher than in the previous study (lifetime use: 10.5% vs 8.8%; last year use: 3.9% vs 2.6%; past-month use: 2.5% vs 1.9%), but not for marijuana addiction (0.6% vs 1.2%).

The III LNUD also indicated that marijuana use is more prevalent among men, in the age group between 18 and 34 years old, and among people with a college degree. These data are in line with the highest prevalence of marijuana use among university students (lifetime use: 26.1%; past-year use: 13.8%; past-month use: 9.1%; and scoring at high risk for marijuana addiction: 0.6%) (Andrade et al. 2010). It is also worth noting that individuals between 12 and 17 years old presented lower use of marijuana in life according to the III LNUD. This result also corroborates the lower prevalence of marijuana use among students of EHS (Carlini et al. 2012).

Cocaine, Crack, and Similar Drugs

In 2017, about 18 million people aging between 15 and 64 years old reported having used cocaine or its derivatives in the last 12 months, which is equivalent of 0.4% of the world population (UNODC 2019). According to the World Drug Report (UNODC 2019), the world regions with the highest prevalence of cocaine use are Oceania (2.2%), North America (2.1%), Europe (1.3%), and South America (1%), areas showing a slight increase in the prevalence compared to the previous year's report.

Cocaine is the second most frequently consumed illicit drug in Brazil, according to the III LNUD. It is estimated that about 4.7 million (3.1%) people have already used cocaine in their lives, while 0.9% and 0.3% of the population reported past-year and past-month use, respectively. As for marijuana, when only the 108 largest Brazilian municipalities are considered, the prevalence of lifetime use, past-year, and past-month use were slightly higher than those of the II household survey. Men than women more frequently reported cocaine use, likewise the 18–34 age group, regardless of the pattern of use. Use in the previous year and month was more frequent among people with no or incomplete elementary education. Dependence was estimated at 0.18% by III LNUD. It is worth of noticing that although the prevalence of dependence is lower than that of marijuana, the treatment access among cocaine or crack users is more common than among marijuana users, denoting the more significant impact of such drugs on user's lives and the prominent need for therapeutic intervention.

The major study on crack-cocaine use in Brazil was conducted in 2012 in the 26 state capitals and Brazil's capital (Bastos and Bertoni 2014), estimating that there were about 370,000 regular users (use for at least 25 days in the last 6 months) of crack-cocaine or similar (cocaine paste, merla, and oxi), corresponding to a prevalence of 0.81% of the population. This prevalence is similar to that estimated for lifetime use in other national studies in the household population (0.9%) (Bastos et al. 2017), university students (1.2%) (Andrade et al. 2010), and EFM students (0.6%) (Carlini et al. 2012). Clearly, the low and uniform prevalence in studies with different methodologies and populations enable us to state that the crack-cocaine use in Brazil is significantly lower compared to alcohol and tobacco.

Non-prescribed Use of Drugs

Some controlled substances, indicated for therapeutic use, are also widely consumed by the world population in a non-prescribed or altered from the prescribed manner. This is the case of opioids and their derivatives. For example, about 53 million people between 15 and 64 years old make use without a prescription, the equivalent of 1.1% of the world population. Although the prevalence is lower compared to other drugs, the consumption of opioids is a cause of great concern due to its health consequences and a high degree of mortality. In 2017, opioids were responsible for 66% of deaths due to substance use, and it is now an epidemic in the USA. North America is currently the region with the highest concentration of non-prescribed users of opioids, with 4% of its population between 15 and 64 years old, corresponding to a quarter of the total number of users in the world (UNODC 2019).

Sedatives and tranquilizers, such as Benzodiazepines and Z-drugs, make up another class of drugs widely consumed in the world, in which prolonged and non-prescribed use is also observed, especially among women and poly users of substances (UNODC 2019). Global estimates of the non-prescribed use of this class of drugs are not yet available. Still, the latest World Drug Reports (UNODC 2018, 2019) show that the most recent surveys from countries in Central and South America indicate a prevalence of more than 2% of the general population of the nations, with a higher prevalence among women and significant use among students.

In North America, the USA has the highest prevalence of non-prescribed use of sedatives and tranquilizers (2.2% of the population), with no evidence on gender differences. The pattern of use shows a quite diverse prevalence among European countries, ranging from less than 1% in Portugal to 19.5% in the Czech Republic. However, all countries reported higher prevalence among women and higher prevalence among students. Data from Africa and Asia are more limited, but in these regions, no state reported a prevalence higher than 2.3% of the population.

The non-prescribed use of drugs is also part of the Brazilian reality, and the last year use is reported by 3% of the Brazilian population between 12 and 65 years (Bastos et al. 2017). The III LNUD shows that 94% of the non-prescribed use of drugs is made by adults (17–65 years), with women reporting twice the prevalence in relation to men as to the past-year use (4%) and past-month use (1.5%) (Bastos et al. 2017). Benzodiazepines and opioids are the substances with the highest prevalence of use, with 3.9% and 2.9% of the population having used them in life, respectively. Concerning past-month use, opioids had a slightly higher prevalence than benzodiazepines (0.6% and 0.4% respectively) and, although this difference has no statistical significance, it may serve as a warning for a potential increasing trend, as observed in North America (Bastos et al. 2017).

Drug Use Consequences

One of the leading indicators for measuring the consequences of health events is DALY (Disability-Adjusted Life Years), which considers not only mortality but disability and life expectancy of a given population, creating a comparable parameter. In the last two decades, alcohol abuse has risen in the ranking of the main factors that have contributed to DALYs worldwide, occupying ninth position in 2015 (WHO 2019a, b). Ranking from 2017 shows that alcohol is the fifth risk factor for DALYs in Brazil, with smoking being the first (HME 2017). The use of other drugs does not appear in the list of the ten most contributing risk factors for DALY globally, nor when analyzed exclusively in Brazil.

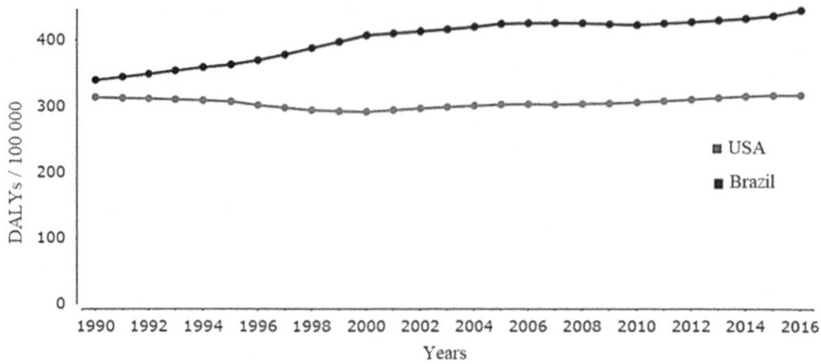

Fig. 2.3 Years of life lost due to death or disability (DALY) per 100 thousand inhabitants caused by alcohol use disorder, both sexes and all age groups between 1990 and 2016. Graph prepared by the authors with data from the Global Burden of Diseases, available at: http://www.healthdata.org/results/country-profiles

These parameters are as essential as consumption measures since they indicate how society has been impacted by substance use. For comparison, the prevalence of alcohol use disorders in the USA for both genders and population 15 years and older was 7.4% in 2010, the year in which the same report indicated a lower prevalence in the same parameters for Brazil of 5.6% (WHO 2019a, b). However, Fig. 2.3 shows the DALY per 100,000 inhabitants of both countries for alcohol use disorders over time, indicating a significant impact of alcohol use disorders on DALYs among the Brazilians compared to the U.S. population.

Observing the relationship between such indicators raises a series of questions about which factors influence the progression of the problematic use of a substance until it presents critical consequences for the subject, impacting its functionality and causing premature death. Measures such as restrictions on drinking and driving and increased therapeutic and social support are examples that may be a differential for a population that even abusing a substance, contribute to decrease the impact of this consumption on the consequences over oneself and others.

On the other hand, even a relatively small use from an epidemiological standpoint may result in dramatic consequences for the individual, sometimes higher from a social point of view than necessarily health. This is the case with the consumption of crack-cocaine, which in the Brazilian context researched is closely related to a series of structural inequalities, creating a cyclical pattern: social vulnerability can induce the onset of use, which implies an increase in social risks for the individual such as imprisonment or homeless situation, which contributes to the maintenance of consumption (Souza 2016).

It is also worth perceiving that despite a reduction in tobacco consumption in recent years, smoking is currently the leading risk factor for DALY in Brazil. This is indicative of the late effects this drug has on the health of users, especially for lung cancer and chronic obstructive pulmonary disease. The impact of the successful strategies enforced by the Brazilian government in recent years to reduce smoking will probably reflect on future generations in terms of disability and mortality.

Final Considerations

The data described here drew upon a brief scenario of drugs use in Brazil and worldwide. Data clearly show that licit drugs (alcohol and tobacco) are the most frequently used among the Brazilian population and that they also have a significant social and health impact. However, the complexity of the subject does not allow us to ignore the impact that other drugs also cause on users and society, no matter due to legal issues, social vulnerability, or even the drugs misuse without adequate medical monitoring. Unfortunately, despite the importance of epidemiological surveys to diagnose and monitor the consumption of substances in the country, there is still a gap in terms of research in the field, the systematization of research and the consequent guidance of public policies based on such findings. This should be a major goal for various sectors directly involved in the issue, such as, but not exclusively, universities, civil society entities, and different government levels.

References

Andrade, A. G., Duarte, P. C. A. V., & Oliveira, L. G. (2010). *I Levantamento Nacional sobre o Uso de Álcool, Tabaco e Outras Drogas entre Universitários das 27 Capitais Brasileiras*. Brasília: SENAD.

Araújo, Á., & Lotufo, F. N. (2014). A nova classificação Americana para os Transtornos Mentais - o DSM-5. *Revista Brasileira De Terapia Comportamental E Cognitiva, 16*(1), 67–82.

Bastos, F. I. P. M., & Bertoni, N. (2014). *Pesquisa Nacional sobre o uso de crack: Quem são os usuários de crack e/ou similares do Brasil? Quantos são nas capitais brasileiras?* Rio de Janeiro: ICICT.

Bastos, F. I. P. M., Vasconcellos, M. T. L., De Boni, R. B., Reis, N. B., Coutinho, C. F., Niquini, R. P., et al. (2017). *III Levantamento Nacional sobre o uso de drogas pela população brasileira*. Rio de Janeiro, Brazil: FIOCRUZ/ICICT.

Carlini, E. A., Galduróz, J. C., Noto, A. R., Carlini, C. M., Oliveira, L. G., & Nappo, S. A. (2006). *II Levantamento domiciliar sobre o uso de drogas psicotrópicas no Brasil: estudo envolvendo as 108 maiores cidades do país*. São Paulo, Brazil: SENAD.

Carlini, E. A., Noto, A. R., Sanchez, Z. M., Carlini, C. M. A., Locatelli, D. P., Abeid, L. R., et al. (2012). *VI Levantamento Nacional sobre o Consumo de Drogas Psicotrópicas entre Estudantes do Ensino fundamental e Médio das Redes Pública e Privada de Ensino nas 27 Capitais Brasileiras*. Brasília: SENAD.

Galduróz, J., Noto, A., Fonseca, A., & Carlini, E. (2004). *V Levantamento sobre o consumo de drogas psicotrópicas entre estudantes do ensino fundamental e médio da rede pública de ensino nas 27 capitais brasileiras - 2004*. São Paulo, Brazil: UNIFESP/CEBRID.

Jekel, J. F., Katz, D. L., & Elmore, J. G. (2006). *Epidemiologia, bioestatística e medicina preventiva* (2nd ed.). Porto Alegre, Brazil: Artmed.

Levy, D., de Almeida, L. M., & Szklo, A. (2012). The Brazil SimSmoke policy simulation model: The effect of strong tobacco control policies on smoking prevalence and smoking-attributable deaths in a middle income nation. *PLoS Medicine, 9*(11), e1001336. https://doi.org/10.1371/journal.pmed.1001336.

Miller, P. G., Strang, J., & Miller, P. M. (2010). *Addiction research methods*. West Sussex, UK: Wiley.

Noto, A. R., Galduróz, J. C. F., Nappo, A. S., Fonseca, A. M., Carlini, C. M. A., Moura, Y. G., & Carlini, E. A. (2004). *Levantamento Nacional sobre o Uso de Drogas entre Crianças e Adolescentes em Situação de Ruas nas 27 Capitais Brasileiras – 2003*. São Paulo, Brazil: UNIFESP/CEBRID.

Oliveira, L. G., Eckschmidt, F., & Wagner, G. A. (2017). A caracterização da dependência química. In A. L. M. Andrade & D. De Micheli (Eds.), *Inovações no tratamento de dependência de drogas* (pp. 3–17). Rio de Janeiro, Brazil: Atheneu.

Sanchez, Z. M., Locatelli, D. P., Noto, A. R., & Martins, S. S. (2013). Binge drinking among Brazilian students: A gradient of association with socioeconomic status in five geo-economic regions. *Drug and Alcohol Dependence, 127*(1–3), 87–93. https://doi.org/10.1016/j.drugalcdep.2012.06.018.

Sodré, F. F., Souza, G. B., Feitosa, R. S., Pereira, C. E. B., & Maldaner, A. O. (2017). Illicit drugs, metabolites and adulterants in wastewater: Monitoring community drug abuse in the Brazilian Federal District during the 2014 soccer world cup. *Journal of the Brazilian Chemical Society, 28*(11), 2146–2154. https://doi.org/10.21577/0103-5053.20170063.

Souza, J. (2016). *Crack e exclusão social*. Brasília: Ministério da Justiça e Cidadania, Secretaria Nacional de Política sobre Drogas.

The Institute for Health Metrics and Evaluation (IHME). (2017). *Global burden of diseases*. Retrieved from http://www.healthdata.org/brazil

United Nations Office on Drugs and Crime (UNODC). (2018). *World drug report 2018*. Vienna, Austria: UNODC.

United Nations Office on Drugs and Crime (UNODC). (2019). *World drug report 2019*. Vienna, Austria: UNODC.

World Health Organization (WHO). (2014). *WHO global status report on alcohol and health* (p. 2014). Geneva, Switzerland: World Health Organization.

World Health Organization (WHO). (2015a). *WHO global report on trends in prevalence of tobacco smoking 2015*. Geneva, Switzerland: World Health Organization.

World Health Organization (WHO). (2015b). *WHO report on the global tobacco epidemic, 2015: Raising taxes on tobacco*. Geneva, Switzerland: World Health Organization.

World Health Organization (WHO). (2018a). *International classification of disease for mortality statistics*, eleventh revision. Retrieved from https://icd.who.int/en

World Health Organization (WHO). (2018b). *Global status report on alcohol and health* (p. 2018). Geneva, Switzerland: World Health Organization.

World Health Organization (WHO). (2019a). *Management of substance abuse, country profiles*, Retrieved from http://www.who.int/substance_abuse/publications/global_alcohol_report/profiles

World Health Organization (WHO). (2019b). *WHO report on the global tobacco epidemic, 2019: Offer help to quit tobacco use*. Geneva: World Health Organization.

Chapter 3
Anthropological Studies in Drug Use Contexts: An Introduction to Theoretical, Methodological, and Ethical Aspects

Ygor Diego Delgado Alves and Pedro Paulo Gomes Pereira

Introduction

Ethnographic studies on drug use began as a consequence of the use of substances by original peoples who were the object of study par excellence of the anthropology. However, urban anthropology has had a wide development, especially after William Foote Whyte's study of boys in a poor neighborhood in Boston in the late 1930s (Whyte 1939). And from the 1950s on, and more precisely after the publication of *Outsiders,* 1963, by social scientist Howard Becker (2008), a seminal work analyzed in Alves (2017), that research on drug use has gained its own character. The emergence of neighborhoods with a significant young population and users of substances, especially heroin, causes the emergence of small open scenes of drug consumption. However, it is the social workers who are the first to witness and conduct research on these people and gradually are developing the skills of true ethnographers and a gaze that is increasingly broadening to encompass different aspects of the issue such as values and way of life.

The AIDS epidemic brings a new urgency to ethnographic studies of injecting drug use. The risks of transmitting the disease make the ritual of drug consumption and the management of paraphernalia of use, as well as the values involved and the networks of people formed around an illegal activity become essential. Ethnographic research is capable of demonstrating the evils of prohibitionism and justifying harm reduction policies. We will be sticking almost exclusively to a small portion of US production on the subject here.

Y. D. Delgado Alves (✉) · P. P. Gomes Pereira
Universidade Federal de São Paulo, São Paulo, SP, Brazil

D. De Micheli et al. (eds.), *Drugs and Human Behavior*,
https://doi.org/10.1007/978-3-030-62855-0_3

Historical Overview

We intend to provide a brief historical overview of ethnographic research with drug users from the US academic production, which we believe to be the most influential in this specific subject in our country, since there is little national production of this study model and in this subject. For this, we will go back to the beginning of the 40s of last century when authors such as La Barre (1942, p. 202), after ethnographic research in Bolivia, exposed the extent of the "*materia medica*" of the Aymara peoples, who inhabited the surroundings of Lake Titicaca. The author published an interesting paper in *The Journal of American Folklore* entitled *Folk medicine and folk science* in which he cites, among others, the uses of mercury to cure syphilis, seaweed for goiter, quinine for malaria, and "cocaine" as a palliative for pain. These observations were published after field research carried out in 1937, which provided extensive ethnobotanical material to the anthropologist. Ethnography can then provide us with rich material on the uses that people, groups, or even persons make of substances. However, if we made use of researches that require the coexistence in the field, for a period that usually exceeds some months, just to know which plants are used for certain purposes, we would only be taking advantage of a portion of the potential of the ethnographic method.

In an article published in 1959 by the *Archives of General Psychiatry of* the *American Medical Association*, Canadian American anthropologist Anthony Wallace of the University of Pennsylvania studies what he considers to be the cultural determinants of the response to the hallucinatory experience caused by mescaline consumption. The author notes that psychiatrists and anthropologists alike often expect some influence from the social environment on the variability of the manifest content of hallucinations, as well as on any behavior. After analyzing multiple studies on the effects of mescaline on Native Americans and undiagnosed white people with mental problems, Wallace concludes that the tone of subjective feeling and the content of hallucinations are strongly influenced by the cultural environment. Wallace considers the possibility that the negative attitude towards any distortion of the normal sensory and cognitive experience, which many members of North American society shared, may influence the subjective experience and even the physiological reactions to mescaline to an unknown degree. In addition, white people used the drug generally as part of academic experiments performed in a hospital setting, while Indians took mescaline in a religious and solemn environment. Whites took the drug once or twice in their lives, for experimental or clinical purposes within a scientific investigation, without any interest in its religious aspect. Indigenous peyote users take mescaline repeatedly, to accompany a serious ritual, with, according to the author, hope of personal salvation of which visions are the evidence. Attempts, apparently in vogue at the time, by white people to ban peyotism would have to take into account propositions of scholars on the subject such as Slotkin (1956), the most relevant anthropologist to study peyotism so far, according to Wallace (1959), for whom the answers obtained in clinical experiments with white people differ so much from indigenous peyotism that they should be considered in completely different categories.

We saw it then, how some ethnographic studies were able to point out the substances consumed and their medicinal purposes; and we were also able to realize how fundamental the cultural environment is for the hallucinogenic and even physiological effects of mescaline. But what about researching drug use in cities, would ethnography lend itself to studying urban drug use? The answer is yes.

Edward Preble (1966) will perform an ethnography in an area smaller than half a square mile, about 1.2 square kilometers, in New York City. A neighborhood mostly occupied by black populations, but with a strong Puerto Rican presence; and it is precisely the social and cultural factors related to drug use among the latter that will interest Preble. To access the field and the people he was interested in, this urban ethnographer spent the first month of research visiting the community to become known on the streets. He attended cafes, bars, shoeshine shops, candy stores, and barbershops. He thus obtained the cooperation of individuals representing the main non-Puerto Rican cultural groups: Jews, Irish, blacks, Russians, and Italians; who provided Preble with information about the neighborhood and about the Puerto Ricans themselves. Contact and research with these subjects were made possible by two key informants, one of them in his twenties and the other at 17 years of age. The first was described as the leader of one of the most important street gangs in the neighborhood, the youngest was a high school student and was not involved in criminal activities. Through them it was possible to access a large family and every block in which they lived, together with their friends. All together they were the main source of material about life stories and aspects of Puerto Rican culture there. But the question is: what will the ethnographer observe as social and cultural factors that may be associated with drug use? Because, once in the field, the researcher will direct his or her gaze or attention to certain aspects previously defined in a research project; until from the quality of the relationships established in the field, this gaze can be expanded, deepened, and even redirected.

After tracing a brief history of Puerto Rican presence in New York, Preble notes that the influx of these people into the most miserable areas of the Bronx and Brooklyn neighborhoods has attracted the hostile attention, materialized in the gang fights, of previously established cultural groups such as the Black, Irish, and Italian. The introduction of heroin use by Puerto Rican gang leaders quickly spread to other members, causing these gangs to fall apart; and young people to form new partnerships, which were commonly established between pairs of drug users. Now, dedicated to fundraising and substance acquisition activities, with no more interest in violent conflict.

With their mass arrival, Puerto Ricans became the target of immense distrust because they speak an incomprehensible language and are accused of stealing the jobs of the elder inhabitants. Racial identification has become a major problem for these people, targets of immense hostility. Teenagers proved to be especially sensitive to social suffering; and one of the adaptive alternatives to the new environment in which they were inserted was to adopt the style of the American street youth, with a certain behavior prone to delinquency. A way of life known at the time as "hip"

(Preble 1966, p. 9) linked to drug use. Young people who did not adopt this new style began to be ridiculed by members of their own community, having to isolate themselves and relegated to a marginal existence in the city. Moreover, of all the young Puerto Ricans in that region, who the ethnographer's interlocutors calculated to be around 400, about half would be unoccupied, without study or work: the part with the highest risk of heroin addiction. The author considers his data reliable due to the low variability between independent estimates made by his interlocutors; and the fact that it is a small community in which the private life of each one is usually of general knowledge.

The aforementioned author also noticed how the family life of Puerto Ricans influences the risk of dependence. The first significant aspect is the disadvantage of adult men in terms of social acceptance and the possibility of finding work. With the low income, both spouses need to work, leaving the children to move between relatives and neighbors, often without supervision after school hours. By forcing women to work, the new family situation, different from Puerto Rico in which a man's value is linked to his ability to support the home, maims the father's confidence and self-esteem. The frequent result is the abandonment of the home, voluntary, or under pressure from the wife. The collapse of traditional paternal authority, even though it may mean initial relief and greater freedom for the woman, ends up charging a high price in terms of structuring and control over the individual behavior of young people, which usually results in uncertainty, confusion, and conflict. For which heroin consumption seems to adjust, by replacing seemingly insoluble problems of adaptation to a totally new, hostile urban environment in frankly unfavorable conditions with a routine dedicated to the daily acquisition of a valuable product.

Preble's work, besides bringing to the urban environment the concern with the study of drug consumption, shows us a series of procedures. First, the author is concerned with delimiting a certain area of the city. Next, he describes his strategy to access the field and tries to delimit and specify who will be his interlocutors, inside and outside the specific group of his interest. He then drafts the major outlines of those people, in this case divided into ethnic groups, and the deleterious influences they will bring on this specific part he intends to study: the young Puerto Ricans. These newly arrived immigrants will try to adapt themselves to the new hostile environment, through the incorporation of a way of life close to the American one and associated with the consumption of drugs. In the family, the difficulties in employment imposed on men and the need for the wife to work also end up putting the male role in check, leading to the dissolution of part of the marriages. The lack of professional perspective in adult life causes young men to suffer extra pressures, in an environment marked by idleness and family dissolution. Thus, a broad spectrum of socio-cultural variables (immigration, urbanism, employability, division into ethnic groups, masculinity, dress, lifestyle, values) are found in the ethnographer's effort to understand drug use.

The trade in these psychoactive substances will also be the subject of description and analysis by contemporary researchers of Preble: how heroin was introduced in a certain neighborhood, who the first sellers were, how these pioneers incorporated other young people into the business and how they made the drug become something attractive, are topics that certainly emerged from living with drug users. Feldman (1968) was a social worker in the same New York City neighborhood, the Lower East Side, which Preble and used 6 years of living with young people, and other professionals who dealt with these people, to observe and gather information. We see, therefore, that professional daily life can be an important space for observation and interlocution, even more so if the researcher is aware of his condition: *Because I was an adult, and, more pertinently, a social worker from a middle-class world, the boys colluded to keep their behavior a secret from me* (Feldman 1968, p. 134). Even so, by working in the streets, Feldman could witness all the excitement of the young people around the arrival of this new habit in his surroundings. Then this young social worker worried about the visible consequences of heroin consumption could observe that the boys shared certain values around a lifestyle defined by their ideal type: the stand-up cat. To be a stand-up cat, for these young men in the mid-1960s, was to enjoy a certain reputation. It required facing fortuitous situations in which he could prove his boldness, strength, adventurous character, in short, to be tough. Identifying and understanding these values were fundamental to the kind of analysis the author came to make. The ideal stand-up cat also understood a certain corporeality, with its mannerisms, slang, clothing, and appropriate haircut, in addition to the attitude of those who are after action all the time. All these aspects then become interesting to understand the consumption of drugs, because the introduction of this habit in the neighborhood was given by its most experienced and successful young people in adopting this lifestyle. Those with the greatest reputation are the first heroin users and dealers who, because of their ascendancy over others, quickly recruit new dealers. The newcomers start to occupy the statement immediately below, but in the hope that in the future they will be able to earn the same highly significant monetary profits as their supplier.

The stand-up cat ideal was also important for Feldman (1968) to be able to understand the resilience of heroin consumption, even in the face of the damage observed by young people in their fellow users. By seeing their old models of behavior: older, successful boys in their ideal way of life marked by a constant search for action; by glimpsing them for a handful of money to buy heroin, the younger ones could simply conclude, from the abundant decadent evidence wandering the neighborhood, that they should not go in the same direction. But this was not the case; on the contrary, heroin consumption continued to attract new followers. What the coexistence for many years, six in total, with these young people revealed to the attentive look of the researcher was that the more dangerous the drug was shown, the more challenging it was to control its effects in the medium term; and the greater the challenge, the more attractive its consumption was shown to boys eager to show bravery. In addition, his use was considered something glamorous, done by some artists of the time and the most successful people among those young men. Heroin consumption, in the words of an intern at Wiltwyck's reformatory, where Preble and Feldman worked, was a novelty that everyone was talking about and that seemed to have taken over everything. According to the young man, who was black, all the cool people (hip) were using and having this new cheap (high).

> To know what was going on and to be in on things, you had to do that. And the only way I could come out of Wiltwyck and be up to date, the only way to take up where I had left off and be the same hip guy I was before I went to Wiltwyck, was to get in on the hippest thing, and the hippest thing was horse.[1] (Feldman 1968, p. 134).

The consumption of heroin revealed itself to the young social worker and researcher, after spend a lot of time close to his interlocutors, to be a doorway to a boring daily life lived in the reformatory. At the same time, it served as an instrument for the affirmation of boys guided by an adventurous lifestyle, in which reputation in front of peers was fundamental to not have a life marked by humiliation and violence. Because it was a drug of destructive effects perfectly perceived by boys, and precisely because of this, the dominion over its most deleterious effects was proof of courage, something fundamental for those who lived under the ideal of *stand-up cat*.

The author also intended to overcome some difficulties faced by research conducted in an institutional environment, often dedicated to the treatment of drug users, who therefore took biased statements. Because they accessed institutionalized people who were at that moment seeking to abandon problematic use, the interviews ended up gathering entirely negative testimonies about the drug experience since its beginning. Stereotypical views, such as that the first dose would have been unbelievably pleasurable, and that all subsequent years of drug use would have been just a vain attempt to relive that idyllic and unique first moment could also be the fruit of institutional culture.

Certain ideas present at the time, and possibly even today, that using drugs would be a behavior linked to psychic problems of adaptation to the environment and that they were insufficient to explain, for example, why other individuals with the same problems did not use drugs, could now be confronted with the street culture of these young people who used substances to enjoy a better reputation.

Two decades after the publication of the Lower East Side heroin users' study, Harvey W. Feldman is confronted with the possibility of the AIDS epidemic, which in the USA was until then confined to New Jersey City, in addition to New York, reaching San Francisco, on the west coast of the country. Injecting drug users (IDUs) run the risk of being contaminated with the HIV virus by sharing syringes and having unprotected sex. Therefore, ethnographies become more applied in seeking to describe a culture of use with important public health implications. And it is to this new task that Feldman will devote himself.

Prohibitionism is now identified as a policy that not only hinders access to information about IDUs, but also has harmful effects on HIV infection. Ethnographic studies begin to question strongly the prohibition of drugs and the limitations imposed on the trade of fundamental items of paraphernalia of use such as syringes. The difficulty in gaining access to these items eventually leads to their sharing and

[1] To know what was going on and to be in on things, you had to do that. And the only way I could come out of Wiltwyck and be up to date, the only way to take up where I had left off and be the same hip guy I was before I went to Wiltwyck, was to get in on the hippest thing, and the hippest thing was horse.

consequently to contamination. Let us remember that during the 1970s, US President Nixon had initiated his policy of war on drugs. Not only did this policy fail to discourage the old ones and prevent the emergence of new illicit drug users, it created an aura of excitement and adventure around drugs that, as the studies of the previous decade had shown, ended up motivating the use rather than discouraging it. Drug use did not increase "[...] despite official attempts to discourage them, but because of them" (Feldman, Biernacki 1988, p. 29). The spirit of ethnography would now be back to understanding how repressive policies created a social context, with clandestine networks of users, that favored the efficient and rapid spread of HIV.

Research is now funded by public health departments to identify the most relevant characteristics of injecting drug use scenes; and thus be able to: (1) typify its users; (2) verify whether there was concern about HIV; (3) identify the factors that led to sharing needles; (4) determine the extent to which precautions were taken against contamination; and (5) examine how much the two highest risk populations, gay men, and IDU were in contact.

In short, we can say that the IDUs were mostly people who were strayed from their family and friends, with low income, but who cared about their health and did not want to get sick. It was found that the stereotyped view of the drug user in search of certain death was wrong; but that he shared syringes because of the difficulty in obtaining them and because he usually lived in hotels where the frequency to each other's rooms to use drugs was common. They did not clean their syringes properly before sharing them because they were uninformed and had no incentive to do so. An aggravating factor was that gay men and IDUs shared the same environments and had common interests in drug use.

We have seen how the goals of the research have broadened and how they have come to position themselves within something much wider: drug policy. But in the 1990s, other substances would impose new approaches and this is the case with crack. Bourgois (1997) publishes in the collection *Crack in America: Demon drugs and social justice* important research on people very similar to those studied by Preble (1966) and Feldman (1968): Puerto Ricans around a Spanish Harlem crack house. However, the change in method and results is brutal. So much so that after the first 13 months of a total period of 5 years in which Bourgois will reside in *El Barrio*, the anthropologist is able to describe scenes and characters that enable him to make a quality leap in academic production about that context.

Like the classical ethnographer, the anthropologist will take up residence in the field and will assume, as far as possible, the way of life of the people with whom he intends to work. The experience of the field is shown in its fullness as the most powerful instrument to access a culture that has in the consumption and trade of drugs one of its characteristics. Thus, it is capable of dismantling certain current interpretations about the poor people who inhabit the miserable neighborhoods of New York, such as the culture of poverty: that derived the situation of the lower strata of the working class from their bad socialization in the values of the wider society. On the contrary, adhering to drug trafficking was an attempt to rise up in the social hierarchy in the only way that presented itself to those descendants of immigrants. Individuals who had experienced low-skill employment and low pay, experiences described as daily humiliation, in addition to providing insufficient income for family support.

Participating in drug trafficking was the available and most rational means to conquer the material goods that define a successful person. In addition, symbolic goods could also be earned in this way, and the most important of these was respect. A drug dealer is harassed all the time by sycophants, people seeking to please those who have some money in the midst of poverty. From being a low skilled worker he is treated as a boss, but in an informal economy where respect is fundamental not to be passed on: victim of default, delusion, or theft. To this end, a whole culture of violence and terror develops, and knowing how to exercise terror is fundamental to having the desired success. Thus, the community is immersed in a daily reality of violence that can only be understood by the clandestine drug economy. For its users, immersed in daily humiliation, hopelessness, and insecurity, and there the original and devastating conclusion of Bourgois (1997) on crack consumption, using drugs produces not only relief, but sense in a daily life marked by the rituals of consumption and obtaining funds to acquire the drug. For the author, this reminds us of ancient religions and their effectiveness in preventing the revolt of colonized peoples. Crack users transform from unemployed and failed students, victims according to official explanations of their own stupidity and laziness, into masses of palpitating pleasure, briefly followed by a fall and immediate warning: " [...] that fills their life with concrete and compelling purpose: get more crack—fast!" (Bourgois 1997, p. 74).

The kind of approach we have seen here has had a great influence on Brazilian drug production from an anthropological point of view.

Current Surveys

Philippe Bourgois remains the most prolific reference in the US context of anthropological research on drug use and trade. The maturity of his research has led him to position his ethnographic work in an even broader historical and economic context. He notes how since the beginnings of commercial capitalism, the trafficking of pleasurable substances has caused havoc. The periods of increased consumption in certain localities or regions have served as an alarm that can help us expose the violent contradictions between " [...] power, social inequality, vulnerability and resistance both within local communities and across large-scale social formations" (Bourgois 2018, p. 386). Imperial power is exercised via prohibitionism; and these periods of greater consumption " [...] almost inevitably generate moral panics and predictably mobilize nationalist xenophobic, messianic and socio-biological racist discourses [...]" (Bourgois 2018, p. 387). Not by chance, the USA has led the hypocritical prohibitionist drug policy in the last century; even with direct interventions in the internal affairs of countries like Mexico and Colombia, just to stay in the most glaring cases in Latin America. As is also the case in Brazil, the industrial production of psychoactive substances made illegal breaks the normal process with which societies dealt with drug consumption; especially among the most vulnerable lumpesinato. Still according to Bourgois (2018, p. 388), a review of the literature on hyperprofitable drug trafficking suggests its historical importance for what Karl Marx called the primitive accumulation of capital. Thus, the challenge posed to researchers would be to seek " [...] even more ambitious critical questions around what new perspectives on illegal psychoactive drugs in the Global South can reveal about our moment in history [...]" (Bourgois 2018, p. 389). Questions that take into account an illicit and predatory economy where illegality allows the development of a certain primitive accumulation industry with clandestine cocaine and heroin laboratories for export and hyper-profits; in the midst of ultra-neoliberal policies that produce immense reservoirs of a lumpenized (Bourgois 2011) population that becomes available as a client or workforce to be exploited in the illegal narcotics production process. That it uses the financialization of the global economy to launder and transfer its money and the modern techniques of flexible export platforms to distribute the drug.

In Brazil, the context of crack consumption was the object of exposure in Alves' research (Alves 2016). The author dedicated himself to outlining the paraphernalia, the techniques and rituals of use, and the effects perceived. Fromm (2017), in his ethnographic research, entered the use scene of the neighborhood of Luz, in São Paulo, by following the paths of three characters, through the programs Cristolândia, De Braços Abertos (DBA), and Recomeço. The author sought to draw attention to the strategies for survival in daily life, in the face of what she believed were attempts to put an end to Cracolândia in the city of São Paulo-Brazil. A description of the DBA can be found in Alves (2017), from the articulations between municipal secretariats, to the beginning of the program, to a description of how it works. It is also by the same author a criticism of the biomedical concept of dependence from what he calls an anthropology of the "flow," as the movements and paths around the consumption of crack in Cracolândia (Alves and Pereira 2019). In addition to the routes around drug use, the ethnography of Malheiro (2019), who participates in the National Network of Antiprohibitionist Feminists (Renfa), describes racial, class, and gender violence. In her work with women who smoked crack in the old center of Salvador, the author pointed out how the construction of a feminist and antiprohibitionist camp has been organizing politically women victims of the war on drugs.

Ethical and Methodological Aspects of Ethnographic Research with Drug Dealers Users

Ethical issues should be central when researching people who are put at risk by their habit, including incarceration and even death. In the book *In search of respect: selling crack in El Barrio*, Bourgois comments on his difficulties as a white man in *El Barrio*, New York area, and the location of his research. As he was often approached by police on suspicion of being a drug user, or simply a guy lost in an inappropriate location to someone of his *status*, Bourgois, in his research with crack users, had legal constraints a constant concern. The mere presence of researchers was thought by him to be something possibly dangerous to drug users. His 5-year ethnographic career had serious consequences for conjugal and family life: the end of the research in *El Barrio* coincides with the end of his marriage (Bourgois 2003).

In research in contexts of illegal practices, entering and remaining in the field are always a challenge. In this sense, the symbolic exchange of material goods enters as a fundamental element of inclusion and exclusion of individuals, including ethnographers, in the community of drug users; and was widely discussed in research by Bourgois and Schonberg (2009) with heroin users in the USA. Anthropologists found that the user community was maintained through a moral economy of exchange, this economy involves them in a network of mutual relationships, and defines the boundaries of the community. In other words, those who exchange are part of it. Not to exchange is to be antisocial and to risk being ostracized. The authors were worried about not buying information, or becoming bosses, but they could not remain unaware of the usual way (exchange of food, money, and drugs) of defining and expressing friendship, organizing hierarchies, and excluding undesirable outsiders. They had to learn when to give and when to deny, and they concluded with the important observation of the inadequacy of the most dogmatic rules of research to the reality of the streets.

David Moore (1993) did an ethnographic study among recreational users of illicit drugs in the city of Perth, Western Australia. After discussing methodological aspects of sampling, data collection, and access to the field, the author makes interesting ethical and even moral considerations about ethnography with drug users. The first is whether there is any obligation on the part of the researcher to report criminal activities related to the trade and consumption of drugs. The answer is no. Only in extreme cases, where we are all obliged to act as citizens, can a radical decision be made such as contacting the police. But in the absence of such a situation, we must respect the Free and Clarified Consent Term (FCCT). This leads us to the following discussion: the meaning of the FCCT for ethnographic research.

For MacRae and Vidal (2006) ethnographers do not have sufficient guidance when making their ethical choices in research with interlocutors whose activities include illegal acts such as the consumption of illicit substances. Procedures such as signing a FCCT become unrealistic with people wanted by the police, for example. In a field situation, the ethnographer is under the rules of his interlocutors, in a situation reverse to that experienced in the laboratory, hospital, or clinic. As the very insertion in the field is negotiated, the subsequent dialogues would be allowed by definition (Oliveira 2004). Consent to self-incrimination makes no sense. Finally, this paperwork for the protection of human beings is aimed more at safeguarding research institutions and less at research subjects, in their interests and dignity (Bourgois and Schonberg 2009).

Another interesting question in Moore (1993) is whether or not ethnographers should use illicit drugs during field work. It can happen that the decision not to participate in drug use prevents them from staying with users, especially in environments more exclusively oriented to their consumption where the presence of a non-user can cause more discomfort. Researchers from the Ayahuasca traditions used the tea during their ethnographies (see, for example, Groisman 2000). It makes no sense to practitioners of the cults that include Santo Daime, for example, for people who have not ingested the tea to participate in the ceremonies. If you want to access, for a reasonably long period, the rituals where the Daime is drunk is almost like an imposition to consume it. Something similar happens with the crack users. In order for Alves (2017) to be part of them, it was necessary to smoke crack. This allowed a rich sharing of experiences. Not only on the effects, but on the history of each interlocutor and of the ethnographer.

References

Alves, Y. D., & Pereira, P. G. (2019). Uma antropologia do "fluxo": reflexões sobre dependência no contexto do crack. *Revista Internacional Interdisciplinar Interthesis, 16*(1), 121–142. https://doi.org/10.5007/1807-1384.2019v16n1p121.

Alves, Y. D. D. (2016). O uso do crack como ele é: o cachimbo, o "bloco" e o usuário. *Etnográfica, 20*(3), 495–515. https://doi.org/10.4000/etnografica.4640.

Alves, Y. D. D. (2017). *Jamais fomos zumbis: contexto social e craqueiros na cidade de São Paulo.* Salvador, Brazil: EDUFBA. https://doi.org/10.7476/9788523218591.

Becker, H. (2008). *Outsiders: Estudos de sociologia do desvio.* Rio de Janeiro, Brazil: Zahar. (Obra original publicada em 1963).

Bourgois, P. (1997). In search of Horatio Alger: Culture and ideology in the crack economy. In C. Reinarman & H. Levine (Eds.), *Crack in America: Demon drugs and social justice.* Berkeley, CA: University of California Press.

Bourgois, P. (2003). *In search of respect: Selling crack in El Barrio.* Berkeley, CA: Cambridge University Press.

Bourgois, P. (2011). Lumpen abuse: The human cost of righteous neoliberalism. *City & Society, 23*(1), 2–12. https://doi.org/10.1111/j.1548-744x.2011.01045.x.

Bourgois, P. (2018). Decolonising drug studies in an era of predatory accumulation. *Third World Quarterly, 39*(2), 385–398. https://doi.org/10.1080/01436597.2017.1411187.

Bourgois, P., & Schonberg, J. (2009). *Righteous dopefiends.* Los Angeles, CA: University of California Press.

Feldman, H. W. (1968). Ideological supports to becoming and remaining a heroin addict. *Journal of Health and Social Behavior, 9*(2), 131–139.

Feldman, H. W., & Biernacki, P. (1988). The ethnography of needle sharing among intravenous drug users and implications for public policies and intervention strategies. *NIDA Research Monograph, 80*, 28–39.

Fromm, D. (2017). Percursos e refúgios urbanos. *Ponto Urbe: Revista do Núcleo de Antropologia Urbana da USP, 2017*, 21. https://doi.org/10.4000/pontourbe.3604.

Groisman, A. (2000). *Santo Daime in the Netherlands: An anthropological study of a new world religion in a European setting* (Doctoral dissertation in Social Anthropology), University of London, London, UK.

La Barre, W. (1942). Folk medicine and folk science. *The Journal of American Folklore, 55*(218), 197–203.

MacRae, E., & Vidal, S. (2006). A Resolução 196/96 e a imposição do modelo biomédico na pesquisa social: dilemas éticos e metodológicos do antropólogo pesquisando o uso de substâncias psicoativas. *Revista de Antropologia, 49*(2), 645–666. https://doi.org/10.1590/s0034-77012006000200005.

Malheiro, L. S. B. (2019). *Tornar-se mulher usuária de crack: trajetória de vida, cultura de uso e políticas sobre drogas no centro de Salvador-BA* (Masters's thesis), Universidade Federal da Bahia, Salvador, Brazil. Retrieved from https://repositorio.ufba.br/ri/handle/ri/28468

Moore, D. (1993). Ethnography and illicit drug use: Dispatches from an anthropologist in the "field". *Addiction Research, 1*(1), 11–25. https://doi.org/10.3109/16066359309035320.

Oliveira, R. C. (2004). Pesquisa em versus pesquisa com seres humanos. In C. Víctora, R. G. Oliven, M. E. Maciel, & A. P. Oro (Eds.), *Antropologia e ética: o debate atual no Brasil* (pp. 33–44). Niterói, Brazil: Editora da Universidade Federal Fluminense.

Preble, E. (1966). Social and cultural factors related to narcotic use among Puerto Ricans in new York City. *International Journal of the Addictions, 1*(1), 30–41. https://doi.org/10.3109/10826086609072269.

Slotkin, J. S. (1956). *The peyote religion: A study in Indian-white relations*. Glencoe, Scotland: Free Press.

Wallace, A. (1959). Cultural determinants of response to hallucinatory experience. *Archives of General Psychiatry, 1*(1), 58. https://doi.org/10.1001/archpsyc.1959.03590010074009.

Whyte, W. (1939). Race conflicts in the north end of Boston. *The New England Quarterly, 12*(4), 623. https://doi.org/10.2307/360446.

Chapter 4
Neuroanthropology of Drugs: Relations Between the Brain, Social Context, and Use of Psychoactive Substances

Richard Alecsander Reichert

Introduction

The human being is part of nature; he is an organism interacting with the world around him. To understand this dynamics it is necessary to recognize the complexity and the need for constant scientific innovations to unveil its mysteries and transformations (Zimmermann and Torriani-Pasin 2011). Among the various human activities is the use of psychoactive substances, present in virtually all of human history. This is an ancient and universal social practice (Bergeron 2012; Guimarães 2013). Over the years, researchers from various fields of knowledge have developed different theories to explain the need and use of substances that alter the state of mind. Many of them, however, do not take into account the multiplicity of factors that surround them. Faced with the complexity and variability of personal and social situations, the union of different scientific fields is necessary, especially because, as several references have already pointed out, there is no way to approach them in a reductionist or simplified manner. It is essential to recognize their multifactoriality and to maintain a progressive endeavor to identify and understand the various dimensions involved.

The idea of dependence was, at first, a biomedical concept understood as a chronic disease with harmful consequences. Today, after much debate between the humanities and biomedical sciences, there are broader differentiations and models that consider psychosocial factors beyond biological ones. The most accepted definition in science today is that described by the Diagnostic and Statistical Manual of Mental Disorders (DSM), which speaks of continued use despite the adverse effects on the person, which include criteria such as interference with vital functioning, family,

In memorian of Alba Zaluar

R. A. Reichert (✉)
Universidade do Vale do Itajaí, Itajaí, SC, Brazil

D. De Micheli et al. (eds.), *Drugs and Human Behavior*,
https://doi.org/10.1007/978-3-030-62855-0_4

academic, professional, and social losses, exacerbated dedication of time and energy to substance use activities, unsuccessful attempts at cessation or reduction of use, development of tolerance (when the person has to administer increasing doses to have the same initial effect), and symptoms of physiological abstinence when the use is stopped (APA 2014). Experts state that in addition to the physiological aspects, cognitive, social, and emotional characteristics should also receive credit for the compulsive disposition to use drugs, play or buy impulsively. That is why people sometimes exchange one medicine for another, or even the drug for behaviors unrelated to their use, such as shopping or playing compulsively, despite the damage they bring.

Velho (1998), Zaluar (2004), and MacRae (2008) stated that experiences related to the use of psychoactive substances could only be understood from a dialectic between the subjective state of individuals and the pharmacological effects of drugs. Thus, they can only be understood in the socio-cultural context of use. That is, for social scientists, social relations have always been what matters. Anthropologists have always been more interested in the changing meanings of pleasure and risk associated with drugs and their social context. Today, in the social sciences, the discussion of substance use and dependence has an expanded focus of studies that now include urban settings and the growing process of globalization that has provoked many changes in traditional or stateless societies, affecting social organization, hierarchies, the mode of production of goods, the different positions in the labor process, affected by the broad markets for the sale and purchase of contemporary psychoactive drugs (Goody 1982; Singer 2012). The exclusion of users in the urban space, abuse, and the negative effects on the family, the neighborhood, and on the user's own person have all come to be addressed by social scientists.

This paradigm shift is an important step for drug research, although it initially remained at the microsocial level, even when they consider that there is a political dimension intrinsic to this issue, since people and social groups are subject to a series of threats and insecurity in their daily lives (Velho 1998). Only when the spectrum of investigations for the macrosocial plan is broadened, is it possible to understand the transformations that have occurred between the ritual use of psychoactive drugs in stateless societies and the market for use in societies with a market. This understanding is fundamental to avoid the errors that Hart (2017) points out when describing that, in fact, drug policies and law enforcement are influenced by the erroneous interpretation of data. Misguided drug policies are enacted based on distorted information that results, for example, in actions like those of Philippine President Rodrigo Duterte, who was responsible for the deaths of thousands of people on charges of using and selling illegal drugs with the excuse that methamphetamine would be responsible for shrinking the brains of users, who then could no longer be rehabilitated. According to Hart (2014), current drug policies are based largely on fiction and ignorance. There is emotional hysteria caused by the spread of false information about drugs, a factor that contributes to serious misunderstandings in public policy formulation and misuse of resources. It is essential that science be used for drug policy making, for health promotion and for the guarantee of human rights.

This is why these and other scientists pay attention to the social and political implications of scientific knowledge, especially with regard to the subject that is so mobilizing and focused on drug use and abuse. A multidisciplinary approach enables a comprehensive overview of the issue and the formulation of more effective public policies. In this sense, biopsychosocial models of drug use and dependence, as in the emerging field of neuroanthropology, are essential for a more comprehensive understanding of the subject. For this, as Alves proposed (Alves 2017, p. 25), "the intention is to have a dialogue between theories."

Drugs: Definitions, Classifications, and Neurobiological Aspects

The human brain consists of billions of cells named neurons, among others, but which have prolongations that conduct nerve impulses. Between the neurons, there are spaces called synapses. The nervous impulses are responsible for the release of chemical substances that travel through the synaptic spaces, called neurotransmitters. There are different types of neurotransmitters in charge of different functions. Psychotropic substances operate on these neurotransmitters, interfering in their functioning, generating certain sensations and perceptions (Masur and Carlini 2004; Guimarães 2013). In short, these substances refer to chemical compounds that alter mood, behavior, and cognition when ingested (Wadley 2016) and are commonly categorized as depressants, stimulants, and hallucinogens. These definitions take into account their effects on the central nervous system.

In neuroscience, the idea that the brain is at the center of the interaction between the person and the world of which it becomes the mediator is factual. On the one hand, it is known that a great part of brain development is influenced by the experiences lived by the individual and, on the other hand, by the coordinated action of numerous genes that can be organized or enter into different synergies according to the external stimulus and individual action. Although, for neuroscientists, the function of the brain is that of mediator between the individual organism and the external world, the duality between the internal nature and the external creation cannot be undone, since they are facets of a persistent interaction that makes them inseparable (Guimarães and Zaluar 2015). For this reason, neuroscientists currently recognize that it is not enough to study only the functioning of the brain and that it is necessary to consider the psychological structure of the user as well as the social context through which the catalyzers of recognition and reward also pass. That is, it is necessary to consider the psychological dimensions of the person and the social contexts of the use of psychoactive substances (Bedendo et al. 2013; De Micheli et al. 2016).

Use and Dependence on Substances: A Historical-Anthropological View

Initially, social scientists who wrote about behavior-changing and hypothetically addictive substances emphasized the long human interaction with such drugs, dating the use at about 10,000 years ago, without explaining pathological use. On the contrary, they described how the consumption of alcohol and other psychoactive drugs was restricted to festive occasions that demanded more sociability, increased solidarity, and diminished social conflicts among participants, that is, the use took place in temporary and socially controlled ritual contexts. These rituals were usually performed after a period of hard work and served to celebrate success in hunting, planting, or harvesting food, in addition to other extraordinary events such as weddings, coronation of monarchs, rituals of passages for men and women, etc. (Singer 2012). They did not record the problematic or uncontrolled use of these substances, therefore without pathology or even social problem. For them, the use of psychoactive drugs was restricted to specific people for a limited period for certain ritual purposes. Their approach was holistic, treating cultures as delimited units with collective values and rules that had to be understood according to the perspective of cultural relativism. Even when they studied societies where excessive consumption was observed, they did not study the effects on health and social relations for fear of practicing ethnocentrism.

The first psychoactive substance mentioned in the literature of social sciences was alcohol. The processing and consumption of beer, according to these studies, permeated many cultures since the Neolithic period, which fostered a debate about whether primitive peoples were taming grain, a crucial change in human history, to make beer or bread. In addition to being an important beverage in Egypt for more than 5000 years, alcohol was used by people on all continents during rituals to honor the dead, for the health and fertility of people, land, and nature, and for exchanges based on reciprocity. Anthropologists agree that beer brings people together and serves to reinforce social hospitality and communitarianism during ceremonial and daily activities. It is a common cultural marker of wealth and status; it can represent a payment of tribute to chiefs and is essential in the redistribution of wealth (Arthur 2014). Beer is consumed for many reasons, but it is primarily a drink for cooperative work. Many people prefer to plant and harvest their crops or build houses with shared work, and beer is part of the pay for this work. In urban environments, beer is considered the most appropriate beverage for informal, relaxation-oriented occasions, especially in non-domestic settings.

However, although social scientists have observed that there is much cultural and religious disagreement about alcohol, they say little about its excessive consumption. Even so, the literature on male violence analyzes how it explodes in the places where men usually meet—bars, bars, pubs, taverns—and where drunkenness usually occurs.

Wine, whose history goes back at least 8000 years, is also drunk widely on the planet, but with varied meanings depending on time and place. Pots used to drink it have been found in China, Iran, and Georgia, in addition to European countries. Like other drinks used in religious rituals, wine had strong spiritual significance. Associated with blood by the ancient Egyptians and incorporated into the Eucharist by Christianity in the beverage identified with the blood of Christ, wine represented metaphorically the masculine, the potent, the spiritual side of the ritual. On the contrary, in the Greek cult of Dionysius and in the Bacchanalias of the Romans, wine represents the festive worldly pleasure, used exaggeratedly by all the participants.

Despite its historical connection with religion, wine is also an unholy food whose production and consumption have changed significantly. It is said that a new culture of wine emerged in the 1980s, as it became a subject for discussion and evaluation by experts in increasingly numerous publications and places dedicated to consumption, consumer associations, festivals, and wine drinking clubs were created. The success of such initiatives illustrates the decline of traditional family wine culture and the emergence of a new, emblematic and fragmented culture in the context of a disintegrated and more individualistic society. What these wine drinkers have in common is the need to express their knowledge of the beverage and share the pleasures associated with its consumption. From this exclusive place for such symbolic exchanges, a wine culture was generated that separated connoisseurs from amateurs, thus excluding ordinary drinkers (Crenn et al. 2004). The democratization of wine consumption in taverns during nineteenth century France was followed by a culture and consumption that contributed to the hierarchization of society, but not to dependence. However, Roland Barthes (Barthes 1972), analyzing French popular culture, describes wine as a totemic drink, a symbol of French identity, in which "drunkenness is a consequence, not the goal; the drink is used to be appreciated and is not an end in itself." However, drunkenness has not ceased to occur in elegant environments, probably only because someone has let himself be carried away by Bacchus (god of wine). In this social context, there is no concern with alcohol abuse.

Some social researchers have distinguished European societies in respect to alcohol consumption. In certain southern European countries, alcohol, especially wine, is traditionally an accepted, morally neutral element of everyday life, and the place of consumption overlaps and merges with the everyday world, just as alcohol consumption is integrated into common behaviors such as sleeping or eating (Martinez and Martín 1987). In northern European countries, where there is an ambiguous, ambivalent, or troubled relationship with alcohol, especially beer and distilled beverages, due to the moral condemnation of drinking, the places of consumption are more likely to be closed establishments, with heavy walls and doors, in order to keep the activities of customers confidential (Campbell 1991). Social scientists have not evaluated the different prevalences of abuse in these types of societies. But a report to the European Commission (Social Issues Research Centre 1998) stated that the "integrated" cultures of the Mediterranean presented significantly fewer alcohol-related problems. Conversely, negative or inconsistent beliefs and expectations found mainly in "dry," "Nordic," or "morally ambivalent" drinking cultures are associated with higher levels of alcohol-related problems. The contagion of unbalanced beer and distillate drinking styles has also been analyzed: the influence of "ambivalent" northern cultures on beer or wine drinkers in southern "integrated" cultures is increasing and is associated with potentially harmful changes in attitudes and behavior (e.g. the adoption of more abusive behavior among young males in Spain). Historical evidence suggests that attempts to curb the antisocial excesses associated with an "alien" beverage through draconian alcohol restrictions alone are likely to result in the association of such behavior with "benign" native drinking and a general increase in its intake (Social Issues Research Centre 1998).

The macrosocial and political approach to psychoactive drugs that are now considered illegal focuses on other issues will make up the historical picture of their use. Since the nineteenth century, as a consequence of colonialism, ritually used drugs have been produced on a large scale and began to exist as global commodities, sold as medicines or pleasure drugs, sometimes even sponsored by colonial power. Geopolitical issues became important to understand what was happening at the local level, that is, how the meaning of some drugs changed due to the ideological and political interference on their connotation. The problem of drug use and dependence then became political and ideological, requiring a broader scope than that generally given for microsocial ethnographic studies. The political problem of drugs, from this perspective, requires a careful analysis of the ideological discourses that have gained general support and become naturalized, so to speak, in the definitions of the substances in question (MacRae 2008).

The social meaning of opium, for example, according to this current, has changed. From a way of paying workers for their labor during the fifteenth century, as well as a medicine prescribed by doctors during the nineteenth century, it became a dangerous drug defined by politicians in powerful countries, who included its derivatives in the new definition: heroin, morphine, codeine, etc. Anthropologists who studied the change in the meaning of the drug over time and space tell this story that ends in the twentieth century with a hybrid substance: a remedy against pain that could cause addiction and a politicized drug that is a threat, becoming a geopolitical issue. The economic and political processes that took place in the mid-nineteenth century, including British mercantile colonialism, made opium a saleable substance and, consequently, opium production increased. Consumption thrived in China after the Opium War during which Britain imposed the use of opium to ensure the sale of the product from its Asian colonies.

Anthropologists, who have taken a critical view and are against the global war on drugs, have focused their analysis on the disintegratory effects of the destruction of opium plantations among residents. According to them, in areas of Southeast Asia, opium has introduced a new and relatively stable source of wealth, easily stored or converted into money, granting small-scale peasants great autonomy as to when and where to sell their products. After the ban on planting the poppy from which opium is extracted, they were persuaded to cooperate with the government and began to proclaim the evils of poppy cultivation and expel "opium addicts" from their villages. The social effects were considered disastrous because of the amount of wealth previously available to the farmers: the villagers' chances of getting a wife through the dowry, the difficulties of finding another plantation that would grow well in the mountains and, above all, the military presence in the villages and their fields (Gillogly 2008).

Other enlightening questions therefore come from the political economy of drugs and addictions from the perspective of critical sociology. For Jack Goody (1982) the importance of culture must be recognized, but the study of food and drink must involve historical research and the approach to political economy, both at the micro level of the family and neighborhood, and at the macro level that includes markets and the state.

To curb the uncontrolled use allowed by the market, a continuous effort was made to control the European and American workforce through deterrent policies, and concern about addiction emerged. During the twentieth century, the prohibition of various drugs was implemented, starting with alcohol in the USA. Drugs were then in the process of becoming widely available commodities sold in formal or informal markets, and used by anyone who could buy them everywhere. The seizure with uncontrolled use and its consequences on study, family, and work generated laws to restrict or even criminalize the trade and use of psychoactive substances that provoked the desire for repeated use.

According to the perspective of interactionism that studies small groups in a highly differentiated modern society, that is, subcultures or social ethos, the act of consuming drugs is a social action. And learning through group socialization with whom, what, how, and when to use is the best way to control consumption and prevent abuse. In recent urban ethnographic studies, such as Howard Becker's, the argument is that users learn within the group when, where, and how much to use the drug, avoiding inconvenient behaviors that are not socially approved (Becker 2008). People learn to use drugs according to certain rules that include the ingestion of a certain limit and the condition that drugs, even illegal ones, do not affect their professional and private life. They would simply get on with their lives without problems. If someone in the user group exceeded the limit, others would have the means to deal with this unwanted situation.

An epidemiological study comparing alcohol consumption practices between two ethnic groups—the Navajo and the Hopi—went against intuitive evidence, since mortality rates from cirrhosis were lower among the Navajo, where men were expected to be heavy drinkers, than among the Hopi, where alcohol consumption was condemned and addicts were rejected. These effects were associated with the latter's disapproval of drinking behavior and the exclusion of users from social coexistence (Kunitz et al. 1970; Kunitz and Levy 1994; Levy and Kunitz 1974). In other words, individual disobedience to socially shared restrictions regarding alcoholic beverages results in the exclusion of offenders, which is more dangerous and leads to more excessive consumption of alcohol and consequently liver diseases than the socially expected collective consumption with the acceptance of heavy drinkers.

Another famous study demonstrating the influence of the environment on drug use is the experiment known as "Rat Park," conducted by Alexander et al. (1978). The researchers realized that the animals used for laboratory research were kept in conditions very discrepant from their natural habitat, which was an important predictor for high rates of substance use by animals. They then sought to find out if alternative boosters could interfere with the choices as to whether or not to use drugs. To make this possible, different environment were built: one was enriched, similar to the natural habitat of experimental subjects, with the presence of other animals for social interacting and mating, toys for physical exercise, among other stimuli; the other was a cage where the animals were isolated and unable to access any alternative source of pleasure. Both compartments had the arrangement of water with morphine that had been sweetened so that the rats would not be repelled by the bitter taste of morphine. The aim was to compare the levels of morphine use between the two groups: (1) rats isolated in laboratory cages and (2) rats socially living in a large open box. The results showed that the isolated rats ingested considerably higher amounts of morphine solution compared to animals in the other group. A possible explanation for this effect is the increased morphine booster potential by relieving the discomfort caused by spatial confinement, social isolation, and deprivation of stimuli. These data allow us to reflect on the role of environmental conditions in determining the self-administration of psychoactive substances. Several other researches, with animals and human beings, keep showing similar results. These studies suggest that dependence is a multifactorial issue, which goes beyond purely biological responses, that is, it is caused by a wide variety of individual risk factors (genetic and environmental) within a larger social system. The main contribution of these investigations to prevention and treatment policies is to show that the availability of natural enhancers, such as social relationships and pleasant living conditions, enables a significant reduction in drug use (Alexander et al. 1978; Gage and Sumnall 2018; Hart 2014).

Norman Zinberg (1984) observed that in Great Britain there were two types of drug dependents that differed from US dependents. The first group functioned well, while the second behaved in a more uncontrolled way generating harm to itself, but this did not characterize a motive for social unrest, moral panic, crime, or public hysteria. Thus, he understood that the distinctions regarding the behavior of dependents in both countries were related to their different social contexts. In England, where the use of heroin was not an illegal act, users had their needs met legally and were free from legal restrictions and possible punishment, and were not considered deviant from social norms. The people of this country could then accept or not the use of drugs as one of the possible particularities of life and continue their daily activities normally.

The case of the U.S. soldiers who were deployed to Vietnam was also analyzed and reported by Zinberg, who explains the attraction to drugs as a way to soften the unpleasant sensations elicited by the stressful and anxiogenic environment, described as "strange" and "frightening." The author says that he advised the withdrawal of users from the war scene, a suggestion that was initially rejected, but which, sometime later, came to be heeded. Studies later showed that the decision to withdraw the soldiers from the adverse circumstances in which they found themselves resulted in the almost complete cessation of heroin use, a fact that ratified the relevance of the environment in the effects and control of drug use.

Thus, Zinberg concluded that to understand drug-related experiences one could not only take into consideration the pharmacological aspects of the substances and the personality of the users, but also the physical and social environment in which they were inserted. So, his theoretical model considers the interrelationship of three variables: (1) Drug, which refers to the active principles and pharmacological aspects of the substances; (2) Set, which refers to the personality characteristics, attitudes, purposes, and expectations of the users; and (3) Setting, which refers to the environmental stimuli, the physical and social context where the use occurs. The setting or social context, through the establishment of sanctions and rituals, acts in the control of drug use behavior by users. More specifically, it refers to the social controls that are organized around what Zinberg calls “social sanctions” and “social rituals,” that is, the norms that define whether and how a given drug should be used. These sanctions and rituals would include both values and rules of conduct shared informally and tacitly by groups, and the formal laws and institutional policies that regulate drug use in the country.

In accordance with the interactionist perspective and the studies presented, the ethnographic research of Alves (2017) on the scenes of drug use in São Paulo found that the pleasures of using crack depend on what is called “tuning” among users, which concerns the establishment of good relations with each other and, therefore, pleasant effects provided by the use of the substance. These characteristics have been defined as empathogenic and refer to the association of drugs with feelings such as love and empathy. Having said this, the author concludes that the encounter between the living organism and the substance occurs in a physical and social environment capable of giving meaning to the use (Silva et al. 2019). This study also verified the use of the substance as a strategy to confront the dangers of life on the streets and analyzed the functioning and effectiveness of intervention programs with the objective of reinforcing self-control abilities in the use of alcohol and other drugs from changes in the structure of life of users. Regarding the concept of “chemical dependency,” the author suggests a complementary idea of “social dependency,” since in addition to dependency related to pharmacological effects, there is a range of relationships, links, and practices associated with the consumption of drugs such as crack. In his view, “social dependency fills a gap in the interpretation of drug use and opens new possibilities for its understanding” (p. 174).

Thus, one can conclude that drug use and its effects involve a complex network of factors that, just as they influence the sensations derived from substance use, can also act as social controls through the application of sanctions and promotion of alternative activities, as seen in the research cited. In view of this, some questions remain: what are the limits to community support for people who make excessive use of psychoactive substances? Do public policy makers really seek to understand the interaction between people and the drugs they use and the role they play in their lives? How long will the social context and its implications for substance use and dependence be neglected?

In view of this, Rui and Labate (2016) reiterate the need for empirical methodological paths to analyze drug use in a contextualized manner, considering the interrelationships between consumption, learning, hierarchy, social relations, and social distinction, in order to highlight how control, etiquette, and social rules are associated with the continuity of drug use and its configuration. According to the authors, “the context of drug use is determinant and influences not only the experience itself, but also the distinctions between users and types of consumption” (p. 44). In this sense, drug use can only be interdisciplinary.

Biopsychosocial Models: Perspectives on Drug Use and Dependence

Zaluar and Freitas (2017, p. 285) state that "one cannot conceive of the study of any human being without considering that the world of the subject is always biopsychosocial." In the 1970s, psychiatrist George Engel published an article entitled "The need for a new medical model: a challenge for biomedicine," in which he presented the biopsychosocial model as opposed to the current biomedical model. This model considers the interaction between biological, psychological, and socio-cultural factors as determining features in the health-disease process, as opposed to the biomedical model, characterized as a simplistic reductionism by seeking to explain disease solely through biochemical or neurophysiological factors which ignore psychosocial variables (Engel 1977, 1980).

The traditional (biomedical) model defined drug dependence as a disease resulting from genetic and biochemical causes. Today, with the knowledge in neuroscience, it is based on the dynamics of the brain, whose mechanisms and functions are much better understood. It is known from scientific research that drugs activate the reward system, an area of the brain also recruited with exercise, sex, food, and other activities, altering the levels of neurotransmitters, especially dopamine. Drugs that can induce addiction, such as alcohol, cocaine, heroin, tobacco, among others, act this way. Each of these substances, however, has different mechanisms, creating a greater or lesser possibility of addiction. Dependence on the substance exists when the individual develops compulsive behavior to consume the drug, despite negative effects, such as sickness. Dependency can arise when the neurobiological components adapt to repeated exposure to the drug and only function in its presence. If absent, several physiological reactions occur.

This scientific knowledge has not been sufficient to understand why some people do not develop such mechanisms and remain in control of drug use, without the negative effects of these consequences related to their abuse.

The biopsychosocial model assumes, then, that biological-genetic, psychological, and socio-cultural variables interact and influence the use and development of substance dependence. According to this model, this set of variables must be taken into account in the formulation and application of prevention and treatment programs (Skewes and Gonzalez 2013) (Fig. 4.1).

Therefore, the neurophysiological effects resulting from the use of psychoactive substances are not only determined by the quantity, the form of administration, and its action in the body, but also by the context in which consumption occurs. Environmental factors significantly influence the effects generated by the substances and, therefore, the use cannot be understood in isolation. This is an interaction between biological and contextual variables (Hart 2014). Dalgalarrondo (2011) adds to that understanding by stating that the functioning of the nervous system is only possible by considering the environment in which the organism (subject) is inserted. In view of this, Lende and Downey (Lende and Downey 2012a, b) explain that "for psychoactive substances to become catalysts and objects of pleasure and

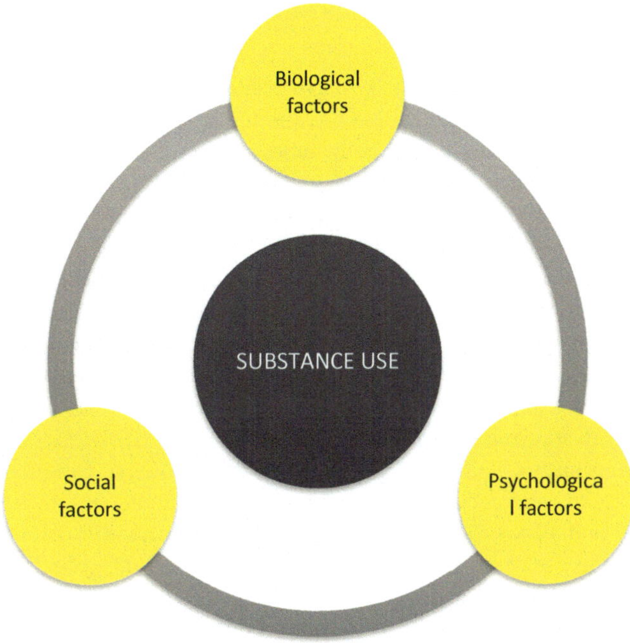

Fig. 4.1 Biopsychosocial model of drug addiction: Source: Skewes & Gonzalez (2013)

desire, they must circulate not only through blood, the brain and other places in the body, but also through social contexts." Alves (2017) reiterates that the experience of use is not limited to pharmacological aspects and says that the change of context is capable of generating expressive modification in the relationship between people and substances. In addition, the author suggests that the effects should be understood not only as derived from the administration of a certain substance in the body in a specific environment, but as the effect of the interaction between all these variables. In his view, however, "very little or almost nothing is said about the user's situation in the environment with which he interacts and the influence that the environment exerts on the effects of the drug and the patterns of its use" (p. 137).

According to Hart (2014), Vallim et al. (2015), and Alves (2017), the reduction of behavior to simplistic terms, without empirical verification, is problematic and can generate even more adverse consequences to the user subjects. Explanations that take only the neurobiological aspects into consideration, for example, fail to consider the context in which the behavior manifests itself. Thus, the focus becomes exclusively on the brain and its biochemical processes, while the understanding of behavior in relation to the context in which it occurs would be more fruitful and would enable more effective interventions.

In view of this, with the purpose of providing an interdisciplinary theoretical model, defend the need for integration of neurosciences and anthropology in favor of the constitution of an integrative field of study, called neuroanthropology.

Neuroanthropology: Reflections and Conceptual Applications

Recently, interdisciplinary approaches have become hegemonic in the literature on drug dependence, with the inclusion of "environmental triggers and experiments," another name for what occurs outside the brain and beyond individual genetics. The idea that social conditions matter, that is, that dependence "runs along the fault lines of society" has reached neuroscientists and a new discipline underway: neuroanthropology (Lende and Downey 2012a, b).

In the last decades, some disciplines have therefore come to integrate knowledge of the neurosciences and the social and human sciences, among them neuroanthropology, to better understand the links between cultural aspects and brain functioning. This is a new approach that aims to establish a dialogue between culture and biology, bringing together theories and methods from different sciences. The neuroanthropological approach aims to fill gaps in reductionist theories that simplify complex issues such as substance dependence, which emerge from the interaction of neurobiological and socio-cultural factors. This discipline has an interdisciplinary character and allows the application of knowledge from different areas to solve problems that impact human life. It is an evidence-based integrated approach that enables not only the understanding of the convergences of brain processes and environmental variables, but can also underpin more effective intervention strategies, such as the arrangement of contingencies conducive to healthy development (Costa 2014; Dias 2010; Domínguez et al. 2009; Duque et al. 2009; Lende and Downey 2012a, b; Ortega and Vidal 2016).

Despite the recent approximation between neuroscience and anthropology, there are divergent theoretical approaches between them, since in anthropology the individual is not placed in a previously organized environment from which he or she receives stimuli as happens in laboratory experiments, but in networks of social interaction already in flux in which, as a result of the symbolic and material exchanges between the people present in them, the environment may have different meanings or scenarios that are always changing. From the common point of view that the brain is the mediator of this interaction between the individual organism or the person, a term most used by anthropologists, with the environment or the social context, which enables two-way traffic that constitutes us as humans, there are clear theoretical differences that need to be better discussed.

Today, neuroscientists know that neural activity depends on both the individual organism and the socio-cultural environment. But it is necessary to clarify how each one of them is conceptualized and how their two-way interaction is conceived. In the current debate in neuroanthropology, the little used anthropological theories of structuralism, culturalism, and functionalism are still successful. In contemporary anthropology, there is no longer a comparison reduced to a few traces between what would be Western culture (individualist) and Eastern culture (relational and hierarchical or holistic). On the contrary, cultures are not rigid systems or defined crystals with clear limits, but dynamic arrangements of orders and conflicts, agreements and constitutive tensions, such as the tension between individual interests and passions and collective assets. Neither does the individual or his or her self becomes the center of reflection any more precisely because the social selves of the same individual are multiple and contextually defined or negotiated in interaction. The forms of reward in the individual brains are therefore multiple and contextual, arising from interpersonal and social interaction.

In adolescence, for example, which is a period of development marked by intense physical, psychological, and social changes, it is natural the presence of some potentially harmful behaviors to the physical and emotional health of individuals, such as the consumption of alcohol and other drugs (Yamauchi et al., 2018). Studies indicate that the brain maturation process is related and explains, in part, the increased involvement in risk situations observed in this age group (Andrade et al. 2017). It is a phase where progressive processes of remodeling, refinement, and neurocognitive maturation take place, following a certain direction: from the most basic to the most complex functions. The brain regions responsible for functions such as emotional regulation, planning, decision making, and behavior control are still developing while altered levels of neurotransmitters such as dopamine and serotonin and regions interconnected to the limbic system mediate behaviors of search for new experiences, sensations, and rewards. Moreover, since they are adolescents, it is normal that they still do not have a developed repertoire of behavioral skills necessary to face daily problems, since they are still experiencing the experiences that life imposes. These characteristics make adolescents more vulnerable to involvement in risk behaviors, stress, and the development of psychological disorders (Andrade et al. 2014; Gipson and Kalivas 2014; Moura et al. 2018; Vitalle 2014; Abrahao et al., 2012; Frade et al., 2013).

The triadic model of the neurobiology of motivated behavior in adolescents describes the main changes that have occurred in the process of maturation of the nervous system and seeks to explain features which are typical of adolescence, such as impulsiveness, search for danger, emotional instability, and social reorientation (Andrade et al., 2018; Andrade et al., 2016; De Micheli et al., 2016). According to this model, (1) the striatum corresponds to the reward system and is associated with the search for new experiences and pleasurable sensations, (2) the amygdala represents the emotional system and is associated with responses to aversive stimuli (fear) and escape behaviors, and (3) the prefrontal cortex acts in the emotional regulation and control of search and escape behaviors. It is important to reiterate that the functions related to regulation and control of behavior are still under development, while the intensity and emotional instability are extreme in adolescence, a phase in which positive reinforcements such as social stimuli, for example, are potentiated (Ernst 2014; Plate et al. 2014). As already mentioned, however, the forms of reward in individual brains are multiple and contextual, and arise from interpersonal and social interaction (Fig. 4.2).

This complex interaction of biological and psychosocial variables relates to behaviors such as drug use, which occurs most often when the user has the company of peers who are involved together in this risk behavior. Mutual support when there is group use becomes a benefit in itself. Having friends who use drugs serves as a powerful cultural force for ongoing experimentation and adaptation of risk

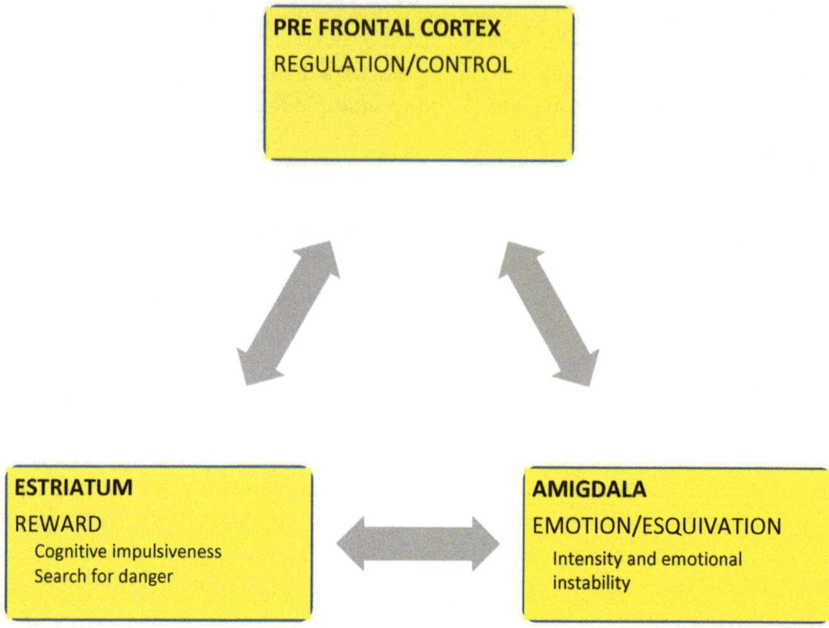

Fig. 4.2 Triadic model of the neurobiology of motivated behavior in adolescents. Source: Ernst (2014)

behaviors (Almeida et al., 2018). Bourgois, studying heroin users in the USA, tells how they have built a precarious balance of mutual solidarity and interpersonal betrayal in what he called the moral economy of sharing (Bourgois and Schonberg 2009). Young people have greater need and sensitivity for bonds, and if drug use is a criterion for belonging to a particular group, many are willing to comply. The behavior of drug use, therefore, is not limited to the pharmacological effects; many times, it has the purpose of affiliation to a group and social position. This is why factors such as social acceptance and links with family and school are related to the reduction of problems associated with substance use (Hart 2014).

Research on resilience and its neural components shows that the environment in which a person's initial development occurs plays a crucial role in the development of vulnerabilities predisposing to risk behaviors such as substance abuse. These studies demonstrate that events in early life can shape the way people respond neurally and physiologically to future events. That is, adverse social contexts and traumatic experiences can affect the development of brain structures and functions and increase the chances of behavioral problems during life. On the other hand, positive environments and caring relationships in early stages of development represent protective factors in relation to disorders such as those related to drug abuse (Bick and Nelson 2015; McCrory and Mayes 2015; Woods-Jaeger et al. 2018).

These risk behaviors are predisposed by the interaction between biological and social factors. For example: monoamine oxidase A (MAOA) is an enzyme that degrades several neurotransmitters essential for impulse control, attention, and other cognitive functions, including dopamine, noradrenaline, and serotonin (Andrade et al., 2011). The absence of MAOA generates effects such as interruption of the normal functioning of other neurotransmitters and therefore increases the probability of a series of problems such as attention deficit and hyperactivity disorder, impulsiveness, harmful use of substances, among others. An important finding was the correlation between low levels of MAOA and severe childhood maltreatment. Vulnerabilities such as genetic inheritance, malnutrition, brain trauma resulting from aggression in the first years of life, neglect, humiliation, family rejection, extreme poverty, prenatal exposure and early induction to the use of alcohol, tobacco and other drugs, complete absence of care, among other factors can generate a series of other structural and functional changes in the brain, modify the functioning of neurotransmitters, impair cognitive functions and thus predispose people to behaviors that are harmful to physical and psychological health and can cause harm to society in general. That is, adverse experiences in early life are associated with increased risk of drug abuse and other disorders in adult life, since they occur at a time when brain regions important for executive functioning are still in development. The biological sciences are important in understanding these problems, since genetic and neurobiological variables are involved; and the social sciences, in turn, are important to the extent that social factors can produce biological changes. In terms of prevention and treatment, given that the social environment moderates or alters the action of biological factors, the key is to find out which environmental influences interact with which biological factors cause behaviors (Baker et al. 2006; Cervera-Juanes et al. 2015; Forster et al. 2018; Tikkanen et al. 2010; Verdejo-García et al. 2013).

It is worth noting that issues that impact human life cannot be credited to any gross reductionism. In addition, the complexity of human actions and the fact that they cannot be explained by simplistic theses, such as the vulnerabilities that lead young people to become involved in risky situations and behaviors such as drug use and trafficking, must be considered. That said, Zaluar and Freitas (2017) payed attention to youth and the new discoveries of neuroscience and remind us that this is a phase of life of extreme importance and that it can be the focus of interventions with the objective of establishing good relations with the world and building alternative and healthy perspectives for the future.

In general, public policies for prevention and treatment of drug use and dependence are not formulated taking into consideration the complexity of the subject and may aggravate existing problems (Alves 2017; Hart 2014; Vallim et al. 2015). And, until recently, the influence of organism–environment interaction and the role of culture in brain development were little recognized (Duque et al. 2009). Therefore, MacKinnon (2014) considers it important to move towards a more integrative scientific field.

Research in neurosciences involves laboratory experiments with the aim of exploring correlations between cognitive functions and structural and functional components of the brain, using methods such as observation, functional magnetic resonance imaging, electroencephalography, among others. In neuroanthropology, studies can address scientific and humanistic issues to discuss the implications of socio-cultural factors on brain development and function (and can investigate, for example, transcultural similarities and differences). For this, one can use the methodological repertoire of fields such as social and cultural neuroscience, which includes comparative transcultural studies, longitudinal research, etc. or even the combination of these strategies. These studies can elucidate the correlations between neuroanatomic and functional structures and the socio-cultural experiences to which subjects are exposed throughout their lives (Duque et al. 2009).

Neuroanthropology recognizes the complexity and multifactoriality of human actions and, therefore, seeks to gather evidence from different fields to enable a global view of the phenomena. To do so, it adopts an integrationist conception with the objective of assimilating how the socio-cultural context shapes the brain and vice versa, considering subject–environment interaction as a way to understand and explain human behavior and its nuances. The understanding of this neurocultural dynamic facilitates the identification of vulnerabilities that may predispose to certain problems (such as, for example, the effects of stress during childhood and its consequences on the long-term development process) and the elaboration of more efficient social, psycho-behavioral, and pharmacological technologies. That is, from the understanding of the variables associated with the phenomena, neuroanthropologists can help in the development of proposals for more beneficial approaches to solving problems at individual and collective levels (Lende and Downey 2012a, b; Dias 2010).

Final Considerations

Nowadays, social scientists agree that a change has occurred in the last decades regarding the studies on the human being: the researches started to adopt a more balanced perspective, considering the reciprocal relations between biogenetic and environmental factors in order to obtain wider explanations regarding the observed variations in behavior. This approach also applies to other areas of health and has collected a series of evidences that both genetic and environmental influences, especially their interaction, are essential to explain behavioral differences and issues such as dependencies in general. This new perspective, which opposes reductionist and simplistic theses, enables the development of protection, prevention, and treatment strategies at individual and community levels (Baker et al. 2006).

Sciences such as sociology and anthropology analyze the way societies and cultures are constituted and impact human life and vice versa. The neurosciences have been elucidating the way the brain interacts with environmental stimuli and behaviors are produced from this complex mutual relationship. Behavioral psychology, in turn, brings together a range of evidence that demonstrates the complexity of the interaction between phylogenetic, ontogenetic, and socio-cultural variables, considering behaviors as products of multiple genetic and environmental contingencies. In the meantime, neuroanthropology emerges. These approaches direct the eye to context as the focus of more effective interventions. The union of these fields of studies and their respective theoretical perspectives provide a broader understanding of issues such as use and dependence on substances, instrumentalize and enable changes in contingencies that influence human actions and decisions in order to provide environments conducive to the installation and maintenance of new behaviors and cultural practices.

These areas of knowledge have developed several researches that reveal the complexity of the drug issue and counteract reductionist and simplifying paradigms. Myths have been elucidated, discoveries made and psychological and pharmacological technologies developed in search of effective interventions.

Theoretical models such as Becker (2008) and Zinberg (1984) and a series of current researches demonstrate that changes in the patterns of licit and illicit drug use are influenced by the social context and not only by the pharmacological aspects of the substances and the personality characteristics of individuals. Recently, Hart (2014), Vallim et al. (2015), Rui and Labate (2016), and Alves (2017), among several other authors, have shown how socio-economic factors and changes in the structure of life of users are able to generate changes in the relationships established with drugs and warn that public policies do not fully address the issue, which requires a multidisciplinary approach in order to encompass the knowledge of biological, psychological, and social sciences.

These theoretical reflections allow the formulation of alternative intervention strategies to punitive policies and compulsory admissions in closed institutions under repressive surveillance. To this end, it is necessary to integrate various bodies and approach the issue from an integral perspective, which is the way most consistent with respect for human rights and effectiveness in achieving the proposed goals.

References

Abrahao, K. P., Quadros, I. M. H., Andrade, A. L. M., & Souza-Formigoni, M. L. O. (2012). Accumbal dopamine D2 receptor function is associated with individual variability in ethanol behavioral sensitization. Neuropharmacology, 62(2), 882–889. https://doi.org/10.1016/j.neuropharm.2011.09.017.

Alexander, B. K., Coambs, R. B., & Hadaway, P. F. (1978). The effect of housing and gender on morphine self-administration in rats. *Psychopharmacology, 58*(2), 175–179. https://doi.org/10.1007/BF00426903.

Alves, Y. D. D. (2017). *Jamais fomos zumbis: contexto social e craqueiros na cidade de São Paulo*. Salvador, Brazil: EDUFBA.

Almeida, D. E. R. G., Andrade, A. L. M., Cruz, F. D., & Micheli, D. D. (2018). Perception of freedom in leisure among substance users and nonusers. Psico-USF, 23(1), 13–24. https://doi.org/10.1590/1413-82712018230102.

American Psychiatric Association. (2014). *Manual de Diagnóstico e Estatístico dos Transtornos Mentais* (5th ed.). Porto Alegre, Brazil: Artmed.

Andrade, A. L. M., De Micheli, D., Silva, E. A., Souza-Formigoni, M. L. O., & Goeldner, F. O. (2014). Desenvolvimento neural na adolescência. In D. De Micheli, A. L. M. Andrade, E. A. Silva, & M. L. O. Souza-Formigoni (Eds.), *Neurociências do abuso de drogas na adolescência: o que sabemos?* (pp. 21–30). São Paulo, Brazil: Atheneu.

Andrade, A. L. M., & De Micheli, D. (2017). Inovações no Tratamento de Dependência de Drogas. 1. ed. Rio de Janeiro: Atheneu.

Andrade, A.L.M., Bedendo, A., Enumo, S.R.F., Micheli, D. (2018) Brain development in adolescence: general aspects and update. Adolescência e Saude. 2018;15(Supl. 1):62–67. Retrieved from: https://www.adolescenciaesaude.com/detalhe_artigo.asp?id=759#

Andrade, A. L. M. & De Micheli, D. (2016). Innovations in the Treatment of Substance Addiction. 1. ed. New York: Springer International Publishing. https://doi.org/10.1007/978-3-319-43172-7

Andrade, A. L. M., Abrahao, K. P., Goeldner, F. O., & Souza-Formigoni, M. L. O. (2011). Administration of the 5-HT2C receptor antagonist SB-242084 into the nucleus accumbens blocks the expression of ethanol-induced behavioral sensitization in Albino Swiss mice. Neuroscience, 189, 178–186. https://doi.org/10.1016/j.neuroscience.2011.05.028

Arthur, J. M. (2014). *Beer through the ages: The role of beer in shaping our past and current worlds*. Retrieved from http://anthronow.com/print/beer-through-the-ages-the-role-of-beer-in-shaping-our-past-and-current-worlds

Baker, L. A., Bezdjian, S., & Raine, A. (2006). Behavioral genetics: The science of antisocial behavior. *Law and Contemporary Problems, 69*(1–2), 7–46.

Barthes, H. (1972). *Mythologies*. London: Paladin.

Becker, H. (2008). *Outsiders: Estudos de sociologia do desvio*. Rio de Janeiro, Brazil: Zahar. (Obra original publicada em 1963).

Bedendo, A., Opaleye, E. S., Andrade, A. L. M., & Noto, A. R. (2013). Heavy episodic drinking and soccer practice among high school students in Brazil: the contextual aspects of this relationship. *BMC Public Health, 13*(1), 247. https://doi.org/10.1186/1471-2458-13-247.

Bergeron, H. (2012). *Sociologia da droga*. Aparecida, Brazil: Idéias & Letras.

Bick, J., & Nelson, C. (2015). Early adverse experiences and the developing brain. *Neuropsychopharmacology, 41*(1), 177–196. https://doi.org/10.1038/npp.2015.252.

Bourgois, P., & Schonberg, J. (2009). *Righteous Dopefiend*. Berkeley, CA: University of California Press.

Campbell, M. A. (1991). Public drinking places and society. In D. J. Pittman & H. R. White (Eds.), *Society, culture and drinking patterns reexamined*. New Brunswick, Canada: Rutgers Center for Alcohol Studies.

Cervera-Juanes, R., Wilhem, L., Park, B., Lee, R., Locke, J., Helms, C., et al. (2015). MAOA expression predicts vulnerability for alcohol use. *Molecular Psychiatry, 21*(4), 472–479. https://doi.org/10.1038/mp.2015.93.

Costa, O. (2014). O que é a Neuroantropologia Afinal? Considerações e Contribuições de uma Ciência Pouco Conhecida. *Revista Neurociências, 22*(01), 149–157. https://doi.org/10.4181/RNC.2014.22.795.9p.

Crenn, C., Demossier, M., & Techoueyres, I. (2004). *Wine and globalisation: Foreword*. Retrieved from https://journals.openedition.org/aof/308

Dalgalarrondo, P. (2011). *Evolução do cérebro: sistema nervoso, psicologia e psicopatologia sob a perspectiva evolucionista*. Porto Alegre, Brazil: Artmed.

De Micheli, D., Andrade, A. L. M., Silva, E. A., & Souza-Formigoni, M. L. O. (2016). Drug Abuse in Adolescence (1st Ed.). New York: Springer International Publishing. https://doi.org/10.1007/978-3-319-17795-3

Dias, A. M. (2010). The foundations of neuroanthropology. *Frontiers in Evolutionary Neuroscience, 2*, 5. https://doi.org/10.3389/neuro.18.005.2010.

Domínguez, D. J. F., Lewis, E. D., Turner, R., & Egan, G. F. (2009). The brain in culture and culture in the brain: a review of core issues in neuroanthropology. *Progress in brain research, 178*, 43–64. https://doi.org/10.1016/S0079-6123(09)17804-4.

Duque, J. F. D., Turner, R., Lewis, E., & Egan, G. (2009). Neuroanthropology: A humanistic science for the study of the culture–brain nexus. *Social Cognitive and Affective Neuroscience, 5*(2–3), 138–147. https://doi.org/10.1093/scan/nsp024.

Engel, G. (1977). The need for a new medical model: A challenge for biomedicine. *Science, 196*(4286), 129–136. https://doi.org/10.1126/science.847460.

Engel, G. (1980). The clinical application of the biopsychosocial model. *American Journal of Psychiatry, 137*(5), 535–544. https://doi.org/10.1176/ajp.137.5.535.
Ernst, M. (2014). The triadic model perspective for the study of adolescent motivated behavior. *Brain and Cognition, 89*, 104–111. https://doi.org/10.1016/j.bandc.2014.01.006.
Forster, G., Anderson, E., Scholl, J., Lukkes, J., & Watt, M. (2018). Negative consequences of early-life adversity on substance use as mediated by corticotropin-releasing factor modulation of serotonin activity. *Neurobiology of Stress, 9*, 29–39. https://doi.org/10.1016/j.ynstr.2018.08.001.
Frade, I. F., De Micheli, D., Andrade, A. L. M., & de Souza-Formigoni, M. L. O. (2013). Relationship between stress symptoms and drug use among secondary students. The Spanish journal of psychology, 16, e4. https://doi.org/10.1017/sjp.2013.5
Gage, S. H., & Sumnall, H. R. (2018). Rat Park: How a rat paradise changed the narrative of addiction. *Addiction, 114*(5), 917–922. https://doi.org/10.1111/add.14481.
Gillogly, K. (2008). Opium, power, people: Anthropological understandings of an opium interdiction project in Thailand. *Contemporary Drug Problems, 35*(4), 679–715. https://doi.org/10.1177/009145090803500409.
Gipson, C. D., & Kalivas, P. W. (2014). Bases neurais da dependência de drogas. In D. De Micheli, A. L. M. Andrade, E. A. Silva, & M. L. O. Souza-Formigoni (Eds.), *Neurociências do abuso de drogas na adolescência: o que sabemos?* (pp. 34–51). São Paulo, Brazil: Atheneu.
Goody, J. (1982). *Cooking, cuisine and class*. Cambridge, UK: Cambridge University Press.
Guimarães, F. S. (2013). Substâncias psicoativas. In R. Lent (Ed.), *Neurociência da mente e do comportamento* (pp. 323–348). Rio de Janeiro, Brazil: Guanabara Koogan.
Guimarães, M., & Zaluar, A. (2015). *A neurociência encontra antropologia* (pp. 46–51). São Paulo, Brazil: Neuroeducação. Retrieved from https://www.researchgate.net/publication/292156482_Cultura_e_Aprendizagem_a_Neurociencia_encontra_a_Antropologia.
Hart, C. (2014). *Um preço muito alto: a jornada de um neurocientista que desafia nossa visão sobre as drogas*. Rio de Janeiro, Brazil: Zahar.
Hart, C. (2017). Reply to 'addiction as a brain disease does not promote injustice'. *Nature Human Behaviour, 1*(9), 611–611. https://doi.org/10.1038/s41562-017-0216-0.
Kunitz, S., Levy, J., & Everett, M. (1970). Alchoholic cirrhosis among the Navajo. *Quarterly Journal of Studies on Alcohol, 30*, 672–685.
Kunitz, S., & Levy, J. (1994). Drinking careers: A twenty-five year study of three Navajo populations. New Haven, CT: Yale University Press.
Lende, D., & Downey, G. (2012a). Neuroanthropology and its applications: An introduction. *Annals of Anthropological Practice, 36*(1), 1–25. https://doi.org/10.1111/j.2153-9588.2012.01090.x.
Lende, D., & Downey, G. (2012b). *The Encultured brain: An introduction to Neuroanthropology*. Cambridge, MA: MIT Press.
Levy, J., & Kunitz, S. (1974). *Indian drinking*. New York, NY: Wiley.
MacKinnon, K. (2014). Contemporary biological anthropology in 2013: Integrative, connected, and relevant. *American Anthropologist, 116*(2), 352–365. https://doi.org/10.1111/aman.12102.
MacRae, E. (2008). The religious uses of licit and illicit psychoactive substances in a branch of the Santo Daime religion. *Fieldwork In Religion, 2*, 3. https://doi.org/10.1558/firn.v2i3.393.
Martinez, R. M., & Martín, L. (1987). Patrones de consumo de alcohol en la comunidad de Madrid. *Comunidad y Drogas, 5*(6), 39–62.
Masur, J., & Carlini, E. (2004). *Drogas: subsídios para uma discussão*. São Paulo, Brazil: Brasiliense.
McCrory, E., & Mayes, L. (2015). Understanding addiction as a developmental disorder: An argument for a developmentally informed multilevel approach. *Current Addiction Reports, 2*(4), 326–330. https://doi.org/10.1007/s40429-015-0079-2.
Moura, L., Torres, L., Cadete, M., & Cunha, C. (2018). Fatores associados aos comportamentos de risco à saúde entre adolescentes brasileiros: uma revisão integrativa. *Revista da Escola de Enfermagem da USP, 52*, e03304. https://doi.org/10.1590/s1980-220x2017020403304.

Ortega, F., & Vidal, F. (2016). Culture: By the brain and in the brain? *História, Ciências, Saúde-Manguinhos, 23*(4), 965–983. https://doi.org/10.1590/s0104-59702016000400002.
Plate, R. C., Richards, J. M., & Ernst, M. (2014). Modelo triádico da neurobiologia do comportamento motivado em adolescentes. In D. De Micheli, A. L. M. Andrade, E. A. Silva, & M. L. O. Souza-Formigoni (Eds.), *Neurociências do abuso de drogas na adolescência: o que sabemos?* (pp. 99–118). São Paulo, Brazil: Atheneu.
Rui, T., & Labate, B. C. (2016). Psicoativos, cultura e controles: contribuições da antropologia ao debate público no Brasil. In B. C. Labate, F. Policarpo, S. L. Goulart, & P. O. Rosa (Eds.), *Drogas, políticas públicas e consumidores* (pp. 37–64). Campinas, Brazil: Mercado de Letras.
Silva, R. A., Messias, J. C. C., Andrade, A. L. M., Souza, J. C. R. P., & Guimarães, L. A. M. (2019). The perception of truck drivers on the use of psychoactive substances at work: an ethnographic study. SMAD. *Revista Eletrônica Saúde Mental Álcool e Drogas, 15*, 1–8. https://doi.org/10.11606/issn.1806-6976.smad.2019.150461.
Singer, M. (2012). Anthropology and addiction: An historical review. *Addiction, 107*(10), 1747–1755. https://doi.org/10.1111/j.1360-0443.2012.03879.x.
Skewes, M., & Gonzalez, V. (2013). The biopsychosocial model of addiction. *Principles Of Addiction, 1*, 61–70. https://doi.org/10.1016/B978-0-12-398336-7.00006-1.
Social Issues Research Centre. (1998). *Social and cultural aspects of drinking, a report to the European Commission*. London, UK: Social Issues Research Centre.
Tikkanen, R., Ducci, F., Goldman, D., Holi, M., Lindberg, N., Tiihonen, J., & Virkkunen, M. (2010). MAOA alters the effects of heavy drinking and childhood physical abuse on risk for severe impulsive acts of violence among alcoholic violent offenders. *Alcoholism: Clinical and Experimental Research, 34*(5), 853–860. https://doi.org/10.1111/j.1530-0277.2010.01157.x.
Vallim, D., Zaluar, A., & Sampaio, C. (2015). Uma etnografia das cenas de uso de crack no Rio de Janeiro e seus efeitos nos usuários. In M. Teixeira & Z. Fonseca (Eds.), *Saberes e praticas na atenção primária à saúde: cuidado à população em situação de rua e usuários de álcool, crack e outras drogas* (pp. 201–216). São Paulo, Brazil: Hucitec.
Velho, G. (1998). *Nobres & anjos: um estudo de tóxicos e hierarquia*. Rio de Janeiro, Brazil: Fundação Getúlio Vargas.
Verdejo-García, A., Albein-Urios, N., Molina, E., Ching-López, A., Martínez-González, J., & Gutiérrez, B. (2013). A MAOA gene*cocaine severity interaction on impulsivity and neuropsychological measures of orbitofrontal dysfunction: Preliminary results. *Drug and Alcohol Dependence, 133*(1), 287–290. https://doi.org/10.1016/j.drugalcdep.2013.04.031.
Vitalle, M. S. S. (2014). Sistema neuro-hormonal da adolescência. In D. De Micheli, A. L. M. Andrade, E. A. Silva, & M. L. O. Souza-Formigoni (Eds.), *Neurociências do abuso de drogas na adolescência: o que sabemos?* (pp. 3–10). São Paulo, Brazil: Atheneu.
Wadley, G. (2016). How psychoactive drugs shape human culture: A multi-disciplinary perspective. *Brain Research Bulletin, 126*, 138–151. https://doi.org/10.1016/j.brainresbull.2016.04.008.
Woods-Jaeger, B., Cho, B., Sexton, C., Slagel, L., & Goggin, K. (2018). Promoting resilience: Breaking the intergenerational cycle of adverse childhood experiences. *Health Education & Behavior, 45*(5), 772–780. https://doi.org/10.1177/1090198117752785.
Yamauchi, L. M., Andrade, A. L. M., Pinheiro, B. O., Enumo, S. R. F & De Micheli, D. (2018). Evaluation of the social representation of the use of alcoholic beverages by adolescents. Estudos de Psicologia (Campinas), 36, e180098. http://dx.doi.org/10.1590/1982-0275201936e180098
Zaluar, A. (2004). *Integração perversa: pobreza e tráfico de drogas*. Rio de Janeiro, Brazil: Editora FGV.
Zaluar, A., & Freitas, L. A. P. (2017). *Cidade de deus: a história de Ailton Batata, o sobrevivente*. Rio de Janeiro, Brazil: Editora FGV.
Zimmermann, A., & Torriani-Pasin, C. (2011). Filosofia e neurociência: entre certezas e dúvidas. *Revista Brasileira De Educação Física E Esporte, 25*(4), 731–742.
Zinberg, N. (1984). *Drug, set, and setting: The basis for controlled intoxicant use*. New Haven, CT: Yale University.

Chapter 5
Substance Use Among Older Adults: Epidemiological Aspects, Associated Variables, and Organic Risks

Camila Chagas, Tassiane Cristine Santos de Paula, and Cleusa Pinheiro Ferri

Introduction: Aging in Brazil and the World

The population is aging, and this has often appeared in the media recently. However, it is still difficult to estimate the scale and consequences of this process for individuals and society as a whole. Rather, it is necessary to differentiate between the aging population and the individual. Population aging is marked by an increase in the number of older adults in the general population, a consequence of the increase in life expectancy of the population. Individual aging, on the other hand, reflects the different trajectories that affect the progressive loss of functions and social roles, depending on biological, social, and economic conditions, among others (Camarano and Kanso 2013).

By 2050, the world population over 60 could reach 2 billion (World Health Organization (WHO) 2018) (this is equivalent to approximately twice the world's largest population—China). Among people over 80 years old, by 2020, it will exceed the number of children under 5 years old. This proportion has never occurred in world history. Moreover, for the first time, people can expect to live at least 60 years (WHO 2018).

Brazil is in line with this trend. According to IBGE, if in 1940 the average life expectancy was 45 years; in 2019, it will grow to 76 years and may reach 81 years in 2050, that is, one in three Brazilians will be over 60 years old (Brazilian Institute of Geography and Statistics—(IBGE 2019)). Currently, the number of older Brazilian people over 60 is approximately 28 million. In 2050, it may reach the mark of 67 million (IBGE 2019). This high contingent reflects, among other aspects, the increase in life expectancy (reduction in infant mortality and improved access to health care) added to the drop in the fertility rate (WHO 2010).

C. Chagas (✉) · T. C. S. de Paula · C. P. Ferri
Universidade Federal de São Paulo, São Paulo, SP, Brazil

D. De Micheli et al. (eds.), *Drugs and Human Behavior*,
https://doi.org/10.1007/978-3-030-62855-0_5

With this increase, the problems arising from drug use, generally observed in younger populations, become a concern also in the older population. Since the older adult may experience more intense physical, social, and psychological impacts. These aspects will be explored in more detail in the next topic.

Older Adult and Substance Use

Physical, Social, and Psychological Differences

The aging process brings changes in several areas of life. It is worth mentioning that, like many things, it has a positive and negative side. For example, the older adult may begin to deal with everyday situations more maturely or may present a decrease in social networking. They may also experience retirement in a positive way (by doing pleasurable activities) or negative (feeling lonely). However, such benefits and losses are relative, as they depend on social and psychological conditions, among others. However, there is a process that affects the older adult in general. This process is linked to the aging of the human body. Thus, it is important to remember that, although it also depends on previous issues (biological, psychological, social, and economic), it will affect all people to some degree, regardless of social class.

Therefore, when we enter the field of drug action in the body of the older adult, we add damage that goes beyond that of the younger adult population. Among the physiological changes are: Harms in pharmacokinetic processing (the path that the drug makes inside the body) as *absorption*—this process tends to slow down or reduce the action of the drugs, due to the reduction in visceral blood flow and decrease in the speed of gastric emptying; *distribution*—due to changes in body composition, such as the reduction in the volume of water in the body added to the increase in body fat, the body has less water to distribute the alcohol, consequently the elimination of the drug will be slower; *metabolism*—metabolization is affected with the decrease of enzymes in the liver, this can result, for example, in the increase of the half-life of the drugs, in which case the duration of the effect can be prolonged (Ramos et al. 2013).

Among the pharmacodynamic changes (related to drug–receptor interaction and observed effects) are *homeostatic mechanisms*: the organs, in general, contribute to keep the body in balance. However, with aging occurs the gradual decrease of physiological functions that contribute to homeostasis, resulting in increased vulnerability to disease and lower tolerance to the effects of drugs. An example is the sedative effect of alcohol and benzodiazepine, which may not be relevant in a young adult, but in the older adult it contributes to increased risk and falls; *receptors and sites of action*—change in the number and sensitivity of receptors that may contribute to greater sensitivity to drugs (Dowling et al. 2008; Ramos et al. 2013). In addition, if at younger ages women already have less body water and more fat when compared to men, at later ages these characteristics become more pronounced. Besides, additional damage emerges from menopausal hormonal transitions (Moore et al. 2007).

Regarding alcohol, since it is one of the substances most consumed by this population (Fig. 5.1), advances in the field of research are more robust. For example,

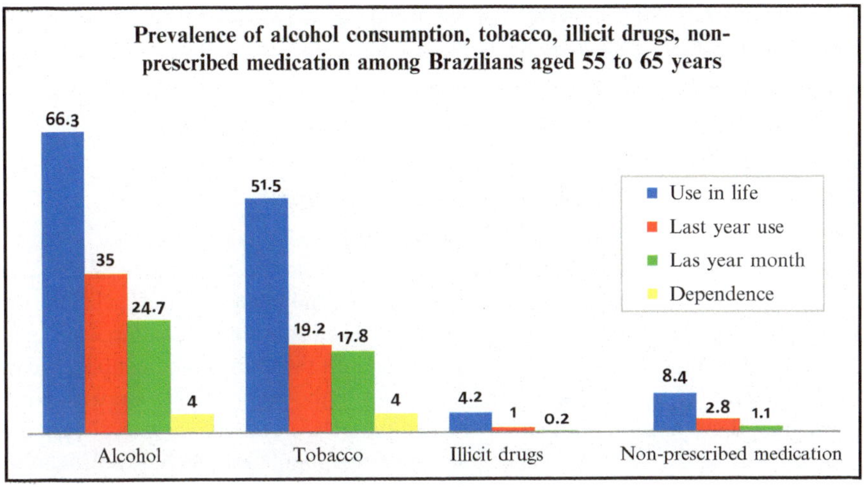

Fig. 5.1 Prevalence of consumption of alcohol, tobacco, illicit drugs, and non-prescribed medication among Brazilians aged 55–65 years. Source: Figure elaborated by the authors based on data from the III LNUD—National Survey on Drug Use by the Brazilian Population (Bastos et al. 2017)

there is evidence that alcohol consumption is associated with the cognitive decline with aging. A 30-year follow-up study found associations between alcohol consumption and cognitive decline and hippocampus atrophy, even with moderate alcohol consumption. The authors found that those who drink between 14 and 21 units per week were three times more at risk for cognitive decline (Topiwala et al. 2017). The World Health Organization (WHO) recommends that alcohol risk prevention projects, which warn of the risks of cognitive decline and/or dementia, should also be directed at younger adults to prevent such harm at a later age (WHO 2019).

In the social and psychological field, several variables emerge. This is because a risk factor for one older person will not necessarily be for the other. However, events such as retirement, widowhood, death of friends, or relatives are important factors to be considered in the consumption of drug risks, especially alcohol. Therefore, the retirement condition has been investigated as a correlate of the harmful use of alcohol by this population. Some studies show that although there is no direct effect of retirement on alcohol consumption, the fact that retirement is voluntary or not in conjunction with people's social network after retirement seems to affect the amount of alcohol consumed and its problems (Seibel and Toscano Junior 2001).

Similarly, excessive alcohol consumption may be associated with comorbidities such as depression and anxiety (Vink et al. 2008). In older people, this consumption is often accompanied by depression due to stressful events such as bereavement (Fox and Wilson 2011). Other clinical conditions such as anxiety, insomnia, falls, and auto negligence, often attributed to the aging process, may be related to the consumption of alcohol or other drugs (Vink et al. 2008). In addition, it is not uncommon for alcohol abstinence to be confused with signs of Parkinson's disease.

Once these questions have been raised, we intend to present the reader with some data that may help him understand the current context of drug use in the older population.

Epidemiology of Drug Use Among Older Adult People

Due to the population over 60, problems related to the use of substances can also expand. According to the latest Brazilian survey conducted by FIOCRUZ, the III LNUD (Bastos et al. 2017), the most commonly used substance among people aged 55–65 years is alcohol, followed by tobacco and non-prescribed medications, and to a lesser extent the use of illicit drugs, as shown in the graph (Fig. 5.1). It is worth noting that these data do not include the population over 65 years of age. Thus, the panorama of drug use by the older portion of the population becomes difficult to scale. On the other hand, this was the first Brazilian survey that stratified the sample among older adults (55–65 years). The other previous Brazilian surveys by CEBRID (Carlini et al. 2005) and LENAD (Laranjeira et al. 2012) did not present data separated by age, which made it impossible to compare data between the surveys. Furthermore, studies on substance use among older people are still limited, and most have been conducted in developed countries such as the USA and European countries, which makes the comparison with Brazil difficult.

Alcohol

Alcohol is the most consumed drug in Brazil and is present in festive moments, celebrations, and among the options to relax. However, it is associated with health problems (heart disease, cancer, dependency, and dementia), mortality, and increased risk of accidents and injuries (RCP 2018). In addition to these losses, there are other risks in the consumption of alcohol by an older adult, as we saw at the beginning of this chapter. This, together with the fact that it is one of the substances most consumed by this population, contributes to alcohol consumption being, without a doubt, one of the greatest concerns when one thinks about substance consumption in the older adult. Other factors are also worthy of attention, among them:

- Underreporting of alcohol-related problems in the older adult. This is because it is not uncommon for alcohol-related complications to be masked by frequent aging problems such as diabetes, falls, depression, or dementia.
- Many older people drink alone at home and this is often not identified by professionals, making it difficult to prevent possible problems.
- Diagnostic criteria may not be appropriate for this population, as they are created based on the needs of the young adult.
- Older people may continue their pattern of drinking when they are younger, and not realize that the consequences of this pattern may be different in this period of life.

The prevalence of alcohol consumption in Brazil among people aged 55 to 65 years is higher (Fig. 5.1) compared to all other substances. A systematic review of the prevalence of current alcohol consumption in Brazilians over 60 found: excessive alcohol consumption of 10.3–27%, heavy consumption of 2.9–7.3%, and dependence of 3.8–9.2% (Chagas et al. 2019).

Thus, the recommendations for low-risk consumption among young and older adults differ significantly. While low-risk consumption for young adults comprises up to 21 doses of alcohol per week and no more than 5 doses on a single occasion (*binge) for* men and up to 14 doses of alcohol per week and no more than 4 doses on a single occasion (*binge*) for women, on the other hand, for older adult this low-risk consumption is lower: no more than 7 doses per week and no more than 3 doses on a single occasion (*binge*). Besides, these definitions refer to healthy older adult people, i.e., those who do not present health problems and use medication, which further restricts the amount of alcohol consumed defined as low risk (NIAAA 2008).

Tobacco

Due to the aging process, tobacco consumption also adds negative consequences for the older adult. This is because older adults have a greater number of physical diseases (stroke, heart disease, cancer) than the young adult (Østbye et al. 2002). Besides, mortality rates among current and former smokers are higher than among those who have never smoked (Østbye et al. 2002).

The prevalence of tobacco consumption in Brazil among people aged 55–65 is also relatively high (Fig. 5.1). However, there are few differences in consumption between men and women, one of which is the diagnosis of tobacco dependence, which is higher among men. It is worth noting that tobacco consumption among people between 55 and 65 years of age is higher when compared with younger age groups. This could be justified by the reflection of the changes that the past generations have experienced since the specific Brazilian legislation for tobacco use control is relatively recent (the 1980s) and has shown positive results in the rates of cigarette use by the younger population. In addition, research suggests that older adults are less likely to try to quit smoking and less likely to quit (Givel 2015). Other Brazilian surveys with people over 60 years of age present prevalence of tobacco use between 9% and 24% (Barbosa et al. 2018; Madruga et al. 2010).

Illicit Drugs

The most consumed illicit substance in Brazil, among people between 55 and 65 years old, is marijuana, the other drugs such as cocaine, crack, hallucinogens are almost not present. These data are in line with international studies presented in the *World Drug Report* 2018 (UNODC 2018).

Although illicit drug use among the population above 55 is low, the higher prevalence of marijuana use can be justified by the idea that sporadic consumption of marijuana does not pose any health risks compared to other illicit drugs. However, the low consumption of illicit drugs by the population over 55 is also justified by the greater perception that there are health risks in the consumption of any illicit drug when compared to younger age groups.

Medicines

Medicines are the substances most consumed by the older adult. However, in addition to the population over 65 years old receiving more prescription medication from their doctor, this same population adds self-medication to a greater proportion than the young. It is worth noting that women are more likely to self-medicate than men (Rao and Crome 2016).

Although aging is characterized by several health issues that often require the use of medications, several problems emerge, among them:

- Older adults may go through several specialists who often prescribe new drugs without checking the interaction with the drugs that are already consumed by the patient.
- The use of benzodiazepines (medication for depression, anxiety, and insomnia) increases with age, which can increase the probability of accidents, falls, fractures, and losses in cognitive functions.
- The combination of alcohol with medications can be dangerous, as it can impact at high risk of liver damage (e.g. analgesic), dizziness, and falls (e.g. antihypertensive), until the sedative effect is increased (e.g. anxiolytic).
- The body of older adult has more difficulty in processing many medications, this can be accentuated by the polypharmacy (concomitant use of various medications) that is common in this population.
- The adverse effects of medication are more likely to occur in older adults.

In Brazil, among people aged 55 and 65, the most commonly used non-prescribed medications are benzodiazepines, followed by opiates, and to a lesser extent barbiturates, amphetamines, anabolic agents, and anticholinergics. The prevalence of the consumption of more than one substance was also identified in the last Brazilian survey (Bastos et al. 2017), highlighting the concomitant consumption of alcohol plus tobacco, and then alcohol plus medication. A national survey of people aged 60 and over found that 83% of the older adults used medicines. In addition, older people aged 60 and overused an average of 3.3 medications and in older people over 70 the average was 4.4 medications (Silva et al. 2012).

Sorting and Evaluation Instruments

Most of the instruments used to screen or evaluate problems related to alcohol consumption and dependence were created for the young adult population. Some of these instruments are used in studies with an older population such as AUDIT

(Alcohol Use Disorders Identification Test) (Babor et al. 2001) and CAGE (Cut-Annoyed-Guilty-Eye) questionnaire (Ewing 1984). However, there are already tools developed, adapted, or validated especially for the older adult population: AUDIT-C (Short version) (Bradley et al. 2007), SMAST-G (*Short Michigan Alcoholism Screening Test - Geriatric version*) (Blow et al. 1998), SHARPS (*Short version of the Alcohol-Related Problems Survey*), and CARET (*Comorbidity-Alcohol Risk Evaluation Tool*) (Fink et al. 2002; Moore et al. 2002).

Shorter versions of the instruments have proven effective in detecting drinking patterns and addiction, and are often used in research. The AUDIT-C (3 items) evaluates the drinking pattern (Bradley et al. 2007), the SMAST-G (10 items) focuses on the psychosocial aspects of aging (e.g., drinking to cope with loss and loneliness) (Blow et al. 1998), but does not include information on quantity and frequency of use, while SHARPS (32 items) and CARET (26 items) in addition to addressing alcohol consumption in the past 12 months, quantity and frequency of alcohol, combine these results with the presence of comorbidities and medication use (Fink et al. 2002; Moore et al. 2002).

It is worth mentioning that the instruments developed for an older adult may increase the recognition of this population with problems related to the use of alcohol in a fast way, but they do not replace a complete evaluation. These instruments can provide decision support to health professionals who need to assess older adult and treat medical conditions efficiently.

Diagnosis

Considering that what has been said in that chapter, thinking about the differential diagnosis for older adults seems urgent. However, the diagnosis of substance use disorder for this population still faces its challenges. Table 5.1 presents some limitations found in the current diagnostic manual, DSM-V.

Types of Treatment and Other Interventions

Faced with all the particularities of drug consumption by older population, the treatment for older adult users and/or substance dependents brings numerous challenges. One of them is precisely the simultaneous presence of a range of health conditions (inherent to aging), combined with psychiatric problems (depression and anxiety), as well as negative long-term social consequences (lack of social support, loneliness) (UNODC 2018).

However, treatment for problems related to alcohol, tobacco, and medication use has been carried out in different contexts (primary care, hospitals, community centers, and general practice) and approaches (short interventions, multi-component interventions, education, and counselling), with diverse results, but in general with

Table 5.1 Limitations of diagnostic criteria of DSM-5. Source: Adapted from Wilson et al. (2015), Moore et al. (2017), and APA (2014)

DSM-V diagnostic criteria for substance use disorder (TUS) The presence of at least 2 symptoms indicates a Substance Use Disorder (SUD). Severity is defined as mild (2–3 symptoms), moderate (4–5 symptoms), or severe (6 or + symptoms).		
	Criteria	Limitations
1	Consumption of the substance in larger quantities or for a longer period than intended	Cognitive damage can interfere with proper self-monitoring
2	Persistent desire or unsuccessful efforts to reduce or control the use of the substance	There may be no incentive to reduce harmful use, which includes less social, personal, and family pressures secondary to age
3	Much time is spent on activities necessary to obtain or recover from the effects of the substance	Negative effects can occur at relatively low levels of use for older adults, as well as their recovery
4	Cracking or a strong desire to use the substance (*craving*)	Older people may not recognize impulses as desires, or they may attribute it to something like anxiety, depression, or boredom
5	Use of recurrent substances, resulting in non-compliance with obligations (work, school, or home)	The roles and expectations of older people and their families change with the transition of life stages and this may not be recognized as a problem
6	Continued use despite persistent or recurrent social or interpersonal problems caused or exacerbated by substance use	Older people deny or may not realize that problems are associated with substance use
7	Important occupational or recreational social activities are abandoned or reduced due to substance use	Older people may have decreased activities due to psychiatric comorbidities or "lentification." Social isolation and disabilities can make detection difficult
8	Recurrent use in situations where physical danger exists	Older people may deny or not realize that a situation that was once safe has become physically dangerous. (e.g. higher risk of falling)
9	The use of substances is continued despite knowledge of having a persistent or recurrent physical or psychological problem which has probably been caused or exacerbated by substances	Older adult may deny or not realize that these symptoms are related to the substance Older adult may not attribute some or all of the problems to the substance

(continued)

Table 5.1 (continued)

DSM-V diagnostic criteria for substance use disorder (TUS) The presence of at least 2 symptoms indicates a Substance Use Disorder (SUD). Severity is defined as mild (2–3 symptoms), moderate (4–5 symptoms), or severe (6 or + symptoms).		
	Criteria	Limitations
10	Tolerance	Due to increased sensitivity to alcohol with age, older adults may have decreased tolerance Older people may not develop a dependency
11	Abstinence	Withdrawal symptoms can manifest themselves in more subtle and prolonged ways in the older adult

beneficial effects for reducing the consumption of these substances and on the health of users (Bhatia et al. 2015).

Still, the most solid and promising results for older adult refer to treatment for problems specifically related to alcohol, and that these are due to issues such as the desire for abstinence, capacity for change, good response to brief intervention and motivational improvement therapy, better results, and greater prospects for long-term recovery when compared to younger groups (Bhatia et al. 2015; Crome and Crome 2018).

Although there are numerous forms of treatment for substance use problems, few studies have been carried out specifically with the older population to compare the effectiveness of these approaches. In addition, studies on treatment in older people focus on alcohol, and few studies include treatment for other drugs such as tobacco and medications among older adult, as well as illicit drugs.

Besides the treatments studied, one of the strategies that have stood out as a successful resource in reducing alcohol consumption among older adult, especially in primary care, is the brief intervention. Brief intervention is a structured technique that aims to identify and guide harmful drinkers to reduce harmful behaviors, which can be adapted to different contexts and needs of professionals (Babor and Higgins-Biddle 2001). This type of intervention includes information material, personalized *feedback*, brief, and telephone counselling, and has shown significant results in reducing alcohol consumption among older adult when compared to other more complex types of intervention (Paula et al. 2019).

Final Considerations

Substance use is a reality among older adult and, although it is a vulnerable group for the consumption of these substances, there is little evidence to measure the consequences. Although diagnosis rates related to substance use disorders are lower, the increase in comorbidities and other health conditions in this age group puts this issue on the public health priority agenda as the older population grows.

No doubt the relevance of attention to drug use among older adult will assume greater importance over time. Meanwhile, to address the special needs of older people with substance use-related problems, it is imperative that health and social services, primary and specialized care professionals, learn to recognize signs and symptoms of the risky consumption alcohol and other drugs in this age group. This recognition is the first step for older adult substance user to benefit from existing interventions and to promote a better overall quality of life among older adult.

References

American Psychiatric Association (APA). (2014). *Manual diagnóstico e estatístico de transtornos mentais* (5th ed.). Porto Alegre, Brazil: Artmed.

Babor, T. F., & Higgins-Biddle, J. C. (2001). *Brief intervention for hazardous and harmful drinking: A manual for use in primary care*. Geneva, Switzerland: World Health Organization. Retrieved from https://apps.who.int/iris/handle/10665/67210.

Babor, T. F., Higgins-Biddle, J. C., Saunders, J. B., & Monteiro, M. (2001). *The alcohol use disorders identification test (AUDIT): Guidelines for use in primary care* (2nd ed.). Geneva, Switzerland: World Health Organization.

Barbosa, M., Pereira, C., Cruz, D., & Leite, I. (2018). Prevalence and factors associated with alcohol and tobacco use among non-institutionalized older adult persons. *Revista Brasileira De Geriatria E Gerontologia, 21*(2), 123–133. https://doi.org/10.1590/1981-22562018021.170185.

Bastos, F., Vasconcellos, M., De Boni, R., Reis, N., & Coutinho, C. (2017). *III Levantamento Nacional sobre o Uso de Drogas pela População Brasileira*. Rio de Janeiro, Brazil: ICIT/FIOCRUZ.

Bhatia, U., Nadkarni, A., Murthy, P., Rao, R., & Crome, I. (2015). Recent advances in treatment for older people with substance use problems: An updated systematic and narrative review. *European Geriatric Medicine, 6*(6), 580–586. https://doi.org/10.1016/j.eurger.2015.07.001.

Blow, F. C., Gillespie, B. W., Barry, K. L., Mudd, S. A., & Hill, E. M. (1998). Brief screening for alcohol problems in elderly populations using the short Michigan alcoholism screening test-geriatric version (SMAST-G). *Alcoholism: Clinical and Experimental Research, 22*(Suppl), 131A.

Bradley, K. A., DeBenedetti, A. F., Volk, R. J., Williams, E. C., Frank, D., & Kivlahan, D. R. (2007). AUDIT-C as a brief screen for alcohol misuse in primary care. *Alcoholism, Clinical and Experimental Research, 31*(7), 1208–1217. https://doi.org/10.1111/j.1530-0277.2007.00403.x.

Camarano, A. A., & Kanso, S. (2013). Envelhecimento da População Brasileira: Uma Contribuição Demográfica. In E. V. Freitas & L. Py (Eds.), *Tratado de geriatria e gerontologia* (3rd ed., pp. 133–152). Rio de Janeiro, Brazil: Guanabara Koogan.

Carlini, E., Galduróz, J., Noto, A., Carlini, C., Oliveira, L., & Nappo, A. (2005). *II Levantamento Domiciliar sobre o uso de drogas psicotrópicas no Brasil: Envolvendo as 108 maiores cidades do país*. Brasília: Centro Brasileiro de Informações sobre Drogas Psicotrópicas –CEBRID.

Chagas, C., Paula, T., Machado, D., Martins, L., Opaleye, D., Piedade, T., et al. (2019). Alcohol consumption by older people in Brazil. *Addictive Disorders & Their Treatment, 18*(4), 229–237. https://doi.org/10.1097/adt.0000000000000168.

Crome, I., & Crome, P. (2018). Alcohol and age. *Age and Ageing, 47*(2), 164–167. https://doi.org/10.1093/ageing/afx191.

Dowling, G. J., Weiss, S. R., & Condon, T. P. (2008). Drugs of abuse and the aging brain. *Neuropsychopharmacology, 33*(2), 209–218. https://doi.org/10.1038/sj.npp.1301412.

Ewing, J. A. (1984). Detecting alcoholism. The CAGE questionnaire. *JAMA, 252*(14), 1905–1907. https://doi.org/10.1001/jama.252.14.1905.

Fink, A., Morton, S. C., Beck, J. C., Hays, R. D., Spritzer, K., Oishi, S., & Moore, A. A. (2002). The alcohol-related problems survey: Identifying hazardous and harmful drinking in older primary care patients. *Journal of the American Geriatrics Society, 50*(10), 1717–1722. https://doi.org/10.1046/j.1532-5415.2002.50467.x.

Fox, M., & Wilson, L. (2011). Depression and alcohol. In M. Fox & L. Wilson (Eds.), *Counselling older people with alcohol problems* (pp. 163–178). London, UK: Jessica Kingsley Publishers.

Givel, M. (2015). Proposals for policy development: Tobacco. In I. B. Crome, L. T. Wu, P. Crome, & R. Rao (Eds.), *Substance use and older people* (pp. 372–378). Hoboken, NJ: Wiley.

Instituto Brasileiro de Geografia e Estatística (IBGE). (2019). *Projeção da população do Brasil e das Unidades da Federação*. Retrieved from https://www.ibge.gov.br/apps/populacao/projecao/

Laranjeira, R., Madruga, C. S., Pinsky, I., Caetano, R., Mitsuhiro, S. S., & Castello, G. (2012). *II Levantamento Nacional de Álcool e Drogas (LENAD)*. São Paulo, Brazil: Instituto Nacional de Ciência e Tecnologia para Políticas Públicas de Álcool e Outras Drogas (INPAD).

Madruga, C. S., Ferri, C. P., Pinsky, I., Blay, S. L., Caetano, R., & Laranjeira, R. (2010). Tobacco use among the elderly: The first Brazilian National Survey (BNAS). *Aging & Mental Health, 14*(6), 720–724. https://doi.org/10.1080/13607860903586177.

Moore, A. A., Beck, J. C., Babor, T. F., Hays, R. D., & Reuben, D. B. (2002). Beyond alcoholism: Identifying older, at-risk drinkers in primary care. *Journal of Studies on Alcohol, 63*(3), 316–324. https://doi.org/10.15288/jsa.2002.63.316.

Moore, A. A., Kuerbis, A., Sacco, P., Chen, G. I., & Garcia, M. B. (2017). Screening and assessment of unhealthy. Alcohol use in older adults. In A. Kuerbis, A. A. Moore, P. Sacco, & F. Zanjani (Eds.), *Alcohol and aging: Clinical and public health perspectives* (pp. 169–180). Cham, Switzerland: Springer.

Moore, A. A., Whiteman, E. J., & Ward, K. T. (2007). Risks of combined alcohol/medication use in older adults. *The American Journal of Geriatric Pharmacotherapy, 5*(1), 64–74. https://doi.org/10.1016/j.amjopharm.2007.03.006.

National Institute on Alcohol Abuse and Alcoholism (NIAAA). (2008). *Older adults*. Retrieved from https://www.niaaa.nih.gov/alcohol-health/special-populations-co-occurring-disorders/older-adults

Østbye, T., Taylor, D. H., & Jung, S. H. (2002). A longitudinal study of the effects of tobacco smoking and other modifiable risk factors on ill health in middle-aged and old Americans: Results from the health and retirement study and asset and health dynamics among the oldest old survey. *Preventive Medicine, 34*(3), 334–345. https://doi.org/10.1006/pmed.2001.0991.

Paula, T., Chagas, C., Souza-Formigoni, M., & Ferri, C. P. (2019). Alcohol and ageing: Rapid changes in populations present new challenges for an old problem. *Substance Use & Misuse, 54*(9), 1580–1581. https://doi.org/10.1080/10826084.2019.1592196.

Ramos, M. G., Hara, C., & Rocha, F. L. (2013). Princípios do Uso dos Psicofármacos em Idosos. In E. V. Freitas & L. Py (Eds.), *Tratado de geriatria e gerontologia* (3rd ed., pp. 538–555). Rio de Janeiro, Brazil: Guanabara Koogan.

Rao, R., & Crome, I. (2016). Alcohol misuse in older people. *Bjpsych Advances, 22*(2), 118–126. https://doi.org/10.1192/apt.bp.115.014480.

Royal College of Psychiatrists (RCP). (2018). *Our invisible addicts* (2nd ed.). London, UK: Royal College of Psychiatrists.

Seibel, S. D., & Toscano Junior, A. (2001). *Dependência de drogas*. São Paulo, Brazil: Atheneu.

Silva, A., Ribeiro, A., Klein, H., & Acurcio, F. (2012). Utilização de medicamentos por idosos brasileiros, de acordo com a faixa etária: um inquérito postal. *Cadernos de Saúde Pública, 28*(6), 1033–1045. https://doi.org/10.1590/S0102-311X2012000600003.

Topiwala, A., Allan, C. L., Valkanova, V., Zsoldos, E., Filippini, N., Sexton, C., et al. (2017). Moderate alcohol consumption as risk factor for adverse brain outcomes and cognitive decline: Longitudinal cohort study. *BMJ, 357*, j2353. https://doi.org/10.1136/bmj.j2353.

United Nations Office on Drugs and Crime (UNODC). (2018). *World drug report*. Retrieved from https://www.unodc.org/wdr2018/.

Vink, D., Aartsen, M. J., & Schoevers, R. A. (2008). Risk factors for anxiety and depression in the elderly: A review. *Journal of Affective Disorders, 106*(1–2), 29–44. https://doi.org/10.1016/j.jad.2007.06.005.

Wilson, D., Jackson, S., Crome, I. B., Rao, R., & Crome, P. (2015). Comprehensive geriatric assessment and the special needs of older people. In I. B. Crome, I. L. T. Wu, P. Crome, & R. Rao (Eds.), *Substance use and older people* (pp. 173–179). Hoboken, NJ: Wiley.

World Health Organization (WHO). (2010). *Population ageing. Ageing and health*. Geneva, Switzerland: World Health Organization. Retrieved from https://www.who.int/features/qa/72/en/.

World Health Organization (WHO). (2018). *Ageing and health*. Geneva, Switzerland: World Health Organization. Retrieved from https://www.who.int/news-room/fact-sheets/detail/ageing-and-health.

World Health Organization (WHO). (2019). *Risk reduction of cognitive decline and dementia*. Geneva, Switzerland: World Health Organization.

Part II
Biological Aspects

Chapter 6
Genetic Aspects of Substance Use Disorders

Daniel da Silva e Silva and Fabrício de Araújo Moreira

Introduction: Substances of Abuse

The use of substances to obtain pleasure and to modify sensory perception, state of alert, and behavior has accompanied mankind since its early days. The effects of such substances can be of a psychostimulant, depressant, or hallucinogenic nature (more than one of these effects being possible for a given substance). Among the many known, the main ones used in western societies are alcohol, tobacco (nicotine), caffeine, marijuana, cocaine, opioids, amphetamines, LSD, and there are variations between them according to culture and historical moment.

The use of some of these substances can result in pleasurable effects, which leads to a desire to use them again, even when the use results in clearly deleterious consequences for the individual or for others. They therefore have reinforcing effects and are called "abuse drugs" or "psychotropic substances." The neural processes related to these effects are multiple and complex. However, experimental approaches in pharmacology and neuroscience suggest that the different drugs of abuse recruit some common neural pathways in the brain, with particular emphasis on via of dopamine called mesolimbic (Koob and Volkow 2010) (Fig. 6.1).

The use and abuse of these substances make increasingly larger doses necessary, characterizing the phenomenon of tolerance. In addition, various adaptations make the interruption of use result in a set of aversive manifestations, characterizing the abstinence syndrome. Frequently, this triggers a compulsive drug seeking which perpetuates its use, a phenomenon called relapse. Together, the impulsive and compulsive desire for the use of a substance (use despite the deleterious consequences),

D. da Silva e Silva (✉)
National Institute on Alcohol Abuse and Alcoholism, Rockville, MD, USA
e-mail: daniel.dasilvaesilva@nih.gov

F. de Araújo Moreira
Universidade Federal de Minas Gerais, Belo Horizonte, MG, Brazil

D. De Micheli et al. (eds.), *Drugs and Human Behavior*,
https://doi.org/10.1007/978-3-030-62855-0_6

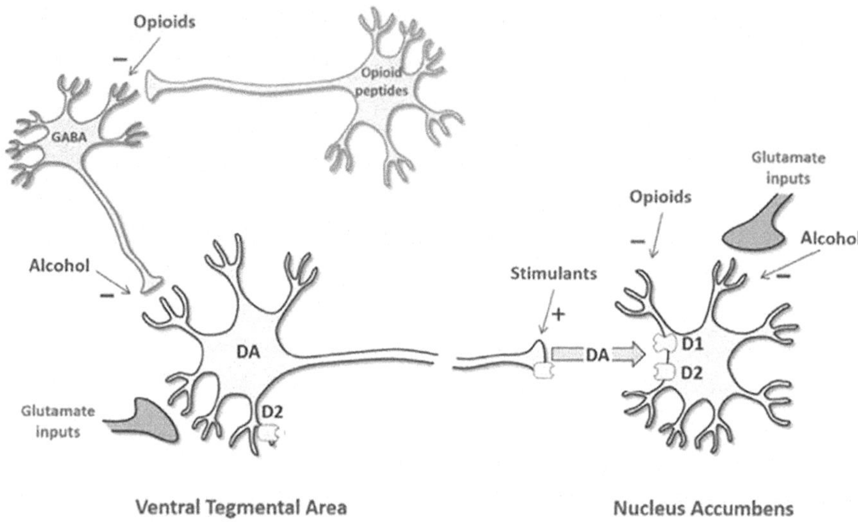

Fig. 6.1 Places of action of some drugs of abuse in the mesolimbic dopaminergic pathway. Although they act by different molecular targets, several drugs of abuse can facilitate, although indirectly, the activity of the mesolimbic dopaminergic pathway. Released dopamine (DA) can act on dopaminergic receptors of types D1 and D2. This route is modulated by other neurotransmitters, particularly glutamate and gamma-aminobutyric acid (GABA) (adapted from Moreira and Dalley 2015)

the occurrence of tolerance, the abstinence syndrome, and other associated factors characterize the psychiatric disorder called substance use disorder.

Alcohol as an Example of Drug Abuse

Ethanol, ethyl alcohol, or simply alcohol is one of the substances most used by mankind and is consumed through so-called alcoholic beverages. Alcohol occupies a central position in the culture of most civilizations. Its consumption is not only legalized, but widely encouraged through advertisements and pressure from social groups. Due to this, it represents one of the greatest health problems nowadays (Degenhardt et al. 2018). In addition to the harm to the individual, it stands out for the potential harm to others, as it causes behavioral disinhibition, increased aggressiveness, and impaired driving ability (Nutt et al. 2007). Some of the best known alcoholic beverages in our culture are beer, wine, and liquor. These are obtained by a process of fermentation of fruits or cereals containing, initially, sugar or starch (for example, grapes to obtain wine or barley to obtain beer), which results in an alcohol concentration of approximately 5% to 15%. The material obtained can be distilled to obtain more concentrated beverages containing 40% to 50% alcohol (in the case of Brazilian cachaça and whiskey, for example).

Archeological research suggests that the fermentation process for obtaining beverages was already known about 7000 years ago (McGovern et al. 2004). Apparently, all civilizations, even those that originated in countries where alcohol is currently prohibited, already consumed it in antiquity (Dietler 2006). The probable origin of the word *alcohol* is in the Arabic language (*al-kuhl*), meaning something like "the essence in powder." "*Kohl*" is a material used as an eyebrow eyeliner. Chemically, it consists of antimony trisulfide (Sb2S3), which can be in the form of a crystalline mineral (stibine mineral), the alcohol being used in the process to transform it into powder by sublimation. Alcohol was considered the essence or "spirit" of this mineral. The word alcohol was later used to refer to any product obtained by sublimation and distillation (in fact, the term "spirit" is still used to refer to some alcoholic beverages, particularly distilled ones). The distillation process was widely used by alchemists in the Middle Ages and spread from the Middle East to Europe. In the modern age, alcohol became the most consumed psychoactive substance in all Western societies, being of immense social, political, and economic relevance (Dietler 2006).

Alcohol can induce a variety of effects that are rare for a substance, particularly because it is a molecule of simple structure. Another interesting feature is its ability to induce effects in high amounts (of the order of grams), compared to most substances (which exert effects in doses of the order of milligrams). The effects of its acute consumption are characteristic of depression of central nervous system functions, reducing anxiety, and promoting behavioral disinhibition, amnesia, impairment of motor coordination, sedation, and hypnosis. In higher doses, general anesthesia and fatal effects of respiratory depression and hypoglycemia occur.

Pharmacokinetic studies show that alcohol is widely absorbed, especially in the small intestine. The peak plasma concentration occurs about 30 min after ingestion, and the speed of absorption is reduced in the presence of food. Part of the alcohol is metabolized in the liver by first-pass metabolism. Once in the bloodstream, it is rapidly distributed to various organs and tissues. People with a higher percentage of fat tissue are more susceptible to the effects of alcohol, as it is distributed less to that tissue, becoming more concentrated in the blood and brain. The elimination of alcohol from the body occurs mainly by metabolism, particularly in the liver, into aldehyde and acetic acid. The unpleasant sensation that can occur after a few hours of consuming a large amount of alcohol (hangover) results from the accumulation of some of these metabolites, particularly acetic aldehyde (or acetaldehyde). Alcohol is metabolized to acetaldehyde by means of the enzyme alcohol dehydrogenase. This, in turn, is transformed into acetic acid under the action of aldehyde dehydrogenase. The alcohol metabolism is saturable and very sensitive to individual genetic variations. Part of the alcohol is also excreted, including through the respiratory tract, and can be detected for consumption estimation (by means of devices called breathalyzers). If consumed in the long term, alcohol presents an enzymatic inducing effect, so that its chronic use can increase its own metabolism (Chan and Anderson 2014).

Regarding the pharmacodynamic aspects, alcohol acts through multiple mechanisms of action. In accordance with its effects of depression of the central nervous system, it can facilitate the action of inhibitory neurotransmitters and attenuate excitatory neurotransmitters. An important molecular target seems to be the receptor of gamma-aminobutyric acid GABA-A, a channel permeable to chloride anions and which has its opening facilitated by alcohol. Another possibility is the blocking of N-methyl-D-aspartate (NMDA) type glutamate receptors, with reduced influx of sodium and calcium cations (Spanagel 2009).

The use of alcohol, therefore, can lead to abuse, i.e. the consumption of the substance in an inappropriate pattern. This can evolve to alcohol use disorders, which includes the compulsive desire for the consumption of the substance in spite of harmful consequences; the need for ever greater doses (tolerance); the aversive sensation when the use of the substance is interrupted (abstinence syndrome). Associated with alcohol use disorders may be Wernicke-Korsakoff Syndrome, cirrhosis of the liver (Kranzler and Soyka 2018).

Genetic Aspects of Substance Use Disorders

Box 6.1. What Is Heritability?

Heritability is a measure of how much variability in a given characteristic such as height, body mass (as well as complex disorders such as SUD, autism, and Parkinson's disease) is directly attributed to genetic factors. In scientific terms, heritability (represented as h2) refers to the proportion of the variation among individuals in a given population that can be explained by genetic and non-environmental variations. This index can range from 0 (when one characteristic has no genetic influence at all) to 1 (when all of the variability associated with one characteristic has an underlying genetic cause, which hardly occurs in practice). Thus, when we say that the heritability for predisposition of cocaine abuse is h2 = 0.7, we are inferring that, in that population under study, among all the variability associated to that characteristic, 70% can be exclusively attributed to genetic variations.

Since this index is calculated on the basis of a specific population and is subject to specific environmental factors, it can be concluded that the inheritability of a given characteristic may vary between different populations or even over time. In general, although it carries valuable information about a given biological trait, heritability is an exploratory and limited measure and cannot be fully extrapolated to different populations or different environments.

It is estimated that during 2017 271 million people, or 5.5% of the global population between 15 and 64 years of age, have used some type of drug. Of these, 35 million, about 13%, have some disorder related to their consumption, including misuse (UNODC 2019). This numerical discrepancy between the use and development of SUD highlights the existence of an important and striking genetic factor regulating the vulnerability to the abusive of these substances.

In fact, substance use disorders (SUD) have an inherent and inseparable environmental factor linked to their etiology, since previous exposure to the drug is the fundamental and triggering factor of the disease. However, hereditary factors also represent an important risk factor for the development of such disorders. Thus, if on the one hand genetic elements contribute with approximately 50% to the susceptibility to alcohol abuse (h2 = 0.5), on the other hand prolonged drug use is an indispensable condition for the initial development of the disease. This paradox between a strong genetic component (or high heritability) tied to an indispensable environmental trigger (or initial voluntary exposure to the drug) emphasizes that despite being genetically modulated, SUD depend greatly on the lifestyle of the individual in question.

Regardless of the drug's pharmacological class, in most cases SUD have a high degree of heritability and are among the highest considering all psychiatric diseases. Studies suggest that the size of the genetic contribution in these disorders varies not only because of the drug itself, but also regarding the population studied and the methodology used. In general, cocaine (h2 = 0.42–0.79) and opioid (h2 = 0.43–0.60) misuse are among the disorders with the highest degree of heritability, while hallucinogens (h2 = 0.25–0.39), stimulants (h2 = 0.40–0.44), and cannabis (h2 = 0.29–0.51) misuse have a smaller but not negligible genetic component attached. Inheritability of legalized drugs with great social appeal such as nicotine (0.59–0.71) and alcohol (0.29–0.51) also has an important genetic influence on their etiology (Agrawal et al. 2012; Tsuang et al. 2001; Verweij et al. 2010; Wang et al. 2012). This high heritability among SUD is ratified by epidemiological data demonstrating that the risk of SUD is 4.5 times higher among first-degree relatives of individuals diagnosed with the same disorder when compared with the general population (Merikangas et al. 1998). Other studies also demonstrate that this number can reach 3 or 8 times when only alcohol use disorders are considered.

Besides the specific heritability of each individual drug, a large portion of the genetic factors that predispose to SUD are shared among different classes of drugs. Studies also show that genetic factors specific to a given drug are rare, thus supporting the idea that different classes of drugs can act on common neural substrates and share similar biological mechanisms (Di Chiara and Imperato 1988). This genetic overlap in the mechanisms of predisposition to SUD can also explain the high degree of co-abuse observed among different drugs such as alcohol, nicotine, cocaine, and cannabis. For example, while approximately 85% of individuals diagnosed with alcohol use disorders also misuse nicotine, it is believed that these two comorbidities share about 50% of their total heritability (Swan et al. 1997).

SUD also share an important part of their genetic basis with several other psychiatric diseases through common neurobiological pathways. Thus, it is not surprising that patients diagnosed with SUD invariably present some degree of psychiatric comorbidity associated with their initial diagnosis. It is estimated that while 37% of patients diagnosed with alcohol use disorders have some other psychiatric comorbidity. This number is close to 50% among those dependent on other drugs (Regier et al. 1990). For example, while Prescott and collaborators estimate that about 60%

of covariance between SUD and depression can be explained purely by genetic factors (Prescott et al. 2000), Fu and collaborators (Fu et al. 2007) also demonstrated a strong and significant genetic correlation between depression and nicotine or cannabis dependence. Additionally, genetic predispositions to stress, impulsivity, anxiety, and dysphoria can also share genetic bases and thus contribute to the development of SUD through common biological substrates. For example, the prevalence of nicotine dependence is about 13% in the general population, but it can reach 30 or 70% in the presence of another psychiatric disorder (Grant et al. 2004).

Although valuable for epidemiological and diagnostic purposes, heritability in isolation does not provide crucial information about the trait under study, such as which genes or biological pathways are involved with that particular trait or even how important the genetic-environmental association is for that trait. It should be noted that like any complex disease, substance use disorders have a polygenic nature, that is, different genes (and their different alleles) interact with each other (and with the environment) in a complex way to express and control a certain characteristic. In addition to the complex genetic architecture of these disorders, several genes can also control biological factors indirectly related to vulnerability to drugs of abuse, such as changing the response to stress or modulating circuits related to decision making, factors directly related to the initiation of drug use and the development of dependency. Thus, genetic analyses of a strictly monogenic nature, although partly valuable, limit the global biological understanding of these disorders and, therefore, the use of large-scale analyses that employ techniques that allow us to understand how these different sets of genes and their different alleles interact with each other is of enormous value.

One such global approach is called Genome Wide Association Studies (GWAS). In this strategy, certain genetic variations called single nucleotide polymorphism (SNPs) are compared between different individuals expressing a specific common trait in search of a positive association between these genetic variants and the trait under study. In general, these studies are conducted comparing patients (positive individuals for a certain trait—SUD, for example) and controls (negative individuals for the same trait) and using a panel of thousands (or millions) of distinct genetic variants. Then, the genetic similarities found within a group and the genetic differences found between different groups are evaluated through statistical tests that measure the power of these associations (Fig. 6.2).

Despite numerous association studies examining possible candidate genes for SUD-related characteristics, few genes have been proven to be associated with these disorders. Among these, many correspond to biological pathways and processes common to different drugs of abuse, while others are specific to certain drugs and seem to depend on the mechanism of action of each substance.

Among the genetic variants positively associated with alcohol abuse, those linked to ethanol metabolism genes and belonging to the family of aldehyde dehydrogenases (*ALDH2*, *ADH1B*) and alcohol dehydrogenases (*ADH1C)* are the ones that present the most robust results and seem to protect against alcohol abuse; others such as those linked to genes belonging to the GABAergic (*GABRA2, GABRG1*), dopaminergic (*DRD2/ANKK1),* and serotonergic (*SLC6A4)* pathways also show

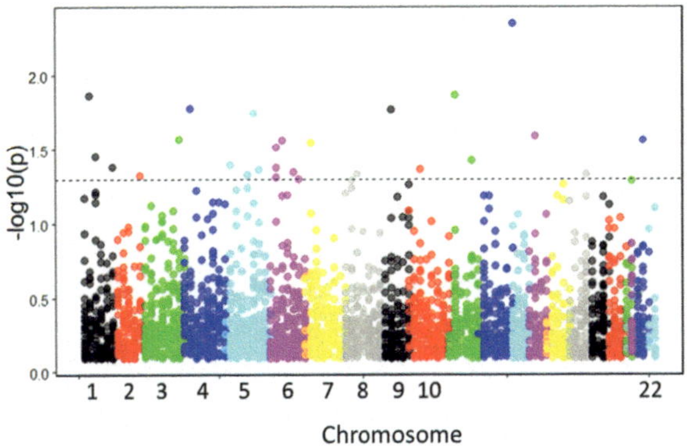

Fig. 6.2 Example of a hypothetical genetic association study. Each point on the graph represents a specific genetic variant (SNP). The Y axis corresponds to the statistical value p and represents how consistent that genetic variant is associated with the characteristic under study, while the X axis corresponds to the location of that genetic variant in the genome. Each of the 22 blocks with distinct colors corresponds to one of the 22 human autosomal chromosomes. The dashed line represents the cut off p-value for an association to be considered true. Thus, in this example, of all the 3000 SNPs tested, 24 distributed along 15 chromosomes were positively associated with the characteristic in question. In the continuation of the analysis, the list of candidate genes will be generated from the evaluation of which genes are linked to those 24 genetic variants.

consistent results and appear to be related to drug misuse predisposition (Edenberg 2007; Enoch 2008; McHugh et al. 2010). Studies also show consistent and robust genetic associations with respect to nicotine abuse, including mostly genes for the different subunits of nicotine receptors such as *CHRNA4* and the *CHRNA5/CHRNA3/CHRNB4 gene* cluster (Saccone et al. 2009) and genes responsible for drug metabolism such as *CYP2A6* (Bloom et al. 2011). Several genes are also effectively associated with different aspects of cocaine abuse, among them some of those also common to other drugs such as *DRD2/ANKK1, COMT,* and *POMC* and others related to specific aspects of cocaine abuse such as the dopamine-related genes *NCAM*, *TTC12*, *CALY,* and *DBH* (Gelernter et al. 2006; Ittiwut et al. 2011; Kalayaesiri et al. 2007; Luo et al. 2004; Zhang et al. 2009; Zuo et al. 2009).

Despite the significant improvement in the detection power of genetic variants achieved in recent years and the growth in sample size obtained through large genetic consortia and meta-analyses studies, according to Agrawal and collaborators genetic association studies still explain only about 2% of the total variance found in endophenotypes associated with SUD (Agrawal et al. 2012). This low detection power corroborates the idea that these disorders are highly heterogeneous diseases, influenced by a large number of genes, each contributing individually with a small biological effect, but which together account for a great biological complexity. In addition, studies of genetic association in essence do not have a causal nature, that is, a positive association between a genetic variant and any characteristic does not imply that variant is the biological cause behind the characteristic in question. In fact, epidemiological and genetic association studies represent only the part of the arduous task of unveiling the biological and genetic nature underlying complex diseases such as SUD.

Another strategy commonly used in the genetic study of complex diseases is transcriptomics. In this approach, the global set of RNA molecules transcribed into a given tissue is evaluated under certain circumstances of interest. In an oversimplified way, it can be said that RNAs are the molecular intermediaries between genes and their final product, the proteins. Thus, the comparative analysis of the total set of RNA molecules (transcriptomic) allows the identification of those genes differently expressed between two distinct conditions, for example, patients with and without SUD. However, unlike DNA, RNAs are versatile molecules and their expression varies substantially between different cells, tissues, and organs. Due to this particular nature, transcriptomic analyses should be performed in a tissue-specific manner. Thus, transcriptomic studies generally use brain biopsies or, more commonly, necropsies of patients previously diagnosed with the characteristic under study. Due to this limitation and also taking advantage of the great flexibility of animal models, many transcriptomic studies use animal models that emulate certain characteristics of SUD such as abusive, compulsive use, craving, and relapse. For example, both rats and mice can be artificially selected to express a high or low preference for alcohol (Crabbe et al. 2010), evaluated for their acute or chronic response to a given drug, or even trained to voluntarily consume alcohol, cocaine, or other drugs (Blegen et al. 2018; Bock et al. 2013).

The results of these studies corroborate many findings found in genetic association studies, mainly identifying genes and biological pathways related to dopamine (DRD1, DRD2, COMT, *PPP1R1B, SLC6A3*), GABA (GABRB1, GABRB2, GABRB3, GABRD, GABRG1, GABRG2), glutamate (GRIA1, GRIN1), GRIK1, GRIK5, GRM5), and serotonin (SLC6A4) as well as so many other individual genes that vary according to the drug under study or even the animal model used, thus usually representing genes with small additive effects and reflecting specific aspects of these disorders (da Silva e Silva et al. 2016; Ferguson et al. 2019; Warden and Mayfield 2017).

References

Agrawal, A., Verweij, K., Gillespie, N., Heath, A., Lessov-Schlaggar, C., Martin, N., et al. (2012). The genetics of addiction—A translational perspective. *Translational Psychiatry, 2*(7), e140–e140. https://doi.org/10.1038/tp.2012.54.

Blegen, M. B., da Silva e Silva, D., Bock, R., Morisot, N., Ron, D., & Alvarez, V. A. (2018). Alcohol operant self-administration: Investigating how alcohol-seeking behaviors predict drinking in mice using two operant approaches. *Alcohol (Fayetteville, NY), 67*, 23–36. https://doi.org/10.1016/j.alcohol.2017.08.008.

Bloom, J., Hinrichs, A. L., Wang, J. C., von Weymarn, L. B., Kharasch, E. D., Bierut, L. J., et al. (2011). The contribution of common CYP2A6 alleles to variation in nicotine metabolism among European-Americans. *Pharmacogenetics and Genomics, 21*(7), 403–416. https://doi.org/10.1097/FPC.0b013e328346e8c0.

Bock, R., Shin, J. H., Kaplan, A. R., Dobi, A., Markey, E., Kramer, P. F., et al. (2013). Strengthening the accumbal indirect pathway promotes resilience to compulsive cocaine use. *Nature Neuroscience, 16*(5), 632–638. https://doi.org/10.1038/nn.3369.

Chan, L., & Anderson, G. (2014). Pharmacokinetic and pharmacodynamic drug interactions with ethanol (alcohol). *Clinical Pharmacokinetics, 53*(12), 1115–1136. https://doi.org/10.1007/s40262-014-0190-x.

Crabbe, J. C., Phillips, T. J., & Belknap, J. K. (2010). The complexity of alcohol drinking: Studies in rodent genetic models. *Behavior Genetics, 40*(6), 737–750. https://doi.org/10.1007/s10519-010-9371-z.

da Silva e Silva, D. A., Frozino Ribeiro, A., Damasceno, S., Rocha, C. S., Berenguer de Matos, A. H., Boerngen-Lacerda, R., et al. (2016). Inflexible ethanol intake: A putative link with the Lrrk2 pathway. *Behavioural Brain Research, 313*, 30–37. https://doi.org/10.1016/j.bbr.2016.07.001.

Degenhardt, L., Charlson, F., Ferrari, A., Santomauro, D., Erskine, H., Mantilla-Herrara, A., et al. (2018). The global burden of disease attributable to alcohol and drug use in 195 countries and territories, 1990–2016: A systematic analysis for the global burden of disease study 2016. *The Lancet Psychiatry, 5*(12), 987–1012. https://doi.org/10.1016/s2215-0366(18)30337-7.

Di Chiara, G., & Imperato, A. (1988). Drugs abused by humans preferentially increase synaptic dopamine concentrations in the mesolimbic system of freely moving rats. *Proceedings of the National Academy of Sciences, 85*(14), 5274–5278. https://doi.org/10.1073/pnas.85.14.5274.

Dietler, M. (2006). Alcohol: Anthropological/archaeological perspectives. *Annual Review of Anthropology, 35*(1), 229–249. https://doi.org/10.1146/annurev.anthro.35.081705.123120.

Edenberg, H. J. (2007). The genetics of alcohol metabolism: Role of alcohol dehydrogenase and aldehyde dehydrogenase variants. *Alcohol Research & Health: The Journal of the National Institute on Alcohol Abuse and Alcoholism, 30*(1), 5–13.

Enoch, M. A. (2008). The role of GABA(A) receptors in the development of alcoholism. *Pharmacology, Biochemistry, and Behavior, 90*(1), 95–104. https://doi.org/10.1016/j.pbb.2008.03.007.

Ferguson, L. B., Zhang, L., Kircher, D., Wang, S., Mayfield, R. D., Crabbe, J. C., et al. (2019). Dissecting brain networks underlying alcohol binge drinking using a systems genomics approach. *Molecular Neurobiology, 56*(4), 2791–2810. https://doi.org/10.1007/s12035-018-1252-0.

Fu, Q., Heath, A. C., Bucholz, K. K., Lyons, M. J., Tsuang, M. T., True, W. R., & Eisen, S. A. (2007). Common genetic risk of major depression and nicotine dependence: The contribution of antisocial traits in a United States veteran male twin cohort. *Twin Research and Human Genetics, 10*(3), 470–478. https://doi.org/10.1375/twin.10.3.470.

Gelernter, J., Yu, Y., Weiss, R., Brady, K., Panhuysen, C., Yang, B., et al. (2006). Haplotype spanning TTC12 and ANKK1, flanked by the DRD2 and NCAM1 loci, is strongly associated to nicotine dependence in two distinct American populations. *Human Molecular Genetics, 15*(24), 3498–3507. https://doi.org/10.1093/hmg/ddl426.

Grant, B. F., Hasin, D. S., Chou, S. P., Stinson, F. S., & Dawson, D. A. (2004). Nicotine dependence and psychiatric disorders in the United States. *Archives of General Psychiatry, 61*(11), 1107. https://doi.org/10.1001/archpsyc.61.11.1107.

Ittiwut, R., Listman, J. B., Ittiwut, C., Cubells, J. F., Weiss, R. D., Brady, K., et al. (2011). Association between polymorphisms in catechol-O-methyltransferase (COMT) and cocaine-induced paranoia in European-American and African-American populations. *American Journal of Medical Genetics Part B: Neuropsychiatric Genetics, 156*(6), 651–660. https://doi.org/10.1002/ajmg.b.31205.

Kalayaesiri, R., Sughondhabirom, A., Gueorguieva, R., Coric, V., Lynch, W. J., Lappalainen, J., et al. (2007). Dopamine β-hydroxylase gene (DβH) -1021C→T influences self-reported paranoia during cocaine self-administration. *Biological Psychiatry, 61*(11), 1310–1313. https://doi.org/10.1016/j.biopsych.2006.08.012.

Koob, G. F., & Volkow, N. D. (2010). Neurocircuitry of addiction. *Neuropsychopharmacology: Official Publication of the American College of Neuropsychopharmacology, 35*(1), 217–238. https://doi.org/10.1038/npp.2009.110.

Kranzler, H. R., & Soyka, M. (2018). Diagnosis and pharmacotherapy of alcohol use disorder: A review. *JAMA, 320*(8), 815–824. https://doi.org/10.1001/jama.2018.11406.

Luo, X., Kranzler, H., Lappalainen, J., Rosenheck, R., Charney, D., Zuo, L., et al. (2004). CALCYON gene variation, schizophrenia, and cocaine dependence. *American Journal of Medical Genetics, 125B*(1), 25–30. https://doi.org/10.1002/ajmg.b.20092.
McGovern, P., Zhang, J., Tang, J., Zhang, Z., Hall, G., Moreau, R., et al. (2004). Fermented beverages of pre- and proto-historic China. *Proceedings of the National Academy of Sciences, 101*(51), 17593–17598. https://doi.org/10.1073/pnas.0407921102.
McHugh, R. K., Hofmann, S. G., Asnaani, A., Sawyer, A. T., & Otto, M. W. (2010). The serotonin transporter gene and risk for alcohol dependence: A meta-analytic review. *Drug and Alcohol Dependence, 108*(1–2), 1–6. https://doi.org/10.1016/j.drugalcdep.2009.11.017.
Merikangas, K. R., Stolar, M., Stevens, D. E., Goulet, J., Preisig, M. A., Fenton, B., et al. (1998). Familial transmission of substance use disorders. *Archives of General Psychiatry, 55*(11), 973. https://doi.org/10.1001/archpsyc.55.11.973.
Moreira, F. A., & Dalley, J. W. (2015). Dopamine receptor partial agonists and addiction. *European Journal of Pharmacology*, 752, 112-115. https://doi.org/10.1016/j.ejphar.2015.02.025
Nutt, D., King, L., Saulsbury, W., & Blakemore, C. (2007). Development of a rational scale to assess the harm of drugs of potential misuse. *The Lancet, 369*(9566), 1047–1053. https://doi.org/10.1016/s0140-6736(07)60464-4.
Prescott, C. A., Aggen, S. H., & Kendler, K. S. (2000). Sex-specific genetic influences on the comorbidity of alcoholism and major depression in a population-based sample of US twins. *Archives of General Psychiatry, 57*(8), 803–811. https://doi.org/10.1001/archpsyc.57.8.803.
Regier, D. A., Farmer, M. E., Rae, D. S., Locke, B. Z., Keith, S. J., Judd, L. L., & Goodwin, F. K. (1990). Comorbidity of mental disorders with alcohol and other drug abuse. Results from the epidemiologic catchment area (ECA) study. *JAMA, 264*(19), 2511–2518.
Saccone, N. L., Saccone, S. F., Hinrichs, A. L., Stitzel, J. A., Duan, W., Pergadia, M. L., et al. (2009). Multiple distinct risk loci for nicotine dependence identified by dense coverage of the complete family of nicotinic receptor subunit (CHRN) genes. *American Journal of Medical Genetics. Part B, Neuropsychiatric Genetics: The Official Publication of the International Society of Psychiatric Genetics, 150B*(4), 453–466. https://doi.org/10.1002/ajmg.b.30828.
Spanagel, R. (2009). Alcoholism: A systems approach from molecular physiology to addictive behavior. *Physiological Reviews, 89*(2), 649–705. https://doi.org/10.1152/physrev.00013.2008.
Swan, G. E., Carmelli, D., & Cardon, L. R. (1997). Heavy consumption of cigarettes, alcohol and coffee in male twins. *Journal of Studies on Alcohol, 58*(2), 182–190. https://doi.org/10.15288/jsa.1997.58.182.
Tsuang, M. T., Bar, J. L., Harley, R. M., & Lyons, M. J. (2001). The Harvard twin study of substance abuse: What we have learned. *Harvard Review of Psychiatry, 9*(6), 267–279.
United Nations Office on Drugs and Crime (UNODC). (2019). *World drug report 2019*. Retrieved from https://wdr.unodc.org/wdr2019/
Verweij, K. J. H., Zietsch, B. P., Lynskey, M. T., Medland, S. E., Neale, M. C., Martin, N. G., et al. (2010). Genetic and environmental influences on cannabis use initiation and problematic use: A meta-analysis of twin studies. *Addiction, 105*(3), 417–430. https://doi.org/10.1111/j.1360-0443.2009.02831.x.
Wang, J.-C., Kapoor, M., & Goate, A. M. (2012). The genetics of substance dependence. *Annual Review of Genomics and Human Genetics, 13*, 241–261. https://doi.org/10.1146/annurev-genom-090711-163844.
Warden, A. S., & Mayfield, R. D. (2017). Gene expression profiling in the human alcoholic brain. *Neuropharmacology, 122*, 161–174. https://doi.org/10.1016/j.neuropharm.2017.02.017.
Zhang, H., Kranzler, H. R., Weiss, R. D., Luo, X., Brady, K. T., Anton, R. F., et al. (2009). Pro-opiomelanocortin gene variation related to alcohol or drug dependence: Evidence and replications across family- and population-based studies. *Biological Psychiatry, 66*(2), 128–136. https://doi.org/10.1016/j.biopsych.2008.12.021.
Zuo, L., Kranzler, H. R., Luo, X., Yang, B., Weiss, R., Brady, K., et al. (2009). Interaction between two independent CNR1 variants increases risk for cocaine dependence in European Americans: A replication study in family-based sample and population-based sample. *Neuropsychopharmacology, 34*(6), 1504–1513. https://doi.org/10.1038/npp.2008.206.

Chapter 7
Neuroscience, Epigenetics, and Psychotropic Substances

Luana Martins de Carvalho

Introduction

The use of psychotropic substances, those with direct effects on the central nervous system and potential for abuse and dependence, has been taking place since the time of ancient civilizations. Currently, the abuse of these substances has become a worldwide problem with the estimate that in the year of 2019, 35 million people worldwide suffered from the disorders associated with the use of substances (SUDs) (UNODC 2019). According to the *National Institute on Drug Abuse*—NIDA (2020), among the main drugs used are alcohol, marijuana, cocaine, opioids, and methamphetamines. It is known that several factors contribute to the abuse of these substances. Biological factors such as genetics, gender, age, ethnicity, and the diagnosis of mental disorders interact with environmental factors with which individuals are inserted, such as economic status, family nucleus, and emotional experiences, making them more prone or not to drug abuse. In the last decade, epigenetic changes have also been proposed as an important factor in the transition from recreational to compulsive use of abusive drugs.

Fortunately, understanding about substance abuse advances significantly every day. Due to the progress of scientific research in genetics and neuroscience and the development of new technologies that provide effective tools for high throughput studies, such as the analysis of molecular changes in specific neuronal populations, every day it is possible to assemble new pieces of the addiction puzzle. In addition, the development of neuroimaging technologies allows access to brain function and neurochemical aspects directly *in* humans diagnosed with SUDs, allowing an in vivo view of the brain aspects of this disorder. In this sense, this chapter aims to provide an overview of the neurobiological aspects of drugs of abuse and how epigenetic changes are involved in this context.

L. M. de Carvalho (✉)
University of Illinois at Chicago, Chicago, IL, USA

D. De Micheli et al. (eds.), *Drugs and Human Behavior*,
https://doi.org/10.1007/978-3-030-62855-0_7

Neurobiology of Drugs of Abuse

Clinically, according to the Diagnostic and Statistical Manual of Mental Disorders (DSM-5), SUDs can be defined as a chronically relapsing disorder, characterized by compulsion to seek and take the drug, loss of control in limiting intake, and emergence of a negative emotional state such as anxiety and irritability, in the absence of drug use (APA 2014).

In general, SUDs is characterized by the deregulation of motivational brain circuits, known as reward system, whose role is to regulate motivated behaviors that are evolutionarily important for the perpetuation and maintenance of species, such as food seek and reproduction (Kelley and Berridge 2002). These behaviors are accompanied by an *incentive salience*, a process of integration through which objects and stimuli from outside capture our attention, gain relevance, and influence thoughts and behaviors. Food seeking is an example of motivated behavior, where the individual execute a goal-directed behavior: the search for food to promote satiety and the inherent generation of rewarding feeling. The association between behavior (search for food) and consequence (satiety) is called *positive reinforcement* and is important for the learning process that consolidates the association between action and reward. This process is the result of a balanced brain circuit where the proper functioning of motivation, decision making, inhibitory control, and reward is achieved. Interestingly, the same brain circuits involved in this process are also recruited in the use of drugs of abuse. Contrary to natural behaviors, in the SUDs we observe the deregulation of these circuits that is characterized by the exacerbation of the *incentive salience* and habits formation, deficits in reward, increased stress and the compromise of executive function (Koob 2013).

For a better understanding of the deregulation of these processes and brain circuits, Koob and Volkow (2010) proposed the addiction as a three-stage cycle: (1) *binge/intoxication stage*; (2) withdrawal/*negative affect stage;* and (3) preoccupation/*anticipation stage* (Koob and Volkow 2010). Figure 7.1 represents the processes and regions involved in these cycles.

In the first stage, *binge/intoxication*, it is postulated that the use of the drugs occurs through the search for their pleasurable (rewarding) effects. Studies with rodents and neuroimaging studies in humans point to the Ventral Tegmental Area (VTA) and the Nucleus Accumbens (NAc) as the main regions that regulate *incentive salience*, drug seeking, and reward (Koob and Volkow 2016). At the molecular level, brain reward signaling occurs through activation of the mesolimbic dopaminergic pathway (ML-DA), composed of dopaminergic neurons connecting VTA and NAc (Wise 2008). Alcohol intake, for example, promotes the activation of dopaminergic neurons in VTA, resulting in the rapid and increasing release of dopamine (DA) in NAc, consolidating the rewarding feeling related to its consumption (Volkow and Morales 2015).

Although each type of drug present a different mechanism of action, the final effect for all of them is the activation of the ML-DA pathway (Volkow and Morales 2015). For example, heroin and morphine act as antagonists to opioid

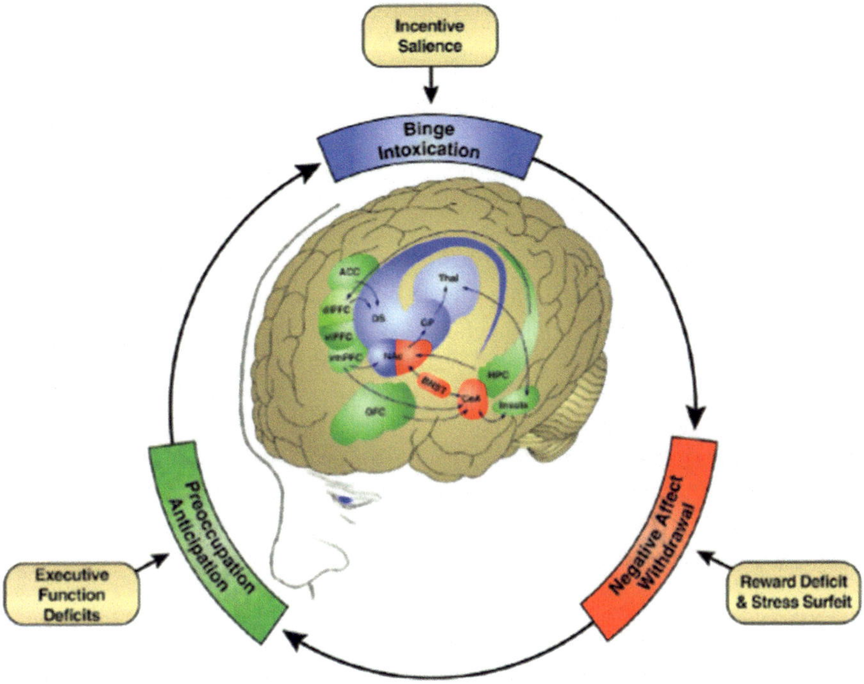

Fig. 7.1 Schematic representation of the neural substrates involved in the different cycles of addiction: binge/intoxication, in blue; abstinence/negative affect, in red; preoccupation/anticipation, in green. Source: Reproduced from Koob and Schulkin (2019). *DS* Dorsal Striated, *GP* Pale Globe, *NAC* Accumbens Nucleus, *Thal* Thalamus, *BNST* Amygdala Terminal Stria, *CeA* Amigdala Central Core, *ACC* Anterior Cingulate Cortex, *dlPFC* Pre-Frontal Dorsolateral Cortex, *vlPFC* Pre-Frontal Ventrolateral Cortex, *vmPFC* Pre-Frontal Ventromedial Cortex, *OFC* Orbitofrontal Cortex, *HPC* Hippocampus

receptors and activate the ML-DA through the disinhibition of GABA receptors. Cocaine increases the concentrations of DA by blocking its transporter and preventing its reuptake in the synaptic cleft. Alcohol, on the other hand, interacts with a variety of receptors, such as opioids and cannabinoids, in addition to GABA and glutamate receptors of the AMPA type, triggering the activation of ML-DA and the release of DA (Abrahao et al. 2017; Adinoff 2004).

In the second stage of addiction, withdrawal/*negative affect stage*, the consumption of the drug is no longer directed by positive reinforcement, but by negative reinforcement (Koob and Volkow 2010). In this context, negative reinforcement can be understood as actions that seek to relieve negative emotional states (e.g. anxiety, discomfort, and tensions). These emotional states emerges during withdrawal temptatives, and it is a result of neurobiological adaptations triggered by chronic use of a drug (Koob and Volkow 2016). At this stage, a loss of function of the reward system is followed by a hyporegulation of the dopaminergic response and the recruitment of brain systems involved in stress modulation, such as the hypothalamic-pituitary-adrenal axis (HPA), the system mediated by the corticotropin release factor (CRF), and the amygdala (Koob 2015). Thus, the combination of the loss of function of the reward system and the recruitment of brain systems involved in stress leads to the drug seeking and consumption, triggering the third cycle of addition.

The third and last stage of addiction, named of *preoccupation/anticipation* is characterized by the emergence of the fissure (or *craving*), defined as an uncontrollable desire to consume the drug, which originates even after long periods of abstinence, leading the individual to relapse episodes (Koob and Volkow 2010). It is proposed that the pre-frontal cortex (PFC) is the main brain substrate of this stage, due to its role in controlling the cognitive and emotional processes that drive the *incentive salience*, and the decision making over drug seeking and consumption (Koob and Volkow 2016). Specifically, it is suggested that the glutamatergic neurons projections between the medial PFC and the ventral striatum are modulated by dopamine activity (via mesocortical dopamine) through dopamine receptors (DRD1 and DRD2), being one of the mechanisms involved in relapse episodes. Additionally, the connectivity between PFC and basolateral amygdala seems to play an important role in the cue-induced relapse (Koob and Volkow 2016).

In summary, the transition from controlled to compulsive drug consumption and eventually to addiction involves neurological adaptations in ML-DA. Although the VTA, NAc, and PFC regions are described as the main regions involved in the above stages, it is important to note that these regions receive and send projections to other brain areas involved, for example, with the regulation of mood (Amygdala, Hypothalamus, and Habenula) and with interoception (Insula and Anterior Cingulate Cortex), which allows, for example, the awareness of negative states, such as anxiety and irritability, which end up leading to relapse.

Epigenetics and Drugs of Abuse

As explained in the previous section, the chronic use of drugs of abuse leads to neurological adaptations in several brain regions, with the reward system being one of the major targets. In the scientific literature on addiction, the term "neuroadaptation" is used to refer to brain neuroplasticity triggered by drug use (Seo and Sinha 2015). Neuroplasticity, in turn, also referred to as brain plasticity or neural plasticity, characterizes the brain's ability to change and adapt in response to environmental stimuli. During this process, synapses are strengthened or weakened, resulting in the increase or decrease of their activities. Finally, these adaptations can be consolidate into long-term changes due to changes in gene expression (Gulyaeva 2017; Kalivas and O'Brien 2008).

It is proposed that the use of drugs of abuse leads to changes in gene expression, directly or indirectly, via increased release of DA and the consequent activation of its receptors and their *downstream* signaling cascades. The stimulation of these cascades in turn causes activation or inhibition of transcription factors (e.g. ΔFOSB

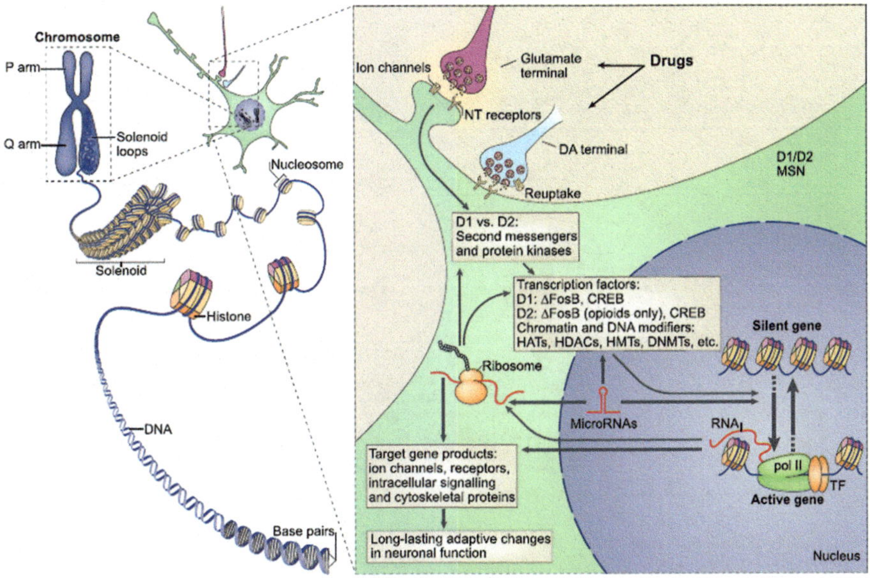

Fig. 7.2 Schematic representation of the mechanisms involved in the changes in the regulation of gene transcription, triggered by drugs of abuse. Source: Reprinted from Nestler and Lüscher (2019). *ΔFOSB* FOS transcription factor, *CREB* cAMP responsive binding protein, *DNMTs* DNA methyltransferase, *HATs* histone acetyltransferase, *HDACs* histone acetylase, *HDMs* histone demethylase, *HMT* histone methyltransferase, *D1 and D2* dopamine receptor 1 and 2

and CREB) and other targets such as chromatin structure modifying enzymes (HDACs, HAT, HMT) that regulate the induction or suppression of genes involved in addiction (Ron and Barak 2016). In this context, epigenetics is considered as one of the probable mechanisms involved in changes in gene transcription regulation (Fig. 7.2). While many of these modifications are transient, some may be stable and inheritable, thus contributing to cellular plasticity and the emergence of maladaptive behaviors observed in addiction (Nestler and Lüscher 2019).

In a broad definition, epigenetics describes a series of biochemical processes that lead to alteration of gene expression, but without causing changes in DNA nucleotide sequence (Jaenisch and Bird 2003). To recall, our DNA is organized and compressed into a structure called chromatin where the fundamental unit is the nucleosome. This in turn is composed of the histone octamers (two copies of each histone H2A, H2B, H3, and H4) in which approximately 147 pairs of DNA bases are wrapped (Fig. 7.3). Basically, epigenetic mechanisms control the space between the nucleosomes and the levels of their condensation, determining the activity of genes. The control of this conformation involves several types of histone modifications, the DNA methylation, and the activity of non-coding RNAs (*microRNAs* (miRNA) and *long non-coding* RNAs (lncRNAs) (Allis and Jenuwein 2016).

The existence of a wide range of post-translational modifications of histones and their combinations makes this epigenetic mechanism extremely complex. Different

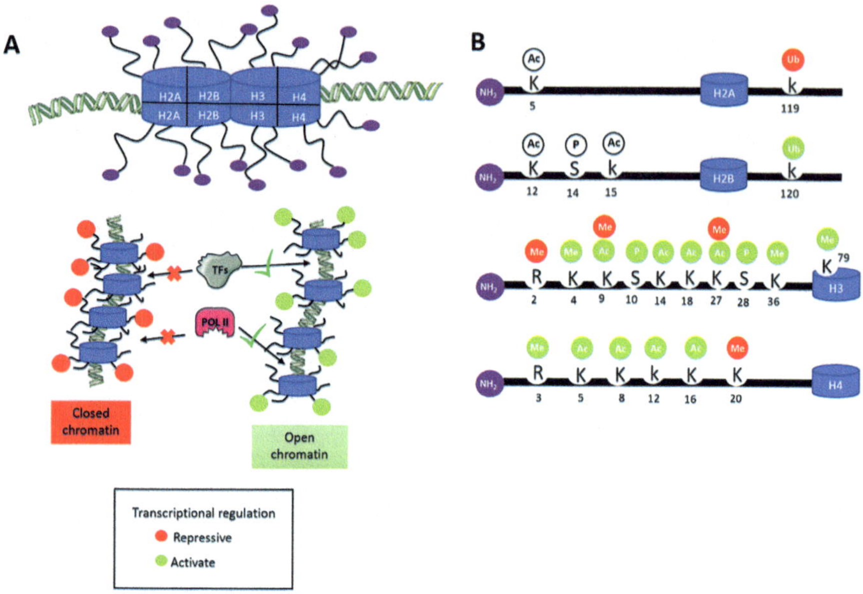

Fig. 7.3 Representation of the structure of the nucleosome (**a**) and the modifications in the amino acid residues of the histones (**b**). Modifications: acetylation (Ac), methylation (Me), phosphorylation (P), and ubiquitination (Ub). Amino acid residues: lysine (K); serine (S), and arginine (R). Histone octomers: H2a, H2b, H3, and H4. The function of each of these modifications in the transcriptional regulation of genes is represented by the colors green (transcription activation) and orange (transcription repression)

chemical groups can be covalently added to the different amino acid residues of the N-terminal tails of each of the histones, naming the changes in chromatin structure—acetylation, methylation, phosphorylation, ubiquitination, sumoylation, citrullination, among others (Fig. 7.3) (Allis and Jenuwein 2016). Such epigenetic marks are added or removed by a group of enzymes known as "*writers*" or "*erasers,*" making the epigenetic modifications reversible and dynamic (Allis and Jenuwein 2016). Although all these modifications contribute to the acquisition and maintenance of addiction, acetylation and methylation of histones are the most studied post-translational modifications in the field of addiction (Mews et al. 2018).

Acetylation involves the participation of the histone acetyltransferase (HAT) and histone deacetylase (HDAC) enzymes, which are responsible for adding and removing, respectively, acetyl groups from histones. The HDACS are divided into 4 classes, where classes I (HDAC1–3 and 8), II (HDAC 4–7 and 9–10), and IV (HDAC 11) are zinc dependent and class III (HDACS sirtuins—Sirt1–7) needs the NAD+ protein as cofactor (Gräff and Tsai 2013). Acetylation of lysine residues (represented by the letter K) removes positive charges reducing affinity between histones and DNA. This process takes chromatin to a permissive state, where access to transcription factors and RNA polymerase to DNA is facilitated. For this reason, acetylation, for example, of histone 3 in lysine residues 9 and 14 (H3K9 and H3K14) is associated with transcriptional gene activation (Fig. 7.3) (Allis and Jenuwein 2016).

The process of methylation of the histones occurs in a similar way, in which the lysine and arginine residues (represented by the letter R) are methylated by the lysine's (KMTs) and arginine's (PRMTs) methyltransferases, respectively, also known as methyltransferase histones (HMT). These enzymes can catalyze the transfer of 2 or even 3 methyl groups to the same histone residue. However, demethylase enzymes (KMD) whose function is to catalyze the removal of methyl groups from these histones may reverse this process. Unlike acetylation, histone methylation can result in both activation and transcriptional repression of genes depending on the histone residue to which the methyl groups have been added. For example, the trimethylation of histone 3 in lysine residue 4 (H3K4), as well as in H3K36 and H3K79 residues, is associated with activation of the gene transcription. In contrast, methylation of the H3K9, H3K27, and H4K20 residues are associated with transcriptional repression (Fig. 7.3) (Alam et al. 2015).

Most studies investigating the epigenetic modifications related to the use of drugs of abuse are conducted in animal models, mainly in rodents, which allows the study of the effects of drugs under controlled conditions of genetic and phenotypic variability (Nestler 2014). These studies focus on brain regions important for reward processing, with PFC, VTA, and NAc being the main regions studied. While some studies examine epigenetic changes in individual candidate genes using, for example, microarray technologies, others use methodologies such as chromatin immunoprecipitation (ChIP) followed by high-performance sequencing to access global changes in chromatin (Maze et al. 2014a, b).

Changes in Histone Acetylation and Methylation

Studies in animal models show that exposure to cocaine results in an overall increase in acetylation, regulating the transcription of genes related to neuroplasticity (De Sa Nogueira et al. 2019; Kumar et al. 2005; Wang et al. 2010). For example, intraperitoneal injections (IP) of cocaine (20 mg/kg) in Sprague-Dawley rats lead to hyperacetylation of H3 and H4 histones in the promoters of *cFos*, *BDNF*, and *Cdk5* genes in striatal neurons (Kumar et al. 2005). A second study showed that self-administration of cocaine (0.5 mg/kg for 12 days) in Wistar rats followed by a short abstinence period (3 days) causes changes in the expression of chromatin remodeling genes (e.g. *Kdm6a, Smarcc2, Dot1l, Brd1)* in the PFC. However, these genes return to their baseline transcription levels after a longer period of abstinence (10 days), confirming the hypothesis that epigenetic changes may be reversible (Sadakierska-Chudy et al. 2017). Also in the same study, although an increase in acetylation of H3K9 and H4K8 histones was observed, no significant global change in methylation levels of histone 3 in lysine residues 4, 9, 27, and 79 were observed (Sadakierska-Chudy et al. 2017).

The use of other psychostimulant drugs such as amphetamine and methamphetamine can also trigger epigenetic changes (Godino et al. 2015). Specifically, a single injection of methamphetamine (20 mg/kg) in rats can induce global changes in acetylation, increasing the acetylation of H4K5 and H4K8 histones and reducing the acetylation of H3K9, H3K18, and H4K16 histones in the NAc of these animals (Martin et al. 2012). These changes are accompanied sequentially by increases and decreases in HDAC1 and HDAC2 proteins levels, and consequently by changes in the transcriptional regulation of genes involved in the rewarding effects of acute and chronic exposure to psychostimulants (*c-fos, phosB, Crf, Cck, and Npas4*) (Martin et al. 2012). Another study using the conditioned place preference test for methamphetamine showed the importance of methylation levels of histone H3K4 for the acquisition and consolidation of methamphetamine-associated memory, one of the main aspects that increase relapse vulnerability (Aguilar-Valles et al. 2014). While the KO of the methyltransferase Mll1 in the NAc of C57BL/J6 mice led to a reduction in methylation in histone H3K4me3 and stopped the acquisition of drug-related memory, the KO of lysine-specific demethylase 5C (Kdm5c) resulted in hypermethylation of histone H3K4 and blocked drug-related memory expression. These results highlight the enzymes "writers" and "erasers" as potential therapeutic targets to be considered for the treatment of SUDs (Aguilar-Valles et al. 2014).

Morphine, a potent opioid used for pain relief, is a drug with great potential for abuse, and like other drugs its abuse can also lead to epigenetic changes. A study with class III HDACs, sirtuins (Sirt), showed that chronic (7 days) administration of morphine (20 mg/Kg) causes a specific increase in Sirt1 expression in NAc of C57BL/J6 mice. Additionally, virus-induced over-expression of Sirt1 increases the rewarding effects of morphine in these animals, while the KO of this protein decreases these effects. Such changes also lead to changes in the regulation of several synaptic proteins, indicating the role of Sirt1 as a possible mediator of molecular and cellular plasticity triggered by morphine abuse (Ferguson et al. 2013).

Studies investigating the effects of alcohol exposure on the genome have shown that its consumption is able to change the chromatin structure in two directions. Through gene activation or repression, alcohol can induce anxiety in addition to other negative symptoms, contributing to an increase in drug use and dependence (Pandey et al. 2017). In this sense, clinical and pre-clinical studies have demonstrated that alcohol consumption can trigger changes in the transcriptional regulation of HDAC coding genes (López-Moreno et al. 2015; Pascual et al. 2012; Sakharkar et al. 2014; Warnault et al. 2013). For example, both alcohol binge drinking in humans and daily alcohol self-administration in rats increases the gene transcription of HDACs class I, II and IV, in peripheral blood in both species (López-Moreno et al. 2015).

A second study using alcohol-preferring rats (P rats) versus nonpreferring rats (NP rats), showed that, at baseline, P rats had an upregulation of HDAC2 and a higher nuclear activity of this enzyme in the central nucleus of the amygdala when compared to NP rats. However, since these P rats were subjected to acute exposure to alcohol (1 g/kg of alcohol via IP), the results observed were opposite: hyporegulation of HDAC2 levels and inhibition of its nuclear activity. Additionally, the KO of HDAC2 in the amygdala of these animals led to a reduction in the anxiety-like behavior and in the voluntary consumption of alcohol, when compared to NP animals. Together, these results suggest that the innate anxious-like behavior observed in P rats may be related to high nuclear activity of HDAC2 in the amygdala, and that the anxiolytic effects obtained with acute alcohol exposure may be related to inhibition of this activity (Moonat et al. 2013). Another study, also on the investigation of histone modifications and the development of anxiety triggered by alcohol exposure, showed that intermittent administration of alcohol (2 mg/kg) in rats during adolescence triggers anxious-like behaviors, increase nuclear and cytosolic activity of HDAC, increase protein levels of HDAC2 and HDAC4 and decrease levels of acetylation of H3K9 histones in the central and medial amygdala of these animals. Interestingly, some of these changes persist until the adult life of the animal, contributing to the increase of alcohol consumption in this phase (Pandey et al. 2015).

The use of HDAC inhibitors has been an important pharmacological tool for the functional validation of the different classes of HDACs in the addiction and maladaptive behaviors that characterize this disorder (Bourguet et al. 2018). For example, the use of HDAC inhibitors has been shown to be effective in preventing changes in the expression of HDAC enzymes and consequently of genes involved in the processing of alcohol rewarding effects, such as the Gabra receptor1 (Bohnsack et al. 2018). In addition, the use of these inhibitors is able to attenuate and/or block anxious-like behaviors related to alcohol consumption and reduce voluntary consumption in rats (Bohnsack et al. 2018; Pandey et al. 2008). For other drugs, such as morphine, the use of the HDAC inhibitor SAHA attenuates tolerance to the use of this drug in animal bone cancer models (He et al. 2018). For nicotine, the administration of the sodium butyrate inhibitor (Nab), besides extinguishing the preference for this drug, analyzed by the conditioned place preference test, is also efficient in blocking the reestablishment of its self-administration in rats (Castino et al. 2015). Similarly, for cocaine, the use of the RGFP966 inhibitor, specific for HDAC3, is also effective in extinguishing the behavior of preference for the drug as well as in blocking the reestablishment of its use (Hitchcock et al. 2019).

Final Considerations

In summary, it can be concluded that most of the drugs of abuse are capable of modulating target genes by modifying histones in different brain regions involved in addiction. Many of these drugs have common targets, such as transcription factors (e.g., *FosB*) and neurotrophic factors (e.g., *Bdnf*) (Mews et al. 2018). Interestingly, while some studies show that these changes can be reversible, others show that they can be persistent, lasting, for example, the entire adult life cycle of the animal. Although the studies used here as examples have reported results in the same direction, for example, the increase in global acetylation congruent with transcriptional activation of specific genes, it is important to note that these changes can be observed in opposite directions. Thus, although the transcriptional effects of most histone modifications are known, it is still difficult to predict the effects of each type of modification on gene expression and behavior (Lawrence et al. 2016).

Much work has been done so far contributing to the understanding of the epigenetic modifications triggered by the different drugs of abuse. However, considering the different brain areas and networks of gene expression recruited and involved in the development of addiction, as well as the specific mechanisms of action of each drug, we are still far from a detailed understanding of the mechanisms involved in these changes. Thus, it is of extreme importance the development of studies that access the different types of epigenetic modifications in different animal models of addiction. All variations included in these models, such as the time and method of drug administration, the species and strains of animals used, age and sex, are factors that can influence the epigenetic modifications and the results interpretation (Becker and Chartoff 2019).

As already mentioned, the several brain areas involved in the development of addition make the study of the genesis of this disorder complex. However, even focusing on a single region it is important to take into consideration that this specific region is formed by several types of neural and non-neuronal cells that perform specific functions, and at some moments, opposite effects in the addiction. For example, the activation of dopaminergic neurons D1 and D2 in NAc results in different actions in the reward processing of cocaine (Lobo et al. 2010). Therefore, it is important to consider the use of technologies that allow the investigation of molecular mechanisms in isolated cells to avoid non-specific results during data analysis.

Finally, the results obtained so far strengthen the role of epigenetic changes in addiction and their consequences for emotional states and the perpetuation of maladaptive behaviors related to drug use. Additionally, the use of HDAC inhibitors and their results in the manipulation of drug seeking and consumption behaviors in animal models suggest epigenetic modulation as a possible therapeutic target for the treatment of SUDs.

References

Abrahao, K. P., Salinas, A. G., & Lovinger, D. M. (2017). Alcohol and the brain: Neuronal molecular targets, synapses, and circuits. *Neuron, 96*(6), 1223–1238. https://doi.org/10.1016/j.neuron.2017.10.032.

Adinoff, B. (2004). Neurobiologic processes in drug reward and addiction. *Harvard Review of Psychiatry, 12*(6), 305–320. https://doi.org/10.1080/10673220490910844.

Aguilar-Valles, A., Vaissière, T., Griggs, E. M., Mikaelsson, M. A., Takács, I. F., Young, E. J., et al. (2014). Methamphetamine-associated memory is regulated by a writer and an eraser of permissive histone methylation. *Biological Psychiatry, 76*(1), 57–65. https://doi.org/10.1016/j.biopsych.2013.09.014.

Alam, H., Gu, B., & Lee, M. G. (2015). Histone methylation modifiers in cellular signaling pathways. *Cellular and Molecular Life Sciences: CMLS, 72*(23), 4577–4592. https://doi.org/10.1007/s00018-015-2023-y.

Allis, C. D., & Jenuwein, T. (2016). The molecular hallmarks of epigenetic control. *Nature Reviews Genetics, 17*(8), 487–500. https://doi.org/10.1038/nrg.2016.59.

American Psychiatric Association (APA). (2014). *Manual diagnóstico e estatístico de transtornos mentais* (5th ed.). Porto Alegre, Brazil: Artmed Editora.

Becker, J. B., & Chartoff, E. (2019). Sex differences in neural mechanisms mediating reward and addiction. *Neuropsychopharmacology: Official Publication of the American College of Neuropsychopharmacology, 44*(1), 166–183. https://doi.org/10.1038/s41386-018-0125-6.

Bohnsack, J. P., Hughes, B. A., O'Buckley, T. K., Edokpolor, K., Besheer, J., & Morrow, A. L. (2018). Histone deacetylases mediate $GABA_A$ receptor expression, physiology, and behavioral maladaptations in rat models of alcohol dependence. *Neuropsychopharmacology: Official Publication of the American College of Neuropsychopharmacology, 43*(7), 1518–1529. https://doi.org/10.1038/s41386-018-0034-8.

Bourguet, E., Ozdarska, K., Moroy, G., Jeanblanc, J., & Naassila, M. (2018). Class I HDAC inhibitors: Potential new epigenetic therapeutics for alcohol use disorder (AUD). *Journal of Medicinal Chemistry, 61*(5), 1745–1766. https://doi.org/10.1021/acs.jmedchem.7b00115.

Castino, M., Cornish, J., & Clemens, K. (2015). Inhibition of histone deacetylases facilitates extinction and attenuates reinstatement of nicotine self-administration in rats. *PLoS One, 10*(4), e0124796. https://doi.org/10.1371/journal.pone.0124796.

De Sa Nogueira, D., Merienne, K., & Befort, K. (2019). Neuroepigenetics and addictive behaviors: Where do we stand? *Neuroscience & Biobehavioral Reviews, 106*, 58–72. https://doi.org/10.1016/j.neubiorev.2018.08.018.

Ferguson, D., Koo, J. W., Feng, J., Heller, E., Rabkin, J., Heshmati, M., et al. (2013). Essential role of SIRT1 signaling in the nucleus accumbens in cocaine and morphine action. *The Journal of Neuroscience: The Official Journal of the Society for Neuroscience, 33*(41), 16088–16098. https://doi.org/10.1523/JNEUROSCI.1284-13.2013.

Godino, A., Jayanthi, S., & Cadet, J. L. (2015). Epigenetic landscape of amphetamine and methamphetamine addiction in rodents. *Epigenetics, 10*(7), 574–580. https://doi.org/10.1080/15592294.2015.1055441.

Gräff, J., & Tsai, L. H. (2013). Histone acetylation: Molecular mnemonics on the chromatin. *Nature Reviews Neuroscience, 14*(2), 97–111. https://doi.org/10.1038/nrn3427.

Gulyaeva, N. V. (2017). Molecular mechanisms of neuroplasticity: An expanding universe. *Biochemistry (Moscow), 82*(3), 237–242. https://doi.org/10.1134/S0006297917030014.

He, X. T., Zhou, K. X., Zhao, W. J., Zhang, C., Deng, J. P., Chen, F. M., et al. (2018). Inhibition of histone deacetylases attenuates morphine tolerance and restores MOR expression in the DRG of BCP rats. *Frontiers in Pharmacology, 9*, 509. https://doi.org/10.3389/fphar.2018.00509.

Hitchcock, L. N., Raybuck, J. D., Wood, M. A., & Lattal, K. M. (2019). Effects of a histone deacetylase 3 inhibitor on extinction and reinstatement of cocaine self-administration in rats. *Psychopharmacology, 236*(1), 517–529. https://doi.org/10.1007/s00213-018-5122-2.

Jaenisch, R., & Bird, A. (2003). Epigenetic regulation of gene expression: How the genome integrates intrinsic and environmental signals. *Nature Genetics, 33*(S3), 245–254. https://doi.org/10.1038/ng1089.

Kalivas, P. W., & O'Brien, C. (2008). Drug addiction as a pathology of staged neuroplasticity. *Neuropsychopharmacology: Official Publication of the American College of Neuropsychopharmacology, 33*(1), 166–180. https://doi.org/10.1038/sj.npp.1301564.

Kelley, A. E., & Berridge, K. C. (2002). The neuroscience of natural rewards: Relevance to addictive drugs. *The Journal of Neuroscience: The Official Journal of the Society for Neuroscience, 22*(9), 3306–3311. https://doi.org/10.1523/JNEUROSCI.22-09-03306.2002.

Koob, G. F. (2013). Addiction is a reward deficit and stress surfeit disorder. *Frontiers in Psychiatry, 4*, 72. https://doi.org/10.3389/fpsyt.2013.00072.

Koob, G. F. (2015). The dark side of emotion: The addiction perspective. *European Journal of Pharmacology, 753*, 73–87. https://doi.org/10.1016/j.ejphar.2014.11.044.

Koob, G. F., & Schulkin, J. (2019). Addiction and stress: An allostatic view. *Neuroscience and Biobehavioral Reviews, 106*, 245–262. https://doi.org/10.1016/j.neubiorev.2018.09.008.

Koob, G. F., & Volkow, N. D. (2010). Neurocircuitry of addiction. *Neuropsychopharmacology: Official Publication of the American College of Neuropsychopharmacology, 35*(1), 217–238. https://doi.org/10.1038/npp.2009.110.

Koob, G. F., & Volkow, N. D. (2016). Neurobiology of addiction: A neurocircuitry analysis. *The Lancet Psychiatry, 3*(8), 760–773. https://doi.org/10.1016/S2215-0366(16)00104-8.

Kumar, A., Choi, K. H., Renthal, W., Tsankova, N. M., Theobald, D. E., Truong, H. T., et al. (2005). Chromatin remodeling is a key mechanism underlying cocaine-induced plasticity in striatum. *Neuron, 48*(2), 303–314. https://doi.org/10.1016/j.neuron.2005.09.023.

Lawrence, M., Daujat, S., & Schneider, R. (2016). Lateral thinking: How histone modifications regulate gene expression. *Trends in Genetics: TIG, 32*(1), 42–56. https://doi.org/10.1016/j.tig.2015.10.007.

Lobo, M. K., Covington, H. E., Chaudhury, D., Friedman, A. K., Sun, H., Damez-Werno, D., et al. (2010). Cell type-specific loss of BDNF signaling mimics optogenetic control of cocaine reward. *Science, 330*(6002), 385–390. https://doi.org/10.1126/science.1188472.

López-Moreno, J. A., Marcos, M., Calleja-Conde, J., Echeverry-Alzate, V., Bühler, K. M., Costa-Alba, P., et al. (2015). Histone Deacetylase gene expression following binge alcohol consumption in rats and humans. *Alcoholism, Clinical and Experimental Research, 39*(10), 1939–1950. https://doi.org/10.1111/acer.12850.

Martin, T. A., Jayanthi, S., McCoy, M. T., Brannock, C., Ladenheim, B., Garrett, T., et al. (2012). Methamphetamine causes differential alterations in gene expression and patterns of histone acetylation/hypoacetylation in the rat nucleus accumbens. *PLoS One, 7*(3), e34236. https://doi.org/10.1371/journal.pone.0034236.

Maze, I., Noh, K. M., Soshnev, A. A., & Allis, C. D. (2014a). Every amino acid matters: Essential contributions of histone variants to mammalian development and disease. *Nature Reviews Genetics, 15*(4), 259–271. https://doi.org/10.1038/nrg3673.

Maze, I., Shen, L., Zhang, B., Garcia, B., Shao, N., Mitchell, A., et al. (2014b). Analytical tools and current challenges in the modern era of neuroepigenomics. *Nature Neuroscience, 17*(11), 1476–1490. https://doi.org/10.1038/nn.3816.

Mews, P., Walker, D. M., & Nestler, E. J. (2018). Epigenetic priming in drug addiction. *Cold Spring Harbor Symposia on Quantitative Biology, 83*, 131–139. https://doi.org/10.1101/sqb.2018.83.037663.

Moonat, S., Sakharkar, A. J., Zhang, H., Tang, L., & Pandey, S. C. (2013). Aberrant histone deacetylase2-mediated histone modifications and synaptic plasticity in the amygdala predisposes to anxiety and alcoholism. *Biological Psychiatry, 73*(8), 763–773. https://doi.org/10.1016/j.biopsych.2013.01.012.

National Institute on Drug Abuse (NIDA). (2020). *Commonly abused drugs charts*. Retrieved from https://www.drugabuse.gov/drugs-abuse

Nestler, E. J. (2014). Epigenetic mechanisms of drug addiction. *Neuropharmacology, 76*, 259–268. https://doi.org/10.1016/j.neuropharm.2013.04.004.

Nestler, E. J., & Lüscher, C. (2019). The molecular basis of drug addiction: Linking epigenetic to synaptic and circuit mechanisms. *Neuron, 102*(1), 48–59. https://doi.org/10.1016/j.neuron.2019.01.016.

Pandey, S. C., Kyzar, E. J., & Zhang, H. (2017). Epigenetic basis of the dark side of alcohol addiction. *Neuropharmacology, 122*, 74–84. https://doi.org/10.1016/j.neuropharm.2017.02.002.

Pandey, S. C., Sakharkar, A. J., Tang, L., & Zhang, H. (2015). Potential role of adolescent alcohol exposure-induced amygdaloid histone modifications in anxiety and alcohol intake during adulthood. *Neurobiology of Disease, 82*, 607–619. https://doi.org/10.1016/j.nbd.2015.03.019.

Pandey, S. C., Ugale, R., Zhang, H., Tang, L., & Prakash, A. (2008). Brain chromatin remodeling: A novel mechanism of alcoholism. *The Journal of Neuroscience: The Official Journal of the Society for Neuroscience, 28*(14), 3729–3737. https://doi.org/10.1523/JNEUROSCI.5731-07.2008.

Pascual, M., Do Couto, B. R., Alfonso-Loeches, S., Aguilar, M. A., Rodriguez-Arias, M., & Guerri, C. (2012). Changes in histone acetylation in the prefrontal cortex of ethanol-exposed adolescent rats are associated with ethanol-induced place conditioning. *Neuropharmacology, 62*(7), 2309–2319. https://doi.org/10.1016/j.neuropharm.2012.01.011.

Ron, D., & Barak, S. (2016). Molecular mechanisms underlying alcohol-drinking behaviours. *Nature Reviews Neuroscience, 17*(9), 576–591. https://doi.org/10.1038/nrn.2016.85.

Sadakierska-Chudy, A., Frankowska, M., Jastrzębska, J., Wydra, K., Miszkiel, J., Sanak, M., & Filip, M. (2017). Cocaine administration and its withdrawal enhance the expression of genes encoding histone-modifying enzymes and histone acetylation in the rat prefrontal cortex. *Neurotoxicity Research, 32*(1), 141–150. https://doi.org/10.1007/s12640-017-9728-7.

Sakharkar, A. J., Tang, L., Zhang, H., Chen, Y., Grayson, D. R., & Pandey, S. C. (2014). Effects of acute ethanol exposure on anxiety measures and epigenetic modifiers in the extended amygdala of adolescent rats. *The International Journal of Neuropsychopharmacology, 17*(12), 2057–2067. https://doi.org/10.1017/S1461145714001047.

Seo, D., & Sinha, R. (2015). Neuroplasticity and predictors of alcohol recovery. *Alcohol Research: Current Reviews, 37*(1), 143–152.

United Nations Office on Drugs and Crime (UNODC). (2019). *World drug report 2019*. Retrieved from https://wdr.unodc.org/wdr2019/

Volkow, N. D., & Morales, M. (2015). The brain on drugs: From reward to addiction. *Cell, 162*(4), 712–725. https://doi.org/10.1016/j.cell.2015.07.046.

Wang, L., Lv, Z., Hu, Z., Sheng, J., Hui, B., Sun, J., & Ma, L. (2010). Chronic cocaine-induced H3 acetylation and transcriptional activation of CaMKIIα in the nucleus accumbens is critical for motivation for drug reinforcement. *Neuropsychopharmacology, 35*(4), 913–928. https://doi.org/10.1038/npp.2009.193.

Warnault, V., Darcq, E., Levine, A., Barak, S., & Ron, D. (2013). Chromatin remodeling--a novel strategy to control excessive alcohol drinking. *Translational Psychiatry, 3*(2), e231. https://doi.org/10.1038/tp.2013.4.

Wise, R. A. (2008). Dopamine and reward: The anhedonia hypothesis 30 years on. *Neurotoxicity Research, 14*(2–3), 169–183. https://doi.org/10.1007/BF03033808.

Chapter 8
Pharmacology of Drugs of Abuse: Pharmacokinetics and Pharmacodynamics of Psychotropic Compounds

Marília Zaluar Passos Guimarães and Gilda Ângela Neves

Introduction: Drugs of Abuse, Dopamine, and the Reward System

Contrary to what Aristotle said, sensations and feelings are brain's attributions and not heart's. In the human brain there are almost 100 billion neurons, whose functions are to receive, integrate, and transmit information to the next neuron. Each neuron makes around 10,000 connections with other neurons, the so-called synapses. In these synapses "information" is passed from one neuron to another through the release of chemical messengers. The arrival of a nerve impulse in the first neuron (called pre-synaptic) triggers the release of a chemical compound: the neurotransmitter. These are small molecules capable of mediating communication between nerve cells. There are several such messengers, like dopamine, serotonin, glutamate, GABA, among others (Brady et al. 2012).

However, the next neuron (called postsynaptic) has to be able to "recognize" this molecule for successful communication. Therefore, there are proteins inserted on the surface of the neuron called receptors, which bind to these molecules, are changed by them and "tell" the postsynaptic neuron about the neurotransmitter presence. In a simplified view, these proteins can belong to two main families: the ion channel and the metabotropic receptor family (von Zastrow 2018). As the name implies, when activated by neurotransmitters, ion channels form pores in the cell membrane which allow ions to flow in or out of the neuron. They are considered fast response receptors. On the other hand, metabotropic receptors are proteins that cross the neuronal membrane and activate other proteins in the intracellular space, initiating a signaling pathway that involves other intracellular messengers. Thus,

M. Z. P. Guimarães (✉) · G. Â. Neves
Instituto de Ciências Biomédicas, Universidade Federal do Rio de Janeiro, Rio de Janeiro, RJ, Brazil
e-mail: marilia@icb.ufrj.br

D. De Micheli et al. (eds.), *Drugs and Human Behavior*,
https://doi.org/10.1007/978-3-030-62855-0_8

when activated by the neurotransmitters, the metabotropic receptors initiate this cascade of signals, resulting in a relatively slow response. There are specific receptors for dopamine (so-called dopaminergic receptors), which do not recognize other neurotransmitters (such as serotonin, for example). This diversity of receptors and neurotransmitters allows the fine communication control between brain cells and, thus, the information is accurately transmitted (Brady et al. 2012).

The neurotransmission, that is, the communication between one neuron and another, must take place in a temporally and spatially controlled way. Consequently, all cellular activities that precede and follow the release of the neurotransmitter are tightly regulated. For example, once the neurotransmitter is released into the synaptic space, it is crucial that it is quickly removed or degraded. If the neurotransmitter remains there longer than necessary, the signal detected by the next neuron will be different. One important way to remove the neurotransmitter from the synaptic space, called synaptic cleft, is reuptake. The neurotransmitter is thrown back into the pre-synaptic neuron via a protein that spams the membrane, meaning that the neurotransmitter is taken away from the synaptic cleft, thus ceasing to perform its function. Another form is degradation, in which extremely specialized proteins (called enzymes) are able to destroy the neurotransmitter molecule still in the cleft and stop its action (Brady et al. 2012).

One neurotransmitter stands out when it comes to drug abuse: dopamine (Volkow et al. 2019). The human brain is not a homogenous mass, but composed of regions specialized in certain functions. One of these regions is the mesolimbic pathway, very rich in dopamine. It is formed by several structures such as the nucleus accumbens and the ventral tegmental area (VTA) (Fig. 8.1). The cell bodies of dopaminergic neurons containing their nuclei are found in the VTA, and, when activated, they release dopamine in the accumbens. Dopamine is released in response to situations such as eating food or an orgasm. But what would be the function of dopamine in this region? Dopamine is considered the chemical equivalent of pleasure and satisfaction, and this route described above, where these sensations are generated, is also known as the reward system (Di Chiara and Bassareo 2007). By performing functions essential to our survival as a species, we are rewarded with a pleasant feeling, which we owe to dopamine. Thus, food, water, sex, among others, bring us this pleasant sensation on different scales. Other activities not so essential to survival, like watching your football team win or playing a video game, also bring us similar sensations. Naturally, due to their pleasant nature, even unconsciously, we seek and wish to feel these sensations whenever possible.

Another important function of dopamine is motivation to go after these feelings of pleasure (Di Chiara and Bassareo 2007; Volkow et al. 2019). The smell or simply recalling the memory of our favorite food is enough to cause dopamine release in the accumbens. This dopamine directs our actions to seek pleasure, in this case, our favorite food. Therefore, we can conclude that the mesolimbic dopaminergic (dopamine-releasing) pathway is involved in feelings of pleasure, motivation, and euphoria.

Evolutionary, these reward feelings were fundamental for the survival of individuals and of species, since due to them there was motivation for feeding and

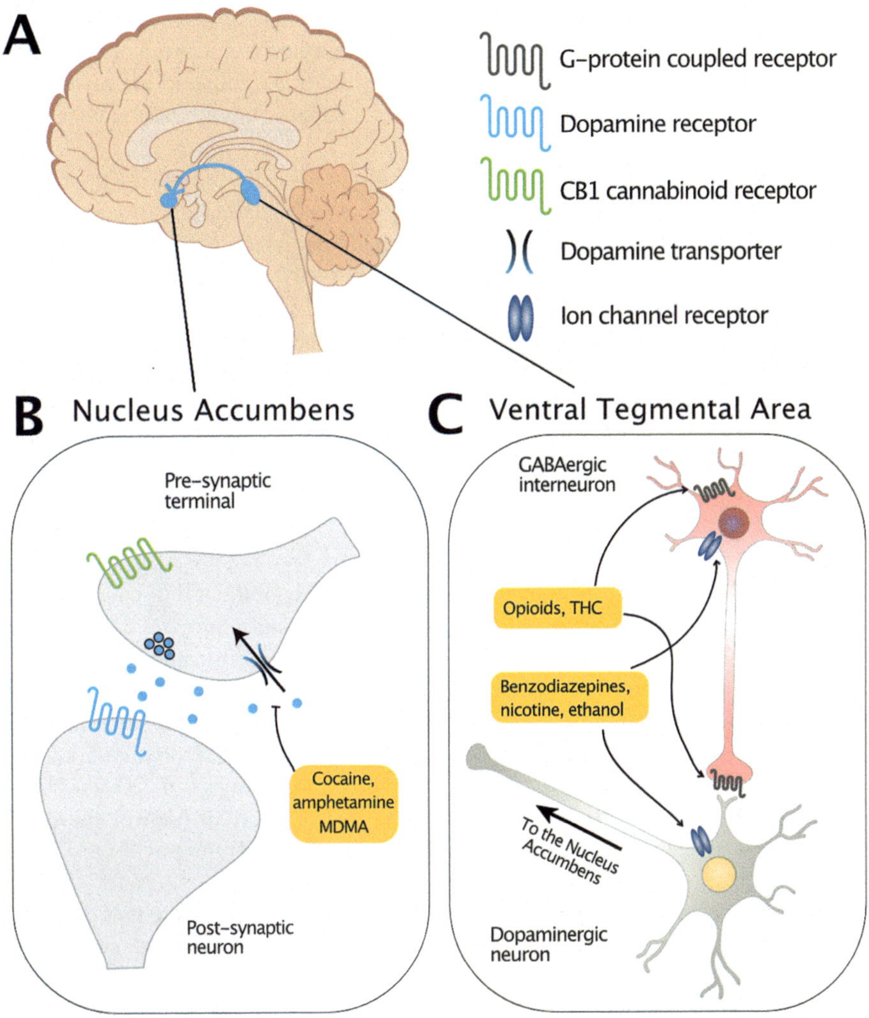

Fig. 8.1 Midbrain dopamine synapse. **A**) Schematic diagram showing the location of the Ventral Tegmental Area (VTA) and projections to the Nucleus Accumbens. This projection is made by neurons that release dopamine. **B**) Dopaminergic synapse in the Nucleus Accumbens, where VTA neurons constitute the pre-synaptic terminal element which release dopamine. Depicted in this figure is the dopamine transporter, which can be inhibited by cocaine, amphetamine and MDMA. **C**) Inhibitory circuity within the VTA. Neurons that release GABA are negative regulators of the activity of VTA-projecting dopaminergic neurons. Opiods and THC inhibit these GABAergic neurons, thereby releasing dopaminergic neurons from GABA inhibition. Benzodiazepines, nicotine and ethanol act on both neuronal types, with a net effect of also causing increased dopamine release

reproduction. On the other hand, we know today that our brain learns to expect a certain pleasurable sensation and, if this good feeling does not come, we feel not only its absence but a negative sensation called dysphoria (feeling of dissatisfaction with life, discomfort; opposite of euphoric) (Volkow et al. 2019; Wise and Koob 2014).

All drugs of abuse have in common the ability to directly or indirectly increase dopamine release in the reward system. The propensity to abuse a drug is closely linked to this phenomenon. After taking the drug, there is an increase in dopamine release, giving the user that feeling of pleasure and motivation. It is the same feeling that naturally occurs, but much more intense or faster with the drug. Thus, the sensation after drug intake can be much greater than natural, leading the person to desire it even more. And, in the absence of the drug, the individual misses that great amount of dopamine, which translates into strong dysphoria (Swift and Lewis 2014).

History of Psychotropic Drug Use

There are numerous historical and archeological records of the use of psychoactive substances by human beings. Evidence of the manufacture and use of alcoholic beverages as food can be found from 7000 BC in records originating from China, Sumeria, Egypt, Persia, and Mesopotamia, among others (Khaderi 2019). The use of plants capable of altering behavior is also reported in historical documents. For example, the plant *Cannabis sp.*, native to Central and South Asia, popularly known as marijuana, has been used for at least 4000 years (Murray et al. 2007). Older records show it was used to obtain fibers for the manufacture of pots, clothes, and paper. This application is due to the fact that the plant, or hemp, quickly produces large amounts of mass (25 tons/ha, while most plants stay between 2.5 and 3.5 tons/ha). Records not so old, dating from 2.5 thousand years ago, indicate that the parts of the plant with high psychoactive substance content had been burned, suggesting that people might have inhaled the smoke produced. In fact, there are many records of *cannabis* being burned in association with religious or medicinal rituals (Ren et al. 2019).

The *Cannabis sp.* plant has dozens of bioactive substances. The best known and also the most abundant is Δ^9-tetrahydrocannabinol, better known as THC. THC is a hydrophobic (not "water like" substance) or lipophilic (oil like) substance. Due to its physicochemical properties, THC was isolated only in the 1960s and synthesized in the laboratory by Prof. Raphael Mechoulam team's in Israel. Since its isolation and study, it became clear that the psychoactive effects of marijuana were mainly due to THC (Murray et al. 2007).

The coca plant (*Erythroxylum coca*), from which the alkaloid cocaine is extracted, has also been used for religious and medicinal purposes in the Americas for thousands of years. When cocaine was isolated in the nineteenth century, its local anesthetic properties were also discovered. In the same century, it was used to treat patients who abused morphine. Sigmund Freud, in his book *Über Coca*, described its euphoric properties and that he himself used and prescribed it to his patients. Freud describes the sensation of cocaine use:

> [The effects were] fun and lasting euphoria, which in no way differs from the normal euphoria of a healthy person... You notice an increase in your self-control and have more vitality and ability to work... Absolutely no desire to continue using cocaine appears after the first, or even repeated, use of the drug (Kalivas et al. 1998, p. 49).

At that time, Freud overestimated the safety and benefits of cocaine by prescribing it for morphine abuse treatment. One of his patients even developed a cocaine-induced psychosis and died soon after.

Another group of plants of American origin are the *Nicotiana* species (*N. tabacum, N. rustica*), popularly known as tobacco. They were used by Native American populations in religious rituals. After the leaves had dried, the smoke from burning them was inhaled. There are reports that tobacco was one of the components of ceremonial pipes used by North American tribes, among them the so-called peace pipe (Dani and Balfour 2011). Tobacco plants were first taken to Europe in the sixteenth century by Christopher Columbus, where they were initially used to decorate environments. Soon they began to be cultivated in Spain, Portugal, and France for medicinal purposes and for use as an insecticide. The habit of smoking tobacco only became frequent among European elites when it was introduced to the court of Queen Elizabeth I in England. And from there it spread to the rest of the world as a symbol of luxury and glamor. Meanwhile, tobacco growing has become one of the main crops and sources of income in the colonial United States (Castaldelli-Maia et al. 2016).

The main component of *Nicotiana spp.* leaves is the alkaloid nicotine (from 0.6 to 3.0% of leaf weight). It was isolated, characterized, and synthesized between the end of the nineteenth century and the beginning of the twentieth century by German researchers (Dani and Balfour 2011). At the same time, the study of the effects of nicotine on heart rate was part of a set of classical works led by Cambridge physiologist John N. Langley. These works are considered the basis of what is now called pharmacology (Maehle 2004). Although the effects of nicotine on behavior are remarkable, its effects on the brain were more meticulously studied only in the 1980s only (Boulter et al. 1986). Nowadays nicotine is recognized as responsible for tobacco addiction and as one of the most addictive substances known.

General Aspects of Pharmacodynamics of Drugs of Abuse

Pharmacodynamics is the area of pharmacology that studies the effects that drugs induce in our body. As written in the introduction, the immediate effect of most drugs of abuse is the rapid increase in dopamine levels in the reward system. However, each drug acts in a different way to induce this effect. Some act directly on the nucleus accumbens, where the terminals of dopaminergic neurons are located. For example, nicotine activates receptors of the family of ion channels (so-called nicotinic receptors) located in the terminals of dopaminergic neurons. Once activated, these receptors stimulate the rapid release of that dopamine stored at the terminals, generating a sensation of pleasure (Wonnacott et al. 2000). Cocaine, on the other hand, has a different action: it is extremely potent on inhibiting the reuptake process, that is, the removal of dopamine from the synapse (Uhl et al. 2002). Thus, once dopamine is released, it remains longer in the synapse cleft, enhancing its rewarding effect.

Other drugs, however, have their main site of action in the VTA, the region of the reward system where the bodies of dopaminergic neurons are located. The activity of dopaminergic neurons in the VTA is finely controlled by a "brake" mechanism. This "brake" is formed by interneurons that release the neurotransmitter GABA, the main inhibitory mediator of the brain. GABA acts on ion channel-type receptors that will cause a decrease in the activity of dopaminergic neurons, leading them to release less dopamine (Stahl 2002). In general, drugs that act on the VTA do the opposite: they increase the activity of dopamine neurons. One example is alcohol (ethanol). One of the actions of alcohol is to decrease the activity of the interneurons that produce GABA, leading to a decrease of GABA release in the VTA and, thus, to the disinhibition of dopaminergic neurons (Abrahao et al 2012; Abrahao et al. 2017). THC acts in a similar way. It directly inhibits the release of GABA at the nerve endings of interneurons, through activation of specific receptors, the so-called cannabinoid type 1 (CB1) receptors. Once again: less GABA, less inhibition of neurons that produce dopamine, more dopamine released in the reward system.

These rapid actions of drugs on dopamine are the main triggers for addiction and the development of drug abuse disorders. However, each particular drug has other specific effects in the brain and other organs of our body. A summary of these effects for some drugs can be seen in Table 8.1.

After experiencing the intense and immediate feeling of pleasure after drugs, several factors may lead to the development of addiction. Two mechanisms are worth highlighting: positive reinforcement and negative reinforcement (Wise and Koob 2014). Positive reinforcement is based on the search for the sensation of well-being itself, that is, the individual uses the drug again in an attempt to repeat the pleasurable sensation. This seems to be one of the mechanisms that triggers drug craving, that is, the urgent and irresistible need to repeat its use (Sinha 2013). With repeated use, the individual begins to experience the effects of the lack of the drug in the body, what we call withdrawal syndrome. The appearance of abstinence symptoms already shows the beginning of physical dependence on the drug (Swift and Lewis 2014). It is a demonstration that the organism is "getting used to" the presence of the drug, adapting and "missing" it. Thus, between one "dose" and another, the individual feels the result of this adaptation: signs and symptoms that are usually the opposite of those caused by the drug. Thus, if the drug makes someone more relaxed and "feeling good," during abstinence he will become nervous and have a feeling of discomfort (for example, see Table 8.1). This is where the mechanism of negative reinforcement comes in: the individual starts to look for the drug not only for the sensation of pleasure, but also to avoid the unpleasant effects of its lack. How much each of these mechanisms contributes to the development of

Table 8.1 Examples of effects and symptoms of abstinence of some selected abuse drugs. Source: Stahl (2002) and Swift and Lewis (2014)

Drug abuse	Effects on the brain (central nervous system)	Effects on other organs and tissues of the human body	Signs and symptoms of withdrawal
Alcohol (ethanol)	Euphoria Muscle relaxation Decrease in anxiety Sedation Induction of sleep Alcoholic coma Death by respiratory depression	Recurrent gastritis and diarrhea, makes it difficult to absorb vitamins; Increased diuresis (inhibition of the release of the antidiuretic hormone) Loss of muscle strength; Impotence and loss of libido Increased blood pressure, may be toxic to the heart with prolonged use Fat accumulation in the liver (steatosis), which may develop into cirrhosis of the liver	Tremors, irritability Nausea Sleep disorders Tachycardia Hypertension Sudoresis Distorted perception Convulsions Auditory and visual hallucinations
Cocaine	Euphoria and intense sense of well-being Feeling of self-confidence Stereotypical behavior (repetitive movements) Pupil expansion Increased anxiety Emotional instability (depression) Paranoia and panic Body temperature increase Hallucinations Memory loss Seizures	Increased blood pressure Tachycardia Vascular spasms Acute myocardial infarction Brain stroke	Dysphoria Heavy depression Sensation of tiredness (fatigue), insomnia Decrease in heart rate Intense craving More serious cases can lead to suicidal ideation

(continued)

Table 8.1 (continued)

Drug abuse	Effects on the brain (central nervous system)	Effects on other organs and tissues of the human body	Signs and symptoms of withdrawal
Marijuana	Euphoria Relaxation Change in perception Distortion of the feeling of time Intensification of sensory experiences (such as eating, watching a film, enjoying nature, listening to music, etc.) Short-term memory and attention are impaired Compromised motor coordination Increased appetite Decrease of seizures High doses: visual hallucinations, depersonalization and psychotic episodes	Mitigation of nausea Decreased intraocular pressure Pain relief	Restlessness Irritability Gentle agitation Insomnia Sleep disorder Nausea, colic
Tobacco (nicotine)	Complex effects depending on the user's baseline state It calms down when they are tense Wakes up when they are sleepy Improves attention and memory	Tachycardia Increased blood pressure Reduction of gastrointestinal tract motility Muscle relaxation	Irritability, impatience and hostility Increased anxiety Dysphoric or depressive mood Restlessness Bradycardia Increased appetite and weight gain

addiction varies between drugs and between individuals, being unclear which one is more important.

Another common feature among all drugs of abuse is the development of tolerance (Volkow et al. 2019). With long-term use, the individual becomes tolerant, that is, more "resistant" to the effects of the drug. This causes him to use increasing amounts or to use the drug in shorter intervals, which can reach several times a day. This characteristic increases the risk of overdosing, since the amount of drug needed for the individual to "feel good" is increased, but the fatal amount (dose) remains the same. Thus, in the incessant search for feeling well, the individual may accidentally end up fatally intoxicated with the drug.

In addition to the reward system, other brain areas are also affected by drugs of abuse and directly contribute to the development of addiction. Regions responsible for memory processes play a very important role (Kutlu and Gould 2016). For example, one area of the brain called hippocampus is responsible for acquiring and storing memories of places or situations where/when the individual uses the drug (contextual memory). Thus, when present in those places again or going through similar situations, he will remember the drug feeling and want to use it. It is not surprising that most relapses in patients trying to quit drugs happen in places or situations similar to those in which they have used the drug before. Another important brain area is the amygdala: it is part of the pathway that regulates emotions in our brain (called limbic system) and has an important role in the "affective" or "emotional" value attributed to the drug (Wassum and Izquierdo 2015). It is not uncommon to hear smokers referring to their morning cigarette as a "great friend." Finally, areas of the cerebral cortex related to decision making are also affected (Koob and Volkow 2016). This results in the inability of the individual to "resist" the drug, thus, even recognizing that drug use does more harm than good, users cannot stop. Therefore, drug use over months or years causes extremely complex changes in our brain, which are still very poorly understood. And this only makes it more difficult to seek treatments or approaches that help these patients to quit.

The Importance of Pharmacokinetics in Drug Abuse

Pharmacokinetics comprises aspects of pharmacology ranging from absorption, i.e. the arrival of exogenous compounds in the systemic circulation, to their excretion or of its metabolites through urine, mainly. Between absorption and excretion, there is also the distribution of these compounds in different tissues and body compartments, and the biotransformation or metabolism of these compounds. In general, the route of administration of the drug (oral, nasal, intravenous, among others) may have a great impact on the speed, intensity, and duration of its effects. Cocaine and crack provide an excellent example to illustrate the impact of pharmacokinetics on the final effect of a drug.

Cocaine is a weak base isolated from coca leaves in the form of a salt (hydrochloride), which is used by nasal route (snorting) or intravenous injection. In this formulation, the cocaine molecule is in its charged form, which makes it soluble in water. This means that, in its neutral (non-charged) form, cocaine would not dissolve in water as easily. After snorting the powder of cocaine in acid form, this substance will be absorbed through the intranasal vessels and will fall into the blood circulation. The blood from the nose circulates first to the heart and from there to the lungs (O'Brien 2018). Then, it is pumped back to the heart and from there to the rest of the body, including the brain. Therefore, by the nasal route, about 10 min can pass without any effect of cocaine, and such effect can last between 20 and 40 min, depending on the dose. By intravenous injection, the effects are practically immediate since the drug reaches the brain much faster.

Seeking faster and more intense effects, it was discovered that the basic (non-charged free base) form of cocaine, crack cocaine, can be heated and smoked. These two forms of cocaine (acid salt or free base) react differently when heated in a pipe, for example. If we use the cocaine salt for smoking, it would not vaporize but rather burn, so it would not reach the circulation and consequently have no effects on the body. However, the basic form of cocaine when heated becomes vapor that can then be inhaled. When it enters the lungs, the vaporized cocaine is quickly and efficiently absorbed, due to the extensive lung surface area (compared to the inside of the nostrils, for example). Once in the pulmonary circulation, cocaine is transported by the blood to the heart and from there directly to the rest of the body (O'Brien 2018). Notice that through the intranasal route (nose), cocaine must travel a longer "way" than through inhalation (lungs). In addition, there is the question of how fast the drug goes from the tissues to the blood. Because of the larger contact surface of the lungs, the effects of smoked cocaine are much faster than those of snorting. While the effects of snorting cocaine take an average of 14 min to appear, smoked crack takes only 1.5 min. The effect of the latter lasts around 15 min (Bradberry 2002).

Another factor also contributes to making crack even more dangerous from the point of view of drug abuse. Because of its fast effect, it is more efficient than the same snorted amount. In other words, smoked cocaine will generate a greater increase in dopamine levels in the accumbens than the same amount of snorted cocaine (Bradberry 2002). For example, it was experimentally shown in monkeys that, to obtain the same amount of dopamine in the brain, it would require a dose 15 times higher via the nasal route, through the blood vessels of the nose, than via the inhalation route, which goes directly to the lung. Therefore, crack causes a stronger effect per unit of cocaine and consequently per unit of money, making it much cheaper.

Experimental assays performed with monkeys show that drug craving is directly related to the speed of drug effect. In these experiments, animals learned to press a lever to receive cocaine directly into their brains. It was observed that animals receiving a higher dose of cocaine pressed the lever more often. On the other hand, if an intravenous infusion of cocaine is made without varying the dose but varying the infusion time, those animals whose dose is infused more quickly press the lever more than those who received the same dose over a longer period. Thus, since crack exerts effects that are more intense in relatively lower doses, but faster, we can conclude that it will cause a much stronger craving than snorted cocaine (Bradberry 2002).

Another interesting example is nicotine (Benowitz 1988). The main form of nicotine use is smoking, whether in the form of cigarettes, pipes, cigars, hookahs or, more recently, electronic cigarettes. All these forms have in common the rapid arrival of nicotine in the brain through the lungs. As a lipophilic substance, nicotine quickly passes through the wall of the lung alveoli. A large amount of blood passes through the lungs and carries this nicotine quickly to the brain. On the other hand, there are medicines used in smoking cessation (as smoking cessation aids) that contain nicotine themselves as the active ingredient. These medicines are chewing gums or adhesive patches. What is the difference? The absorption and, consequently, the arrival of nicotine to the brain is much slower with these formulations. By using a chewing gum, nicotine must be absorbed from the intestines along with food and drinks consumed by the individual, and only then it reaches the blood. In patches, the process is even slower: nicotine literally has to cross the "barrier" of the skin to reach the deepest tissues (subcutaneous) where the blood vessels are. These slow-absorbing formulations prevent the brain from associating the use of the patch or gum with the feeling of quick pleasure (unlike with cigarettes). Thus, they are used to help those individuals who have decided to quit smoking to cope with withdrawal symptoms.

In addition to the short effect latency, the time needed to eliminate the drug from the body also influences the development of addiction. The faster the drug is eliminated, i.e. it leaves the body of the individual, the more intense the symptoms of abstinence will be. And these more severe unpleasant symptoms will lead to a greater need to use the drug again. Nicotine, for example, is quickly eliminated from the human body through urine (Benowitz 1988). The concentration of nicotine in the blood drops rapidly (2 h to decrease by half the initial level) and within 10 h it is completely eliminated. This makes the symptoms of nicotine withdrawal strong and frequent, causing the individual to "light" another cigarette. Conversely, THC is a slow eliminating drug. After smoking a marijuana cigarette, THC concentration in the blood drops slowly (30 h to halve), taking about six and a half days for it to be completely eliminated (Sharma et al. 2012). For this reason, users rarely report the occurrence of abstinence from marijuana consumption and thus this factor has little influence on the development of THC dependence.

Current and Selected Topics on Drugs

Medicinal Properties and Risks of Cannabis

Despite the millenary use of marijuana, only in 1988 it was discovered that there were receptors in the brain that would be activated by THC. These receptors were isolated in 1990 and called cannabinoid type 1 (CB1) receptors. The CB1 receptors are of the G protein-coupled subtype of metabotropic receptors. Among all these type of receptors, CB1 is one of the most abundant in the brain, if not the most abundant of all. This gives us an idea of the wide range of effects THC can have on the central nervous system. But why would we have a receptor for something we do not produce, but is produced by a plant? The answer is that the receptor does not only recognize THC, but also some molecule synthesized by the brain itself. In search of this molecule, the first endocannabinoid (or endogenous cannabinoid) was discovered in 1992 and called anandamide (Murray et al. 2007). Anandamide comes from the word "ananda" which in Sanskrit means joy, bliss, delight. This raises the question of why we are not constantly intoxicated, since our brain produces molecules similar to THC. Basically, the effects of THC last longer because we are not able to degrade it like we break down endocanabinoids. That is, anandamide and other endocanabinoids are degraded very quickly. In this way, our CB1 receptors are activated more intensely and for a much longer period by THC.

Animal Studies: The Cannabinoid Tetrad

Like us, mice, rats, and monkeys used in scientific research have CB1 receptors. These animals served as models to understand many of the effects of marijuana on the body. In rodents, four main effects were characterized that were named the "cannabinoid tetrad." All substances capable of activating CB1 receptors exhibit these effects in animals: (1) Analgesia in pain models; (2) Hypolocomotion (animals move less in an open field, without obstacles or visual cues that cause interest); (3) Hypothermia (decrease in body temperature); (4) Catalepsy (when placed by the front paws on a thin platform, the animals stay absolutely immobile for a long time, something that a normal animal does not) (Pertwee et al. 2010).

Another very important group of studies started from the use of animals whose CB1 receptors were genetically removed, thus losing their function. These mice have decreased fertility and their pups show high mortality. It was found that mice pups lacking the CB1 receptor suckled less than the normal pups, which explained at least in part this mortality. In fact, nowadays we know that there are cannabinoid substances in breast milk that stimulate newborns to suckle, acting at various levels (stimulation of sucking, appetite, among others). In addition, animals without CB1 receptor do not exhibit the cannabinoid tetrad when given THC, for example. Thus, it was possible to confirm these effects of marijuana and to detect previously unknown effects such as decreased fertility and modulation of food intake.

Effects of Cannabis and Its Medicinal Interest

Among the effects caused by marijuana in humans (Table 8.1), there are some that make this plant of great clinical interest for the treatment of chronic pain, epilepsy, anorexia, and nausea resulting from chemotherapy treatment, among many others. It is no coincidence that many countries in the world have now made the medicinal use of *cannabis* legal, including Brazil (December 2019). As mentioned earlier, *cannabis* has several bioactive compounds in addition to THC. Another cannabinoid that has been intensively researched for its medicinal properties is cannabidiol, which has the advantage of not being psychotropic. Thus, cannabidiol can and has been used to treat some types of refractory epilepsies (which do not respond to usual drugs) that affect children (Friedman et al. 2019).

Unpleasant Effects of Cannabis

Some marijuana users, especially in their first experiences with the drug, may experience anxiety and panic. This is due to the vasodilating effects of THC, which, in individuals with specific cardiovascular characteristics, can lead to a drop in blood pressure. A factor that also contributes to this sensation is hypothermia. The body responds to these drops in blood pressure and temperature by increasing the heart rate (tachycardia). This tachycardia can cause a feeling of discomfort, such as in a situation of great anxiety (tremor, tachycardia, increased respiratory rate, sweating, among others) (Jordt and Guimarães 2006).

Another important issue is the higher likelihood of traffic accidents of individuals under the effects of drugs. Studies carried out in this regard have to be very careful to separate users who have concomitant use of alcohol. However, there seems to be a correlation, which can be explained by the role that CB1 receptors have in motor coordination control. As mentioned above, animal studies already pointed to a regulatory role on motor activity via CB1.

Research on the cellular mechanisms of the effects of cannabinoids on the brain has focused mainly on memory. Endocannabinoids have been shown to play a role in facilitating the acquisition of new short-term memories, as well as helping to eliminate aversive memories (Lisboa et al. 2019). These effects are due to the massive presence of CB1 in brain areas involved in memory. However, when THC is given to animals, these memory-modulatory systems are disturbed, since the spatial and temporal resolution of CB1 activation is lost. Thus, some of the balance of signaling that occurs in those synapses is lost.

It is observed that chronic users of marijuana, even though not under the effect of the drug, have a diminished ability to establish new memories and to remember past facts. These findings are similar to the effects seen in acute marijuana intoxication. The sequelae in the memory of chronic users are related to the duration, frequency, dose, and age of onset of marijuana use. In fact, there are meta-analyses comparing several studies conducted with chronic *cannabis* users which point out deficits in executive and cognitive aspects, besides memory. Therefore, one should consider the impact of marijuana use on learning, a process closely related to memory (Figueiredo et al. 2020).

Use of Marijuana During Adolescence and the Risk of Schizophrenia

The proposal of the induction of behaviors similar to a psychotic episode due to the abuse of marijuana in adults arose in the 1970s (Chopra and Smith 1974). Currently, the occurrence of a transitory behavioral change (characterized by motor agitation, amnesia, delusions and hallucinations) due to intoxication by this plant is recognized, i.e., it is possible to have a THC overdose (Leweke et al. 2004).

The estimated annual prevalence of marijuana use in the Brazilian population is 2.1% and studies indicate a growing consumption among adolescents (De Micheli and Formigoni 2004). A recent meta-analysis (Marconi et al. 2016) indicates an increase of up to 6 times in the risk of developing schizophrenia (a chronic, uncurable psychiatric disorder) by adolescents who use marijuana. This risk is higher in those who start using younger (before the age of 12) and/or to those who use it more often and mainly preparations with a high THC content (such as "skank" or "hashish"). However, a minority of individuals develop psychosis only due to the use of marijuana. The greatest concern are adolescents who are already part of risk groups, that is, who have some relative with schizophrenia or other psychiatric disorders, who are constantly exposed to stress or who have experienced trauma. In these cases, the use of marijuana may anticipate and/or aggravate the occurrence of the disorder.

Recently, a warning was given about the increasing use of synthetic cannabinoids in the USA (Yeruva et al. 2019). These substances were developed for use only in research (restricted to laboratories), but ended up reaching the public as an alternative to the use of marijuana or for use in electronic cigarettes. In general, the components of these products are much more powerful than THC, and the risks of their use are not fully known. Several cases of psychotic outbreaks induced by these substances have already been reported, and changes in behavior can last for more than a month. Cases of fatal intoxications have also been reported. A complete picture of the risks of using these formulations by adolescents are currently unknown.

Alcohol, Endorphins, and Endocannabinoids: What is the Relationship?

Alcohol or ethanol is one of the most consumed drugs of abuse and one with the most complex pharmacology (Andrade et al. 2011; Abrahao et al. 2017). It is a small molecule that easily mixes with water (hydrophilic) and thus quickly reaches all organs and compartments of our body. This explains in part the great amount of effects caused by this drug. Subsequently, it is not surprising to find out that ethanol can interact not with one, but with several proteins and receptors in our organism. As already mentioned, it disinhibits dopaminergic neurons from the reward pathway, acting on $GABA_A$-type ion channels (activated by GABA), but other receptors are also involved in this effect. An example is the family of opioid receptors, a group of metabotropic receptors sensitive to endorphins (yes, the same endorphins released during exercise) (Méndez et al. 2019). Animal studies have shown that alcohol is capable of increasing beta-endorphin production in the reward pathway. This endorphin helps to increase dopamine levels in the accumbens and, therefore, the well-being feeling caused by alcohol. Similarly, genetically modified mice that lack beta-endorphin-sensitive receptors (called μ opioid receptors) consume less alcohol than their counterparts who have them. This explains in a certain way the use of naltrexone (a drug with opioid action) in the treatment of alcoholism.

Another brain chemical system involved in the effects of alcohol is the endocannabinoid (Henderson-Redmond et al. 2016). Animal studies have shown that the use of alcohol increases the production of anandamide in several brain regions. This increase is maintained with prolonged use of alcohol, which leads to overactivation of the CB1 receptors. To protect themselves, neurons decrease the number of CB1 receptors in synapses, and this decrease seems to be involved in tolerance development to the relaxing and pleasurable effects of ethanol. The contribution of CB1 receptors to alcohol dependence has also been proven in studies with genetically modified rodents. Alcohol consumption does not increase the release of dopamine in the reward pathway in mice that do not have the CB1 receptor. In studies where they learn to press a lever to receive alcohol, these genetically modified animals seek less alcohol. Under the same conditions these animals have less motivation to receive alcohol: when they need to push the lever several times to gain a dose of alcohol they give up much easier than animals that have intact CB1 receptors. These studies show that compounds that decrease the action of alcohol on the endocannabinoid system could be important aids for patients trying to stop drinking.

The "Flavors of Nicotine"

The smoking habit is one of the main avoidable causes of death in current society, especially when it comes to deaths from respiratory diseases (Prochaska and Benowitz 2019). The use of cigarettes, cigars, pipes, or other forms in which tobacco leaves are burned accounts for about 87% of deaths from lung cancer and 61% of deaths from other chronic lung diseases (emphysema, for example). Although nicotine is the component responsible for addiction, i.e., that sustains tobacco use, other components of cigarettes seem to be more toxic than nicotine and, thus, the main responsibles for lung diseases. This finding led to a marked reduction in the number of smokers in our society: from about 45% of the population at the end of the 1960s to 18% today.

On the other hand, the tobacco industry has found alternatives to promote the use of nicotine. New devices have been developed in which tobacco is not burned, but only heated (so-called smokeless tobacco) and electronic cigarettes (e-cigarettes) that are filled with a liquid that is then transformed into steam at the time of use and inhaled. The use of these e-cigarettes has been growing in recent years, especially among adolescents. One of the factors that make these products very attractive to young people is the mixture of flavorings (different flavors) to the inhalation liquid (DeVito and Krishnan-Sarin 2018). These flavors range from tobacco extract (to imitate the taste of traditional cigarettes) to sweet flavors that resemble fruits or desserts or more refreshing flavors with the use of menthol. These "flavors" are intended to mask the unpleasant taste of nicotine and to prevent the feeling of irritation that nicotine and other vapor components cause in the throat and lungs.

Recent studies show that the presence of "flavors" in electronic cigarettes has influenced the pattern of these products use (DeVito and Krishnan-Sarin 2018). Approximately 95% of adolescent users of electronic cigarettes declare to preferentially use flavored ones, i.e., flavors make them more appealing. In addition, many users report believing that flavored e-cigarettes are less harmful to health than tasteless ones, no matter how much nicotine they have.

But the problem of adding these "flavors" to e-cigarettes goes beyond that: recent research on rodents shows that the chemicals that make up the different "tastes" of cigarettes can potentiate the effects of nicotine in the brain. Works published in 2017 and 2018 have shown that menthol (a component of e-cigarettes and traditional menthol cigarettes) is able to increase the effects of nicotine on the reward system, potentiating the activation of dopamine neurons and increasing the release of dopamine in the accumbens (Henderson et al. 2017; Zhang et al. 2018). These effects are independent of menthol taste, since it was given to rats through injections. Similar effects have also been detected with the use of farnesol in rats (a compound used to simulate the taste of green apples). In addition, menthol seems to decrease the degradation of nicotine in our body, allowing it to reach the brain in higher concentrations. This and other evidence indicates that the different "flavors" of nicotine available today may not only make e-cigarettes more attractive to young people (by increasing their use), but also increase the chance that these adolescents will become addicted to nicotine.

Finally, the components of e-cigarettes are not as well studied as those of traditional cigarettes. Hence, it is not yet certain how much safer they can be considered in comparison to tobacco burning products. New studies are urgently needed to clarify these points and guide policies to potentially restrict the use of these products.

Final Considerations

The study of the pharmacology of drugs of abuse is important to understand how they affect individuals and how it relates to the environmental cues. It is a key tool for proposing new forms of treatment and prevention of addiction. The constant emergence of previously unknown new drugs or new forms of use of known drugs strongly indicates that these studies should continue. However, prohibition or proscription of most of these drugs makes scientific research extremely difficult, delaying the advance of knowledge and the development of potential treatments.

References

Abrahao, K. P., Salinas, A. G., & Lovinger, D. M. (2017). Alcohol and the brain: Neuronal molecular targets, synapses, and circuits. *Neuron, 96*(6), 1223–1238. https://doi.org/10.1016/j.neuron.2017.10.032.

Abrahao, K. P., Quadros, I. M. H., Andrade, A. L. M., & Souza-Formigoni, M. L. O. (2012). Accumbal dopamine D2 receptor function is associated with individual variability in ethanol behavioral sensitization. Neuropharmacology, 62(2), 882–889. https://doi.org/10.1016/j.neuropharm.2011.09.017

Andrade, A. L. M., Abrahao, K. P., Goeldner, F. O., & Souza-Formigoni, M. L. O. (2011). Administration of the 5-HT2C receptor antagonist SB-242084 into the nucleus accumbens blocks the expression of ethanol-induced behavioral sensitization in Albino Swiss mice. *Neuroscience, 189*, 178–186. https://doi.org/10.1016/j.neuroscience.2011.05.028.

Benowitz, N. L. (1988). Drug therapy. Pharmacologic aspects of cigarette smoking and nicotine addiction. *The New England Journal of Medicine, 319*(20), 1318–1330. https://doi.org/10.1056/NEJM198811173192005.

Boulter, J., Evans, K., Goldman, D., Martin, G., Treco, D., Heinemann, S., & Patrick, J. (1986). Isolation of a cDNA clone coding for a possible neural nicotinic acetylcholine receptor alpha-subunit. *Nature, 319*(6052), 368–374. https://doi.org/10.1038/319368a0.

Bradberry, C. W. (2002). Dynamics of extracellular dopamine in the acute and chronic actions of cocaine. *The Neuroscientist, 8*(4), 315–322. https://doi.org/10.1177/107385840200800407.

Brady, S. T., Siegel, G. J., Albers, R. W., & Price, D. L. (2012). *Basic neurochemistry: Principles of molecular, cellular and medical neurobiology*. Oxford, UK: Academic.

Castaldelli-Maia, J. M., Ventriglio, A., & Bhugra, D. (2016). Tobacco smoking: From 'glamour' to 'stigma'. A comprehensive review. *Psychiatry and Clinical Neurosciences, 70*, 24–33. https://doi.org/10.1111/pcn.12365.

Chopra, G. S., & Smith, J. W. (1974). Psychotic reactions following cannabis use in East Indians. *Archives of General Psychiatry, 30*(1), 24–27. https://doi.org/10.1001/archpsyc.1974.01760070014002.

Dani, J. A., & Balfour, D. J. (2011). Historical and current perspective on tobacco use and nicotine addiction. *Trends in Neurosciences, 34*(7), 383–392. https://doi.org/10.1016/j.tins.2011.05.001.

De Micheli, D., & Formigoni, M. L. (2004). Drug use by Brazilian students: Associations with family, psychosocial, health, demographic and behavioral characteristics. *Addiction, 99*(5), 570–578. https://doi.org/10.1111/j.1360-0443.2003.00671.x.

DeVito, E. E., & Krishnan-Sarin, S. (2018). E-cigarettes: Impact of e-liquid components and device characteristics on nicotine exposure. *Current Neuropharmacology, 16*(4), 438–459. https://doi.org/10.2174/1570159X15666171016164430.

Di Chiara, G., & Bassareo, V. (2007). Reward system and addiction: What dopamine does and doesn't do. *Current Opinion in Pharmacology, 7*(1), 69–76. https://doi.org/10.1016/j.coph.2006.11.003.

Figueiredo, P. R., Tolomeo, S., Steele, J. D., & Baldacchino, A. (2020). Neurocognitive consequences of chronic cannabis use: A systematic review and meta-analysis. *Neuroscience and Biobehavioral Reviews, 108*, 358–369. https://doi.org/10.1016/j.neubiorev.2019.10.014.

Friedman, D., French, J. A., & Maccarrone, M. (2019). Safety, efficacy, and mechanisms of action of cannabinoids in neurological disorders. *The Lancet Neurology, 18*(5), 504–512. https://doi.org/10.1016/s1474-4422(19)30032-8.

Henderson, B. J., Wall, T. R., Henley, B. M., Kim, C. H., McKinney, S., & Lester, H. A. (2017). Menthol enhances nicotine reward-related behavior by potentiating nicotine-induced changes in nAChR function, nAChR upregulation, and DA neuron excitability. *Neuropsychopharmacology, 42*(12), 2285–2291. https://doi.org/10.1038/npp.2017.72.

Henderson-Redmond, A. N., Guindon, J., & Morgan, D. J. (2016). Roles for the endocannabinoid system in ethanol-motivated behavior. *Progress in Neuro-Psychopharmacology & Biological Psychiatry, 65*, 330–339. https://doi.org/10.1016/j.pnpbp.2015.06.011.

Jordt, S. E., & Guimarães, M. Z. P. (2006). TRPA1: A sensory channel of many talents. In W. Liedtke & S. Heller (Eds.), *TRP ion channel function in sensory transduction and cellular signaling cascades (frontiers in neuroscience)* (pp. 151–161). Boca Raton, FL: CRC Press. https://doi.org/10.1201/9781420005844.ch11.

Kalivas, P. W., Pierce, R. C., Cornish, J., & Sorg, B. A. (1998). A role for sensitization in craving and relapse in cocaine addiction. *Journal of Psychopharmacology, 12*(1), 49–53. https://doi.org/10.1177/026988119801200107.

Khaderi, S. A. (2019). Introduction: Alcohol and alcoholism. *Clinics in Liver Disease, 23*(1), 1–10. https://doi.org/10.1016/j.cld.2018.09.009.

Koob, G. F., & Volkow, N. D. (2016). Neurobiology of addiction: A neurocircuitry analysis. *The Lancet Psychiatry, 3*(8), 760–773. https://doi.org/10.1016/S2215-0366(16)00104-8.

Kutlu, M. G., & Gould, T. J. (2016). Effects of drugs of abuse on hippocampal plasticity and hippocampus-dependent learning and memory: Contributions to development and maintenance of addiction. *Learning & Memory, 23*(10), 515–533. https://doi.org/10.1101/lm.042192.116.

Leweke, F. M., Gerth, C. W., & Klosterkötter, J. (2004). Cannabis-associated psychosis: Current status of research. *CNS Drugs, 18*(13), 895–910. https://doi.org/10.2165/00023210-200418130-00005.

Lisboa, S. F., Vila-Verde, C., Rosa, J., Uliana, D. L., Stern, C., Bertoglio, L. J., et al. (2019). Tempering aversive/traumatic memories with cannabinoids: A review of evidence from animal and human studies. *Psychopharmacology, 236*(1), 201–226. https://doi.org/10.1007/s00213-018-5127-x.

Maehle, A. H. (2004). "Receptive substances": John Newport Langley (1852-1925) and his path to a receptor theory of drug action. *Medical History, 48*(2), 153–174. https://doi.org/10.1017/s0025727300000090.

Marconi, A., Di Forti, M., Lewis, C. M., Murray, R. M., & Vassos, E. (2016). Meta-analysis of the association between the level of cannabis use and risk of psychosis. *Schizophrenia Bulletin, 42*(5), 1262–1269. https://doi.org/10.1093/schbul/sbw003.

Méndez, M., Hernández-Fonseca, K., & Abate, P. (2019). The enkephalinergic system and ethanol effects. In V. Preedy (Ed.), *Neuroscience of alcohol* (pp. 443–451). Cambridge, MA: Academic Press.

Murray, R. M., Morrison, P. D., Henquet, C., & Forti, M. D. (2007). Cannabis, the mind and society: The hash realities. *Nature Reviews Neuroscience, 8*(11), 885–895. https://doi.org/10.1038/nrn2253.

O'Brien, C. P. (2018). Drug use disorders and addiction. In L. S. Goodman, A. Gilman, L. L. Brunton, R. Hilal-Dandan, & B. C. Knollmann (Eds.), *Goodman & Gilmans the pharmacological basis of therapeutics* (pp. 433–442). New York, NY: McGraw-Hill Education.

Pertwee, R. G., Howlett, A. C., Abood, M. E., Alexander, S. P., Di Marzo, V., Elphick, M. R., et al. (2010). International Union of Basic and Clinical Pharmacology. LXXIX. Cannabinoid receptors and their ligands: Beyond CB_1 and CB_2. *Pharmacological Reviews, 62*(4), 588–631. https://doi.org/10.1124/pr.110.003004.

Prochaska, J. J., & Benowitz, N. L. (2019). Current advances in research in treatment and recovery: Nicotine addiction. *Science Advances, 5*(10), eaay9763. https://doi.org/10.1126/sciadv.aay9763.

Ren, M., Tang, Z., Wu, X., Spengler, R., Jiang, H., Yang, Y., & Boivin, N. (2019). The origins of cannabis smoking: Chemical residue evidence from the first millennium BCE in the Pamirs. *Science Advances, 5*(6), eaaw1391. https://doi.org/10.1126/sciadv.aaw1391.

Sharma, P., Murthy, P., & Bharath, M. M. (2012). Chemistry, metabolism, and toxicology of cannabis: Clinical implications. *Iranian Journal of Psychiatry, 7*(4), 149–156.

Sinha, R. (2013). The clinical neurobiology of drug craving. *Current Opinion in Neurobiology, 23*(4), 649–654. https://doi.org/10.1016/j.conb.2013.05.001.

Stahl, S. M. (2002). *Essential psychopharmacology: Neuroscientific basis and practical application* (2nd ed.). Cambridge, UK: Cambridge University Press.

Swift, R. M., & Lewis, D. C. (2014). Farmacologia da dependência e abuso de drogas. In D. E. Golan, A. H. Tashjian, E. J. Armstrong, & A. W. Armstrong (Eds.), *Princípios de farmacologia: A base fisiopatológica da farmacoterapia* (pp. 260–278). Rio de Janeiro, Brazil: Guanabara Koogan.

Uhl, G. R., Hall, F. S., & Sora, I. (2002). Cocaine, reward, movement and monoamine transporters. *Molecular Psychiatry, 7*(1), 21–26. https://doi.org/10.1038/sj.mp.4000964.

Volkow, N. D., Michaelides, M., & Baler, R. (2019). The neuroscience of drug reward and addiction. *Physiological Reviews, 99*(4), 2115–2140. https://doi.org/10.1152/physrev.00014.2018.

von Zastrow, M. (2018). Drug receptors & pharmacodynamics. In B. G. Katzung (Ed.), *Basic & clinical pharmacology* (pp. 20–40). New York, NY: McGraw-Hill Education.

Wassum, K. M., & Izquierdo, A. (2015). The basolateral amygdala in reward learning and addiction. *Neuroscience and Biobehavioral Reviews, 57*, 271–283. https://doi.org/10.1016/j.neubiorev.2015.08.017.

Wise, R. A., & Koob, G. F. (2014). The development and maintenance of drug addiction. *Neuropsychopharmacology, 39*(2), 254–262. https://doi.org/10.1038/npp.2013.261.

Wonnacott, S., Kaiser, S., Mogg, A., Soliakov, L., & Jones, I. W. (2000). Presynaptic nicotinic receptors modulating dopamine release in the rat striatum. *European Journal of Pharmacology, 393*(1–3), 51–58. https://doi.org/10.1016/s0014-2999(00)00005-4.

Yeruva, R. R., Mekala, H. M., Sidhu, M., & Lippmann, S. (2019). Synthetic cannabinoids-"spice" can induce a psychosis: A brief review. *Innovations in Clinical Neuroscience, 16*(1–2), 31–32.

Zhang, M., Harrison, E., Biswas, L., Tran, T., & Liu, X. (2018). Menthol facilitates dopamine-releasing effect of nicotine in rat nucleus accumbens. *Pharmacology, Biochemistry, and Behavior, 175*, 47–52. https://doi.org/10.1016/j.pbb.2018.09.004.

Chapter 9
Impacts of Drug (Ab)Use on the Development of the Human Central Nervous System

André Bedendo

Introduction

Drugs that can cause addiction such as alcohol, tobacco, some types of medicines, and illicit substances have the potential to affect human functioning in the short and long term. These changes occur at both biological (changing morphology and organ function), psychological/behavioral (affecting cognitive function and behavior expression), and social (changing family and peer relationships) levels. The magnitude of the impact of these drugs is directly associated with the substance use profile. Two patterns of use are particularly associated with more harm: (1) use in large quantities and at high frequency; (2) heavy episodic use, that

Since the human brain is an organ that remains in development even after birth, when drug use occurs during critical phases of development, the damage can be further enhanced. In this chapter you will see how drugs modify the functioning of the Central Nervous System (CNS), affecting the processing of information and the expression of behaviors throughout the development of the CNS.

Neurobiology of Drug Use

The effect of psychotropic drugs (those that have the potential to cause dependence) occurs due to their actions on the CNS. This action happens in the short and long term, altering the normal physiological functioning of the CNS and promoting morphological changes. In the short term, the drugs alter the concentration of neurotransmitters (chemical molecules that transmit information between neurons) in

A. Bedendo (✉)
Universidade Federal de São Paulo, São Paulo, SP, Brazil
e-mail: andre.bedendo@unifesp.br

D. De Micheli et al. (eds.), *Drugs and Human Behavior*,
https://doi.org/10.1007/978-3-030-62855-0_9

several areas of the brain. When these changes are sustained over the long term, they can promote morphological changes such as an increase or decrease in the number of receptors (proteins expressed on the surface of neurons that connect to the neurotransmitters, allowing the transmission of information from the external environment to the internal environment of the cell). This mechanism of altering the quantity of receptors is a process that occurs naturally in the CNS by means of brain plasticity processes and aims to maintain the balance and proper functioning of the system. For example, when there is an excess of dopamine (DA) stimulation in a certain region due to the recurrent use of agents such as drugs, one way to reduce over-stimulation is by reducing the number of receptors. With fewer receptors available for DA binding, there is a consequent reduction in stimulation in the region.

The drugs act on several regions of the CNS changing its normal functioning, but there are some parts that are particularly affected. Among them the *ventral tegmental area* (VTA), the *nucleus accumbens* (Nacc), and the *prefrontal cortex* (PFC). These regions make up the so-called *mesolimbic* and *mesocortical* pathways, also known as the *Brain Reward System* (BRS). This system is of great importance for the understanding the maintenance of use. Below we will see how the drugs affect each of these regions.

Ventral Tegmental Area (VTA)

VTA is located in the mesencephalon and from it originate groups of dopaminergic neurons that connect with other regions of the limbic system, such as the Nacc, amygdala, and hippocampus (mesolimbic pathway), and cortical regions (mesocortical pathway), such as the PFC. The dopaminergic signaling from VTA supports basic behaviors associated with human survival such as feeding, hydration, and sexual behavior. Once stimulated, the mesolimbic and mesocortical pathways promote the release of DA in the Nacc and PFC, respectively. The behavioral consequence of DA release is the increased salience of these stimuli, promoting a rewarding sensation that favors behavior repetition.

The evolutionary relevance of VTA in maintaining basic human survival behaviors associated with feeding and reproduction is quite clear, however, it is also influenced by substance use. Some drugs stimulate VTA neurons and promote DA release, activating the same basic brain system essential to evolution.

Nucleus Accumbens (Nacc) and Mesolimbic Pathway

The Nacc is one of the neuron destinations projecting from VTA which constitutes the mesolimbic pathway. Substance use promotes through different pharmacological effects the rapid increase of DA release in Nacc (Di Chiara 2002; Owesson-White et al. 2009). In particular, DA released in this region is associated with the rewarding aspect of drug use, which reinforces this behavior. Thus, every time a drug is consumed, the release of DA in Nacc signals this behavior as pleasant, acting as an acute reinforcer (Goldstein and Volkow 2002), that is, it increases the chances of this behavior (drug use) occurring again in the future. Therefore, like food, water, and sex, drugs activate a system that will signal to the brain that the behavior should be repeated again.

In addition to the release of DA in Nacc through the action of drugs in the VTA, as in the case of alcohol and opioids, some substances such as cocaine and amphetamines promote the increase of DA concentrations directly in Nacc. This occurs by blocking the reuptake of DA directly in the Nacc or even forcing the release of the neurotransmitter from the synaptic vesicles (World Health Organization 2004).

Through interaction with other regions of the limbic system (responsible for emotional processing) such as the hippocampus and amygdala, the reoccurring drug use and consequent release of DA in Nacc favors the pairing of a stimulus (drug or environmental characteristics present during drug use) with a response (pleasure caused by DA release in Nacc). This promotes the consolidation of drug conditioned memories (Goldstein and Volkow 2002; Volkow et al. 2010). Over time, even in the absence of the drug, environmental clues (walking by places where the drug use previously occurred) or anticipation of situations where use could potentially occur promote the firing of dopamine neurons (Schultz 2002), in a powerful maladaptive memory mechanism that can lead to a new drug use (Volkow et al. 2010).

Prefrontal Cortex (PFC) and Mesocortical Path

The mesocortical pathway, a bundle of neurons that departs from the VTA to the PFC, acts in parallel and interacts with the mesolimbic pathway (Goldstein and Volkow 2002). Studies indicate that the PFC seems to be associated with the craving, drug expectancy, loss of control, compulsive behavior, and drug salience (Koob and Le Moal 2005).

While the action of drugs on the mesolimbic pathway is associated with the rewarding sensation, a *bottom-up* process (processing of sensory information with reduced action of higher cognitive processes), the action on the mesocortical pathway is related to the regulatory control of the behavior. In the latter case, the emphasis is on *top-down* processes (in which complex cognitive processes predominate in behavior regulation) (Wiers and Heinz 2015).

Reoccurring drug use appears to reduce PFC inhibitory control, "releasing" behaviors that would normally be kept under monitoring (Goldstein and Volkow 2002). Thus, drug dependence is a disorder characterized by both increased drug salience (regulated by the mesolimbic pathway) and an executive control deficiency (regulated by the mesocortical pathway) (Wiers and Heinz 2015).

Brain Reward System and the Development of Drug Dependence

For a long time, it was believed that people with drug addiction were more sensitive to the reinforcing effects of drugs and this reinforcing effect would reflect the higher levels of DA (Volkow et al. 2016). However, research has shown this to be incorrect, since people with addiction have lower levels of DA than people without addiction (Volkow et al. 1997, 2014). As we have seen before, the PFC is also related to the attribution of salience to a given stimulus (Goldstein and Volkow 2002; Koob and Le Moal 2005), essential for maintaining goal-oriented behaviors and making the association between stimulus-response more flexible (Koob and Volkow 2016). Consequently, there is a reduction in non-drug related saliency and the self-regulatory ability among people with drug addiction is impaired (Volkow et al. 2016; Volkow and Morales 2015) resulting from the reduction in the normal function of motivational systems (Koob and Le Moal 2008). This helps to understand the reason a person with a substance-related disorder act impulsively (which might lead to relapse), despite deliberately manifesting a desire to stop drug use (Volkow et al. 2016).

Brain Development and Maturation

The human brain is formed by approximately 86 billion neurons and weighs about 1.5 kg (Azevedo et al. 2009; Herculano-Houzel 2009). Communication between neurons occurs through synapses, and it is estimated that there are between one and two hundred trillion synapses in the adult neocortex (Tang et al. 2001), the part of the brain cortex responsible for high-order brain functions such as cognition, sensory perception, and sophisticated motor control. Weighting approximately 2% of total body weight, the brain consumes about 20% of the energy produced by our body (Herculano-Houzel 2011b), and it is estimated that between 60 and 80% of it is used for maintaining neuronal intrinsic communication (Raichle 2006; Raichle and Mintun 2006).

For a long time it was believed that humans' superior cognitive abilities were due to their larger brain size, their relative high brain to body ratio or because they had much more developed neocortex for our body size (Gazzaniga 2008; Herculano-Houzel 2011a). However, the most recent hypotheses suggests that the superior cognitive capabilities of humans refer to the greater number of neurons which generates an excess of cells beyond those needed to operate the body. This overabundance of cells would be available to command cognitive and behavioral processes (Herculano-Houzel 2011a).

All the cognitive capacity of the human brain is not yet fully established during birth, and it takes more than two decades for the organ to fully develop. For this to occur properly, two important maturation processes are necessary: *myelinization* and *synaptic pruning*. This brain maturation occurs in an orchestrated manner, following an order in which some regions finish their maturation before others.

Myelinization and Synaptic Pruning

As we have seen before, the cognitive and behavioral capabilities of the human being seem to be not only related to his size and mass, but his ability to concentrate a large number of cells in a small volume. Obviously, at birth the human brain presents a smaller volume than when it was an adult, but at 6 years of age this volume is about 95% of its maximum (Giedd 2008). So, what would explain the development of various human abilities after that age since the brain has such a similar volume to an adult? The answer can be summed up by the word *refinement*. This refinement refers to maturation processes that will allow the improvement of brain functions without significantly altering the total brain volume.

Before birth the neurogenesis (the process by which new neurons are created) is already completed and will be succeeded by the formation of synapses (synaptogenesis), a process that will remain very active during the first years after birth (Silbereis et al. 2016). This seems to be an important brain task in the postnatal period, since the peak in the number of synapses occurs between the first and second year of life (Huttenlocher 1990; Huttenlocher and Dabholkar 1997), reaching rates of approximately 42 million new synapses per minute (Silbereis et al. 2016). Althought, already formed, many neurons are not fully maturated and still need to undergo a stage known as *myelinization*.

Myelinization is the process by which the myelin sheath is added to the axons of neurons. It acts by isolating the axon and favors the speed and synchronicity of information transmission by neurons, which is important for high-order cognitive, behavioral, and emotional behaviors (Deoni et al. 2011). Thus, the myelin sheath has a function analogous to the sheath of an electrical wire, while the axon would be the conductive part of the wire. The myelinization process takes place more markedly soon after birth and extends into adolescence (Silbereis et al. 2016). Once the neuron is myelinated, the efficiency of communication between different brain regions is favored, being particularly important for the inhibitory control by the PFC, as we will see further on.

In addition to myelinization, *synaptic pruning*, a progressive elimination and reorganization of brain synapses also occurs. Synaptic pruning begins after advanced stages of myelinization, around 4–5 years of age, extending to over 20 years of age, and is considered essential for functional specialization in neocortical areas (Silbereis et al. 2016). The main function of synaptic pruning is to strengthen the most important brain synapses (the ones that are more frequently activated) and to eliminate those considered superfluous (those with less activation). This would allow more nutrients provision to the most activated connections, favoring the development of cognitive skills characteristic of late adolescence.

Maturation Directionality (Posterior-Anterior and Subcortical-Cortical)

Current knowledge in neuroscience indicates that the brain develops in a posterior-anterior (from back to front) and subcortical-cortical (from the innermost regions of the brain—subcortical—to the outermost regions—cortical) manner. Overall, this development directionality is related to the initial development of more basic cognitive abilities (emotional processing, motor behavior, processing of sensory information, speech, and language), followed by the high-order brain functions (executive functioning and inhibitory control).

Between 5 and 20 years of age the brain will undergo a maturation process in which the regions of the *occipital and parietal lobes*, important for visual processing and motor behavior, will develop more rapidly. Thus, the biological substrate needed to perform these capabilities will be more promptly available. In turn, the *frontal lobe,* associated with high-order brain functions, shows signs of more advanced maturation only around 20 years of age (Gogtay et al. 2004; Gogtay and Thompson 2010). Finally, the *temporal lobe,* despite having its poles maturated early, is still under maturing until around 20 years of age, as well as the frontal lobe. The timing differences in the maturation of the temporal lobe seems to be related to the different functions exerted by this area, including the associative function in the integration of memory and sensory information (Gogtay et al. 2004; Gogtay and Thompson 2010). The brain maturation process described here seems to be partially associated with the synaptic pruning mechanism (Giedd et al. 2015; Gogtay and Thompson 2010).

Brain maturation also seems to follow an ordering from "inside out," i.e. from internal regions (subcortical) to external regions (cortical). Connections between *subcortical* areas and *subcortical-cortical* regions, associated with emotional reactivity, reinforcement processing (VTA), anticipation of rewards (ventral striatum), associative learning and emotions (amygdala) develop earlier during childhood and early adolescence. On the other hand, *cortical-subcortical* connections, which start from the PFC to the amygdala and ventral striatum; or *cortical-cortical*, between different areas of the PFC (lateral prefrontal cortex and medial prefrontal cortex) will only be fully developed by the end of adolescence/beginning of adult life (Casey 2015; Casey et al. 2016; Casey et al. 2019). Both *cortical-subcortical* and *cortical-cortical* pathways are related to inhibitory control and executive functions.

In short, from the point of view of brain maturation, we can argue that circuits related to emotional processing are maturated before the connections responsible for control and emotional regulation. Consequently, this would generate an imbalance between emotional reactivity (*bottom-up*) and the ability to regulate those emotions (*top-down*). This imbalance is particularly evident during adolescence and remains until the early adulthood (Casey et al. 2019), when the *top-down* capabilities for self-controlling emotions, desires, and actions would be developed (Casey 2015).

Impact of Drug Use on Development and Maturation of the CNS

At the end of the first month of intrauterine development of a fertilized embryo, it is already possible to observe structures such as the plate, the tube, and the neural groove, which will give rise to the CNS, and which will undergo an intense process of evolution until the birth of the baby (Lent 2010). However, as we have seen before, brain development will take a long time to reach an adequate degree of maturation. During this process, from the embryonic life until the beginning of adulthood, substance use can affect the natural course of brain development by promoting physiological changes. In this section, we present the main impacts of drug use on two critical periods of human development: prenatal and adolescence.

Prenatal Drug Exposure

It is widely known that drug use can cause harm to the user and to others. In this regard, alcohol or other drugs use by a pregnant woman can result in serious neurological and behavioral consequences to offspring. Box 9.1 presents the main consequences of drug use during pregnancy.

Box 9.1 Main Consequences of Drug Use During Pregnancy

Fetal alcohol syndrome
Newborn abstinence syndrome
Premature birth
Low birth weight
Abnormal organ growth
Delayed behavioral development
Cognitive problems (e.g. memory, attention, problem solving)
Increased chance of developing problems associated with drug use during adulthood

Due to its significant problems, guidelines recommend the discontinuation of any drug use among pregnant women or women planning to become pregnant (Carson et al. 2017; Floyd et al. 2008; Ministério da Saúde 2010; National Health Service 2017).

Fetal Alcoholic Syndrome

Alcohol is the world most consumed drug and its teratogenic effects are well established. Therefore, alcohol use during pregnancy receives particular attention from studies and health institutions around the world. In addition to the serious short- and medium-term damages, prenatal exposure to alcohol is associated with long-term damages such as persistent brain abnormalities during adolescence (Sowell et al. 2002) and a higher risk of developing problems associated with alcohol use during adult life (Baer et al. 2003). However, the *fetal alcoholic syndrome* (FAS) is considered one of the most serious consequences associated with drug use during pregnancy.

The FAS is caused exclusively by the mother's alcohol use during pregnancy. The syndrome is characterized by pre and/or postnatal growth deficiency (weight and/or height), craniofacial anomalies, severe CNS problems (including microcephaly), cognitive and behavioral problems (problems of memory, attention, executive function, language and learning, impairment in general intellectual performance, among others). It is also important to note that low-risk alcohol drinking guidelines for the general population does not apply to pregnant women. There is no scientific evidence to support safe or low-risk alcohol use during pregnancy (Carson et al. 2017; Floyd et al. 2008), and total abstinence is recommended.

Drug Use during Adolescence

Adolescence is a period associated with several social and psychological vulnerabilities (Chambers et al. 2003), including higher alcohol or drugs experimentation compared to childhood or adult life (Casey and Jones 2010). During adolescence, physiological changes occur in the CNS and the most prominent ones were previously presented in this chapter. These factors, associated with a number of other psychosocial variables, can increase vulnerability to drug use among adolescents, as well as exposure to risks.

According to the neuroscience findings presented above, there is an overlap of specific brain areas involved with drug use neurobiology and brain maturation. In this regard, the development of regions associated with motivation, impulsivity, and drug dependence coincide. Thus, behaviors characteristic of adolescence, such as impulsivity and sensation seeking can be explained by brain maturation in which an immature control system favors impulsive and risky behaviors (Chambers et al. 2003).

Neurobiological, cognitive, and personality aspects precede alcohol consumption among adolescents, but may be affected by drug use. From the cognitive and personality point of view, low inhibitory cognitive control (greater impulsiveness and sensation seeking behavior) and deficit in executive functions favor alcohol use among adolescents. Studies show brain alterations that precede the alcohol among adolescents, which includes reduced gray matter volumes, less connectivity between PFC and limbic regions, and reduced white matter integrity. On the other hand, alcohol use among adolescents is also associated with attention deficits, verbal learning and memory, lower cognitive flexibility, and disinhibition. This alcohol use is related to the gray matter reduction, lower connectivity between the PFC and limbic regions, and a lower white matter integrity (Spear 2018).

Adolescence is a development stage in which a greater engagement in risk behaviors is observed and sensation seeking in different species (Spear 2013, 2016). These behavior seems to be associated with a more active reward system (associated with Nacc) and a less active avoidance circuitry (associated with amygdala), compared to adults. This would explain risk-taking and reward-seeking behaviors (Ernst et al. 2005). In addition, the peak activation of mesolimbic and mesocortical pathways seems to occur during adolescence, and these pathways are more sensitive to reinforcing events among adolescents than adults (Spear 2018). Additionally, some studies also highlight a reduced PFC *top-down* control (Casey and Jones 2010; Spear 2013). Consequently, there is an imbalance between the inhibitory controlling circuitry and the reward system in the adolescent brain. Finally, evidence suggests that these changes in neural connections are at least partly dependent on the experiences lived (Spear 2018). Thus, adolescence is an adaptive period of relevant importance in the specialization of brain systems that will allow the cognitive control characteristic of later stages of development (Luna et al. 2015).

One of the critical systems for brain development is the endocannabinoid, being related to the neuronal refinement during adolescence (Arain et al. 2013). Alcohol and marijuana are examples of substances that act on this system. Therefore, using these during adolescence may alter the normal CNS development. In fact, evidence suggests that alcohol drinking during adolescence, with or without marijuana, is associated with changes in the trajectories of normal development of white and gray matter (Pfefferbaum et al. 2018). These changes seem to be related particularly to heavy marijuana use and especially *binge drinking* (consumption of five or more standard doses of alcohol among men or four or more among women on the same occasion; which are more prevalent among adolescents) (Squeglia and Gray 2016).

Finally, it is important to highlight that in addition to the neurobiological characteristics associated with risk taking and decision-making among adolescents, adolescents are particularly susceptible to peer influences. In this regard, risky decision-making in groups is particularly frequent among adolescents rather than adults (Gardner and Steinberg 2005). Evidence suggests that this greater susceptibility to peer influence during adolescence is related to a reduced neural connectivity associated with impulse control (Steinberg 2008).

Final Considerations

The long process of brain development and maturation that began in the first weeks after fertilization will take almost three decades to complete. This process will be the result of individual factors (biological, psychological, and social) that are in constant interaction with the environment. This chapter highlighted the neurobiological processes relevant to normal brain maturation, such as myelinization and synaptic pruning. However, due to the drug effects on the CNS, they alter brain normal functioning, and potentially affecting several important regions yet to be maturated. At the same time, substance use is also affected by changes in the normal brain development. In particular, the impact of drug use in two critical periods of human development has been highlighted, emphasizing that any exposure to drugs during pregnancy can cause harms to the unborn and how drug use affects regions of the brain that are both related to normal development and drug use.

References

Arain, M., Haque, M., Johal, L., Mathur, P., Nel, W., Rais, A., et al. (2013). Maturation of the adolescent brain. *Neuropsychiatric Disease and Treatment, 9*, 449–461. https://doi.org/10.2147/NDT.S39776.

Azevedo, F. A., Carvalho, L. R., Grinberg, L. T., Farfel, J. M., Ferretti, R. E., Leite, R. E., et al. (2009). Equal numbers of neuronal and nonneuronal cells make the human brain an isometrically scaled-up primate brain. *The Journal of Comparative Neurology, 513*(5), 532–541. https://doi.org/10.1002/cne.21974.

Baer, J. S., Sampson, P. D., Barr, H. M., Connor, P. D., & Streissguth, A. P. (2003). A 21-year longitudinal analysis of the effects of prenatal alcohol exposure on young adult drinking. *JAMA Psychiatry, 60*(4), 377–385. https://doi.org/10.1001/archpsyc.60.4.377.

Carson, G., Cox, L. V., Crane, J., Croteau, P., Graves, L., Kluka, S., et al. (2017). No. 245-alcohol use and pregnancy consensus clinical guidelines. *Journal of Obstetrics and Gynaecology Canada, 39*(9), e220–e254. https://doi.org/10.1016/j.jogc.2017.06.005.

Casey, B. J. (2015). Beyond simple models of self-control to circuit-based accounts of adolescent behavior. *Annual Review of Psychology, 66*, 295–319. https://doi.org/10.1146/annurev-psych-010814-015156.

Casey, B. J., Galvan, A., & Somerville, L. H. (2016). Beyond simple models of adolescence to an integrated circuit-based account: A commentary. *Developmental Cognitive Neuroscience, 17*, 128–130. https://doi.org/10.1016/j.dcn.2015.12.006.

Casey, B. J., Heller, A. S., Gee, D. G., & Cohen, A. O. (2019). Development of the emotional brain. *Neuroscience Letters, 693*, 29–34. https://doi.org/10.1016/j.neulet.2017.11.055.

Casey, B. J., & Jones, R. M. (2010). Neurobiology of the adolescent brain and behavior: Implications for substance use disorders. *Journal of the American Academy of Child and Adolescent Psychiatry, 49*(12), 1189–1201; quiz 1285. https://doi.org/10.1016/j.jaac.2010.08.017.

Chambers, R. A., Taylor, J. R., & Potenza, M. N. (2003). Developmental neurocircuitry of motivation in adolescence: A critical period of addiction vulnerability. *The American Journal of Psychiatry, 160*, 1041–1052. https://doi.org/10.1176/appi.ajp.160.6.1041.

Deoni, S. C., Mercure, E., Blasi, A., Gasston, D., Thomson, A., Johnson, M., et al. (2011). Mapping infant brain myelination with magnetic resonance imaging. *The Journal of Neuroscience, 31*(2), 784–791. https://doi.org/10.1523/JNEUROSCI.2106-10.2011.

Di Chiara, G. (2002). Nucleus accumbens shell and core dopamine: Differential role in behavior and addiction. *Behavioural Brain Research, 137*(1–2), 75–114.

Ernst, M., Nelson, E. E., Jazbec, S., McClure, E. B., Monk, C. S., Leibenluft, E., et al. (2005). Amygdala and nucleus accumbens in responses to receipt and omission of gains in adults and adolescents. *NeuroImage, 25*(4), 1279–1291. https://doi.org/10.1016/j.neuroimage.2004.12.038.

Floyd, R. L., Jack, B. W., Cefalo, R., Atrash, H., Mahoney, J., Herron, A., et al. (2008). The clinical content of preconception care: Alcohol, tobacco, and illicit drug exposures. *American Journal of Obstetrics and Gynecology, 199*(6 Suppl 2), S333–S339. https://doi.org/10.1016/j.ajog.2008.09.018.

Gardner, M., & Steinberg, L. (2005). Peer influence on risk taking, risk preference, and risky decision making in adolescence and adulthood: An experimental study. *Developmental Psychology, 41*(4), 625–635. https://doi.org/10.1037/0012-1649.41.4.625.

Gazzaniga, M. S. (2008). *Human: The science behind what makes us unique*. New York, NY: Ecco.

Giedd, J. N. (2008). The teen brain: Insights from neuroimaging. *The Journal of Adolescent Health, 42*(4), 335–343. https://doi.org/10.1016/j.jadohealth.2008.01.007.

Giedd, J. N., Raznahan, A., Alexander-Bloch, A., Schmitt, E., Gogtay, N., & Rapoport, J. L. (2015). Child psychiatry branch of the National Institute of Mental Health longitudinal structural magnetic resonance imaging study of human brain development. *Neuropsychopharmacology, 40*(1), 43–49. https://doi.org/10.1038/npp.2014.236.

Gogtay, N., Giedd, J. N., Lusk, L., Hayashi, K. M., Greenstein, D., Vaituzis, A. C., et al. (2004). Dynamic mapping of human cortical development during childhood through early adulthood. *Proceedings of the National Academy of Sciences of the United States of America, 101*(21), 8174–8179. https://doi.org/10.1073/pnas.0402680101.

Gogtay, N., & Thompson, P. M. (2010). Mapping gray matter development: Implications for typical development and vulnerability to psychopathology. *Brain and Cognition, 72*(1), 6–15. https://doi.org/10.1016/j.bandc.2009.08.009.

Goldstein, R. Z., & Volkow, N. D. (2002). Drug addiction and its underlying neurobiological basis: Neuroimaging evidence for the involvement of the frontal cortex. *The American Journal of Psychiatry, 159*(10), 1642–1652. https://doi.org/10.1176/appi.ajp.159.10.1642.

Herculano-Houzel, S. (2009). The human brain in numbers: A linearly scaled-up primate brain. *Frontiers in Human Neuroscience, 3*, 31. https://doi.org/10.3389/neuro.09.031.2009.

Herculano-Houzel, S. (2011a). Brains matter, bodies maybe not: The case for examining neuron numbers irrespective of body size. *Annals of the New York Academy of Sciences, 1225*, 191–199. https://doi.org/10.1111/j.1749-6632.2011.05976.x.

Herculano-Houzel, S. (2011b). Scaling of brain metabolism with a fixed energy budget per neuron: Implications for neuronal activity, plasticity and evolution. *PLoS One, 6*(3), e17514. https://doi.org/10.1371/journal.pone.0017514.

Huttenlocher, P. R. (1990). Morphometric study of human cerebral cortex development. *Neuropsychologia, 28*(6), 517–527. https://doi.org/10.1016/0028-3932(90)90031-i.

Huttenlocher, P. R., & Dabholkar, A. S. (1997). Regional differences in synaptogenesis in human cerebral cortex. *The Journal of Comparative Neurology, 387*(2), 167–178. https://doi.org/10.1002/(sici)1096-9861(19971020)387:2<167::aid-cne1>3.0.co;2-z.

Koob, G. F., & Le Moal, M. (2005). *Neurobiology of addiction*. Cambridge, MA: Academic Press.

Koob, G. F., & Le Moal, M. (2008). Addiction and the brain antireward system. *Annual Review of Psychology, 59*, 29–53. https://doi.org/10.1146/annurev.psych.59.103006.093548.

Koob, G. F., & Volkow, N. D. (2016). Neurobiology of addiction: A neurocircuitry analysis. *Lancet Psychiatry, 3*(8), 760–773. https://doi.org/10.1016/S2215-0366(16)00104-8.

Lent, R. (2010). *Cem Bilhões de Neurônios? - Conceitos Fundamentais de Neurociência* (2nd ed.). Rio de Janeiro, Brazil: Atheneu.

Luna, B., Marek, S., Larsen, B., Tervo-Clemmens, B., & Chahal, R. (2015). An integrative model of the maturation of cognitive control. *Annual Review of Neuroscience, 38*, 151–170. https://doi.org/10.1146/annurev-neuro-071714-034054.

Ministério da Saúde. (2010). *Gestação de Alto Risco - Manual Técnico*. Brasília: Ministério da Saúde. Retrieved from http://bvsms.saude.gov.br/bvs/publicacoes/gestacao_alto_risco.pdf

National Health Service. (2017). *Drinking alcohol while pregnant - your pregnancy and baby guide*. London, UK: NHS. Retrieved from https://www.nhs.uk/conditions/pregnancy-and-baby/alcohol-medicines-drugs-pregnant/.

Owesson-White, C. A., Ariansen, J., Stuber, G. D., Cleaveland, N. A., Cheer, J. F., Wightman, R. M., & Carelli, R. M. (2009). Neural encoding of cocaine-seeking behavior is coincident with phasic dopamine release in the accumbens core and shell. *The European Journal of Neuroscience, 30*(6), 1117–1127. https://doi.org/10.1111/j.1460-9568.2009.06916.x.

Pfefferbaum, A., Kwon, D., Brumback, T., Thompson, W. K., Cummins, K., Tapert, S. F., et al. (2018). Altered brain developmental trajectories in adolescents after initiating drinking. *The American Journal of Psychiatry, 175*(4), 370–380. https://doi.org/10.1176/appi.ajp.2017.17040469.

Raichle, M. E. (2006). The Brain's dark energy. *Science, 314*(5803), 1249–1250. https://doi.org/10.1126/science.1134405.

Raichle, M. E., & Mintun, M. A. (2006). Brain work and brain imaging. *Annual Review of Neuroscience, 29*, 449–476. https://doi.org/10.1146/annurev.neuro.29.051605.112819.

Schultz, W. (2002). Getting formal with dopamine and reward. *Neuron, 36*(2), 241–263.

Silbereis, J. C., Pochareddy, S., Zhu, Y., Li, M., & Sestan, N. (2016). The cellular and molecular landscapes of the developing human central nervous system. *Neuron, 89*(2), 248–268. https://doi.org/10.1016/j.neuron.2015.12.008.

Sowell, E. R., Thompson, P. M., Mattson, S. N., Tessner, K. D., Jernigan, T. L., Riley, E. P., & Toga, A. W. (2002). Regional brain shape abnormalities persist into adolescence after heavy prenatal alcohol exposure. *Cerebral Cortex, 12*(8), 856–865. https://doi.org/10.1093/cercor/12.8.856.

Spear, L. P. (2013). Adolescent neurodevelopment. *The Journal of Adolescent Health, 52*(2 Suppl 2), S7–S13. https://doi.org/10.1016/j.jadohealth.2012.05.006.

Spear, L. P. (2016). Alcohol consumption in adolescence: A translational perspective. *Current Addiction Reports, 3*(1), 50–61. https://doi.org/10.1007/s40429-016-0088-9.

Spear, L. P. (2018). Effects of adolescent alcohol consumption on the brain and behaviour. *Nature Reviews. Neuroscience, 19*(4), 197–214. https://doi.org/10.1038/nrn.2018.10.

Squeglia, L. M., & Gray, K. M. (2016). Alcohol and drug use and the developing brain. *Current Psychiatry Reports, 18*(5), 46. https://doi.org/10.1007/s11920-016-0689-y.

Steinberg, L. (2008). A social neuroscience perspective on adolescent risk-taking. *Developmental Review, 28*(1), 78–106. https://doi.org/10.1016/j.dr.2007.08.002.

Tang, Y., Nyengaard, J. R., De Groot, D. M., & Gundersen, H. J. (2001). Total regional and global number of synapses in the human brain neocortex. *Synapse, 41*(3), 258–273. https://doi.org/10.1002/syn.1083.

Volkow, N. D., Koob, G. F., & McLellan, A. T. (2016). Neurobiologic advances from the brain disease model of addiction. *The New England Journal of Medicine, 374*(4), 363–371. https://doi.org/10.1056/NEJMra1511480.

Volkow, N. D., & Morales, M. (2015). The brain on drugs: From reward to addiction. *Cell, 162*(4), 712–725. https://doi.org/10.1016/j.cell.2015.07.046.

Volkow, N. D., Tomasi, D., Wang, G. J., Logan, J., Alexoff, D. L., Jayne, M., et al. (2014). Stimulant-induced dopamine increases are markedly blunted in active cocaine abusers. *Molecular Psychiatry, 19*(9), 1037–1043. https://doi.org/10.1038/mp.2014.58.

Volkow, N. D., Wang, G. J., Fowler, J. S., Logan, J., Gatley, S. J., Hitzemann, R., et al. (1997). Decreased striatal dopaminergic responsiveness in detoxified cocaine-dependent subjects. *Nature, 386*(6627), 830–833. https://doi.org/10.1038/386830a0.

Volkow, N. D., Wang, G. J., Fowler, J. S., Tomasi, D., Telang, F., & Baler, R. (2010). Addiction: Decreased reward sensitivity and increased expectation sensitivity conspire to overwhelm the brain's control circuit. *BioEssays, 32*(9), 748–755. https://doi.org/10.1002/bies.201000042.

Wiers, C. E., & Heinz, A. (2015). Neurobiology of alcohol craving and relapse prediction: Implications for diagnosis and treatment. In S. J. Wilson (Ed.), *The Wiley handbook on the cognitive neuroscience of addiction* (pp. 219–239). Chichester, UK: Wiley.

World Health Organization (WHO). (2004). *Neuroscience of psychoactive substance use and dependence*. Geneva, Switzerland: World Health Organization.

Chapter 10
Effects of Substance Use on Neural Development

Hudelson dos Passos and Ian Carlos Hübner

Introduction

Teratology refers to the branch of science that studies environmental contributions to prenatal development. Teratology studies began in the second half of the twentieth century when the discovery of congenital rubella showed that the fetus is not fully protected against exogenous organisms (Webster 1998). The most striking period in the history of teratology was the thalidomide tragedy, which occurred in the 1960s and affected thousands of individuals worldwide (Moro and Invernizzi 2017).

Teratogen or teratogenic agent is a given name for any substance, organism, physical agent, or state of deficiency, external to the genome, which when present during the embryonic or fetal period causes changes in the structure or function of the offspring (Dicke 1989), or "any physical, chemical or biological agent that can cause morphofunctional changes to an organism during its embryonic or fetal development" (Sette et al. 2017, pp. 295–296). Thus, psychoactive substances can be considered teratogenic when they produce deleterious effects on the development of the Nervous System (NS) in the prenatal period.

The influence of teratogens on the development of the embryo or fetus will depend on several factors, the most relevant being the stage of development of the concept (variability of susceptibility to teratogenic agents according to the stage of development), the relationship between dose and effect (teratogenic influence increases according to dose and effect criteria), and the maternal–fetal genotype (the genetic heterogeneity of the mother or fetus may suggest greater predisposition

H. dos Passos
Faculdade Guilherme Guimbala, Joinville, SC, Brazil

I. C. Hübner (✉)
Sociedade Educacional de Santa Catarina - Unisociesc, Joinville, SC, Brazil

D. De Micheli et al. (eds.), *Drugs and Human Behavior*,
https://doi.org/10.1007/978-3-030-62855-0_10

or resistance to the influence of a particular agent) (De Micheli et al. 2016; Schüler-Faccini et al. 2011).

The emergence of NS occurs relatively late in the course of embryonic development, the first processes leading to the emergence of NS occur around the third gestational week in which the ectoderm, one of the three embryonic leaflets, begins to differentiate and originates the neural tube through the process of neurulation (Jessel and Sanes 2014), but the nervous system will only complete its maturation process during the second decade of life of individuals through different structural mechanisms of development (Silbereis et al. 2016).

The integral period of structuring and maturation of the nervous system is called neurodevelopment, and it encompasses embryological and fetal processes and goes through phenomena of childhood, adolescence, and the consolidation of maturation in adult life, making NS one of the most complex and time-consuming systems to fully establish itself.

During the gestational period, the most drastic changes in NS occur, originating and maturing in most of the nerve and glial cells and the structuring of the central and peripheral nervous system (Bear et al. 2017), damage to these structural processes of NS can lead to long-term losses, affecting the other development processes (Andrade et al. 2014). In addition to prenatal development processes, several mechanisms of maturation and change continue throughout childhood and adolescence, allowing better adjustment of NS to the environment. These processes of structural and functional modification of NS in response to the environment are called neuroplasticity (Ismail et al. 2017).

Neuroplasticity can be understood in three different types during normal NS development; experience-expectant, experience-dependent, and experience-independent. Experience-independent plasticity occurs by phylogenetic mechanisms and does not depend on external stimuli for it to occur; experience-dependent plasticity requires external but non-specific stimuli and can occur at any time in life, such as modifications that occur in response to learning. Finally, experience-expectant plasticity occurs only in specific periods and requires adequate stimuli, corresponding to critical periods of development (Kolb and Gibb 2014).

Given the changing nature of NS during development, any change leading to a functional or structural change in the brain outside the expected limits can lead to deficits in cognitive, behavioral, and emotional development. Substances such as psychoactive drugs, act in SN and when exposed during their development produce functional changes and can lead to long-term changes in brain structures (Piper and Meyer 2017).

The first years of life are fundamental for the development of skills that will serve as a basis for the emergence of new and more complex ones, which will allow children to adapt to the new environmental demands that will arise over time (Muszkat and Rizzutti, 2018). In the first months of life, human babies are able to respond to maternal facial expressions; at the age of 2 they already show greater abilities to name emotions; at around 3 they are able to report emotional experiences and at 4 they tend to be able to perceive that emotional reactions can vary among people (Muszkat and Rizzutti 2018; Muszkat et al. 2014).

In this period, essential skills are developed, such as broad and fine motor skills, visuospatial skills, self-regulation and self-monitoring, elaboration and generalization of strategies, mathematical skills, reasoning, memory, linguistic and verbal skills, formation of concepts and categories, ability to infer mental states of others, and consciousness and feelings of oneself (Mecca et al. 2014). In a hierarchical process of development, these skills are necessary for later learning of other more complex and elaborate skills, such as Executive Functions (EF).

The EF subcomponents are, among others, planning, decision making, inhibitory control, cognitive flexibility, work memory, and selective attention. One of the theoretical proposals (Diamond 2013) about EF proposes that they are based on three basic skills: (a) Inhibition/inhibitory control: ability to inhibit inappropriate behavior (self-control) and to manage interference, inhibiting attention to distractors (this ability is called selective attention), unwanted memories and thoughts (ability called cognitive inhibition); (b) Working memory: ability to maintain information for a short period of time and manipulate it mentally (updating it, transforming it, etc.); (c) Cognitive flexibility: it is the most complex of them, because it demands the previous ones. It refers to the ability to think from different perspectives, change the focus of attention between tasks, or even think from different perspectives of your own (Dias and Trevisan 2018).

In addition to the prenatal period, exposure to drugs that act on NS during the entire development can lead to functional changes that cause harm to individuals. Adolescence is another period of great importance for neurodevelopment and for exposure to drugs, because in this period the beginning of substance use usually occurs and the effect on psychological aspects may become more evident (Squeglia and Gray 2016). Adolescence is characterized by drastic changes in the brain reward circuit, changing the pattern of release and response to dopamine, an important neurotransmitter for the pleasure process related to the use of substances, facilitating their use as a way to achieve more intense rewards (Galván 2010).

Adolescence is the period in which various psychological and cognitive functions begin to establish and intensify, including EF that allow behavior control and planning of less immediate goals, exposure to drugs in this period, and impairing the normal development of these functions can lead to greater susceptibility to the development of addiction behavior and create problems that last for life (Crews et al. 2007).

Adolescence can be considered a critical period for the development of complex mental functions, in this period a series of neuroplastic changes occurs that allow the maturation of the regions involved in these functions, especially between those associative of the cortex and the prefrontal cortex. It can be highlighted that in this period there is the maturation of inhibitory GABAergic interneuron groups in the cortex, which allows a greater control and response to environmental stimuli, a change in the expression of *neurotrophic* factors such as the *brain-derived neurotrophic factor* (BDNF) in the prefrontal cortex, the maturation of dopaminergic pathways related to learning and reward, and finally, the myelinization of these pathways (Larsen and Luna 2018).

Psychoactive Drugs and the Neurodevelopment

There are several classes of psychoactive drugs with different intrinsic mechanisms which will generate a range of physiological and behavioral responses, but all of which have the ability to functionally alter the central nervous system, in Table 10.1 are the main examples of substances and the summary of their neurophysiological mechanism. As the study on the consequences of the use of some of these substances on neurodevelopment does not yet have robust results, it was chosen to talk about some of the most common abuse drugs, alcohol, marijuana, tobacco, and cocaine.

Prenatal Alcohol Exposure (PAE) is one of the largest preventable causes of intellectual disability in the world and the prevalence of alcohol use during any period of pregnancy exceeds 9%, and in Brazil it can exceed 15% (Popova et al. 2017). Children with PAE can present several alterations in distinct processes of development that include impaired growth, craniofacial abnormalities, behavioral alterations, and in the central nervous system (Lange et al. 2013).

The term Fetal Alcohol Spectrum Disorder (FASD) is used to encompass the wide range of symptoms and differences resulting from exposure to alcohol in different gestational periods and drinking patterns (Andrade et al., 2014; Riley et al. 2011). The most severe form of symptoms caused by PAE is Fetal Alcohol Syndrome (FAS), which has as criteria for diagnosis prenatal and/or postnatal growth failure; Central nervous system dysfunction resulting in cognitive, motor, and behavioral problems; and a characteristic pattern of facial abnormalities such as middle-face hypoplasia, spaced eyes, and smooth filter (Riley et al. 2011).

The effects of the PAE differ by the amount of alcohol consumed and the gestational period in which exposure occurred, and in the first trimester of human pregnancy exposure to alcohol can cause eye malformations (Strömland 2004). Studies

Table 10.1 Summary of pharmacological mechanisms of major psychoactive drugs

Substance	Primary action mechanism	Behavioral effects
Cannabinoids	They activate the cannabinoid receptors. They also increase dopamine activity in the mesolimbic passage	Relaxation, increased sensory perception, decreased short-term memory, motor incoordination, analgesia, antiemetic, and anti-epileptic effects, increased appetite.
Cocaine	Cocaine prevents the recapture of transmitters such as dopamine, thus prolonging its effects.	Increased alertness, energy, and motor activity, sense of competence; euphoria, anxiety, restlessness, paranoia.
Ethanol	It increases the inhibitory effects of GABA and decreases the excitement effects of glutamate.	Sedation, impaired memory, motor incoordination, decreased anxiety.
Nicotine	Activates nicotinic cholinergic receptors. Increases dopamine synthesis and release.	Increased alertness, attention, concentration, and memory; decreased anxiety and appetite; stimulant-like effects.

Source: Adapted from World Health Organization (2006)

in animal models show that PAE can modify the normal development of the tube and neural crest and can lead to the microcephaly observed in humans (Miller 1996) and the facial dysmorphology characteristic of FAS (Sulik et al. 1981). In these models, exposure during the second trimester equivalent was also observed to affect cell migration, proliferation time and reduce the number of neuronal and glial cells in many brain areas (Aronne et al. 2011). Finally, studies in the area still show that during the third trimester exposure to alcohol can increase cell death, compromise synaptogenesis, and lead to persistent deficits in neuronal plasticity, executive functions, and learning and memory processes (Wozniak et al. 2004; Isayama et al. 2009).

Alcohol consumption during adolescence can also lead to changes in the central nervous system and its consequent neurocognitive changes. Alterations in the volume of the hippocampus, prefrontal cortex, and cerebellum were observed in adolescents who consumed alcohol. In addition, alterations in the thickness of the cerebral cortex of adolescents who consumed large amounts of alcohol acutely were found, which may indicate alterations in brain maturation (Squeglia et al. 2014). In addition to brain changes, individuals who make continuous use of alcohol during adolescence also demonstrate cognitive and behavioral changes, such as lower performance in verbal learning and memory, deficits in visuospatial functioning, altered speed of psychomotor response, and decreased performance in working memory (Squeglia and Gray 2016).

Exposure to cannabinoids present in marijuana during pregnancy can also lead to changes in NS development generating neurocognitive changes throughout life. Richardson et al. (2016) evaluating the main longitudinal studies that followed individuals who were exposed to marijuana during pregnancy found cognitive and behavioral changes in childhood such as impaired performance in memory tasks and verbal skills, attentional and reasoning problems, as well as increased hyperactivity and impulsiveness. In adolescence some of these changes have persisted, and the attentional problems have remained, as well as impaired performance in tasks that demand executive functioning, reasoning skills, hyperactivity, and impulsiveness has also been perceived, in addition to the presence of externalizing behaviors such as delinquency.

Individuals who use marijuana during adolescence present cognitive alterations such as attention deficits, learning and memory problems, and perseverance in response, having more difficulties in changing strategies according to the environment, in agreement, adolescents in abstinence from marijuana from 3 to 4 weeks presented deficits in memory, attention, planning, and psychomotor speed compared to adolescents who did not use the substance (Lubman et al. 2015).

Some studies also indicate neuroanatomic changes in the brains of adolescents who use marijuana, smaller volumes of gray matter and total cortex were found, changes in prefrontal and insular cortical thickness, smaller volume of the medial orbitofrontal cortex, asymmetry in the volume of the hippocampus and amygdala, in addition, individuals who make heavy use show greater reduction in the volume of prefrontal cortex regions and the early onset of use was also related to greater changes in the prefrontal cortex (Lubman et al. 2015).

Cocaine also has the capacity to alter the development of individuals exposed during the gestational period, since it is a small molecule with good capacity to cross the placenta and quickly reach the fetus a few minutes after use (Gkioka et al. 2016). Some structural changes were observed in the brains of exposed newborns during pregnancy, the research of the group of Grewen et al. (2014) showed lower volumes of gray matter in the prefrontal and frontal cortical regions of these individuals, these areas being important for executive functions and inhibitory control, and also showed increased cerebrospinal fluid indicating neuronal abnormality.

Behavioral and cognitive alterations can also be observed in these individuals, already in childhood motor alterations can be perceived, such as a lower performance in fine motor skills and greater movement after an initial stimulation, in social relations, individuals exposed to cocaine tend to demonstrate more externalizing problems in school period, in adolescence cognitive alterations become more evident, such as deficits in working memory, learning and visual and verbal memory, visuospatial memory and short-term memory, besides attentional problems (Gkioka et al. 2016).

Animal model studies have shown that exposure of cocaine during adolescence induces prolonged changes in synapses of the medial prefrontal cortex, indicating long-term neuropsychiatric and behavioral changes in adult life. Moreover, in adult life, individuals showed a permanent increase in GABAergic transmission in pyramidal neurons, inhibiting the action of these neurons and consequently contributing to the development of neuropsychiatric disorders (Shi et al. 2019).

The use of tobacco during pregnancy varies widely among countries and regions, with the world prevalence of cigarette use during pregnancy being 1.7%, but with great difference in intensity and frequency of use due to cultural issues in each region of the world (Crume 2019). Exposure to tobacco and its components, including nicotine, affects the development of various physiological systems, but has deleterious effects mainly on the central nervous system (Holbrook 2016).

The use of tobacco in pregnancy is related to several complications at the beginning of life and can even lead to sudden infant death syndrome in more serious situations and can cause changes in cognitive and behavioral development, such as a reduction in IQ scores, greater aggressive and antisocial behavior, which can lead to the appearance of conduct disorder, in addition to greater impulsiveness and higher incidence of diagnosis of attention deficit hyperactivity disorder (ADHD) (Minnes et al. 2011).

Exposure to nicotine during adolescence can lead to attentional and work memory deficits and this seems to be related to altered activity of the prefrontal cortex, in addition, these individuals also exhibit more impulsive behaviors and less inhibitory control and a greater chance of developing lifelong substance use disorders (Counotte et al. 2011).

Final Considerations

In this chapter, it was possible to present some aspects of neurodevelopment (especially the embryonic, fetal, childhood, and adolescent periods), as well as the influence it suffers from the use of some of the main psychoactive drugs. Some of the most common psychoactive drugs, such as cannabinoids, cocaine, ethanol and nicotine, offer different risk potentials for neurodevelopment.

The central nervous system, sensitive to exposure to psychoactive drugs during neurodevelopment, suffers from influences that can lead to various alterations in its maturational and neuroplastic processes, which have repercussions on functional alterations in behavior and cognition throughout the life of individuals, these alterations can occur through the teratogenic effect when exposure occurs during pregnancy or through direct use, especially in adolescence.

The study on psychoactive drugs and neurodevelopment needs more research, especially at the national level, in order to better understand the effect of these substances on neurodevelopment so that prevention, evaluation, and intervention practices become even more effective.

References

Andrade, A. L. M., De Micheli, D., & Fisberg, M. (2014). Cognitive Aspects of Fetal Alcohol Syndrome in Young Adults: Two Case Studies. *Interação em Psicologia, 17*(2), 217–223. https://doi.org/10.5380/psi.v17i2.27359

Aronne, M. P., Guadagnoli, T., Fontanet, P., Evrard, S. G., & Brusco, A. (2011). Effects of prenatal ethanol exposure on rat brain radial glia and neuroblast migration. *Experimental Neurology, 229*(2), 364–371. https://doi.org/10.1016/j.expneurol.2011.03.002.

Bear, M. F., Connors, B. W., & Paradiso, M. A. (2017). Conectando o encéfalo. In M. F. Bear, B. W. Connors, & M. A. Paradiso (Eds.), *Neurociências: desvendando o sistema nervoso* (4th ed., pp. 781–822). Porto Alegre: Artmed.

Counotte, D. S., Smit, A. B., Pattij, T., & Spijker, S. (2011). Development of the motivational system during adolescence, and its sensitivity to disruption by nicotine. *Developmental Cognitive Neuroscience, 1*(4), 430–443. https://doi.org/10.1016/j.dcn.2011.05.010.

Crews, F., He, J., & Hodge, C. (2007). Adolescent cortical development: a critical period of vulnerability for addiction. *Pharmacology Biochemistry and Behavior, 86*(2), 189–199. https://doi.org/10.1016/j.pbb.2006.12.001.

Crume, T. (2019). Tobacco use during pregnancy. *Clinical Obstetrics and Gynecology, 62*(1), 128–141. https://doi.org/10.1097/GRF.0000000000000413.

De Micheli, D. Andrade, A. L. M., Silva, E. A. & Souza-Formigoni, M. L. O. (2016). Drug Abuse in Adolescence. 1. ed. New York: Springer International Publishing. http://doi.org/10.1007/978-3-319-17795-3

Diamond, A. (2013). Executive functions. *Annual Review of Psychology, 64*, 135–168.

Dias, N. M., & Trevisan, B. T. (2018). Como avaliar funções executivas em uma criança pré-escolar? In N. M. Dias & A. G. Seabra (Eds.), *Neuropsicologia com pré-escolares: Avaliação e intervenção* (pp. 119–134). São Paulo: Pearson Clinical Brasil.

Dicke, J. M. (1989). Teratology: principles and practice. *Medical Clinics of North America, 73*, 567–582.

Galván, A. (2010). Adolescent development of the reward system. *Frontiers in Human Neuroscience, 4*, 6. https://doi.org/10.1016/s0025-7125(16)30658-7.
Gkioka, E., Korou, L. M., Daskalopoulou, A., Misitzi, A., Batsidis, E., Bakoyiannis, I., & Pergialiotis, V. (2016). Prenatal cocaine exposure and its impact on cognitive functions of offspring: a pathophysiological insight. *Reviews in the Neurosciences, 27*(5), 523–534. https://doi.org/10.1515/revneuro-2015-0064.
Grewen, K., Burchinal, M., Vachet, C., Gouttard, S., Gilmore, J. H., Lin, W., et al. (2014). Prenatal cocaine effects on brain structure in early infancy. *Neuroimage, 101*, 114–123. https://doi.org/10.1016/j.neuroimage.2014.06.070.
Holbrook, B. D. (2016). The effects of nicotine on human fetal development. *Birth Defects Research Part C: Embryo Today: Reviews, 108*(2), 181–192. https://doi.org/10.1002/bdrc.21128.
Isayama, R. N., Leite, P. E. C., Lima, J. P. M., Uziel, D., & Yamasaki, E. N. (2009). Impact of ethanol on the developing GABAergic system. *The Anatomical Record, 292*(12), 1922–1939. https://doi.org/10.1002/ar.20966.
Ismail, F. Y., Fatemi, A., & Johnston, M. V. (2017). Cerebral plasticity: windows of opportunity in the developing brain. *European Journal of Paediatric Neurology, 21*(1), 23–48. https://doi.org/10.1016/j.ejpn.2016.07.007.
Jessel, T. M., & Sanes, J. R. (2014). A estruturação do sistema nervoso. In E. R. Kandel, J. H. Schwartz, T. M. Jessel, S. A. Siegelbaum, & A. J. Hudspeht (Eds.), *Princípios de Neurociências* (5th ed., pp. 1015–1033). Porto Alegre: AMGH.
Kolb, B., & Gibb, R. (2014). Searching for the principles of brain plasticity and behavior. *Cortex, 58*, 251–260. https://doi.org/10.1016/j.cortex.2013.11.012.
Lange, S., Shield, K., Rehm, J., & Popova, S. (2013). Prevalence of fetal alcohol spectrum disorders in child care settings: a meta-analysis. *Pediatrics, 132*(4), e980–e995. https://doi.org/10.1542/peds.2013-0066.
Larsen, B., & Luna, B. (2018). Adolescence as a neurobiological critical period for the development of higher-order cognition. *Neuroscience & Biobehavioral Reviews*. https://doi.org/10.1016/j.neubiorev.2018.09.005.
Lubman, D. I., Cheetham, A., & Yücel, M. (2015). Cannabis and adolescent brain development. *Pharmacology and Therapeutics, 148*, 1–16. https://doi.org/10.1016/j.pharmthera.2014.11.009.
Mecca, T. P., Antônio, D. A., Rabelo, I. S., Valentini, F., & Macedo, E. C. (2014). Avaliação da inteligência em crianças pré-escolares. In A. G. Seabra, J. A. Laros, E. C. Macedo, & N. Abreu (Eds.), *Inteligência e funções executivas: Avanços e desafios para a avaliação neuropsicológica* (pp. 141–170). São Paulo: Memnon.
Miller, M. W. (1996). Effect of early exposure to ethanol on the protein and DNA contents of specific brain regions in the rat. *Brain Research, 734*(1-2), 286–294. https://doi.org/10.1016/0006-8993(96)00651-8.
Minnes, S., Lang, A., & Singer, L. (2011). Prenatal tobacco, marijuana, stimulant, and opiate exposure: outcomes and practice implications. *Addiction Science and Clinical Practice, 6*(1), 57.
Moro, A., & Invernizzi, N. (2017). A tragédia da talidomida: a luta pelos direitos das vítimas e por melhor regulação de medicamentos. *História, Ciências, Saúde, 24*(3), 603–622. https://doi.org/10.1590/s0104-59702017000300004.
Muszkat, M., Araripe, B. L., Andrade, N. C., & Muñoz, P. d. (2014). Neuropsicologia do autismo. In D. Fuentes, L. F. Malloy-Diniz, C. P. Camargo, & R. M. Cosenza (Eds.), *Neuropsicologia teoria e prática* (pp. 183–191). Porto Alegre: Artmed.
Muszkat, M., & Rizzutti, S. (2018). Desenvolvimento neurológico no período pré-escolar e suas alterações. In N. M. Dias & A. G. Seabra (Eds.), *Neuropsicologia com pré-escolares: Avaliação e intervenção* (pp. 31–58). São Paulo: Pearson Clinical Brasil.
Organização Mundial da Saúde. (2006). *Neurociência do uso e da dependência de substâncias psicoativas*. São Paulo: Roca.
Piper, B. J., & Meyer, J. S. (2017). Developmental Neurotoxicity of Abused Drugs. In *Reproductive and Developmental Toxicology*. Cambridge: Academic Press.

Popova, S., Lange, S., Probst, C., Gmel, G., & Rehm, J. (2017). Estimation of national, regional, and global prevalence of alcohol use during pregnancy and fetal alcohol syndrome: a systematic review and meta-analysis. *The Lancet Global Health, 5*(3), e290–e299. https://doi.org/10.1016/S2214-109X(17)30021-9.

Richardson, K. A., Hester, A. K., & McLemore, G. L. (2016). Prenatal cannabis exposure-The "first hit" to the endocannabinoid system. *Neurotoxicology and Teratology, 58*, 5–14. https://doi.org/10.1016/j.ntt.2016.08.003.

Riley, E. P., Infante, M. A., & Warren, K. R. (2011). Fetal alcohol spectrum disorders: an overview. *Neuropsychology Review, 21*(2), 73. https://doi.org/10.1007/s11065-011-9166-x.

Schüler-Faccini, L., Sansaverino, M. T., Abeche, A. M., Vianna, F. S., & Silva, A. A. (2011). *Manual de teratogênese em humanos*. Rio de Janeiro: FEBRASGO.

Sette, N. L. F., Augusto, M. T., & Matarucco, C. R. (2017). A influência do consumo de substâncias teratogênicas durante o período gestacional na saúde materno-infantil. *Revista UNIFEV: Ciência & Tecnologia, 3*, 211–227.

Shi, J. C., Nie, J., Liu, H., Li, Y., Lu, X., Shen, X., Yuan, T. F., & Guan, X. (2019). Adolescent cocaine exposure enhances the GABAergic transmission in the prelimbic cortex of adult mice. *FASEB J, 33*(7), 8614–8622. https://doi.org/10.1096/fj.201802192rr.

Silbereis, J. C., Pochareddy, S., Zhu, Y., Li, M., & Sestan, N. (2016). The cellular and molecular landscapes of the developing human central nervous system. *Neuron, 89*(2), 248–268. https://doi.org/10.1016/j.neuron.2015.12.008.

Squeglia, L. M., & Gray, K. M. (2016). Alcohol and drug use and the developing brain. *Current Psychiatry Reports, 18*(5), 46. https://doi.org/10.1007/s11920-016-0689-y.

Squeglia, L. M., Jacobus, J., & Tapert, S. F. (2014). The effect of alcohol use on human adolescent brain structures and systems. In E. V. Sullivan & A. Pfefferbaum (Eds.), *Handbook of clinical neurology* (Vol. 125, pp. 501–510). https://doi.org/10.1016/B978-0-444-62619-6.00028-8.

Strömland, K. (2004). Visual impairment and ocular abnormalities in children with fetal alcohol syndrome. *Addiction Biology, 9*(2), 153–157. https://doi.org/10.1080/13556210410001717024

Sulik, K. K., Johnston, M. C., & Webb, M. A. (1981). Fetal alcohol syndrome: embryogenesis in a mouse model. *Science, 214*(4523), 936–938. https://doi.org/10.1126/science.6795717.

Webster, W. S. (1998). Teratogen update: congenital rubella. *Teratology, 58*(1), 13–23. https://doi.org/10.1002/tera.1420310216.

Wozniak, D. F., Hartman, R. E., Boyle, M. P., Vogt, S. K., Brooks, A. R., Tenkova, T., Young, C., Olney, J. W., & Muglia, L. J. (2004). Apoptotic neurodegeneration induced by ethanol in neonatal mice is associated with profound learning/memory deficits in juveniles followed by progressive functional recovery in adults. *Neurobiology of Disease, 17*(3), 403–414. https://doi.org/10.1016/j.nbd.2004.08.006.

Chapter 11
Neuropsychological and Behavioral Aspects of Drug Use and Abuse: Theory, Research, and Intervention

Fernanda Machado Lopes, Flávia Zacouteguy Boos, Adriana Mokwa Zanini, and Fernanda Rasch Czermainski

Introduction

The use of psychotropic substances (PS) is a phenomenon present throughout human history (Carlini et al. 1996). The PS, better known as drugs of abuse, are substances that, when introduced into the body, act in the central nervous system (CNS), altering the brain function and affecting to a greater or lesser degree the perception, mood, behavior, and consciousness. Unlike psychoactive substances (which also act in the CNS), the PS have significant potential to generate abuse and dependence. The variability in the use of PS suffered and still suffers the influence of multiple factors, such as social, cultural, and religious. Historically, the various sociocultural contexts are related to the presentation of substances, dosages, forms, and situations of consumption. Thus, the understanding of the behaviors of use of PS depends on the analysis not only of the pharmacological properties of such substances but also psychological, genetic, and neurodevelopmental aspects, in addition to the sociocultural context of those who consume them (Abreu & Malvasi, 2011).

The consumption of PS can vary from occasional or recreational use to drug abuse and dependence. However, an increasing number of people suffer from substance use disorders (SUDs), which is a significant public health problem. According to the World Drug Report (UNODC), of the 271 million people who took some drug

F. M. Lopes (✉)
Universidade Federal de Santa Catarina, Florianópolis, SC, Brazil

F. Z. Boos
Universidade Federal de São Paulo, São Paulo, SP, Brazil

A. M. Zanini
Instituto Porto Alegre da Igreja Metodista, Porto Alegre, RS, Brazil

F. R. Czermainski
Universidade Estácio de Sá, Rio de Janeiro, Brazil

D. De Micheli et al. (eds.), *Drugs and Human Behavior*,
https://doi.org/10.1007/978-3-030-62855-0_11

worldwide in 2016, 35 million (almost 13%) suffer from SUD; however, prevention and treatment remain insufficient in many parts of the world, and it is estimated that only one in seven people with SUD receives adequate treatment each year (UNODC – United Nations Office on Drugs and Crime 2019).

SUD includes ten distinct classes of drugs (alcohol, caffeine, marijuana, hallucinogens, inhalants, opioids, sedatives, hypnotics and anxiolytics, stimulants, tobacco, and other unknown substances), each with specific diagnostic criteria (American Psychiatric Association, 2014). Although the pharmacological mechanisms of each class of drugs are distinct, all have in common the activation of the brain reward system, associated with the reinforcement of behavior, through the modulation (release/inhibition) of neurotransmitters associated with the sensation of pleasure and relief of displeasure, and this change in brain activation may persist even after detoxification.

In general, SUD is characterized by loss of control over drug use or its exacerbated use, so that the consequences of this consumption begin to affect several areas of the individual's life, as well as its overall functioning (Koob & Volkow, 2010). A set of cognitive, behavioral, and physiological symptoms is usually present and indicates the continuous use by the individual, despite the significant problems resulting from the use of the substance (American Psychiatric Association 2014). As a consequence, the individual begins to manifest a recurrent failure in the mechanisms of control of consumption behavior, despite the negative consequences of great magnitude for his own life (Goodman, 2008; Pedrero-Pérez et al. 2011).

Research has understood SUD as disorders characterized by impulsivity and compulsion. Such studies suggest that individuals with a low level of self-control may be more likely to develop SUD compared to individuals who do not present deficits of this nature. Self-control difficulties may be associated with damage to brain mechanisms of inhibition, an important cognitive component whose deficits may have a meaningful impact on behavior (Fernandez-Serrano et al. 2012; Koob and Volkow, 2010; Volkow & Fowler, 2000). Moreover, studies suggest that SUDs are associated with cognitive and behavioral losses, mainly involving impairment of executive functions, memory, attention, inhibition, and flexibility, in addition to impulsive, compulsive, and aggressive behavior (Czermainski et al. 2017; Pedrero-Pérez & Sánchez de León, 2012; Rigoni et al. 2013; Tavares et al. 2012).

From this brief introduction, the complexity of the SUD study is evident. Multiple factors contribute to the consumption of PS, which is a challenge for researchers seeking to understand this phenomenon (Bedendo et al. 2015; De Micheli et al. 2020). Some of these factors, involving cognitive and behavioral aspects, seem to play an essential role in addictive behaviors and may influence the maintenance of abstinence and treatment success. This chapter aims to address the neuropsychological and behavioral aspects associated with drug use and abuse. Next, the classification of drugs related to the action on the CNS, as well as the main neuropsychological alterations associated with drug abuse, will be presented in a synthetic form.

Neuropsychological Aspects of Psychotropic Drugs

One of the most striking characteristics of addiction is the intense desire to obtain and consume the drug (craving), impulsiveness, compulsion, and difficulty in remaining abstinent despite the adverse physical, emotional, and social consequences this consumption may have. The literature points out that the continued use of drugs in the presence of specific environmental stimuli (such as certain people, paraphernalia of use, among others) can lead to the formation of associative memories, as well as frequent use at certain times (smoking after lunch or with friends) can lead to the formation of habits. Therefore, exposure to cues previously associated with the drug commonly induces craving and facilitates relapses even after long periods of abstinence; in addition, remaining without the drug in typical situations of use becomes much more difficult (Koob & Volkow, 2016; Perry & Lawrence, 2017).

In stock, the drugs of abuse activate the mesocorticolimbic dopaminergic pathway, also known as the reward system. This system is essential for the preservation of behaviors that are essential for maintaining life because, when activated, the individual tends to repeat them. Pleasant/rewarding natural stimuli, such as palatable food consumption and sex itself, activate this pathway (Volkow & Morales, 2015). This circuit is not exclusive to humans; its biological relevance is such that it is conserved in different animals, from invertebrates to other mammals. Thanks to this similarity—at different levels of complexity—many studies have been conducted in preclinical research (with animal models), and nowadays they help to understand better how drugs alter the functioning of the brain and behaviors, as well as can help to seek more effective treatments in the case of problematic drug use.

The mesocorticolimbic pathway consists of dopaminergic neurons of the ventral tegmental area (VTA) that project their axons to limbic regions involved with the detection of reward, such as the nucleus accumbens (NAc), with the emotions and acquisition of memories, such as the amygdala and hippocampus, as well as to cortical regions, such as different portions of the prefrontal cortex (PFC). The dorsal hippocampus and the basolateral amygdala are involved in the acquisition and retrieval of associative memories related to drug use, such as the environmental cues that "remind" the rewarding effects of a substance. The PFC regions, in turn, are involved in assigning value to a stimulus (in this case, the drug and stimuli associated with it, such as environmental cues) and executive functions (planning, inhibitory control, and decision-making). The signaling of reward is done mainly through the increase of dopamine in NAc; drug use, in particular, induces a hyper-stimulation of this system compared to natural rewards and causes positive subjective sensations, such as pleasure and euphoria, increasing the likelihood of behavior repeating itself. With continued use, over-stimulation of this system induces lasting changes in the standard functioning of neurons and brain circuits, with changes in the release of many neurotransmitters (dopamine, glutamate, GABA, serotonin, endogenous opioids, among others), levels of receptors, and in the connection between different brain regions (Koob & Volkow, 2016).

The overvaluation of drugs and their associated stimuli (incentive salience phenomenon—Berridge et al. 2009), to the detriment of other activities that previously generated pleasure, seems to be associated with a dopaminergic hypofunction in NAc. It contributes to the individual's reduction of behaviors related to the so-called natural pleasures and increases the frequency of drug-seeking and consumption behavior since this is the most intense pleasure stimulus. Areas of the PFC (anterior orbitofrontal and cingulate cortex), in turn, are involved in assigning value to drugs and overvaluing them and the environmental cues, which stand out in the environment for some chronic drug users, trigger craving, and facilitate relapses. The anterior cingulate, regions adjacent to the medial PFC next to the dorsal striatum, are related to inhibitory control and decision-making, and this is another impaired circuit in some samples of addicts (Volkow & Morales, 2015; Tang et al. 2015).

Morphofunctional changes in the orbitofrontal cortex can be perceived in cocaine addicts, as exemplified in a study using neuroimaging in which a reduction of the gray substance in this region (related to a hypofunction) was found, associated with the extension of the time of use and also with compulsion by the drug (Ersche et al. 2011). Although at baseline (in rest) the orbitofrontal cortex is hypofunctional in cocaine-dependent individuals, the review of Volkow and Morales (2015) cites studies showing that the activation of this region is increased in cocaine-dependent individuals compared to control subjects when they receive an intravenous dose of the drug or are exposed to associated cues, which classically triggers craving. In consonance, another study with cocaine addicts showed that the attempt to actively suppress craving during the display of a video with drug cues was able to reduce the activity of the orbitofrontal cortex, NAc, and other regions of the limbic system, along with a decrease in craving, which is believed to be related to inhibitory control stimulation (Volkow et al., 2010). Thus, the literature points out that the orbitofrontal cortex is involved in the attribution of salience to stimuli (drugs and related cues) and inhibitory control. In addicts, the morphofunctional impairment of this region has been associated with the propensity to impulsive and compulsive behavior. In addition to this region, craving is associated with the activation of the anterior cingulate, medial PFC, striated areas, and insula (Tang et al., 2015).

Together, studies have shown that motivational and cognitive changes, mainly the executive functions of inhibitory control and decision-making, are associated with the deregulation of neural circuits in drug addiction. Furthermore, frontal, subcortical, and cortical neuroadaptations can contribute to the transition from occasional/controlled use to problematic use and help explain the compulsion and difficulty of these people to remain abstinent (Tang et al., 2015). However, it is essential to note that the development of dependency is quite complex, so that there may be confounding factors that justify neuropsychological changes, such as risk factors associated with drug use (psychiatric comorbidities and genetic factors, for example), rather than a pure consequence of such use (Yücel et al. 2007).

If, on the one hand, drugs can alter the standard functioning of the brain and result in motivational and behavioral changes, on the other hand, their use is not enough for someone to develop SUD. These are multifactorial and complex disorders, so that science still does not fully understand what makes some people to develop dependency while others with the same use pattern do not. It is known that the course of problematic substance use is influenced by multiple variables, such as genetic factors, psychological characteristics such as impulsiveness, presence of comorbidities such as depression and anxiety, emotional self-regulation capacity, socioeconomic aspects, peer pressure, an expectation of the drug effect, sources of reward available, among others. Moreover, the use pattern (quantity per occasion and frequency of consumption) is essential for the development of the SUD, since no drug is capable of generating dependency with only one use or occasional consumption. In turn, some drugs have a higher power to generate dependency, due to their pharmacokinetic properties and mechanism of action, such as nicotine and heroin, for example. Due to all these aspects, statements of causality between drug use and neuroanatomic and functional alterations should be cautious, since many variables are not possible to be controlled in human studies. Thus, we say that the biopsychosocial characteristics of a person may constitute protective factors or risk factors, which decrease or increase, respectively, the chance of developing SUD.

Although drugs have in common the activation of the mesocorticolimbic pathway by different mechanisms of action, they produce different effects on those who consume them. Thus, these substances are grouped into three classes using as criteria their potent effect on the CNS (Chalout, 1971 as cited by Carlini et al. 2001):

- *Depressant drugs:* are substances that reduce the activity of the CNS and have sedative, hypnotic, and anxiolytic effects. Examples of depressants are alcohol, inhalants (glue, shoe polish, poppers), opioids (morphine, heroin, fentanyl, codeine), benzodiazepines (bromazepam, clonazepam, alprazolam), and GHB (gamma-hydroxybutyric acid).
- *Stimulant drugs:* are substances that stimulate the activity of the CNS, increasing agitation, reducing sleep, and appetite. Examples are cocaine/crack/"merla," amphetamines (weight-loss drugs), tobacco/nicotine, and caffeine.
- *Hallucinogen drugs (also referred as psychedelic drugs*): qualitatively alter ("disturb") the way reality is perceived (the self and the environment), as well as thoughts and emotions. They can induce illusions, hallucinations, and delusions. There is no clear evidence that classic psychedelics can increase dopamine release or that they induce addiction (Nichols, 2016). Examples of this class are LSD-25, psilocybin (present in mushrooms), mescaline (found in cacti such as San Pedro and Peyote), and DMT (found in ayahuasca). Marijuana is the most socially relevant representative of this class (although it also has depressing and stimulating properties), it induces an increase of dopamine in NAc and can induce addiction.

As this classification has educational purposes, some drugs have mixed effects and could be classified in more than one class. Marijuana, for example, is classified as a hallucinogen, although it has depressant effects and acts on cannabinoid receptors and not serotonergic, as classical psychedelics do. Another example is MDMA or ecstasy (the latter sometimes does not have MDMA), which can enter the group of stimulants due to the structural chemical similarity with amphetamines as well as some of its effects; however, it also has hallucinogen characteristics.

As previously mentioned, chronic drug users may present changes in executive functions that are indispensable for adaptation to new situations and involve behavior flexibility. These functions, such as attention, working memory, cognitive flexibility, impulse control, decision-making, among others, are associated with therapeutic success or failure (Lopes et al. 2019). Next, we will address specific neuropsychological changes related to the chronic use of some drugs. By the limit of space, an example of each class of drugs according to their social relevance in Brazil will be discussed; these will be alcohol, cocaine/crack, and marijuana. The objective is not to exhaust the literature on the subject, but to highlight the neuropsychological alterations that predominate in the scientific literature on chronic users of these substances, in order to contribute to the choice of the best therapeutic strategy.

Alcohol

Cognitive damage from alcohol use may vary depending on the pattern and time of use. Some studies point out the relationship between frequency and time of use with worse cognitive performance, while others suggest that these deficits are detected only in regular use of at least ten years (Yücel et al., 2007). More severe impairments can be observed in cases of Wernicke's encephalopathy and Korsakoff syndrome, which are associated with extensive alcohol use for several years and induce persistent neuropsychological damage (Rigoni et al., 2013; Perry, 2016). The most consistent findings in chronic alcoholics are in the areas of attention, short-term and working memory, executive functions (logical reasoning, problem-solving, cognitive flexibility, inhibitory control, and decision-making), visuospatial abilities, initial rule learning, emotional stability, and impulsiveness (Yücel et al., 2007; Rigoni et al., 2013).

Magnetic resonance imaging and postmortem analyses indicate that heavy alcohol use is associated with reduced brain volume, which appears to be mainly localized in the frontal lobes, subcortical regions, and cerebellum (Perry, 2016). These changes, specifically in frontal regions, seem to be associated with cognitive impairment, especially in executive functions that are relevant for treatment adherence and maintenance of abstinence. A review study found that from one month of abstinence, there can be at least partial reversal of brain volume, and cognitive aspects can be rehabilitated with abstinence of at least one year (Perry, 2016).

Concerning relapse, meta-analysis evaluated studies that investigated the activation of regions of the brain in the face of alcohol-related cues able to inducing craving (Schacht et al. 2012). The authors found that there was greater activation of parietal and temporal regions, such as posterior cingulate, precuneus, and superior temporal gyrus in heavy drinkers and individuals with SUD when compared to control groups. These regions are involved in different functions, among them memory, processing of the stimulus salience, subjective evaluation of rewards, and decision-making. In heavy drinkers and those with SUD, cues also increased the activation of the ventromedial PFC, anterior ventral cingulate, and ventral striatum; this was correlated with craving, and some studies showed that treatment for alcoholism (without specifying which) was able to reduce this activation. However, the activation of these regions in the presence of cues has also occurred in social drinkers and control groups, which indicates that in the case of alcohol the findings regarding these regions are not evident in the problematic use. At the same time, the posterior cingulate, precuneus, and superior temporal gyrus seem to be more associated with this condition. The loss of decision-making has already been seen in other addictive disorders, such as gambling. The meta-analysis of Kovács et al. (2017) evaluated articles that used formal neuropsychological testing on people with alcohol use and pathological gambling disorders, finding that these two groups have a decision-making deficit compared to groups without the disorders and that they do not differ from each other. The authors reflect that there may be differences in cognitive profiles and personality traits (e.g., impulsiveness and novelty seeking) that are common to these two types of disorders and could mediate their development.

Cocaine/Crack

A systematic review with cocaine and crack addicts indicated that the selected studies provide substantial evidence of inhibitory control, cognitive flexibility, decision-making, and working memory impairment when compared to the control group in formal neuropsychological tests (Czermainski et al., 2017). Such losses were observed by the reviewed studies through a significant variability in response times to neuropsychological tests, i.e., changes in information processing speed, in addition to failure in self-monitoring during test execution, difficulty in adapting responses to negative outcomes (in tasks involving monetary reinforcement), and to changes in rules, showing impairment of these functions.

Regarding neuroanatomic alterations, a sample formed by cocaine addicts (mean of 10 years of use) presented a reduction in the volume of gray matter in the orbitofrontal cortex, cingulate, and insula compared to a group of people with no history of drug abuse, and this reduction was related to the time of substance use. Additionally, an increase in volume was detected in the basal ganglia, of which the striatum is part. The volume reduction in the insula and the increase in the basal ganglia were correlated with the reduction in attentional control, while increased drug compulsion measures were correlated with volume reduction in the orbitofrontal cortex (Ersche et al., 2011).

Regarding changes in the functioning of the reward system in cocaine addicts who maintained use or even abstinence for 3–6 weeks, a reduced release of dopamine in the striatum caused by a (medicin) drug with cocaine/crack-like effect was observed in these groups when compared to a control group (Volkow et al. 2011). Other studies with neuroimaging point a reduction in dopaminergic type D2 receptors in the striatum correlated with a hypoactivation in the orbitofrontal cortex, dorsolateral PFC, and anterior cingulate cortex, regions involved with the incentive salience of drug or drug-related cues, inhibitory control, emotion regulation, and decision-making. In addition, the visualization of cocaine-related cues was able to induce an increase of dopamine in the striatum higher than the drug itself. These changes in the dopaminergic system and cortical circuit seem to be involved with increased motivation to cocaine seeking and compulsion (Volkow et al., 2011).

Conversely, it is important to be cautious in extrapolating these findings, as they have not been confirmed in other studies with different samples of cocaine users or addicts, as exemplified in the work of Volkow et al. (2010) in which the orbitofrontal cortex did not have its activation altered when drug-related cues were presented to addicts, even though they increased craving. Regarding the changes in brain activity during the inhibitory control tests, Czermainski et al. (2017) also point out the inconsistency of the studies, since some verified the hypoactivation of the ventrolateral PFC, anterior cingulate, among other areas, while other studies point out the hyperactivation of these same regions.

Marijuana

The most consistent losses in chronic marijuana users are in the domains of learning/verbal memory and attention (Broyd et al. 2016; Nader, & Sanchez, 2017; Duperrouzel et al. 2019). Conversely, evidence of impairment in executive functions, such as working memory, processing speed, abstraction, planning, reasoning, interference control, and problem-solving (Broyd et al., 2016; Duperrouzel et al., 2019), as well as motor and language skills, are mixed or less consistent (Volkow et al., 2016). This means that not all studies have found an effect of the chronic use of marijuana in these domains, which may point to a more subtle effect of the use of this drug in these functions. In support of this statement, the systematic review and meta-analysis of Duperrouzel et al. (2019) found harm in the executive functions of chronic marijuana users, but with a small difference when compared to the control group (small effect size).

Similarly, regarding decision-making, different papers point out both losses and the absence of effects in different samples of chronic users in neuropsychological tests that evaluate sensitivity to losses and gains (Duperrouzel et al., 2019). The results that verified decision-making losses in the Iowa Gambling Task indicate that chronic users have altered sensitivity to losses and gains, i.e., they tend to make riskier decisions, overestimating gains, and underestimating losses. Conversely, no effect of marijuana on visuospatial functions was found (Volkow et al., 2016; Duperrouzel et al., 2019).

The more intense pattern of use (frequency, amount, and duration of use) and the earlier onset of use also seem to be associated with the worsening performance of marijuana users in neuropsychological tests in several reviewed papers (Broyd et al., 2016; Nader & Sanchez, 2017), although these findings have not been corroborated by the systematic review and meta-analysis of Duperrouzel et al. (2019). The authors of this meta-analysis argue that the effects of early use on adolescence should be further studied, since the brain is in the process of maturation and presents important neurobiological changes, especially in the PFC (Duperrouzel et al., 2019). Therefore, this is a development period that could be quite sensitive to the adverse effects of marijuana with consequences in adulthood, and studies with animal models also support this possibility.

Neuroanatomical changes have been demonstrated in regions with a high concentration of CB1 receptors (cannabinoid receptor type 1), more consistently in the hippocampus and PFC, regions involved with memory and executive functions. High levels of consumption and duration of use seem to be more associated with changes in the hippocampus and PFC, and the age of onset of use seems to be more related to changes in PFC (Lorenzetti et al. 2016). Some studies suggest that learning/verbal memory deficits (Broyd et al., 2016) and neuroanatomical changes (Lorenzetti et al., 2016) may be associated with amounts of THC or the proportion of THC/cannabidiol ingested, pointing to less harmful consequences for marijuana consumption with reduced concentrations of THC and higher concentrations of cannabidiol. Many studies point to the recovery of cognitive and executive functions with one-month abstinence (Nader & Sanchez, 2017; Volkow et al., 2016), although this may not happen in relation to the pattern of brain activation, which indicates that compensatory neural mechanisms may be involved or that the recovery of neural function occurs in time after neuropsychological functions (Lorenzetti et al., 2016). Meta-analyses focused on neuroimaging studies present less consensus regarding brain regions with differences in activation pattern between users and non-users than meta-analyses focused on neuropsychological functions. However, the evidence is more consistent regarding the PFC, hippocampus, and insula regions.

In summary, the literature reflects the variability in cognitive and executive functions in chronic drug users, as well as how much these functions could remain altered after abstinence. This variability reflects the complexity of the phenomenon of drug use in humans, which involves characteristics of the samples studied regarding consumption (pattern, duration, and onset of use), presence of associated risk factors, and use of other substances. Therefore, health professionals must consider all these aspects of the treatment plan.

Explanatory Theoretical Models on SUD

Several theoretical models seek to explain the etiology of SUD, such as the moral, biological, neuropsychological, social, and psychological models, among others (Cordeiro, 2018), and each one can understand the SUD from several aspects. The moral model was the first attempt of contemporary society to explain the use and abuse of substances. In this perspective, individuals were held responsible for the use, understanding that they made a conscious choice to transgress social norms. Thus, users were criticized and blamed for the consequences of their consumption, because "no one told them to drink," and they continued drinking for "lack of willpower." Nowadays, some relatives and laypeople still tend to do this reading, but in the health sciences, the idea predominates that just blaming subjects for their dependence is not therapeutic, so that they should be seen as sick persons in need of treatment (Cordeiro, 2018; Perrenoud & Ribeiro, 2019). Therefore, this model is in disuse in the scientific community, since it neither explains nor complements the others.

According to the biological model, there are people with a genetic predisposition to the inappropriate use of PS. Specifically, regarding the neurobiological perspective, as detailed in the first section of this chapter, PS generates pleasure through stimulation in the limbic brain regions, especially the reward system, which increases the chance of repeated use. From the repetitive use, the organism develops a tolerance to the substance, requiring higher doses to obtain the same pleasurable effects. Moreover, the decrease or lack of the substance induces the abstinence syndrome, and the consumption occurs to relieve the symptoms that cause physiological and emotional suffering (American Psychiatric Association 2014; Perrenoud & Ribeiro, 2019).

The neuropsychological model explains the SUD from deficits in cognitive functions, which may be the origin of PS use and its consequence. The deficits vary according to the substance used, as well as the quantity and frequency. Although there is still no consensus in the literature, this model considers that psychoactive drugs influence the executive function effects, generally through failures in impulse control and decision-making, which can impair treatment and facilitate relapses. This dynamic tends to lead to a growing cycle of deregulation of the brain reward system, resulting in compulsive use (Almeida, 2019; American Psychiatric Association 2014; Garcia et al. 2014).

The social model conceives learning through social interactions, since behavior in general, including the use of PS, is shaped by society's rules and culture. Thus, individuals inserted in a society that values the use of PS learn to use them as a resource in several aspects, either for leisure and social interaction or to deal with suffering, among other possibilities. It is suggested to train social skills to develop their lifestyle more independently from the lifestyle of society (Perrenoud & Ribeiro, 2019).

The psychological model comprises the explanation of SUD through different approaches, which, in turn, may involve several explanatory theories. For the present chapter, four of the approaches most found in the literature were selected: the systemic, the psychoanalytical, the analytic-behavioral, and the cognitive models. The systemic approach comprises the PS user as a spokesperson for the family problem. Thus, the family and the people who have a connection with this individual interfere in their feelings and behavior and may present codependency and feed this self-destructive conduct. By considering drug use as a family symptom, this model suggests that the family should participate in the treatment, as a system that needs help. Otherwise, even unconsciously, the family tends to prevent the individual's treatment progress, avoiding focusing on other issues in the system (Payá, 2019).

Among the several understandings of psychoanalytical approach, it can be highlighted that the individual with SUD has a pathology of emptiness (which is not exclusive to this public), with difficulty to feel pleasure in life, because he did not have good enough parents regarding the care in the early stages of his development. Thus, the subject did not internalize these cares, did not adequately develop the capacity of self-care, and, as a consequence, has low self-esteem. Drug addiction shifts the feeling of emptiness to something achievable, even purchasable, and different from parental functions in childhood. Moreover, this dynamic may be associated with psychiatric symptoms, which leads patients to self-medicate with the PS, in an attempt to deny their suffering. Psychoanalytic psychotherapies are indicated to follow after about one or two years of consolidated abstinence (as sequential psychotherapy) for patients who still refer to emptiness and lack of pleasure, even with their comorbidities treated. Some authors warn that the early use of this approach may induce relapses in situations of minimal frustrations, with treatment withdrawal and increase of risk behaviors (Gabbard, 2016; Kessler et al. 2015; Ramos & Ramos, 2019; Santos, 2007).

The analytic-behavioral approach studies the phenomena generally through the experimental method and focuses on the interaction between the environment (stimuli) and organism (responses to these stimuli, which are observable behaviors). For this aspect, one type of interaction is the classic or respondent conditioning, which considers that day-to-day situations are associated with stimuli (previously neutral, but when paired with the drug, it became appetitive) that facilitate the use of PS as a response. For example, PS users partners and the pub where one usually drinks are stimuli associated with the drug. Therefore, exposure to them triggers craving and increases the risk of consumption. According to this approach, identifying these interactions between stimulus and response helps to modify them. Another type of interaction is operant conditioning, which encompasses, among others, the concepts of positive and negative reinforcement. The sensations of well-being caused by the psychoactive properties of the drug are positive reinforcers to the user behavior, while the withdrawal of malaise (including relief of withdrawal symptoms) acts as negative reinforcement. Thus, both reinforcers increase the frequency of use behavior, which can lead to a dysfunctional pattern of compulsion and characterize dependence (Banaco & Montan, 2018; Cordeiro, 2018).

The cognitive approach contemplates the concepts of reinforcing the analytic-behavioral model related to drug use, but emphasizes the influence of mental processes, especially perception and cognition, on behavior. The underlying assumption of Aaron Beck is that cognition influences behavior, and, as it can be monitored and altered, the desired behavior can be influenced by cognitive change (Beck, 2013). In short, he considers that behaviors are managed by automatic belief and thought systems, derived from one's own mental schema, i.e., the way one represents oneself, others, and the world internally. Regarding the cognitive aspects of the use of PS, these have been well established since the 1990s in Aaron Beck's Cognitive Model for the use of substances (for more information, see Beck et al. 1993).

Depending on the model, relapse risk situations may be external or internal stimuli associated with the use of PS. Exposure to these situations or the appearance of memories or thoughts can activate beliefs about drug use, in addition to the automatic thoughts related to these beliefs, which generate craving. Consequently, permissive beliefs about the use of PS are activated, such as "after such a stressful day,

I deserve to drink a dose," and the individual then articulates a plan of action to obtain and use the substance. This dynamic configures a cycle since the recurrence of the use behavior exposes to new risk situations and generates new associations that activate automatic beliefs and thoughts (Oliveira et al. 2011; Silva, 2018).

Finally, although the models are different in epistemological terms, it is believed that they can be complementary to each other since none is sufficient in isolation considering the complexity of the phenomenon of substance use. Professionals in the field must consider that drug users are heterogeneous people in several aspects; therefore, each one can benefit from different approaches, which can also vary according to the moment of life and motivation for treatment and the therapist–patient relationship (Santos, 2007).

Clinical Interventions for SUD Treatment

As several theoretical models seek to understand and explain the SUD, several are the interventions used to treat this problem. Due to the complexity and multifactorial nature of the aspects involved in drug use/abuse, it is often necessary to integrate intervention strategies, even if they come from different theoretical models. With the objective of contributing to the practice of professionals of health sciences who work in the treatment of drug users, three of the most commonly used non-pharmacological approaches that present at least partial evidence of efficacy and effectiveness in the literature (Cafruni et al. 2014; Pechansky & Baldisserotto, 2014) will be briefly described: motivational interviewing, relapse prevention, and cognitive-behavioral therapy.

Motivational interviewing (MI) is a non-confrontational approach that aims to stimulate the person to make a decision to change his/her behavior. It was developed by Miller and Rollnick (2001) to help assess and resolve ambivalence and promote change in addictive behaviors, initially those related to drugs, and then it was expanded for application in eating disorders, pathologic gambling, and other impulse control problems (Souza & Araújo, 2010). MI considers that change is a process that involves different motivational stages, such as precontemplation (no intention to change), contemplation (ambivalent and aware of the problem, but still no change), determination (decides to change), action (acts towards change), and maintenance (maintains the new behavior), which may include relapse and return to some previous stage (for more details, see the trans-theoretical model of change of Prochaska and DiClemente, 1992). The therapist's interventions should take into account the particularities of the stage in which patients are predominantly present. MI is based on six fundamentals, which form the acronym FRAMES: feedback, to discuss with patients the results of the evaluation and diagnosis of the SUD; responsibility, to emphasize responsibility and patient autonomy in their decisions; advice, through clear, direct, and non-judgmental guidelines; menu, provide the patient with a catalog of alternative treatment actions; empathy, as the therapist's posture; and self-efficacy, which reinforces the optimism and self-confidence of patients in their resources and in their success in search of the assumed goals (Miller & Rollnick, 2001; Souza & Araújo, 2010).

Considered a therapeutic proposal, MI is not a technique, but a posture, a way of acting together with the client. It requires a skillful clinical style that stimulates clients' internal motivations to promote healthier and more adaptive behaviors (Melo et al. 2008; Petry et al. 2011). Its five principles involve expressing empathy, promoting discrepancy, avoiding argumentation, following resistance, and promoting self-efficacy (Pechansky & Baldisserotto, 2014). Thus, the therapist's posture should be empathetic, collaborative, client-centered, and directive, but not confrontational. Skills include flexibility, tolerance to frustration, the ability to evoke from clients their reasons for change, and the ability to work respectfully, i.e., informing, warning, and advising, but aware that the final decision is the clients (Pechansky & Baldisserotto, 2014). It can be used by any therapist, as long as duly trained in its principles, fundamentals, and methods.

The relapse prevention (RP) model aims to evaluate the various aspects that would facilitate the relapse process and to seek strategies for dealing with risk situations with the patient. It was developed by Marlatt and Gordon (1985) with the objective of maintaining the change in behavior of abstinence from the drug and had as a theoretical basis the Theory of Social Learning of Bandura (1969, cited by Marlatt and Donovan, 2009), which understands that behavior is influenced both by the real consequence it brings and the expectation of result (Petry et al., 2011; Souza & Araújo, 2010). Thus, if individuals have an expectation that the use of the drug will bring a sensation of relaxation and stress relief, added to the pleasurable effect of the mechanism of action of the substance in the reward system, it is very likely that the use behavior will continue. Conversely, if they have developed coping strategies for fissure-provoking situations and a high risk of relapse, as well as reformulated their expectations of the drug's effect (e.g., "besides the drug, other things relax me and do not bring harm"), they will increase their chances of staying abstinent and increase their sense of self-efficacy. This model, therefore, advocates that compulsive use behavior can be disrupted and modified through new learning, which includes social and self-knowledge skills. As individuals successfully train and apply coping strategies, they increase their confidence in the possibility of controlling their attitudes and strengthen their purpose to remain abstinent, which reduces the incidence of relapse (Marlatt & Donovan, 2009; Petry et al., 2011). Regarding efficacy, RP has some evidence with patients motivated for treatment; therefore, it is suggested to be applied in an integrated manner with MI and other therapies, such as cognitive-behavioral (Campbell et al. 2018).

Cognitive-behavioral therapy (CBT), also called cognitive therapy, is based on the cognitive model described in the previous section. It follows a structured, collaborative intervention model (patient and therapist with an active posture), aimed at solving current problems and modifying dysfunctional thoughts and behaviors (Beck, 2013; Pechansky & Baldisserotto, 2014). In the treatment of SUD, since the basic premise of CBT is that thoughts influence emotions and behaviors and can be monitored and modified in the desired direction (Beck, 2013), the therapeutic work will involve both cognitive restructuring and the application of behavioral techniques of craving management, problem-solving, and training in social skills. The cognitive restructuring aims to help patients identify, evaluate, and modify the automatic thoughts and dysfunctional beliefs that influence harmful behaviors, such as "I am only happy when I use drugs" or "without the drug my suffering will be unbearable." At SUD, the goal of restructuring will be to weaken addictive beliefs, which can be permissive (e.g., "it was a hard day, I deserve to use just a little"), anticipatory (e.g., "the drug will elevate my mood") or relieving (e.g., "the drug will relieve my stress"), and strengthen those of control (e.g., "I can resist now, and then I will feel better and more confident"). Furthermore, the focus will also be on increasing self-esteem and self-efficacy in several areas of the subjects' life through the analysis of evidence from real situations and cognitive techniques, such as dysfunctional thought record, down arrow, decatastrophization, among others (Beck, 2013; Rangé & Marlatt, 2008).

Behavioral techniques, in turn, will have as their most direct objective the reduction of symptoms, fissure management, and the training of more assertive behaviors. Some of the most used and suggested by Souza and Araújo (2010) are a distraction (shifting attention from their thoughts and sensations related to the fissure); coping cards (cards or tickets that contain phrases or images that motivate the maintenance of abstinence); relaxation (respiratory, by image visualization or muscle distension); and behavioral tests, among others (more details on CBT techniques can be accessed in Abreu & Guilhardi, 2004). It should be noted that both cognitive techniques influence the change to the desired behavior, and behavioral techniques serve as evidence for cognitive restructuring, resulting in altered perception and interpretation of situations that will influence future behaviors. Besides the techniques, the strategy of psychoeducation (described in detail in Chapter III of this book) helps patients to understand the functioning of the treatment, its own disorder, and the techniques used in therapy so that they are continuously self-applied.

Considering evidence-based practice, numerous studies have already been published evaluating the effect of MI and CBT in the treatment of substance-related problems, which made it possible to conduct systematic literature review studies with and without meta-analysis evaluating the consistency of the results found. A meta-analysis study evaluating results from research that applied MI in the period between 2000 and 2016 (3025 participants in total) verified the effectiveness of MI, especially for users of alcohol and other drugs, but also for other problems related to food, sex, and compulsive gambling issues (Magill et al., 2018). In turn, an international study that examined 34 reviews on the topic (including six cochrane-based studies) found strong evidence of the efficacy and effectiveness of MI use for problems related to alcohol, tobacco, and marijuana, some for compulsive gambling, but few for methamphetamine and opioids (DiClemente et al. 2017). In the Brazilian context, although a systematic review study has shown that MI has increased the motivation in the process of change in the analyzed research, the authors suggested further studies to verify the effectiveness of this technique in this country (Andretta et al. 2014).

CBT, for its part, is among the most studied treatment approaches for addict behaviors and has one of the highest levels of empirical support of well-controlled studies (Andrade et al. 2016; Bedendo et al. 2018, 2019; Campbell et al. 2018; Carroll & Kiluk, 2017; Perry & Lawrence, 2017; Rodrigues et al. 2013). However, despite the substantial evidence base of randomized clinical trials, meta-analyses indicate a modest effect size, with evidence of relatively long-lasting effects, but with limited diffusion in clinical practice (Carroll & Kiluk, 2017). There is still no consensus in terms of the effectiveness of treating crack users, for example, Rodrigues et al. (2013). Considering the skills needed to initiate and sustain behavioral changes during the rehabilitation of drug users, new therapeutic developments that seek to improve cognitive functions, such as brain stimulation, physical exercise, and cognitive training should help overcome some of the barriers imposed by the disease itself (more details on neurocognitive interventions can be found in Perry and Lawrence, 2017). In this sense, updated CBT clinical interventions are suggested based on recent findings of cognitive science and neuroscience, seeking to accelerate the understanding of the mechanisms of action to increase the chances of success in the treatment of SUD and reduce the chances of relapses (Campbell et al., 2018; Carroll & Kiluk, 2017).

In addition to the interventions described, systemic approach strategies that seek to involve the family in understanding the pathology and treatment guidelines through psychoeducation, as well as activation of the user support network in recovery, should be encouraged (Payá, 2019). Studies indicate that the family, as well as the network of friends, can act as a risk factor or protection and prevention of drug abuse (Malbergier et al. 2012; Medeiros et al. 2013; Paz & Colossi, 2013). Results of the multicenter study conducted with 741 adults hospitalized or outpatient for intensive treatment revealed that all patients, especially crack users, had family problems such as fights, discussions, and difficulties in relationships with partners (Moura et al. 2014). These data corroborate the indication that Brazilian programs to treat people with SUD should include or improve treatment with family interventions.

Considering the modalities of treatment, there do not seem to be many studies comparing the efficacy of the therapy in group and individual modality for substance users; what is shown is that both have advantages and disadvantages (Oliveira et al. 2017). A literature review study on the efficacy of treatment of alcohol use disorders (Orchowski & Johnson, 2012) revealed that group therapy had a lower treatment dropout rate and longer abstinence time; thus, it is indicated for this population because it provides sharing of experiences and craving management strategies. Other advantages of this modality include the possibility of identifying with people with the same difficulty, the feeling of acceptance and belonging; of mutual support, through the exchange of experiences and strategies for the acquisition and maintenance of abstinence; and of learning new patterns of interpersonal relationships (Oliveira et al., 2017). Still, in terms of a single health system, group care can be an effective strategy in terms of benefits, time, and cost; nevertheless, more studies are needed to evaluate its effectiveness and efficacy in treating people with SUD.

Final Considerations

Finally, it should be noted that this chapter has focused on the neuropsychological and behavioral aspects of SUD and, therefore, contains limitations regarding integral treatment. For example, several clinical treatments can be indicated, besides interventions such as psychopharmacotherapy and psychiatric/hospital internment, which were not addressed here, but should be considered from a multidisciplinary perspective (Ramos & Ramos, 2019). Moreover, interventions with a focus on social aspects, such as community prevention and treatment interventions, were not approached, nor were public policies directed to the street population, for example. However, this theme will be discussed in more detail in other units of this book, such as Chapter IV, which will focus on social aspects and public policies for psychosocial attention to substance use.

This chapter emphasized that the consumption of PS is a complex phenomenon, influenced by multiple factors (such as cultural, genetic, and psychological) and can range from occasional and recreational use to drug abuse and dependence. Given the complexity of the subject, it should be noted that the authors' objective was not to approach it in its entirety but to present theoretical data, research evidence, and possibilities of intervention, which may be useful to all those interested in understanding this phenomenon.

References

Abreu, C. C., & Malvasi, P. A. (2011). Aspectos transculturais, sociais e ritualísticos do consumo de substâncias. In A. Diehl, D. C. Cordeiro, & R. Laranjeira (Eds.), *Dependência química: prevenção, tratamento e políticas públicas* (pp. 67–80). Porto Alegre: Artmed.

Abreu, C. N., & Guilhardi, H. (2004). *Terapia comportamental e cognitivo-comportamental: Práticas clínicas*. São Paulo: Roca.

Almeida, P. P. (2019). Neuropsicologia e reabilitação cognitiva na dependência química. In A. Diehl, D. C. Cordeiro, & R. Laranjeira (Eds.), *Dependência química: prevenção, tratamento e políticas públicas* (2nd ed., pp. 70–74). Porto Alegre: Artmed.

Andrade, A. L. M., Lacerda, R. B., Gomide, H. P., Ronzani, T. M., Sartes, L. M. A., Martins, L. F., et al. (2016). Web-based self-help intervention reduces alcohol consumption in both heavy-drinking and dependent alcohol users: a pilot study. *Addictive Behaviors, 63*, 63–71. https://dx.doi.org/10.1016/j.addbeh.2016.06.027.

American Psychiatric Association. (2014). *Manual diagnóstico e estatístico de transtornos mentais: DSM-5* (5th ed.). Porto Alegre: Artmed.

Andretta, I., Meyer, E., Kuhn, R. P., & Rigon, M. (2014). A entrevista motivacional no Brasil: uma revisão sistemática. *Psicologia da Saúde, 22*(2), 15–21. https://doi.org/10.15603/2176-1019/mud.v22n2p15-21.

Banaco, R., & Montan, R. N. M. (2018). Teoria analítico-comportamental. In N. A. Zanelatto & R. Laranjeira (Eds.), *O tratamento da dependência química e as terapias cognitivo-comportamentais: um guia para terapeutas* (2nd ed., pp. 115–132). Porto Alegre: Artmed.

Beck, A. T., Wright, F. W., Newman, C. F., & Liese, B. (1993). *Cognitive therapy of substance abuse*. New York, NY: Guilford.

Beck, J. (2013). *Terapia cognitiva: Teoria e prática* (2nd ed.). Porto Alegre: Artmed.

Bedendo, A., Andrade, A. L. M., & Noto, A. R. (2015). Sports and substance use in high school students different perspectives of this relationship. *SMAD Revista Eletrônica Saúde Mental Álcool e Drogas, 11*(2), 85–96. https://dx.doi.org/10.11606/issn.1806-6976.v11i2p85-96.

Bedendo, A., Andrade, A. L. M., & Noto, A. R. (2018). Internet-based alcohol interventions for college students: systematic review. *Revista Panamericana de Salud Pública, 42*, e54. https://dx.doi.org/10.26633/RPSP.2018.54.

Bedendo, A., Ferri, C. P., Souza, A. A. L., Andrade, A. L. M., & Noto, A. R. (2019). Pragmatic randomized controlled trial of a web-based intervention for alcohol use among Brazilian college students: Motivation as a moderating effect. *Drug and Alcohol Dependence, 199*, 92–100. https://dx.doi.org/10.1016/j.drugalcdep.2019.02.021.

Berridge, K. C., Robinson, T. E., & Aldridge, J. W. (2009). Dissecting components of reward: 'liking', 'wanting', and learning. *Current Opinion in Pharmacology, 9*(1), 65–73. https://doi.org/10.1016/j.coph.2008.12.014.

Broyd, S. J., Hell, H. H., Beale, C., Yücel, M., & Solowij, N. (2016). Acute and chronic effects of cannabinoids on human cognition—A systematic review. *Biological Psychiatry, 79*, 557–567. https://doi.org/10.1016/j.biopsych.2015.12.002.

Cafruni, K. H., Brolese, G., & Lopes, F. (2014). Tratamentos não farmacológicos para dependência química. *Revista da Sociedade de Psicologia do Rio Grande do Sul, 14*(1), 10–19.

Campbell, E. J., Lawrence, A. J., & Perry, C. J. (2018). New steps for treating alcohol use disorder. *Psychopharmacology, 235*(6), 1759–1773. https://doi.org/10.1007/s00213-018-4887-7.

Carlini, E. A., Nappo, S. A., Gauduróz, J. C., & Noto, A. R. (2001). Drogas psicotrópicas - o que são e como agem. *Revista IMESC, 3*, 9–35. Retrieved from http://10.15.194.22/wp-content/uploads/2019/03/Revista-IMESC-n%C2%BA-3-outubro-2001.pdf

Carlini, E. A., Noto, A. R., Galduróz, J. C. E., & Nappo, S. A. (1996). Visão histórica sobre uso de drogas: passado e presente. *Jornal Brasileiro de Psiquiatria, 45*(4), 227–236.

Carroll, K. M., & Kiluk, B. D. (2017). Cognitive behavioral interventions for alcohol and drug use disorders: Through the stage model and back again. *Psychology of Addictive Behaviors, 31*(8), 847–861. https://doi.org/10.1037/adb0000311.

Cordeiro, D. C. (2018). Transtornos por uso de substâncias – conceituação e modelos teóricos. In N. A. Zanelatto & R. Laranjeira (Eds.), *O tratamento da dependência química e as terapias cognitivo-comportamentais: um guia para terapeutas* (2nd ed., pp. 3–13). Porto Alegre: Artmed.

Czermainski, F. R., Willhelm, A. R., Santos, A. Z., Pachado, M. P., & De Almeida, R. M. M. (2017). Assessment of inhibitory control in crack and/or cocaine users: A systematic review. *Trends in Psychiatry and Psychotherapy, 39*(3), 216–225. https://doi.org/10.1590/2237-6089-2016-0043.

De Micheli, D., Andrade, A., & Galduróz, J. C. (2020). Limitations of DSM-5 diagnostic criteria for substance use disorder in adolescents: what have we learned after using these criteria for several years? *Brazilian Journal of Psychiatry*, in press. https://doi.org/10.1590/1516-4446-2020-1151.

DiClemente, C. C., Corno, C. M., Graydon, M. M., Wiprovnick, A. E., & Knoblach, D. J. (2017). Motivational interviewing, enhancement, and brief interventions over the last decade: A review of reviews of efficacy and effectiveness. *Psychology of Addictive Behaviors, 31*(8), 862–887. https://doi.org/10.1037/adb0000318.

Duperrouzel, J. C., Granja, K., Pacheco-Colón, I., & Gonzalez, R. (2019). Adverse effects of cannabis use on neurocognitive functioning: A systematic review of meta-analytic studies. *Journal of Dual Diagnosis, 22*, 1550–4271. https://doi.org/10.1080/15504263.2019.162-6030.

Ersche, K. D., Barnes, A., Jones, P. S., Morein-Zamir, S., Robbins, T. W., & Bullmore, E. T. (2011). Abnormal structure of frontostriatal brain systems is associated with aspects of impulsivity and compulsivity in cocaine dependence. *Brain, 134*, 2013–2024. https://doi.org/10.1093/brain/awr138.

Fernandez-Serrano, M. J., Perales-López, J. C., Moreno-López, L., Santos-Ruiz, A., Perez-Garcia, M., & Verdejo-Garcia, A. (2012). Impulsividad y compulsividad en individúos dependientes de cocaína. *Adicciones, 24*(2), 105–114. https://doi.org/10.20882/adicciones.102.

Gabbard, G. O. (2016). Transtornos relacionados a substâncias e transtornos aditivos e transtornos alimentares. In G. O. Gabbard (Ed.), *Psiquiatria psicodinâmica na prática clínica* (5th ed., pp. 345–381). Porto Alegre: Artmed.

Garcia, F., Moreira, L., & Assumpção, A. (2014). Neuropsicologia das dependências químicas. In L. Fuentes, L. Malloy-Diniz, C. H. Camargo, & R. Cosenza (Eds.), *Neuropsicologia: teoria e prática* (2nd ed., pp. 241–248). Porto Alegre: Artmed.

Goodman, A. (2008). Neurobiology of addiction. An integrative review. *Biochemical Pharmacology, 75*, 266–322. https://doi.org/10.1016/j.bcp.2007.07.030.

Kessler, F. H., Pechansky, F., Rebouças, D. B., & Piccin, J. (2015). Abordagem psicodinâmica do paciente dependente químico. In C. L. Eizirik, R. W. Aguiar, & S. S. Schestatsky (Eds.), *Psicoterapia de orientação analítica: fundamentos teóricos e clínicos* (3rd ed., pp. 808–830). Porto Alegre: Artmed.

Koob, G., & Volkow, N. D. (2010). Neurocircuitry of addiction. *Neuropsychopharmacology, 35*(1), 217–238. https://doi.org/10.1038/npp.2009.110.

Koob, G. F., & Volkow, N. D. (2016). Neurobiology of addiction: A neurocircuitry analysis. *Lancet Psychiatry, 3*(8), 760–773. https://doi.org/10.1016/S2215-0366(16)00104-8.

Kovács, I., Richmanb, M. J., Jankaa, Z., Maraz, A., & Andóa, B. (2017). Decision making measured by the Iowa Gambling Task in alcohol use disorder and gambling disorder: A systematic review and meta-analysis. *Drug and Alcohol Dependence, 181*, 152–161. https://doi.org/10.1016/j.drugalcdep.2017.09.023.

Lopes, F. M., Andretta, I., & Oliveira, M. S. (2019). Avaliação psicológica dos transtornos relacionados a substâncias psicoativas. In M. N. Baptista et al. (Eds.), *Compêndio de avaliação psicológica* (pp. 692–701). Petrópolis: Vozes.

Lorenzetti, V., Solowij, N., & Yücel, M. (2016). The role of cannabinoids in neuroanatomic alterations in cannabis users. *Biological Psychiatry, 79*(7), e17–e31. https://doi.org/10.1016/j.biopsych.2015.11.013.

Magill, M., Apodaca, T., Borsari, B., Gaume, J., Hoadley, A., Gordon, R., Tonigan, J. S., & Moyers, T. (2018). A meta-analysis of motivational interviewing process: Technical, relational, and conditional process models of change. *Journal of Consulting and Clinical Psychology, 86*(2), 140–157. https://doi.org/10.1037/ccp0000250.

Malbergier, A., Cardoso, L. R., & Amaral, R. A. (2012). Uso de substâncias e problemas familiares. *Cadernos de Saúde Pública, 28*(4), 678–688. https://doi.org/10.1590/S0102311X-2012000400007.

Marlatt, A. G., & Donovan, D. M. (2009). *Prevenção de recaída*. Porto Alegre: Artmed.

Marlatt, A. G., & Gordon, J. (1985). *Relapse prevention: Maintenance strategies in the treatment of addictive behaviors*. New York: Guilford.

Medeiros, K. T., Maciel, S. C., Sousa, P. F., Tenório, F. M., Souza, C., & Dias, C. V. (2013). Representações sociais do uso e abuso de drogas entre familiares de usuários. *Psicologia em Estudo, 18*(2), 269–279. https://doi.org/10.1590/S1413-73722013000200008.

Melo, W. V., Oliveira, M., Araújo, R. B., & Pedroso, R. (2008). A entrevista motivacional em tabagistas: uma revisão teórica. *Revista de Psiquiatria do Rio Grande do Sul, 30*(1 Suppl), 1. https://doi.org/10.1590/S0101-81082008000200001.

Miller, W., & Rollnick, S. (2001). *Entrevista motivacional: preparando as pessoas para a mudança de comportamentos adictivos*. Porto Alegre: Artmed.

Moura, H. F., Benzano, D., Pechansky, F., & Kessler, F. H. (2014). Crack/cocaine family problems. *Clinics, 69*(7), 497–499. https://doi.org/10.6061/clinics/2014(07)10.

Nader, D. A., & Sanchez, Z. M. (2017). Effects of regular cannabis use on neurocognition, brain structure, and function: A systematic review of findings in adults. *The American Journal of Drug and Alcohol Abuse, 12*, 1–15. https://doi.org/10.1080/00952990.2017.1306746.

Nichols, D. E. (2016). Psychedelics. *Pharmacological Reviews, 68*, 264–355. https://doi.org/10.1124/pr.115.011478.

Oliveira, M., Freire, S., & Laranjeira, R. (2011). *Psicoterapias cognitivo-comportamentais: um diálogo com a psiquiatria* (2nd ed., pp. 409–423). Porto Alegre: Artmed.

Oliveira, M., Sartes, L. M., Ribeiro, N., Ismael, S. M., & Cazassa, M. J. (2017). Terapia cognitivo-comportamental em grupo aplicada a usuários de drogas. In C. B. Neufeld & B. P. Rangé (Eds.), *Terapia cognitivo-comportamental em grupos* (pp. 212–235). Porto Alegre: Artmed.

Orchowski, L. M., & Johnson, J. E. (2012). Efficacy of group treatments for alcohol use disorders: A review. *Current Drug Abuse Reviews, 5*(2), 148–157. https://doi.org/10.2174/1874473711205020148.

Payá, R. (2019). Terapia familiar e dependência química. In A. Diehl, D. C. Cordeiro, & R. Laranjeira (Eds.), *Dependência química: Prevenção, tratamento e políticas públicas* (2nd ed., pp. 278–284). Porto Alegre: Artmed.

Paz, F. M., & Colossi, P. M. (2013). Aspectos da dinâmica da família com dependência química. *Estudos de Psicologia, 18*(4), 551–558. https://doi.org/10.1590/S1413294X2013000-400002.

Pechansky, F., & Baldisserotto, C. F. (2014). Tratamentos psicoterápicos utilizados no tratamento de pessoas dependentes de substâncias psicotrópicas. In: M. L. Formigoni. *Modalidades de tratamento e encaminhamento: módulo* 6. (pp. 81–97). SUPERA: Sistema para a detecção do Uso abusivo e dependência de substâncias Psicoativas: Encaminhamento, intervenção breve, Reinserção social e Acompanhamento. Brasil. Brasília, Secretaria Nacional de Políticas sobre Drogas.

Pedrero-Pérez, E., & Sánchez de León, J. (2012). Subtipos de adictos a la cocaína con y sin consumo problemático de alcohol asociado: hacia una neuropsicología de la personalidad aplicada a la clínica. *Adicciones, 24*(4), 291–300. https://doi.org/10.20882/adicciones.79.

Pedrero-Pérez, E. J., Rojo-Mota, G., Sánchez de León, J. M., Llanero-Luque, M., & Puerta-Garcia, C. (2011). Rehabilitación cognitiva en el tratamiento de las adicciones. *Revista de Neurologia, 52*(3), 163–172. https://doi.org/10.33588/rn.5203.2010513.

Perrenoud, L., & Ribeiro, M. (2019). Etiologia dos transtornos relacionados ao uso de substâncias. In A. Diehl, D. C. Cordeiro, & R. Laranjeira (Eds.), *Dependência química: Prevenção, tratamento e políticas públicas* (2nd ed., pp. 9–14). Porto Alegre: Artmed.

Perry, C. J. (2016). Cognitive decline and recovery in alcohol abuse. *Journal of Molecular Neuroscience, 60*(3), 383–389. https://doi.org/10.1007/s12031-016-0798-4.

Perry, C. J., & Lawrence, A. J. (2017). Addiction, cognitive decline and therapy: Seeking ways to escape a vicious cycle. *Genes, Brain and Behavior, 16*, 205–218. https://doi.org/10.1111/gbb.12325.

Petry, M. C., Kolling, N. M., & Melo, W. V. (2011). Atualidade na dependência do crack. In R. Wainer, N. M. Piccoloto, & G. K. Pergher (Eds.), *Novas temáticas em terapia cognitiva* (pp. 39–60). Porto Alegre: Sinopsys.

Prochaska, J. O., & DiClemente, C. (1992). Stages of change in the modification of problem behaviors. In M. Hersen, M. Eiser, & W. Miller (Eds.), *Progress in behavior modification* (pp. 184–214). Sycamore: Sycamore Press.

Ramos, F. P., & Ramos, S. P. (2019). Como nós tratamos pacientes com dependência química? In A. Diehl, D. C. Cordeiro, & R. Laranjeira (Eds.), *Dependência química: Prevenção, tratamento e políticas públicas* (2nd ed., pp. 317–324). Porto Alegre: Artmed.

Rangé, B. P., & Marlatt, G. A. (2008). Terapia cognitivo-comportamental de transtornos de abuso de álcool e drogas. *Revista Brasileira de Psiquiatria, 30*(suppl. 2), S88–S95. https://doi.org/10.1590/S1516-44462008000600006.

Rigoni, M. S., Susin, N., Trentini, C. M., & Oliveira, M. S. (2013). Alcoolismo e avaliação de funções executivas: Uma revisão sistemática. *Psicotecnia, 44*(1), 122–129.

Rodrigues, V. S., Horta, R. L., Szupszynski, K. P., Souza, M. C., & Oliveira, M. S. (2013). Revisão sistemática sobre tratamentos psicológicos para problemas relacionados ao crack. *Jornal Brasileiro de Psiquiatria, 62*(3), 208–216. https://doi.org/10.1590/S004720852013-000300005.

Santos, M. A. (2007). Psicoterapia psicanalítica: aplicações no tratamento de pacientes com problemas relacionados ao uso de álcool e outras drogas. SMAD. *Revista Eletrônica Saúde Mental Alcool e Drogas, 3*(1), 1–15.

Schacht, J. P., Anton, R. F., & Myrick, H. (2012). Functional neuroimaging studies of alcohol cue reactivity: A quantitative meta-analysis and systematic review. *Addiction Biology, 18*(1), 121–133. https://doi.org/10.1111/j.1369-1600.2012.00464.x.

Silva, C. J. (2018). A dependência química e o modelo cognitivo de Aaron Beck. In N. A. Zanelatto & R. Laranjeira (Eds.), *O tratamento da dependência química e as terapias cognitivo-comportamentais: um guia para terapeutas* (2nd ed., pp. 102–114). Artmed: Porto Alegre.

Souza, A. C. F., & Araújo, R. B. (2010). Acompanhamento terapêutico na dependência química. In I. Londero (Ed.), *Acompanhamento Terapêutico: teoria e técnica na terapia comportamental e cognitivo-comportamental* (pp. 127–138). São Paulo: Santos.

Tang, Y., Posner, M. I., Rothbart, M. K., & Volkow, N. D. (2015). Circuitry of self-control and its role in reducing addiction. *Trends in Cognitive Sciences, 19*(8), 439–444. https://doi.org/10.1016/j.tics.2015.06.007.

Tavares, G. P., Scheffer, M., & De Almeida, R. M. M. (2012). Drogas, violência e aspectos emocionais em apenados. *Psicologia: Reflexão e Crítica, 25*(1), 89–95. https://doi.org/10.1590/S0102-79722012000100011.

UNODC – United Nations Office on Drugs and Crime. (2019). *World drug report*. New York: United Nations Publications.

Volkow, N. D., & Fowler, J. S. (2000). Addiction, a disease of compulsion and drive: Involvement of the orbitofrontal cortex. *Cerebral Cortex, 10*(3), 318–325. https://doi.org/10.1093/cercor/10.3.318.

Volkow, N. D., Fowler, J. S., Wang, G., Telang, G., Logan, J., Jayne, M., & Swanson, J. M. (2010). Cognitive control of drug craving inhibits brain reward regions in cocaine abusers. *NeuroImage, 49*, 2536–2543. https://doi.org/10.1016/j.neuroimage.2009.10.088.

Volkow, N. D., & Morales, M. (2015). The brain on drugs: From reward to addiction. *Cell, 162*(4), 712–725. https://doi.org/10.1016/j.cell.2015.07.046.

Volkow, N. D., Swanson, J. M., Evins, A. D., DeLisi, L. E., Meier, M. H., Gonzalez, A., & Baler, R. (2016). Effects of cannabis use on human behavior, including cognition, motivation, and psychosis: A review. *JAMA Psychiatry, 73*(3), 292–297. https://doi.org/10.1001/jamapsychiatry.2015.3278.

Volkow, N. D., Wang, G., Fowler, J. S., Tomas, D., & Telang, F. (2011). Addiction: Beyond dopamine reward circuitry. *PNAS, 108*(37), 15037–15042. https://doi.org/10.1073/pnas.1010654108.

Yücel, M., Lubman, D. I., Solowij, N., & Brewer, W. J. (2007). Understanding drug addiction: A neuropsychological perspective. *Australian and New Zealand Journal of Psychiatry, 41*, 957–968. https://doi.org/10.1080/00048670701689444.

Part III
Psychological Aspects

Chapter 12
Psychological Evaluation in Users of Psychoactive Substances: The Psychodiagnosis Process

Richard Alecsander Reichert, Fernanda Machado Lopes, Júlio Cézar Gonçalves do Pinho, Jamir João Sardá Junior, and Roberto Moraes Cruz

Introduction

Psychoactive drugs are substances that act on the central nervous system (CNS) and generate physical, cognitive, and behavioral changes. Among the various types of classification (licit or illicit, natural, semi-synthetic or synthetic), we can highlight the classification according to their action in the CNS: (a) *depressants*, which reduce the functions, generating sensations of relaxation, sleepiness, among others (e.g., alcohol, inhalants, benzodiazepines, opioids); (b) *stimulants,* which accelerate the activity and cause euphoria, agitation, and other effects (e.g., alcohol, inhalants, benzodiazepines, opioids, amphetamines, caffeine, cocaine/crack, nicotine); and (c) *disturbing,* which modifies the functioning of the CNS, both quantitatively and qualitatively, and may cause perceptual alterations and/or hallucinations (e.g., ecstasy, marijuana, LSD) (Andrade et al., 2016; American Psychiatric Association (APA) 2014; De Micheli et al., 2016; DiClemente, 2018; Lopes, Andretta, & Oliveira, 2019).

A proportion of people who use psychoactive substances develop consumption patterns that can lead to other mental disorders (Frade et al., 2014; Schulden, Lopez & Compton, 2012). These disorders are clinical comorbidities associated with disability in social and occupational activities on a continuous or recurring basis (World Health Organization (WHO) 2019) and identified through significant disorders in mood, cognition, emotional regulation, and/or behavior (American Psychiatric Association (APA) 2014).

R. A. Reichert (✉) · J. C. G. do Pinho · J. J. S. Junior
Universidade do Vale do Itajaí, Itajaí, SC, Brazil

F. M. Lopes · R. M. Cruz
Universidade Federal de Santa Catarina, Florianópolis, SC, Brazil

D. De Micheli et al. (eds.), *Drugs and Human Behavior*,
https://doi.org/10.1007/978-3-030-62855-0_12

Mental disorders consist of patterns of behavior (such as the use of psychoactive substances) that (a) occur at (1) very high frequencies and/or intensities or (2) very low and/or (b) occur in an inappropriate context and therefore generate personal injury and/or harm to the person or others (Bedendo et al., 2017; Banaco, Zamignani, Martone, Vermes, & Kovac, 2015). In this sense, the diagnostic criteria for mental disorders related to the use of psychoactive substances include (a) minimum number of signs and symptoms presented, (b) minimum period of manifestation of the same, and (c) duration of the phenomena reported and/or observed (American Psychiatric Association (APA) 2014; Barlow & Durand, 2015). These criteria for DSM-5 are (American Psychiatric Association (APA) 2014):

1. The substance is often consumed in larger quantities and for longer than expected;
2. There is persistence of a desire or unsuccessful attempts to reduce or control use;
3. Abundant time is dedicated to activities related to obtaining the drug, using it or restoring its effects;
4. There is a crack or a strong desire or need for the use of the substance;
5. There is recurrent use, affecting work, study, interpersonal relations, and family;
6. The use of the substance is continued even in the face of social or interpersonal problems caused or amplified by the effects of the drug;
7. There is the abandonment or reduction of engagement in social, professional, or recreational activities due to drug use;
8. The substance is consumed in situations/contexts that pose risks to physical integrity;
9. The use is maintained even with the presence of physical or psychological problems;
10. Tolerance, defined by:

    a. Requirement of successively greater amounts of the substance to generate intoxication or achieve the desired effects;
    b. The effects are gradually reduced with the continuous use of the same amount of the substance;

11. Abstinence, expressed by:

    a. Abstinence syndrome and/or
    b. The substance (or other, with similar effects) is consumed to ease or avoid withdrawal symptoms.

For the diagnosis of mental disorders due to the use of psychoactive substances, according to DSM-5, it is necessary that at least two of the criteria are manifest, occurring during a period of twelve months. The severity of the disorder should be examined according to the number of symptoms found: (a) mild, with two to three symptoms; (b) moderate, with four to five symptoms; and (c) severe, with six or more symptoms (American Psychiatric Association (APA) 2014). However, it is possible to establish an accurate diagnosis through a series of procedures that in psychology constitutes the field of psychological evaluation or assessment (Araújo, 2007).

Psychological Evaluation

Psychological evaluation is a field of study that focuses on the comprehension of psychological phenomena aiming to establish a diagnosis to subside a therapeutic plan. For this, psychological evaluation uses methods and instruments for the observation and measurement of psychological phenomena, as well as theoretical foundations that aim to explain them (Alchieri & Cruz, 2003; Cruz, 2002). Thus, psychological evaluation is guided by the demand or interest of specific investigation (e.g., executive functions, mood, personality characteristics, emotional states, or cognitive processes), by its purpose (checking aptitude, performance, clinical hypothesis, diagnosis, or prognosis) and based on the state of the art guided by theoretical models and procedures of data and information collection (Cruz & Sardá Jr., 2019; Fernández-Ballesteros, 2014).

The psychological evaluation could be guided, in conceptual terms, by the identification of four elements (Alchieri & Cruz, 2003; Cruz, 2002): (a) the object, which specifies the psychological phenomenon or process to be investigated; (b) the objective, which defines the purpose of the psychological evaluation; (c) the method, which guides the direct or indirect access (procedures) through which it is possible to access the phenomenon or psychological process to be investigated—observation, inquiry techniques, psychological tests, document analysis (Araújo, 2007; Krug, Trentini, & Bandeira, 2016); (d) the theoretical field, which supports the process of comprehension, analysis, and interpretation of the findings. Figure 12.1 summarizes the conceptual framework of psychological assessment (Cruz, 2002), with examples related to the assessment of psychoactive substance use disorders.

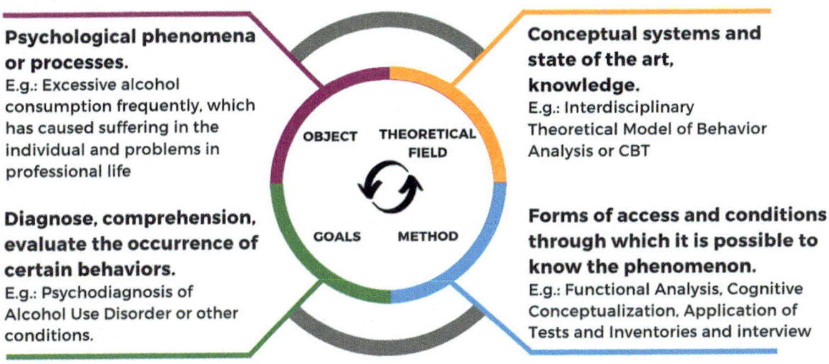

Fig. 12.1 Configuration of the defining scheme of the field of psychological assessment, with examples related to the assessment of disorders due to the use of psychoactive substances. Source: Adapted from Cruz (2002)

In the psychological evaluation process, the psychologist is responsible for identifying the object or demand, drawing up a plan of activities that address the objectives of the evaluation process, examining the presumed hypotheses, describing the psychological characteristics identified, interpreting them in the light of updated scientific knowledge, and, when under clinical demand, presuming diagnosis and supporting possible interventions (Cruz & Sardá Jr. 2019).

Psychological evaluation is understood, therefore, as a scientific-professional activity of psychologists, which involves procedures of collection, analysis, and interpretation of psychological data (Federal Council of Psychology, 2007). These data and information are collected to test hypotheses, elaborate diagnoses, describe cognitive and behavioral aspects, describe profiles, make predictions, and indicate possibilities of interventions. Therefore, psychological evaluation is a modality of professional procedure used in practically all areas of psychology (organizational and work, hospital, school, health and clinical processes, traffic and mobility, legal, sports, among others), for several purposes, either to characterize a professional profile, evaluate the skills needed to drive a vehicle, or examine clinical hypotheses, as in the case of clinical psychodiagnosis.

In relation to the use of psychoactive substances, psychological evaluation assists in the identification of the personal and environmental variables involved and also of potential losses in terms of cognitive functioning, emotional disorders, humor alteration, and maladaptive behavior (Almeida et al. 2017; Andrade et al. 2016, 2017a b; Barbosa et al. 2018; Lopes et al. 2019; Santos, Santiago, Oliveira, Lima, & Melo, 2018). In this sense, it is important to define the objectives of the evaluation process, which is permeated by the different dimensions of the object to be evaluated and its characteristics (Table 12.1).

By understanding the dimensions involved in mental disorders through the use of substances described in the scientific literature, the objectives of the evaluation process can be more clearly defined. For example: if one wants to investigate the presence of psychiatric comorbidities, or if the focus of evaluation is the functioning of cognitive processes in an individual (e.g.: executive functions) or, still, the presence of dysfunctional beliefs or thoughts that sustain the use of psychoactive substances. In addition, it is relevant to investigate the presence of risk and protective factors,

Table 12.1 Dimensions of the object of evaluation and repercussions on mental health

Dimensionality	Repercussions on mental health
Humoral/affective	Mood, depression, anxiety, psychophysiological reactivity
Cognitive	Attentional, cognitive, and belief dysfunctions in the use of psychoactive substances Dysfunctions in the processing of executive functions/memory
Functional capacity	Low self-efficacy, adaptive and stress management constraints, social isolation, loss of autonomy, and quality of life management
Risk factors	Chronic diseases, precarious health care structure
Social and family factors	Restrictions on social skills and family relationships, low social and family support for health care and treatment

Source: the authors

such as the absence/presence of a support network. Conversely, not every evaluation process of psychological problems related to drug use is aimed to assess quality of life. Therefore, it is important that in each context, or even based on a theoretical model of drug dependence, the objective of the psychological evaluation process is defined.

Different methods are needed to evaluate psychological phenomena and their various forms of manifestation and association with other phenomena (biological or social, for example). Adopting more than one method, technique, or instrument allows to access different or complementary dimensions of the phenomena, covering the accessed object in a whole. The methodological rigor and the use of different data collection procedures are necessary to ensure the quality of the gathered information. The use of valid and reliable psychological measures, techniques, and instruments widens the possibilities of access to the analyzed phenomena and, at the same time, reduces the probability of errors or operational biases.

The Psychodiagnosis Process

Psychodiagnosis is a modality of psychological evaluation for clinical purposes (Cruz, 2002) and is of paramount importance for decision-making in terms of clinical picture framing, treatment conduct, and case evolution. The process of psychodiagnosis promotes the detection of clinical complaints, psychological compromises, or mental comorbidities associated with disorders in general which may interfere with health care and treatment (Krug et al., 2016). This process of evaluation may include personal, family, and social information regarding the health conditions of patients. Thus, once the evaluation process has been carried out, specific interventions can be performed (Capitão, Scortegagna, & Baptista, 2005).

In order to discuss and highlight the importance of reliability in psychodiagnosis, an example is given: a psychology professional receives a call to attend to a 30-year-old individual, who requests an appointment to do a psychological evaluation. In the first meeting, it is observed that the individual presents communicational skills, is lucidity, presents good eye contact and absence of signs of confusion or psychotic symptoms, but complains of intense psychological suffering. There is an attempt to establish a *rapport* for the initial interview for data collection. At the end of the first session, the brief formulation of the case identified several symptoms initially reported by the individual: reduced willingness to leave home and perform daily activities, apathy, and frequent concern when remembering that there are college work to be done, emotional reaction to minimal signs of stress, thoughts of self-injury, discouragement, and sense of failure when noticing that his grades are decreasing during the semester, marked difficulties in making new friendships, feeling of hopelessness, sadness most of the day in the last 6 months, and deep-rooted beliefs that he will never be able to complete graduation.

What should the psychologist's attitude be in the face of this information? Systematize the symptoms and relate them in terms of a diagnostic hypothesis?

Summarize the evaluation process, with a view to the possible framing in a diagnostic picture? What about the important information that the individual consumes between four and six beers a day, throughout the week, and possibly other alcoholic beverages, since the age of seventeen? Would this information be relevant when associated with the symptoms presented?

Despite the available knowledge about contemporary psychopathological theories, many professionals tend to conclude with erroneous or hasty diagnoses. Considering the example, despite a few symptoms described, the technical knowledge would lead to believe that the diagnostic hypothesis of the exemplified case could be that of major depression disorder (MDD). However, with the inclusion of information on alcohol use for almost thirteen years, the initial hypothesis of MDT may not be as appropriate, i.e., incomplete. Thus, it is clear that there is a need to deepen the examination/comprehension of the case, with a psychological interview and/or anamnesis, as well as the use of psychological tests or screening instruments to produce a more comprehensive psychodiagnosis and a conclusion with a higher degree of assertiveness. In general, this is one of the problems encountered when relying only on isolated aspects for conducting a psychodiagnosis: the difficulty of perceiving the function that these symptoms have in the context in which the individual is inserted (Cunha, 2003). So, we return to the milestone of the concept of psychodiagnosis.

In general, psychodiagnosis refers to a set of procedures that aim to decode in a systematic, orderly, scientific, and comprehensive way the cognitive-behavioral, psychosocial, and functional functioning of an individual, in order to, later, and from the formulation of the case, draw a treatment plan focused on solving problems and improving the quality of life of the subject (Krug et al., 2016). It is, therefore, a psychological evaluation oriented to the characterization of a diagnosis, prognosis, and possible referral to treatments directed to the identified needs.

Although it is a traditional definition in psychology, there are conceptual misunderstanding about the definition of psychodiagnosis and psychological evaluation. Several authors in the Brazilian scenario (Castro et al. 2009; Cunha 2003; Castro, Campezatto & Saraiva, 2009; Krug et al., 2016; Ocampo & Arzeno, 2009) suggest that, as a priority, a psychodiagnosis should involve interview techniques and psychological tests validated by the psychological test evaluation system (SATEPSI), while psychological evaluation is more comprehensive, i.e., it can have different goals, be used in different areas of psychology, and need not involve the application of tests, or at least not exclusively those validated by SATEPSI. Thus, for didactic and organizational purposes, when referring to psychodiagnosis we are referring to a process of psychological evaluation for clinical purposes.

It is understood therefore that psychodiagnosis is not a process that should be carried out in a simplistic, intuitive, and restricted manner. The brief example of case X, described above, portrays the situation of other individuals who are diagnosed on the basis of limited or shallow investigation procedures. The detailed search for personal, family, clinical, conduct, and social habits data, in the case of disorders associated with the use of psychoactive substances, requires the joint use of technical resources and specialized materials (survey techniques, screening, psychological tests, functional and cognitive analyses, scientific literature of similar cases) that enable not only a diagnostic reading, but also training procedures or modification of attitudes and strategies to confront the patient in the face of the problems experienced, which, therefore, could generate greater probabilities of efficacy in the medium/long term treatment.

To understand the stages of the process of psychodiagnosis it is strictly necessary to understand the most assertive concept of psychopathology. Although the term itself generates the notion of illness, Dalgalarrondo (2018) defines psychopathology, in the broadest sense, as a grouping of knowledge regarding people's mental health, to the extent that this knowledge is not permissive to inference by dogmas or truths, but rather, in a systematic and elucidative manner, being permanently open to the changes brought about by scientific findings. This notion reflects directly on the path of psychodiagnosis, allowing the dynamism and flexibility necessary for this practice.

In this sense, when examining at the substance use disorders criteria, both in DSM-5 and ICD 10, an accurate look should be taken about the diagnostic criteria related to the amount of the drug ingested, since this aspect is extremely variable and is related to genetic, environmental, functional, and learning differences (American Psychiatric Association (APA) 2014; World Health Organization (WHO) 2019). Even so, although there are guidelines, there are several means that end up becoming causal arguments among health professions, one of the most recurrent are the socio-cultural aspects (Dalgalarrondo, 2018; Whitbourne & Halgin, 2015). These influences can be treated as social stigmas, that is, labels that segregate people who have some body variation, or those who express behaviors, cognition, and wills discrepant from others. Conversely, these socio-cultural arguments are commonly used in the daily practice of many professionals, a paradigm that needs to be shifted when practices based on scientific evidence are highlighted. This is a caution that any health professional, with the power of decision to define a diagnostic hypothesis, should pay attention to (Cunha, 2003).

In psychotherapy practice, signs and symptoms expressed by an individual are categorized into two major groups: syndromes and nosological entities. Syndromes are characterized mainly by constant groupings of stable signs and symptoms; however, these cannot yet be etiologically identified as a result of a pathological process. In general, syndromes are a recurrent and momentary grouping of signs and symptoms, which may or may not be associated with a mental disorder. Conversely, nosological entities are states from which one can presume, from the semiology presented, their path in general and the possible treatments. This predictability is possible due to their genetic, neurological, biochemical, and psychological mechanisms that are known, that is, they have a well-defined etiology (Assumpção, 2008).

Briefly, there is an effort to identify these nosological entities concisely, because it is possible to apply potential treatments and measure their effectiveness in a more precise manner, making their generalization presumed for other cases, and thus advance the construction of interventional practices based on scientific data (Dalgalarrondo, 2018). However, this is not an easy task. In general, cases in which cognitive-behavioral and psychosocial changes are exacerbated, intense and maintain a stable course are not difficult for the development of a diagnostic hypothesis; however, there are cases in which the delineation of these boundaries is complex, especially when it comes to the manifestation of behaviors considered pathological and the ways of "feeling normal," such as the cases related to disorders by the use of psychoactive substances (Whitbourne & Halgin, 2015).

Independently of the disorder, this discussion leads to a sandy field of health areas in general, the dichotomy between what is normal and what is pathological. This theme has been fostered for decades and has led to the construction of diversified criteria related to normality/abnormality, outlined from ideological, philosophical, and functional positions.

Specifically, in psychopathology, nine are the criteria usually used to characterize the concept of normality: normality as absence of illness, ideal normality, statistical normality, normality as well-being, functional normality, normality as process, subjective normality, and normality as freedom and operational normality (Dalgalarrondo, 2018; Whitbourne & Halgin, 2015).

Far from being a simple subject, it is possible to observe the complexity of conforming psychodiagnosis, especially in its practical application, after all, there are human beings who depend on the results of this reflection. It is important to point out that we would prefer the use of the term dysfunction, which could be defined as the loss of function of an organ or system. Thus, the diagnostic process is a dialectic relationship between the particular and the universal, so that the conceptual conception of diagnosis must be understood from basic general constructs for scientific work (Whitbourne & Halgin, 2015).

With this in mind, it becomes essential to understand the basic outline in order to reach a psychodiagnosis that precisely helps in the formulation of TUS cases and in the occasional interventions for each individual, since this is the main objective of a psychodiagnosis: to design a treatment plan focused on problem-solving and changes in the general functioning of the subject (Krug et al., 2016).

The Psychological Interview as a Methodological Resource

Silvares and Gongora (1998) define interview as a verbal interaction between people. From the clinical point of view, the interview is a method used to obtain information that enables a later effective intervention, taking into account the complexity and particular characteristics of the subjects and also psychological disorders (Macedo & Carrasco, 2005). In view of this, the procedure aims at collecting data that make possible a thorough analysis of cases and situations.

Table 12.2 presents some aspects listed by Silvares and Gongora (1998) to be addressed during the psychological evaluation, more specifically during the initial clinical interview. The content of the chart was adapted for the assessment in users of psychoactive substances.

The aspects presented in Table 12.2 are important for a thorough assessment in the field of substance dependence. General health conditions, for example, need to

Table 12.2 Aspects to be considered in the initial clinical interview for the description and application of criteria related to substance use disorders

Items	Description and application to substance use disorders
General health conditions	One of the diagnostic criteria for substance use disorders is continuity of use despite physical or psychological problems (American Psychiatric Association (APA) 2014). In addition, studies indicate that there is a high prevalence of psychiatric comorbidities associated with substance use (Schulden et al., 2012; Vujanovic et al., 2017). Therefore, it is essential to evaluate the general health of the subjects in order to verify and perform a differential diagnosis. The investigation of possible comorbidities is determinant for more assertive diagnosis, treatment, and prognosis
Biography	The etiology of substance use disorders involves a complex interaction of factors (Schulden et al., 2012). The evaluation of phylogenetic, ontogenetic, and cultural variables is necessary for the understanding of behaviors (Barlow & Durand, 2015; Marçal, 2010). For this, the subjects' life history must be investigated
Historical data of the phenomena	Historical data include when and how the use and the resulting problems associated with the use of substances began, in what context and under what conditions, what factors were associated with the installation of this behavior, what were the positive and negative reinforcing consequences, etc. This information is important to understand the behavior from a molar functional analysis[a] (macroanalysis), i.e., to understand it from the function it acquired during the history and the experiences of the subjects
Dimensions	Information related to the intensity, frequency, and duration of the phenomena is essential for both the diagnosis and the measurement of the severity of the picture (American Psychiatric Association (APA) 2014; Barlow & Durand, 2015). In relation to substance use, the dimensions measured can be the amount of time devoted to use, the frequency (number of times it occurs), the magnitude of the covert responses that predispose to use and the feelings after behavior, etc.
Related events	It refers to a molecular functional analysis (microanalysis) with the objective of identifying and describing specific contingencies (Nery & Fonseca, 2018)—contexts, circumstances, environmental conditions, i.e., the discriminatory stimuli predisposing to the use of substances
General consequences caused	Behavior is maintained to the extent that it produces positive consequences or avoids negative consequences for subjects. In this sense, it is valid to state that every behavior has a function (corresponding to the consequences derived from actions). The use of substances provides access to positive (pleasurable sensations and greater social interaction, for example) and negative (such as the relief of unpleasant feelings) reinforces. In other words, the behavior of using substances is functional and is maintained because it generates adaptive effects to the subjects, despite possible adverse consequences (which also need to be raised to reach a psychodiagnosis)

(continued)

Table 12.2 (continued)

Items	Description and application to substance use disorders
Potential boosters	Functional analysis is used to identify the function of behaviors (Nery & Fonseca, 2018). Thus, we try to identify the strengthening potentials (stimuli that increase the probability of responses), responsible for maintaining the target behaviors. Regarding the use of drugs, we seek to identify the consequences that maintain their occurrence (examples: relaxation, relief of anxiety, proximity and contact with people, sense of well-being, etc.)
Positive and negative points of the environment	Environmental (variable) stimuli that influence the recurrence of substance use should be identified, as well as factors related to the reduction or cessation of use. According to Monteiro (2010, p. 130), "*it is necessary to discriminate the healthy and unhealthy, adaptive and nonadoptive aspects of the patient, as well as his parents and relatives*." For example: family conflicts increase the probability of recurrence of drug use by Y (fictional person); conversely, involvement in academic activities, harmony within the family, and interpersonal relationships in other contexts help to control this behavior. The identification of these positive and negative points (which refer to whether or not they contribute to the emission of problem behaviors, and not to moral judgments) facilitates the intervention, the psychoeducation process, and the management of contingencies that maintain the behavior
Perceptions and reactions of others	Substance use disorders are characterized by harm (e.g., reduction, abandonment) at work, in studies, in interpersonal relationships, among other activities (check all diagnostic criteria in the introduction of this chapter). Thus, knowing the perception of spouses, relatives, friends, and work colleagues, for example, is one of the possible means to understand the impacts of substance use on the functioning of the subjects' lives and also to ascertain the severity of the condition
Associated emotional responses/ perception of the subjects themselves	Emotional responses must be considered in the evaluation process, since the definition of psychological disorders includes clinically significant suffering on the part of the subjects. This item also avoids classifying common behaviors as "abnormal" or pathological without considering people's own perception of them. In view of this, it should be evaluated whether the recurrent use of substances is associated with aversive feelings, i.e., whether adverse consequences are perceived and felt. It is worth noting, however, that in some cases there may be no awareness of possible harm. Positive responses associated with the use should also be considered, as they allow the identification of possible functions that the behavior performs (for example: feeling relaxed or happy)

Source: Based on Silvares and Gongora (1998)
[a]For more information on molecular and molar functional analysis, see Nery and Fonseca (2018)

be assessed, as they can influence differential psychodiagnosis. For example, Beck (2013) cites cases of hyperthyroidism that are confused with depression; and in cases of substance use disorders, psychiatric comorbidities are common. The evaluation of these comorbid problems contemplates cognitive-affective processes underlying substance use disorders and enables a more effective clinical approach (Vujanovic et al., 2017). Therefore, the subjects' life history needs to be carefully evaluated, listing the genetic, ontogenetic, and social factors involved and potentially determining the installation and maintenance of problem behaviors. When not observed correctly and not taken into account such aspects may lead to erroneous diagnosis, treatment, and prognosis, so as to generate more damage to individuals and others involved.

Barlow and Durand (2015) propose an integrated approach in the investigation of psychological phenomena, as well as psychopathologies, in order to cover their biopsychosocial variables. Regarding substance use disorders, the authors consider the following aspects: *biological*: genetics, heredity, neurobiology; *psycho-behavioral*: positive and negative reinforces; *cognitive*: expectations, beliefs; *social*: exposure in the family, peer influence; and *cultural*: traditions, values. Therefore, a careful analysis of the phenomenon and associated factors is required, in addition to a theoretical explanatory model and a set of techniques that consider relevant information and results to a greater accuracy and effectiveness in diagnosis, treatment, and prognosis (Araújo, 2007; Santos et al. 2018).

Instruments for the Evaluation of Substance Use Disorders

Due to the complexity involved in behavioral dependencies, a complete psychological evaluation should include the investigation of predisposing factors (genetics), precipitants (triggers of use), and behavioral maintainers (role of the drug in the life of individuals, in the network of friends, etc.), as well as cognitive, emotional, and socio-environmental aspects, such as intellectual resources, socio-emotional abilities, ease of access to the drug and resources to acquire it (De Micheli et al. 2020). It is also suggested that other aspects of the patient's functioning that may be related to drug use be investigated, such as family, relational, or occupational aspects (Petry, Kolling, & Melo, 2011).

Considering the ambivalence present in the thought/conduct of substance use disorder (SUD) patients, who are often referred to psychodiagnosis against their own will, instruments such as scales and psychological tests can help the professional to obtain information that complements the interview and contribute to referral to a more personalized treatment (Lopes et al., 2019). Table 12.3 presents the main scales used in Brazil (adapted or validated for use at the national level) in order to investigate patterns of consumption, cleftness, motivation for cessation and expectations of drug effects, aspects that are relevant when working with psychological evaluation of patients with problems due to the use of psychoactive substances.

A fairly frequent issue among users of substances who want to stop consumption is relapses. In the evaluation that precedes treatment, it is important, therefore, that "trigger" situations (crack triggers, which is the intense desire to consume the drug) and coping strategies are identified. In this sense, tools such as the *temptation use drugs scale* (TUD), *drug abstinence self-efficacy scale* (DASE), and the Knapp and Bertolote (1994) may be useful (Lopes et al., 2019). The TUD and DASE, adapted for Brazilian samples (Freire, Silva, Ávila, DiClemente, & Oliveira, 2017), are

Table 12.3 Tools for evaluating aspects of drug use

Instrument	Objective	Development or adaptation to Brazil
Alcohol, smoking, and substance involvement screening test (ASSIST)	To evaluate the frequency and problems related to the use of nine classes of psychoactive substances (tobacco, alcohol, marijuana, cocaine, stimulants, sedatives, inhalants, hallucinogens, and opiates)	Henrique et al. (2004)
Addiction severity index (ASI-6)	Assess the severity of alcohol and other drug dependence in a multidimensional manner, including medical history, employment, involvement with legal issues, family and social history	Kessler (2011)
Teen addiction severity index (Teen-ASI)	Evaluate the use of alcohol and other drugs by adolescents, including school status, employment/support, family relationships, friends/social relationships, legal status, and psychiatric status	Sartes et al. (2009)
Drug use screening inventory (DUSI)	To evaluate the frequency and problems related to the consumption of alcohol and other drugs by adolescents, including evaluation of behavior, health, psychiatric disorders, sociability, family system, school, work, relationships, and leisure	Micheli and Formigoni (2000)
Cutting down, annoyance by criticism, guilty feeling, and eye-openers (CAGE)	Perform screening for alcohol abuse or dependence	Gaya (2011)
Short-form alcohol dependence data (SADD)	Assess the severity of alcohol dependency	Jorge and Mansur (1986)
Alcohol use disorder identification test (AUDIT)	Perform a tracking of problematic alcohol use	Santos et al. (2012)
Fagerström test for nicotine dependence (FTND)	Assess the severity of nicotine dependence	Carmo and Pueyo (2002)
Questionnaire of smoking urges-brief (QSU-B)	Assess the crack in smokers	Araujo et al. (2007)
Modified smoking reasons (EMF) scale	Evaluate seven domains of smoking behavior: addiction, pleasure of smoking, tension reduction or relaxation, social interaction, activation or excitability, habit or automatism, and hand-to-mouth movement	Souza et al. (2009)
Marijuana expectancy questionnaire (MEQ)	To evaluate beliefs regarding the use of marijuana, including cognitive and behavioral impairment, reduction of tension and relaxation, social and sexual facilitation, increased perception and cognition, negative global effects, cracking, and physical effects	Pedroso et al. (2004)

(continued)

Table 12.3 (continued)

Instrument	Objective	Development or adaptation to Brazil
Marijuana users expected results inventory (IERUM)	Evaluate expectations of results regarding marijuana use, including emotional aspects, perception, sexuality, cognitive aspects, and cleft	Pedroso et al. (2010)
Cocaine craving questionnaire-brief (CCQ-B)	Assess the intensity of the desire (crack) to use crack	Araujo et al. (2011)
Cocaine selective severity assessment (CSSA)	Assess crack and symptoms related to cocaine/crack abstinence	Kluwe-Schiavon et al. (2015)
Crack use relapse scale (CURS)	Evaluate family and relational conflicts, negative feelings, pleasurable feelings, crack for crack, crack after using another drug, and other losses related to crack use	Pedroso et al. (2016)

composed of 24 items each, in which subjects must mark how tempted they feel to use the drug in certain situations (TUD) and how confident they feel about resisting the drug (DASE), on a numerical scale ranging from one (minimum) to five (maximum), providing data on self-efficacy.

The ability to deal with risk situations inventory aims to identify the most dangerous situations and assess the individual's most prominent vulnerabilities to drug use. Several situations of risk to abstinence are listed and the patient must score how self-efficacy he or she considers to face each one. The situations mix external stimuli, such as "going to parties," and internal stimuli, such as "being anxious or depressed," being important to record the most difficult times of the day and/or week. Such diagnosis of situations will serve for the development of personalized coping strategies to maintain abstinence (Knapp & Bertolote, 1994; Souza & Araújo, 2010).

In addition to the instruments specifically aimed at investigating aspects related to the use/abuse of substances presented in Table 12.3, others instruments that evaluate cognitive functions and executive functions may also be useful, considering that studies have shown a relationship between behavioral dependencies and harm to these functions (REF). Table 12.4 presents some of the instruments that can be indicated when there is suspicion of damage in cognitive functions (such as memory, attention, intelligence) or executive functions, such as judgment, decision-making, cognitive flexibility, and impulsiveness control.

From the instruments described in Tables 12.3 and 12.4, it can be seen that there is a relatively significant variety of measurement instruments useful for investigating aspects related to substance use and dependence. It is important to emphasize the importance of paying attention to the psychometric properties of these instruments and their standardization process. Finally, it is important to emphasize that the application of the instruments described in this section involves specialized

Table 12.4 Cognitive function evaluation tools and executive functions

Instrument	Objective	Development or adaptation in Brazil
Montreal cognitive assessment (MOCA)	Evaluate mild cognitive impairment through the analysis of eight cognitive domains: short-term memory, visuospatial abilities, executive functions, attention, concentration, work memory, language, and orientation	Memória et al. (2013)
Wechsler intelligence scale for adults (WAIS-III)	Assess intellectual capacity and overall cognitive functioning in adults between 16 and 89 years	Nascimento (2000)
Iowa gambling task	Evaluate decision-making capacity	Schneider and Parente (2006)
Rey's complex figures test	Evaluate planning ability, perception, organization, fine motor skills, and immediate reproduction memory	Oliveira and Rigoni (2010)
Trail testing	Assess complex visual processing, motor speed, inhibitory control, and cognitive flexibility	Rabelo et al. (2010)
Wisconsin letters classification test (WCST)	To evaluate the capacity of abstract reasoning and cognitive flexibility; to trace lesions in the frontal lobe	Miguel (2005)

training, as well as it is recommended that none of them be used in isolation, but in a complementary manner to the clinical interview.

The Returning Interview

In the scientific literature that underlies the professional performance in psychology, the relevance of the clinical interview in the processes of psychological evaluation and psychodiagnosis, as well as a variety of psychological examination techniques, is highlighted. Regardless of the process and the number of stages of a psychodiagnosis, it is important to communicate the results produced. A devolutive interview is called the *feedback of the* psychodiagnosis process, a way of returning the results obtained, as well as the understanding of the aspects evaluated, to the patients and other interlocutors (Araújo, 2007; Silvares & Gongora, 1998).

It is even considered that the devolutive interview in psychodiagnosis is crucial for the following stages of the therapeutic process (Ocampo and Arzeno 2009). Thus, the devolutive interview marks the transition from evaluation and psychodiagnosis to the process of communicating the conclusions obtained to the subjects and then the necessary referrals. This stage is extremely relevant to demonstrate to those involved the importance of the aspects evaluated and the analysis of the situation, as it influences the assertiveness of diagnosis, prognosis, and guidance to those involved (Marques, 2005). For Monteiro (2010, p. 129), the devolutive interview has the role of "contextualizing the lived experience" in psychodiagnosis.

Ocampo and Arzeno (2009) highlight some important issues in the devolutionary process. Among them (a) "If information is not returned, the fantasies of illness, gravity, incurability, madness, etc. intensify" and (b) "If we return information, we give the patient an opportunity to see himself with more criteria of reality, with less idealizing or derogatory distortions" (p. 318). They also consider it essential to return information to family members whenever possible. According to them, it is important that they know the professional's opinion to avoid possible distortions about the case. In addition, it is also important to stress that the devolutive interview, especially when carried out with the involvement of third parties, enables more people to know the situation, who may cooperate in the treatment and help in relation to the patients' complaints, contributing to the resolution of the problems and the reduction of suffering.

During the return, the topics in Table 12.2 can be used to present and explain the variables and their influence on the installation and maintenance of problem behaviors related to substance use, as well as to signal the focus of future interventions. However, it is necessary to discriminate both the healthier aspects of the subject and his/her family group and the less adaptive ones. Therefore, caution is recommended in selecting the aspects to be reported in the return, taking into account the characteristics of each person involved and a prediction of how they may react to the information provided (Krug et al., 2016; Ocampo & Arzeno, 2009).

Macedo and Carrasco (2005) characterize the devolutive step as important for the reduction or cessation of distortions in the situation, while it is a process of providing information on the conclusions and explanations of the next steps. Thus, in addition to conclusions (and answers, if there are any doubts) about the psychodiagnosis, it is essential to clarify the prognosis and the exposure of measures and resources that can help in the minimization or resolution of suffering (Marques, 2005).

Finally, the moment of the devolutive interview is an opportunity for the professional to carry out a process of psychoeducation with the patient and family members, making the devolutive interview, as far as possible, a learning activity and change promoters. The psychoeducation strategy includes psychological and pedagogical instruments in order to elucidate the patients and interlocutors the pathology in question and the prognosis, as well as to guide on possible referrals (Lemes & Neto, 2017).

When it comes to substance use and dependence, people significant to them (such as family) often feel confused and pressured, while their basic task is to help care for people who have drug-related problems. When concerns about the adverse consequences of substance use are properly discussed by providing scientifically based information, the chances of promoting the replacement of blaming attitudes with coping strategies increase. Thus, it becomes possible to build a supportive network that contributes to the reduction of possible harm associated with drug use, and the devolutionary interview is a propitious moment for constructive dialogue (Silva, Noto, De Micheli & Camargo, 2015; Silva, Rodrigues, De Micheli & Andrade, 2015). Therefore, the devolutive interview is an opportunity for the development of assertive attitudes towards prognosis and treatment, aiming at solving problems, not only in relation to drug use and dependence, but also in relation to relationships of family and social coexistence.

Final Considerations

Every psychodiagnostic process aims at understanding the human being in its entirety, based on demands related to the clinical conditions of people, usually associated with restrictions in their psychological functioning. In the case of the use of psychoactive substances, in a pathological manner, it is relevant to identify the symptoms or associated disorders or dysfunctions, as well as the psychosocial repercussions and treatment difficulties.

Furthermore, based on the aspects evaluated, it is possible to perceive that there are consistent theoretical models on the understanding of drug dependence that allow us to understand its etiology, present signs and symptoms, as well as risk and protection factors. It is up to psychologists to define the inherent and specific objectives of each situation to be evaluated, since this can vary in a great manner, given the existence of several dimensions of this phenomenon, as well as the dynamics of this process, as well as therapeutic approaches. Certainly, the definition of the theoretical model adopted will largely guide the objectives to be defined.

The availability of instrumental resources is significant, which provides options for examining psychological constructs relevant to the investigation of disorders and/or dysfunctions related to the use of psychoactive substances. But, undoubtedly, it is the investigative attitude and technical skills of the psychologist that can provide a psychodiagnosis that is equal to the need to understand psychological phenomena in their multidimensionality.

References

Alchieri, J. C., & Cruz, R. M. (2003). *Avaliação psicológica: Conceito, métodos e instrumentos*. São Paulo: Casa do Psicólogo.

American Psychiatric Association (APA). (2014). *Manual diagnóstico e estatístico de transtornos mentais* (5th ed.). Porto Alegre: Artmed Editora.

Araújo, M. F. (2007). Estratégias de diagnóstico e avaliação psicológica. *Psicologia: Teoria e Prática, 9*(2), 126–141.

Araujo, R., Castro, M., Pedroso, R., Santos, P., Leite, L., Rocha, M., & Marques, A. C. (2011). Validação psicométrica do cocaine craving questionnaire-brief – versão brasileira adaptada para o crack para dependentes hospitalizados. *Jornal Brasileiro de Psiquiatria, 60*(4), 233–239. https://doi.org/10.1590/S0047-20852011000400001.

Araujo, R., Oliveira, M., Moraes, J., Pedroso, R., Port, F., & Castro, M. G. (2007). Validação da versão brasileira do questionnaire of smoking urges-brief. *Archives of Clinical Psychiatry, 34*(4), 166–175. https://doi.org/10.1590/S0101-60832007000400002.

Assumpção, F. B. (2008). *Psicopatologia evolutiva*. Porto Alegre: Artmed.

Almeida, D. E. R. G., De Micheli, D., & Andrade, A. L. M. (2017). Leisure and substance use among adolescents: a systematic review. Estudos e Pesquisas em Psicologia, 17(3), 970-988. http://dx.doi.org/10.1590/1413-82712018230102

Andrade, A. L., M., & De Micheli, D. (2016). Innovations in the Treatment of Substance Addiction (1st Ed.). New York: Springer International Publishing. http://dx.doi.org/10.1007/978-3-319-43172-7.

Andrade, A. L. M., Scatena, A., & De Micheli, D. (2017a). Evaluation of a preventive intervention in alcoholic and non-alcoholic drivers – a pilot study. SMAD. Revista eletrônica saúde mental álcool e drogas, 13(4), 205–212. https://doi.org/10.11606/issn.1806-6976.v13i4p205-212

Andrade, A. L. M., Teixeira, L. R. D. S., Zoner, C. C., Niro, N. N., Scatena, A., & Amaral, R. A. D. (2017b). Factors associated with postpartum depression in social vulnerability women. SMAD. Revista eletrônica saúde mental álcool e drogas, 13(4), 196–204. http://dx.doi.org/10.11606/issn.1806-6976.v13i4p196-204

Andrade, A. L. M. & De Micheli, D. (2016). Innovations in the Treatment of Substance Addiction. 1. ed. New York: Springer International Publishing. http://dx.doi.org/10.1007/978-3-319-43172-7

Banaco, R. A., Zamignani, D. R., Martone, R. C., Vermes, J. S., & Kovac, R. (2015). Psicopatologia. In M. Hübner & M. Moreira (Eds.), *Temas clássicos da psicologia sob a ótica da análise do comportamento* (pp. 154–166). Rio de Janeiro: Guanabara Koogan.

Barlow, D. H., & Durand, V. M. (2015). *Psicopatologia: uma abordagem integrada* (2nd ed.). São Paulo: Cengage Learning.

Beck, J. S. (2013). *Terapia cognitivo-comportamental: Teoria e prática* (2nd ed.). Porto Alegre: Artmed.

Barbosa, L. A., Andrade, A. L. M., Oliveira, L. G., & De Micheli, D. (2018). Prevalence of psychotropic substance use by urban bus drivers: a systematic review. SMAD. Revista eletrônica saúde mental álcool e drogas, 14(4), 234-244. http://dx.doi.org/10.11606/issn.1806-6976.smad.2018.000400

Bedendo, A., Andrade, A. L. M., Opaleye, E. S., & Noto, A. R. (2017). Binge drinking: a pattern associated with a risk of problems of alcohol use among university students. Revista latino-americana de enfermagem, 25. e2925-e2933. http://dx.doi.org/10.1590/1518-8345.1891.2925

Capitão, C. G., Scortegagna, S. A., & Baptista, M. N. (2005). A importância da avaliação psicológica na saúde. *Avaliação Psicológica, 4*(1), 75–82.

Carmo, J. T., & Pueyo, A. A. (2002). A adaptação ao português do Fagerström test for nicotine dependence (FTND) para avaliar a dependência e tolerância à nicotina em fumantes brasileiros. *Revista Brasileira de Medicina, 59*(1/2), 73–80.

Castro, E. K., Campezatto, P. V. M., & Saraiva, L. A. (2009). As etapas da psicoterapia com crianças. In M. G. K. Castro & A. Stürmer (Eds.), *Crianças e adolescentes em psicoterapia: A abordagem psicanalítica.* Porto Alegre: Artmed.

Cruz, R. M. (2002). O processo de conhecer em avaliação psicológica. In R. M. Cruz, J. C. Alchieri, & J. J. Sardá Jr. (Eds.), *Avaliação e medidas psicológicas: produção do conhecimento e da intervenção profissional* (pp. 15–24). São Paulo: Casa do Psicólogo.

Cruz, R. M., & Sardá, J. J., Jr. (2019). Avaliação psicológica do estresse. In M. N. Baptista & A. E. de Villemor-Amaral (Eds.), *Compêndio de avaliação psicológica* (p. 625). Petrópolis: Vozes.

Cunha, J. A. (2003). *Psicodiagnóstico-V*. Porto Alegre: Artmed.

Dalgalarrondo, P. (2018). *Psicopatologia e semiologia dos transtornos mentais.* Porto Alegre: Artmed.

DiClemente, C. C. (2018). *Addiction and change: How addictions develop and addicted people recover* (2nd ed.). New York: The Guilford Press.

De Micheli, D. Andrade, A. L. M., Silva, E. A. & Souza-Formigoni, M. L. O. (2016). Drug Abuse in Adolescence. 1. ed. New York: Springer International Publishing. http://dx.doi.org/10.1007/978-3-319-17795-3

De Micheli, D., Andrade, A., & Galduróz, J. C. (2020). Limitations of DSM-5 diagnostic criteria for substance use disorder in adolescents: what have we learned after using these criteria for several years? *Brazilian Journal of Psychiatry*, in press. https://doi.org/10.1590/1516-4446-2020-1151.

Federal Council of Psychology (2007). *Resolução CFP N.° 007/2003*. Retrieved from http://www.crpsp.org.br/portal/orientacao/resolucoes_cfp/fr_cfp_007-03.aspx

Fernández-Ballesteros, R. (2014). *Evaluación psicológica*. Madrid: Pirámide.

Freire, S., Silva, D., Ávila, A., DiClemente, C., & Oliveira, M. (2017). Adaptation and validation of the Brazilian DASE and TUD scales for cocaine/crack users. *Paidéia, 27*(67), 93–99. https://doi.org/10.1590/1982-43272767201711.

Frade, I. F., De Micheli, D., Andrade, A. L. M., & de Souza-Formigoni, M. L. O. (2014). Relationship between stress symptoms and drug use among secondary students. The Spanish journal of psychology, 16, e4. https://doi.org/10.1017/sjp.2013.5

Gaya, C. M. (2011). Estudo de validação de instrumentos de rastreamento para transtornos depressivos, abuso e dependência de álcool e tabaco (Doctoral dissertation, Universidade Federal de São Paulo, São Paulo, Brasil).

Henrique, I., De Micheli, D., Lacerda, R., Lacerda, L., & Formigoni, M. L. (2004). Validação da versão brasileira do teste de triagem do envolvimento com álcool, cigarro e outras substâncias (ASSIST). *Revista da Associação Médica Brasileira, 50*(2), 199–206. https://doi.org/10.1590/S0104-42302004000200039.

Jorge, M. R., & Mansur, J. (1986). Questionários padronizados para Avaliação do grau de Severidade da Síndrome de Dependência do Álcool. *Jornal Brasileiro de Psiquiatria, 35*(5), 287–292.

Kessler, F. (2011). Desenvolvimento e validação da sexta versão da Addiction Severity Index (ASI6) para o Brasil e outras análises em uma amostra multicêntrica de usuários de drogas que buscam tratamento no país (Doctoral dissertation, Universidade Federal do Rio Grande do Sul, Porto Alegre, Brazil).

Kluwe-Schiavon, B., Tractenberg, S., Sanvicente-Vieira, B., Rosa, C., Arteche, A., Pezzi, J. C., & Grassi-Oliveira, R. (2015). Propriedades psicométricas da cocaine selective severity assessment (CSSA) em mulheres usuárias de crack. *Jornal Brasileiro de Psiquiatria, 64*(2), 115–121. https://doi.org/10.1590/0047-2085000000066.

Knapp, P., & Bertolote, J. M. (1994). *Prevenção de recaída: um manual para pessoas com problemas pelo uso de álcool e de drogas*. Porto Alegre: Artmed.

Krug, J., Trentini, C. M., & Bandeira, D. R. (2016). Conceituação de psicodiagnóstico na atualidade. In C. S. Hutz, D. R. Bandeira, C. Trentini, & J. S. Krug (Eds.), *Psicodiagnóstico* (pp. 16–20). Porto Alegre: Artmed.

Lemes, C. B., & Neto, J. O. (2017). Aplicações da psicoeducação no contexto da saúde. *Temas Em Psicologia, 25*(1), 17–28. https://doi.org/10.9788/TP2017.1-02.

Lopes, F. M., Andretta, I., & Oliveira, M. S. (2019). Avaliação psicológica dos transtornos relacionados a substâncias psicoativas. In M. N. Baptista et al. (Eds.), *Compêndio de Avaliação Psicológica* (pp. 692–701). Petrópolis: Vozes.

Macedo, M. M. K., & Carrasco, L. K. (2005). A entrevista clínica: um espaço de intersubjetividade. In M. M. K. Macedo & L. K. Carrasco (Eds.), *(Con)textos de entrevista: olhares diversos sobre a interação humana* (pp. 19–32). São Paulo: Casa do Psicólogo.

Marçal, J. V. S. (2010). Behaviorismo radical e prática clínica. In A. De-Farias (Ed.), *Análise comportamental clínica: aspectos teóricos e estudos de caso* (pp. 30–48). Porto Alegre: Artmed.

Marques, N. (2005). Entrevista de triagem: espaço de acolhimento, escuta e ajuda terapêutica. In M. M. K. Macedo & L. K. Carrasco (Eds.), *(Con)textos de entrevista: olhares diversos sobre a interação humana* (pp. 161–180). São Paulo: Casa do Psicólogo.

Memória, C., Yassuda, M., Nakano, E., & Forlenza, O. (2013). Brief screening for mild cognitive impairment: Validation of the Brazilian version of the Montreal cognitive assessment. *International Journal of Geriatric Psychiatry, 28*, 34–40. https://doi.org/10.1002/gps.3787.

Micheli, D., & Formigoni, M. L. (2000). Screening of drug use in a teenage Brazilian sample using the drug use screening inventory (DUSI). *Addictive Behaviors, 25*(5), 683–691. https://doi.org/10.1016/s0306-4603(00)00065-4.

Miguel, F. K. (2005). Teste Wisconsin de classificação de cartas. *Avaliação Psicológica, 4*(2), 203–204.

Monteiro, R. (2010). Relato de uma entrevista de devolução com a criança no psicodiagnóstico. *Estudos Interdisciplinares Em Psicologia, 1*(1), 129–135.

Nascimento, E. (2000). Adaptação e validação do teste WAIS-III para um contexto brasileiro (Doctoral dissertation, Universidade de Brasília. Brasília, Brazil).

Nery, L. B., & Fonseca, F. N. (2018). Análises funcionais molares e moleculares: um passo a passo. In A. K. C. R. de-Farias, F. N. Fonseca, & L. B. Nery (Eds.), *Teoria e formulação de casos em análise comportamental clínica* (pp. 22–54). Porto Alegre: Artmed.

Ocampo, M. L. S., & Arzeno, M. E. G. (2009). Devolução de informação no processo psicodiagnóstico. In M. L. S. Ocampo (Ed.), *O processo psicodiagnóstico e as técnicas projetivas* (11th ed., pp. 315–332). São Paulo: Martins Fontes.

Oliveira, M. S., & Rigoni, M. S. (2010). *Figuras Complexas de Rey: Teste de Cópia e de Reprodução de Memória de Figuras Geométricas Complexas*. São Paulo: Casa do Psicólogo.

Pedroso, R., Castro, M., & Araujo, R. (2010). Inventário de expectativas de resultados em usuários de maconha (IERUM): construção e validação. *Revista de Psiquiatria do Rio Grande do Sul, 32*, 24–29. https://doi.org/10.1590/S0101-81082010000100005.

Pedroso, R., Oliveira, M., Araujo, R., & Moraes, J. (2004). Tradução, equivalência semântica e adaptação cultural do marijuana expectancy questionnaire (MEQ). *Psico-USF, 9*(2), 129–136. https://doi.org/10.1590/S1413-82712004000200003.

Pedroso, R., Zanetello, L., Guimarães, L., Pettenon, M., Gonçalves, V., Scherer, J., Kessler, F., & Pechansky, F. (2016). Confirmatory factor analysis (CFA) of the crack use relapse scale (CURS). *Archives of Clinical Psychiatry, 43*(3), 37–40. https://doi.org/10.1590/0101-60830000000081.

Petry, M. C., Kolling, N. M., & Melo, W. V. (2011). Atualidade na dependência do crack. In R. Wainer, N. M. Piccoloto, & G. K. Pergher (Eds.), *Novas temáticas em terapia cognitiva* (pp. 39–60). Porto Alegre: Sinopsys.

Rabelo, I. S., Pacanaro, S. V., Rosseti, M. O., & Leme, I. F. (2010). *Teste de trilhas coloridas*. São Paulo: Casa do Psicólogo.

Santos, I. M. S., Santiago, T. R. S., Oliveira, J. R. V., Lima, E. D., & Melo, M. R. A. (2018). Avaliação Psicológica com Usuários de Substâncias Psicoativas (SPA): uma Revisão Sistemática da Literatura. *PSI UNISC, 2*(1), 48–60. https://doi.org/10.17058/psiunisc.v2i2.10837.

Santos, W., Gouveia, V., Fernandes, D., Souza, S., & Grangeiro, A. (2012). Alcohol use disorder identification test (AUDIT): Explorando seus parâmetros psicométricos. *Jornal Brasileiro de Psiquiatria, 61*(3), 117–123. https://doi.org/10.1590/S0047-20852012000300001.

Sartes, L. M., De Micheli, D., & Formigoni, M. L. (2009). Psychometric and discriminative properties of the teen addiction severity index (Brazilian Portuguese version). *European Child & Adolescent Psychiatry, 18*(11), 653–661. https://doi.org/10.1007/s00787-009-0021-z.

Schneider, D., & Parente, M. A. (2006). O desempenho de adultos jovens e idosos na Iowa Gambling Task (IGT): um estudo sobre a tomada de decisão. *Psicologia: Reflexão e Crítica, 19*(3), 442–450. https://doi.org/10.1590/S0102-79722006000300013.

Schulden, J., Lopez, M., & Compton, W. (2012). Clinical implications of drug abuse epidemiology. *Psychiatric Clinics of North America, 35*(2), 411–423. https://doi.org/10.1016/j.psc.2012.03.007.

Silva, E. A., Noto, A. R., De Micheli, D., & Camargo, B. M. V. (2015). *Diálogos com a família sobre uso, abuso e dependência de drogas*. São Paulo: Casa do Psicólogo.

Silva, E. A., Rodrigues, T. P., De Micheli, D., & Andrade, A. L. M. (2015). Estratégias utilizadas no tratamento de famílias com usuários de substâncias. *Psicologia Em Pesquisa, 9*(2), 198–204. https://doi.org/10.5327/Z1982-1247201500020010.

Silvares, E., & Gongora, M. (1998). *Psicologia clínica comportamental: A inserção da entrevista com adultos e crianças*. São Paulo: EDICON.

Souza, A. C. F., & Araújo, R. B. (2010). Acompanhamento terapêutico na dependência química. In I. Londero (Ed.), *Acompanhamento terapêutico: Teoria e técnica na terapia comportamental e cognitivo-comportamental* (pp. 127–138). São Paulo: Santos.

Souza, E., Crippa, J. A., Pasian, S., & Martinez, J. A. (2009). Modified reasons for smoking scale: Translation to Portuguese, cross-cultural adaptation for use in Brazil and evaluation of test-retest reliability. *Jornal Brasileiro de Pneumologia, 35*(7), 683–689. https://doi.org/10.1590/S1806-37132009000700010.

Vujanovic, A., Meyer, T., Heads, A., Stotts, A., Villarreal, Y., & Schmitz, J. (2017). Cognitive-behavioral therapies for depression and substance use disorders: An overview of traditional, third-wave, and transdiagnostic approaches. *The American Journal of Drug and Alcohol Abuse, 43*(4), 402–415. https://doi.org/10.1080/00952990.2016.1199697.

Whitbourne, S. K., & Halgin, R. P. (2015). *Psicopatologia: Perspectivas clínicas dos transtornos psicológicos* (7th ed.). Porto Alegre: Artmed.

World Health Organization (WHO). (2019). *International statistical classification of diseases and related health problems, eleventh revision*. Retrieved from https://icd.who.int/browse10/2019/en

Chapter 13
Evidence-Based Psychotherapy for Substance Use Disorder

Jan Luiz Leonardi, Dan Josua, and Cainã Gomes

Introduction

In the early 1990s, Division 12 of the *American Psychological Association* (APA) set up a task force to define and identify empirically supported psychological treatments (Chambless 1993). Two criteria were used: (1) the intervention should be thoroughly described in a manual as a requirement for procedure standardization (the independent variable in question), thus enabling therapists to replicate processes and findings and (2) the intervention should have its efficacy supported by experimental evidence, which could stem from at least two randomized clinical trials or a set of single case trials[1] (Chambless and Ollendick 2001; Task Force on Promotion and Dissemination of Psychological Procedures 1995).

The first Division 12 task force report, published in 1995, listed 18 empirically sustained treatments and received several updates through the following years (e.g., Chambless et al. 1998). More recently, however, Division 12 has replaced the assessment of clinical or single case trials with systematic, meta-analysis reviews (Tolin et al. 2015), a rigorous method used to synthesize the results of clinical research. Currently, researchers and practitioners may refer to the list of empirically supported treatments, their respective manuals, the clinical research on which they are based, the meta-analyses, and training information at www.div12.org/psychological-treatments.

After a long struggle between diverse theoretical, conceptual, methodological, and practical perspectives on empirically sustained treatments (Leonardi and Meyer 2015), the American Psychological Association (APA 2006) defined the concept of *evidence-based practice in psychology* as an individualized clinical

[1] For a brief explanation on different methods in psychotherapy research, see Leonardi (2017).

J. L. Leonardi (✉) · D. Josua · C. Gomes
Instituto de Psicologia Baseada em Evidências, São Paulo, SP, Brazil

D. De Micheli et al. (eds.), *Drugs and Human Behavior*,
https://doi.org/10.1007/978-3-030-62855-0_13

decision-making process that occurs through the integration of the best available evidence (i.e., integrated therapeutic procedures that have provenly produced positive outcomes and minimized negative ones) with clinical expertise (i.e., ability to formulate the case, apply techniques, monitor progress, establish therapeutic relationships, etc.) in the context of patients' characteristics, culture, and preferences (i.e., their objectives, values, beliefs, setting, and clinical status). From this perspective, the three elements of the definition—empirical evidence, professional repertoire, and patient's idiosyncrasies—are fundamental in clinical decision-making, so that a therapy that fails to consider the interrelationship between all three components cannot be seen as evidence-based practice in psychology.

In this sense, to conduct evidence-based psychotherapy for substance use disorder, practitioners must take into account available, empirically supported treatments (i.e., the best available evidence), required therapeutic skills (i.e., clinical expertise), and patients' idiosyncrasies.

This chapter thus aims to present an overview of psychological interventions with greater evidence of effectiveness for substance use disorder, outline the main clinical skills required for therapists to treat this population, and point out important considerations regarding treatments and patients' idiosyncrasies.

Empirically Sustained Treatments

Data from randomized clinical trials and systematic reviews of the meta-analysis literature revealed that the psychological interventions with the greatest evidence of effectiveness are motivational interviewing, motivational enhancement therapy, community reinforcement approach, contingency management, and couple behavioral therapy (Blonigen et al. 2015; Dutra et al. 2008; Klimas et al. 2018; Martin and Rehm 2012). Such treatments are briefly presented below, but the interested reader can find a detailed description in their respective manuals.

Motivational Interviewing

More than a sui generis therapeutic approach, motivational interviewing (MI) is regarded as a way to understand human communication and manage this dialog to favor positive behavioral changes. In the words of its creators:

> MI is a collaborative, goal-oriented style of communication with particular attention to the language of change. It is designed to strengthen personal motivation for and commitment to a specific goal by eliciting and exploring the person's own reasons for change within an atmosphere of acceptance and compassion (Miller and Rollnick 2012, p. 29).

In other words, MI is a dialog conduction method inspired by the tradition of Carl Rogers' *Person-Centered Psychology*, but also aimed at committing to the change of well-established behavior (e.g., reducing or zeroing alcohol intake) (Miller and Rollnick 2012). This proposal is based on a philosophical conception that emphasizes the importance of ensuring an intrinsic motivation for treatment, i.e., departing from patients' self-attributed relevant reasons.

Thus, as opposed to a traditional approach for treating SUD—which often sets problematic character traits as these patients' motivations to seek treatment—MI understands that the difficulties in care are often due to the very way these patients are received in the therapeutic setting. For this reason, MI proposes that instead of bombarding patients with information about the risks of alcohol abuse, for instance, the therapist actively listens as means to help clients articulate how (and if) alcohol proved harmful in their lives. After all, MI assumes that treatment difficulties do not stem from ignorance about the harms of addictive behavior, but from an ambivalence between the inclination to change and the desire to remain engaged in problem behavior.

It may seem obvious in retrospect, but one's motivation to stop smoking, to name one example, does not depend on knowledge about the damage cigarettes cause to the lung. Conversely, they struggle to give up on the effects brought by cigarettes (e.g., the anxiolytic effect of nicotine) even when aware of all the risks offered by smoking. MI addresses such dilemma with a reasonably simple proposition: practitioners must provide a space that favors clients themselves to speak and recognize the reasons for abandoning their addiction.

A therapist with qualified MI training must then operate four basic strategies: (1) open questions, (2) affirmations, (3) reflective listening, and (4) summary reflections (aka OARS). Such strategies must be performed at a 2:1 ratio—that is, two uses of either affirmation, reflective listening, or summary reflection per open question addressed to the patient (Miller and Rollnick 2012).

Open questions are designed to lead patients to engage in more elaborate answers than simply "yes" or "no." For example, "why did you decide to seek therapy?" as opposed to "did you come to treat your substance abuse?" Statements are a direct, simple remark that communicates a quality of the client, such as "you showed courage." Summaries are a therapist's attempt to simplify a longer, more complex chunk of the patient's speech. The conclusion of summaries must focus on change talk (Miller and Rollnick 2012)—as successfully demonstrated in a series of studies that evaluated the effect of the conclusion on narrative perception (cf. Kahneman 2011).

Lastly, perhaps the most important MI strategy is the use of precise summary reflections—affirmative sentences that recapitulate or paraphrase the patient's speech to both to demonstrate understanding and emphasize important details of communication. Summary reflections are a fundamental tool to demonstrate that the client is being heard and that their conception matters for the treatment. In effective summary reflections, a trained MI practitioner usually reiterates a speech section that describes the patient's change, thereby emphasizing such event (Miller and Rollnick 2012).

To date, these principles have been evaluated in more than 200 randomized clinical trials that have demonstrated their efficacy for a variety of psychopathologies, especially those related to substance and alcohol abuse with mild to strong effects

(Blonigen et al. 2015; Miller and Rollnick 2012). A meta-analysis by the *Cochrane Collaboration* reviewed 59 studies that followed more than 13,000 patients with addiction or alcoholism disorders who underwent MI treatment. Data showed strong results in post-intervention and weaker results in medium and long-term follow-up (Smedslund et al. 2011). An additional review study with smokers suggests that MI is especially effective if performed in long sessions (over 20 min) with a total of at least two intervention days; however, the heterogeneity of these studies calls for a careful interpretation of results (Lai et al. 2010).

Motivational Enhancement Therapy

*Motivational enhancement therapy (*MET) is a systematic, brief (around 4 sessions), MI-based intervention for patients with alcohol and drug addiction problems (Blonigen et al. 2015; Miller et al. 1992). At MATCH—a multi-center project funded by the US *National Institute of Mental Health*—MET was evaluated and compared to longer duration interventions (12 sessions of cognitive-behavioral therapy or 12 sessions of *12-step* programs, such as *alcoholics anonymous*) with approximately 1700 alcohol abusers (Project MATCH Research Group 1998). All interventions obtained similar results, which suggests that shorter MET interventions have comparable outcomes to more robust programs. Similar findings were obtained in another study conducted in the United Kingdom (UKATT Research Team 2005).

Following the precepts of MI, MET is a structured way to ensure that patients have intrinsic motivation and argue in favor of positive behavioral changes. In sum, it consists of a non-confrontational model of intervention that, comparable to MI, has demonstrated efficacy in various randomized clinical trials (Miller et al. 1992).

Community Reinforcement Approach

The *community reinforcement approach* (CRA) is a behavioral treatment package aimed at reducing substance abuse. The term CRA was coined in the 1970s by behavioral psychologist Nathan Azrin, although a treatment manual for alcohol abuse was only assembled in the mid-1990s (Hunt and Azrin 1973; Meyers and Smith 1995).

Since then, several literature reviews have placed CRA among the most well documented, effective treatment methods for alcoholism. Patients showed greater treatment adherence, greater pharmacological compliance, lower unemployment rates, enhanced social skills, and longer abstinence periods (Finney and Monahan 1996; Meyers et al. 2011).

Based on the concept of operant behavior (Skinner 1991)—that subsequent events can retroact and alter the likelihood of future behavior occurrences—the authors of CRA sought to understand substance use behavior through functional analysis. In short, it consists of identifying dependent (or contingent) relations between an individual's responses, the context in which they occur (antecedent conditions) and their effects in the world (subsequent conditions) (for more details, see Toscano et al. 2019). Once the individual is aware of risk contexts, they can implement problem-solving strategies aiming at relapse prevention.

One CRA technique involves behavioral experiments of abstinence. Given that complete abstinence may be unattainable—thereby leading to therapy dropouts—the therapist encourages short periods of abstinence. For example, once the patient reaches a 2-day abstinence period, the therapist must value the achievement and encourage longer periods.

CRA also evaluates patients' levels of satisfaction in different life aspects. This facilitates goal-setting to produce reinforcers that compete with the effects of substance use. In addition, often through *role-plays,* therapist and patient also practice communication training (e.g., refusal to drink) and problem-solving skills.

Two additional critical components of CRA are the *Work Club* and the *Fun Club*. Patients receive professional counseling to find sources of income and job satisfaction, which range from seeking skills improvement courses to curriculum development and preparation for job interviews. They are also offered leisure opportunities that wean them from substance abuse. The presence of a new social context promotes reinforcement of alternative behaviors towards a healthier life.

The last noteworthy component of CRA is relationship counseling. Patients commonly have a social environment that has been affected by excessive consumption of alcohol or other drugs. As patients jeopardize relationships due to substance use, they may start approaching other users. Because the desire for social connection can and must be met, a close, non-user is commonly included in the treatment (often the patient's spouse).

CRA programs use a version of the *Happiness Scale* for couples (Meyers and Smith 1995) and each member of the dyad requests a minor change from their partner. Aided by the therapist, the couple practices communication and problem-solving. Finally, the therapist presents the *Daily Reminder to Be Nice* chart (Meyers and Smith 1995) as means foster kind gestures that may have faded over time in the relationship.

CRA has already been adapted to include family members in the treatment course (*Community Reinforcement and Family Training,* CRAFT) and to address substance abuse in adolescents (*Adolescent-Community Reinforcement Approach,* A-CRA).

Contingency Management

Contingency management (CM) arises from the same theoretical perspective as CRA: the environment plays a fundamental role in the acquisition and maintenance of substance consumption. However, instead of alternative behaviors, CM seeks to reinforce incompatible ones (Higgins and Petry 1999).

In summary, the treatment consists of monitoring the patient's abstinence through frequent testing (e.g., urine test) and applying different consequences depending on the result. Thus, if the patient tests negative for a drug, they are allowed access to tangible reinforcers (e.g., money, clothes, movie tickets, etc.). If positive, the reinforcer is retained.

Some versions of CM use vouchers that progressively increase the reinforcement value upon each desired test result. For instance, the three first negative test results are rewarded with a R$10, R$20, and R$40 voucher, respectively, so that after three consecutive desired results, the patient earns a sum of R$70. This aims at presenting consequences for abstinence in a progressive way, thereby avoiding relapses.

Most CM surveys follow a 12-week schedule. Despite its simplicity, CM has demonstrated effective treatment results for various substance use disorders such as cocaine, heroin, alcohol, methamphetamine, marijuana, and tobacco (Lussier et al. 2006; Prendergast et al. 2006). However, a recent meta-analysis (Sayegh et al. 2017) that reviewed follow-up data revealed that CM fails to sustain intervention effects for periods longer than 3 months. Therefore, the question arises whether CM should be used as a stand-alone evidence-based intervention or accompanied by others.

Behavioral Couple Therapy

Behavioral couple therapy (BCT) is an intervention for individuals with alcohol and other drug use disorders and their spouses, who play a central role during treatment. BCT is based on the premise that couples with troubled relationships can unintentionally create contingencies that reinforce substance use. Conversely, intimate partners can play an important role in strengthening abstinence. Another assumption is that positive intimate relationships are an essential source of motivation to change problem behaviors; therefore, reducing relationship-related suffering can lower the risk of relapse. Throughout the treatment, patients learn that the relationship with their partner can be both part of the problem and the solution.

The treatment program consists of about 2 h of evaluation to aid planning, followed by 12–20 weekly therapy sessions with their partner. BCT is recommended for couples who have been together for at least 1 year in which only one party has been involved with alcoholism and/or drug abuse. BCT is ill-advised for couples with a recent history of domestic violence or judicial restraining measures.

The BCT therapist works to encourage the partner's support when the patient presents an effort towards a lifestyle change. Once all parties are aware of the behaviors that contribute to maintaining the problem, a behavior modification contract is made. This jointly made contract consists of a commitment both parties make to lower the rate of undesired behaviors (e.g., verbal assaults, threats) and increase desired ones (e.g., attending a support group). A commitment of recovery is also of critical importance on BCT: the patient states their sobriety daily and declares their intention to remain abstinent, while the spouse expresses support for their efforts.

BCT also strives to increase positive couple interactions through activities and assignments designed to strengthen emotional bonding, such as engaging in a mutually enjoyable activity (e.g., cooking class) or simply manifesting kindnesses and affection towards their partner. In addition, the treatment involves fostering communication and problem-solving: the therapist highlights the importance of mutual speaking and listening, teaches the couple to check understanding of their partner's remarks, teaches direct and clear communication of emotions, and negotiation skills for compromising. At the end of the treatment, a continued recovery plan is made to improve relapse prevention skills. In session, all parties commit to discussing, writing, and rehearsing the plan. This prepares patients, for instance, for a situation in which their partner arrives home drunk. BCT encourages the therapist to maintain sporadic (and increasingly spaced) contact with patients to monitor progress and assess the need for further sessions.

BCT is shown to be more effective for patients who abused alcohol or other drugs when compared to other individual modality treatments (Powers et al. 2008). Post-intervention results indicated lower substance use, happier relationships, lower rates of domestic violence, fewer marital separations, and better functioning children (Epstein and McCrady 1998; Fals-Stewart et al. 2001; Kelley and Fals-Stewart 2002; O'Farrell and Fals-Stewart 2000; Winters et al. 2002).

Clinical Expertise

Clinical expertise consists of different therapists' competencies, such as diagnostic evaluation, case formulation, identification of target behaviors, planning and implementing interventions, monitoring progress, measuring outcomes, interpersonal skills, establishing therapeutic bond, understanding individual and cultural differences, communicating with other professionals, and obtaining and applying the best available evidence for each particular case. Although thoroughly addressing such topics exceeds the scope of the present chapter—especially as other chapters here will do so—we highlight essential clinical expertise in the context of substance use disorder.

Firstly, the aforementioned empirically sustained treatments emphasize the importance of a solid therapeutic alliance. It consists of the emotional bond and collaborative relationship between patient and therapist, which includes agreement on the objectives of the intervention. Meier et al. (2005) reviewed articles in English published between 1985 and 2005 on the relation between therapeutic alliance and treatment outcomes for substance use. Although studies vary in methodological terms (type of intervention, time of data collection, type of measurement, etc.), the review concluded that building an effective therapeutic alliance early in the intervention is a predictor of efficacy, lowering the rate of both drug use and treatment dropouts.

However, whether the therapeutic alliance in fact plays a causal role is unclear as the authors only present correlational results between the quality of the alliance and the improvement of the clinical picture (Kazdin 2005). Therefore, a stronger therapeutic alliance may contribute to a decrease in substance use or vice versa.

Another extremely important component of clinical expertise in the treatment of substance use disorder is the therapist's interpersonal style. Several studies (Najavits and Weiss 1994; Najavits et al. 2000) have identified that more empathetic, less confrontational therapists with well-developed social skills tend to have better results with chemical dependents. Notably, conducting treatment with more empathy and less confrontation is the essence of MI—described previously.

In addition, as in any other clinical condition, effective treatment of substance use disorder requires gathering detailed information, formulating the case, and identifying target behaviors. Therefore, practitioners must resort to several tools, namely: clinical interviews (history of substance use; history of treatment; triggers for substance use; rules and beliefs; environmental factors; behavioral deficits; motivation for change; among others), behavioral assessment (e.g., substance use during treatment, self-monitoring diaries, behavioral observation by the therapist and/or other people), and self-reported scales (e.g., *Alcohol, Smoking and Substance Involvement Screening Test,* ASSIST; *Dependency Severity Scale, Addiction Severity Index*, ASI; *Drug Use Screening Inventory,* DUSI). Self-monitoring diaries, behavioral observation, and self-reported scales are especially useful to measure the patient's condition pre- and post-intervention and thus assess the effectiveness of treatment.

Finally, in addition to mastering theory and practice of the chosen empirically supported treatment, the therapist must be willing to stay up to date with clinical research in evidence-based psychotherapy, adapting his practice according to new evidence.

Patient Idiosyncrasies

Finally, therapists must evaluate clients' particularities when considering different empirically sustained treatments for substance use disorders. For example, Rosenblum et al. (2005) point out that patients with a more severe clinical status respond better to CBT, making this modality of intervention more appropriate for patients who struggle to describe feelings. However, CBT requires a substantial cognitive capacity from the patient; therefore, patients with lowered intellectual capacities may not benefit from this program (Maude-Griffin et al. 1998; Smith and McCrady 1991).

Conversely, patients who present less severe substance use disorder and already have coping mechanisms prior to the beginning of treatment seem to obtain better results within less structured intervention models (Gottheil et al. 2002). In addition, patients with weaker social support seem to benefit more from interventions that strengthen their social relations—the findings of Azrin et al. (1982) support this assumption.

More recent studies with alcohol users found significant effects when analyzing the style of interaction between therapist and client (Karno and Longabaugh 2005a, b; Karno et al. 2009). Specifically, patients who were more reactive and prone to anger had worse results when seen by more directive therapists. Admittedly, a patient with oppositional characteristics benefits less from direct instructions. These findings were replicated in a sample of patients being treated for methamphetamine use (Karno et al. 2012).

In summary, these studies—although preliminary—show a growing concern to ensure that not only the treatment offered is empirically sustained, but also that the choice of intervention and the manner in which the therapeutic process is conducted are appropriate to the particularities of the patient. In general, these studies have confirmed a rather logical assumption: more disorganized patients (e.g., patients with depression and low neurophysiological functioning) benefit most from well-structured interventions (Granholm et al. 2011), whereas patients with oppositional and anger tendencies benefit from interventions more focused on promoting motivation, such as MI.

Future research on evidence-based psychotherapy should certainly focus on better integrating patients' idiosyncrasies into empirically sustained treatments, since disregarding their goals, values, context, and clinical status may put any intervention attempt at risk.

References

American Psychological Association (APA). (2006). Evidence-based practice in psychology: APA presidential task force on evidence-based practice. *American Psychologist, 61*, 271–285. https://doi.org/10.1037/0003-066X.61.4.271.

Azrin, N. H., Sisson, R. W., Meyers, R., & Godley, M. (1982). Alcoholism treatment by disulfiram and community reinforcement therapy. *Journal of Behavior Therapy and Experimental Psychiatry, 13*(2), 105–112. https://doi.org/10.1016/0005-7916(82)90050-7.

Blonigen, D. M., Finney, J. W., Wilbourne, P. L., & Moos, R. H. (2015). Psychosocial treatments for substance use disorders. In P. E. Nathan & J. M. Gorman (Eds.), *A guide to treatments that work* (4th ed., pp. 731–761). New York, NY: Oxford University Press.

Chambless, D. L. (1993). *Task force on promotion and dissemination of psychological procedures: A report adopted by the Division 12 Board.* Washington, DC: American Psychological Association. Retrieved from http://www.apa.org/divisions/div12/est/chamble2.pdf.

Chambless, D. L., & Ollendick, T. H. (2001). Empirically supported psychological interventions: Controversies and evidence. *Annual Review of Psychology, 52*, 685–716. https://doi.org/10.1146/annurev.psych.52.1.685.

Chambless, D. L., Baker, M., Baucom, D. H., Beutler, L. E., Calhoun, K. S., Crits-Christoph, P., et al. (1998). Update on empirically validated therapies, II. *The Clinical Psychologist, 51*, 3–16.

Dutra, L., Stathopoulou, G., Basden, S. L., Leyro, T. M., Powers, M. B., & Otto, M. W. (2008). A meta-analytic review of psychosocial interventions for substance use disorders. *The American Journal of Psychiatry, 165*(2), 179–187. https://doi.org/10.1176/appi.ajp.2007.06111851.

Epstein, E. E., & McCrady, B. S. (1998). Behavioral couples treatment of alcohol and drug use disorders: Current status and innovations. *Clinical Psychology Review, 18*(6), 689–711. https://doi.org/10.1016/s0272-7358(98)00025-7.

Fals-Stewart, W., O'Farrell, T. J., & Birchler, G. R. (2001). Behavioral couples therapy for male methadone maintenance patients: Effects on drug-using behavior and relationship adjustment. *Behavior Therapy, 32*, 391–411. https://doi.org/10.1016/S0005-7894(01)80010-1.

Finney, J. W., & Monahan, S. C. (1996). The cost-effectiveness of treatment for alcoholism: A second approximation. *Journal of Studies on Alcohol, 57*(3), 229–243. https://doi.org/10.15288/jsa.1996.57.229.

Gottheil, E., Thornton, C., & Weinstein, S. (2002). Effectiveness of high versus low structure individual counseling for substance abuse. *American Journal of Addictions, 11*, 279–290. https://doi.org/10.1080/10550490290088081.

Granholm, E., Tate, S. R., Link, P. C., Lydecker, K. P., Cummins, K. M., McQuaid, J., et al. (2011). Neuropsychological functioning and outcomes of treatment for co-occurring depression and substance use disorders. *The American Journal of Drug and Alcohol Abuse, 37*(4), 240–249. https://doi.org/10.3109/00952990.2011.570829.

Higgins, S. T., & Petry, N. M. (1999). Contingency management. Incentives for sobriety. *Alcohol Research and Health: The Journal of the National Institute on Alcohol Abuse and Alcoholism, 23*(2), 122–127.

Hunt, G. M., & Azrin, N. H. (1973). A community-reinforcement approach to alcoholism. *Behaviour Research and Therapy, 11*(1), 91–104. https://doi.org/10.1016/0005-7967(73)90072-7.

Kahneman, D. (2011). *Thinking, fast and slow*. New York, NY: Farrar, Straus and Giroux.

Karno, M. P., & Longabaugh, R. (2005a). An examination of how therapist directiveness interacts with patient anger and reactance to predict alcohol use. *Journal of Studies on Alcohol, 66*(6), 825–832. https://doi.org/10.15288/jsa.2005.66.825.

Karno, M. P., & Longabaugh, R. (2005b). Less directiveness by therapists improves drinking outcomes of reactant clients in alcoholism treatment. *Journal of Consulting and Clinical Psychology, 73*(2), 262–267. https://doi.org/10.1037/0022-006X.73.2.262.

Karno, M. P., Longabaugh, R., & Herbeck, D. (2009). Patient reactance as a moderator of the effect of therapist structure on posttreatment alcohol use. *Journal of Studies on Alcohol and Drugs, 70*(6), 929–936. https://doi.org/10.15288/jsad.2009.70.929.

Karno, M., Farabee, D., Brecht, M. L., & Rawson, R. (2012). Patient reactance moderates the effect of directive telephone counseling for methamphetamine users. *Journal of Studies on Alcohol and Drugs, 73*(5), 844–850. https://doi.org/10.15288/jsad.2012.73.844.

Kazdin, A. E. (2005). Treatment outcomes, common factors, and continued neglect of mechanisms of change. *Clinical Psychology: Science and Practice, 12*, 184–188.

Kelley, M. L., & Fals-Stewart, W. (2002). Couples versus individual-based therapy for alcoholism and drug abuse: Effects on children's psychosocial adjustment. *Journal of Consulting and Clinical Psychology, 70*, 427–437.

Klimas, J., Fairgrieve, C., Tobin, H., Field, C. A., O'Gorman, C. S., Glynn, L. G., et al. (2018). Psychosocial interventions to reduce alcohol consumption in concurrent problem alcohol and illicit drug users. *The Cochrane Database of Systematic Reviews, 12*(12), CD009269. https://doi.org/10.1002/14651858.CD009269.pub4.

Lai, D., Cahill, K., Qin, Y., & Tang, J. (2010). Motivational interviewing for smoking cessation. *Cochrane Database of Systematic Reviews, 1*, CD006936. https://doi.org/10.1002/14651858.cd006936.pub2.

Leonardi, J. L. (2017). Métodos de pesquisa para o estabelecimento da eficácia das psicoterapias. *Interação em Psicologia, 21*, 176–186. https://doi.org/10.5380/psi.v21i3.54757.

Leonardi, J. L., & Meyer, S. B. (2015). Prática baseada em evidências em psicologia e a história da busca pelas provas empíricas da eficácia das psicoterapias. *Psicologia: Ciência e Profissão, 35*(4), 1139–1156. https://doi.org/10.1590/1982-3703001552014.

Lussier, J. P., Heil, S. H., Mongeon, J. A., Badger, G. J., & Higgins, S. T. (2006). A meta-analysis of voucher-based reinforcement therapy for substance use disorders. *Addiction, 101*(2), 192–203. https://doi.org/10.1111/j.1360-0443.2006.01311.x.

Martin, G. W., & Rehm, J. (2012). The effectiveness of psychosocial modalities in the treatment of alcohol problems in adults: A review of the evidence. *Canadian Journal of Psychiatry, 57*(6), 350–358. https://doi.org/10.1177/070674371205700604.

Maude-Griffin, P. M., Hohenstein, J. M., Humfleet, G. L., Reilly, P. M., Tusel, D. J., & Hall, S. M. (1998). Superior efficacy of cognitive-behavioral therapy for urban crack cocaine abusers: Main and matching effects. *Journal of Consulting and Clinical Psychology, 66*(5), 832–837. https://doi.org/10.1037//0022-006x.66.5.832.

Meier, P. S., Barrowclough, C., & Donmall, M. C. (2005). The role of the therapeutic alliance in the treatment of substance misuse: A critical review of the literature. *Addiction, 100*(3), 304–316. https://doi.org/10.1111/j.1360-0443.2004.00935.x.

Meyers, R. J., & Smith, J. E. (1995). *Clinical guide to alcohol treatment: The community reinforcement approach*. New York, NY: Guilford Press.

Meyers, R. J., Roozen, H. G., & Smith, J. E. (2011). The community reinforcement approach: An update of the evidence. *Alcohol Research & Health: The Journal of the National Institute on Alcohol Abuse and Alcoholism, 33*(4), 380–388.

Miller, W. R., & Rollnick, S. (2012). *Motivational interviewing: Helping people change*. New York, NY: Guilford Press.

Miller, W. R., Zweben, A., DiClemente, C. C., & Rychtarik, R. G. (1992). *Motivational enhancement therapy manual*. Rockville, MD: National Institute on Alcohol Abuse and Alcoholism.

Najavits, L. M., & Weiss, R. D. (1994). Variations in therapist effectiveness in the treatment of patients with substance use disorders: An empirical review. *Addiction, 89*(6), 679–688. https://doi.org/10.1111/j.1360-0443.1994.tb00954.x.

Najavits, L. M., Crits-Christoph, P., & Dierberger, A. (2000). Clinicians' impact on the quality of substance use disorder treatment. *Substance Use and Misuse, 35*(12–14), 2161–2190. https://doi.org/10.3109/10826080009148253.

O'Farrell, T. J., & Fals-Stewart, W. (2000). Behavioral couples therapy for alcoholism and drug abuse. *Journal of Substance Abuse Treatment, 18*(1), 51–54. https://doi.org/10.1016/s0740-5472(99)00026-4.

Powers, M. B., Vedel, E., & Emmelkamp, P. M. (2008). Behavioral couples therapy (BCT) for alcohol and drug use disorders: A meta-analysis. *Clinical Psychology Review, 28*(6), 952–962. https://doi.org/10.1016/j.cpr.2008.02.002.

Prendergast, M., Podus, D., Finney, J., Greenwell, L., & Roll, J. (2006). Contingency management for treatment of substance use disorders: A meta-analysis. *Addiction, 101*(11), 1546–1560. https://doi.org/10.1111/j.1360-0443.2006.01581.x.

Project MATCH Research Group. (1998). Matching alcoholism treatments to client heterogeneity: Project MATCH three-year drinking outcomes. *Alcoholism, Clinical and Experimental Research, 22*(6), 1300–1311. https://doi.org/10.1111/j.1530-0277.1998.tb03912.x.

Rosenblum, A., Foote, J., Cleland, C., Magura, S., Mahmood, D., & Kosanke, N. (2005). Moderators of effects of motivational enhancements to cognitive behavioral therapy. *The American Journal of Drug and Alcohol Abuse, 31*(1), 35–58.

Sayegh, C. S., Huey, S. J., Zara, E. J., & Jhaveri, K. (2017). Follow-up treatment effects of contingency management and motivational interviewing on substance use: A meta-analysis. *Psychology of Addictive Behaviors: Journal of the Society of Psychologists in Addictive Behaviors, 31*(4), 403–414. https://doi.org/10.1037/adb0000277.

Skinner, B. F. (1991). *The behavior of organisms: An experimental analysis*. Acton, MA: Copley Publishing Group. (Obra original publicado em 1938).

Smedslund, G., Berg, R., Hammerstrøm, K., Steiro, A., Leiknes, K., Dahl, H., & Karlsen, K. (2011). Motivational interviewing for substance abuse. *Cochrane Database of Systematic Reviews, 5*, CD008063. https://doi.org/10.1002/14651858.cd008063.pub2.

Smith, D. E., & McCrady, B. S. (1991). Cognitive impairment among alcoholics: Impact on drink refusal skill acquisition and treatment outcome. *Addictive Behaviors, 16*, 265–274. https://doi.org/10.1016/0306-4603(91)90019-E.

Task Force on Promotion and Dissemination of Psychological Procedures. (1995). Training in and dissemination of empirically-validated psychological treatments: Report and recommendations. *The Clinical Psychologist, 48*, 3–23. Retrieved from https://www.div12.org/wp-content/uploads/2017/07/Original-EST-Documents.pdf.

Tolin, D. F., McKay, D., Forman, E. M., Klonsky, E. D., & Thombs, B. D. (2015). Empirically supported treatment: Recommendations for a new model. *Clinical Psychology: Science and Practice, 22*(4), 317–338. https://doi.org/10.1111/cpsp.12122.

Toscano, M., Macchione, A. C., & Leonardi, J. L. (2019). Análise funcional do comportamento. In W. V. Melo (Ed.), *A prática das intervenções psicoterápicas: Como tratar pacientes na vida real* (pp. 84–101). Novo Hamburgo, Brazil: Sinopsys.

UKATT Research Team. (2005). Cost effectiveness of treatment for alcohol problems: Findings of the randomised UK alcohol treatment trial (UKATT). *BMJ (Clinical Research Edition), 331*(7516), 544. https://doi.org/10.1136/bmj.331.7516.544.

Winters, J., Fals-Stewart, W., O'Farrell, T. J., Birchler, G. R., & Kelley, M. L. (2002). Behavioral couples therapy for female substance-abusing patients: Effects on substance use and relationship adjustment. *Journal of Consulting and Clinical Psychology, 70*(2), 344–355. https://doi.org/10.1037//0022-006x.70.2.344.

Chapter 14
Substance Use Disorders and Psychiatric Multimorbidity

Luís Pereira Justo

Introduction

The use of substances in order to modify the perception of the world or the individual about himself, religious rituals or simply to obtain some kind of pleasure is quite old in the history of being human (Leal-Galícia et al. 2018). There is much diversity in this history as to the types of substances, patterns of consumption, contexts in which they are used and consequences of use both for users and those with whom they live. Most people who at some point come into contact with a substance with potential for changes in psychological/behavioral experience do not become an abusive or dependent user because use is more often sporadic and limited to a phase of life (Xavier da Silveira and Doering Silveira 2017). However, such experimentation or non-problematic mode of consumption always entails major health risks in general. A proportion of these people end up having their lives significantly damaged by the use of such substances.

Throughout the twentieth century and the beginning of the twenty-first, the problems associated with various natural or synthetic exogenous substances such as alcohol, marijuana, cocaine/crack, opioids, tobacco, amphetamines, and others have gained importance never before achieved. Due to the global dissemination of use, easier access, changes in people's lifestyles and forms of social interactions, the appearance of new drugs or changes in the levels of psychoactive components of substances already known, greater visibility of the consequences for behavior and health and possibly still unknown factors, the topic "harm caused by alcohol and other drugs" has come to mobilize more intensely societies and their rulers.

Science has been elucidating aspects of the problems related to substances and their users. However, the accumulated knowledge is still insufficient to take measures well based on the control of these conditions. On the other hand, the

L. P. Justo (✉)
Universidade Federal de São Paulo, São Paulo, SP, Brazil

D. De Micheli et al. (eds.), *Drugs and Human Behavior*,
https://doi.org/10.1007/978-3-030-62855-0_14

elaboration and implementation of successful actions by public administrations has proven to be a challenge of great proportions. This together determines the orphanhood of effective care in this area, no matter how many individuals, groups, and governments try to control inherent problems, which seem to multiply with the facilitation provided by the advance of mobility technologies around the planet. So far there are no pharmacological or psychological treatments, as well as public policies that have been efficacious, effective, and efficient for most of the pathological conditions related to the consumption of substances. Beliefs without closer links with objectively verifiable reality and with evidence produced by quality research have dominated the behavior of individuals and groups engaged in solving problems determined by problematic use of substances. This applies to issues related to drug trafficking, valid knowledge about the consequences of drug use, control of supply and exposure of specific individuals and population sectors, as well as prevention of health problems and treatment of diseases linked to the consumption of alcohol and other drugs. The influence of ideologies has also been relevant in the discussions on the meanings of the relationship between human beings and non-medical drugs for the various societies, often overlapping the practical demands of ethical and effective resolution of dangerous situations for individuals and societies.

In the health dimension, the detection of harm to those who become frequent users of drugs is increasing. Adversities can affect the biological functioning of the body in a variety of ways and also determine damage to personal capabilities and to social functioning. When trying to take individual care of these problems it is essential to approach them in a multidisciplinary as well as an interdisciplinary manner; thinking about measures of broad improvement for the community is fundamental to the broad knowledge of the situations in which the adversities imposed by the use and trade of both illegal and licit psychotropic substances are inserted. Psychiatrist role includes the most objective diagnosis of substance use disorders, their level of severity, their consequences in the lives of the people affected, the identification of comorbidities and multimorbidities, the choice of therapeutic interventions in this area that have the best chances of success, and the performance in concert with other professionals and collaborators for the treatment and prevention of morbidities.

In this chapter, some topics related to possible concomitances between substance use disorders and other psychiatric disorders, while multimorbidities will be discussed.

Comorbidity and Multimorbidity

Although the distinction between these terms is relatively recent in the medical literature, it seems to have meaning and significance, especially in relation to a patient's therapeutic projects or in the development of good public policies to address drug problems such as marijuana, cocaine/crack, tobacco, alcohol, and many others. When the use of more than one substance in the same period of time or throughout life is identified, it can be understood that there is a diagnosis related to the complications of the use of multiple drugs and to treating the individual in order to consider the consumption of each one and the whole. This would not be exactly a comorbidity or a multimorbidity. It is worth taking into account that chemical agents, sometimes called "abuse substances," often involve common neurobiological mechanisms and end up having pathophysiological affinities in establishing vulnerabilities or pathologies. Moreover, psychological and social factors involved should not, in principle, be taken as isolated determinants for substance use disorders. However epidemiological studies have provided the knowledge about the increased frequency of existence of several psychiatric disorders and other types of health damages associated with alcohol, marijuana, cocaine/crack, opioid, amphetamine, etc. use disorders (De Micheli et al. 2020).

The concept of comorbidity refers to the existence of more than one concomitant or subsequent pathological condition in an individual, when we can identify one of them as the most important, the index, and such pathological conditions interfere with each other (Catalá-López et al. 2018; Jakovljevic and Borovecki 2018). The definition of multimorbidity, in spite of the fact that it still lacks consensual robustness, is also linked to the coexistence of two or more pathologies in a person (generally associated with chronicity), but all are considered on the same level, without any of them being prioritized in terms of etiological importance or treatment priority (Catalá-López et al. 2018; Jakovljevic and Borovecki 2018; Xu et al. 2017). In this perspective, when coexisting pathologies are considered as components of a multimorbidity state they should be treated simultaneously, with the same investment and considered in their specificities even if they interinfluence or have etiological links; there is no hierarchy. Individuals with multimorbidities tend to go through more hospitalizations, these are more prolonged; they have more loss of quality of life, take more medications, have more difficulties in adhering to treatments and worse outcomes (Smith et al. 2012).

Alcohol

Based on the prevalence detected in a study that used DSM-5 criteria, as an example to think about the importance of pathological use of alcohol, the diagnostic rates of problematic use were 13.9%, considering the last year of data collection of the survey, and 29.1% over the lifetime in the population sample studied (Grant et al. 2015). Alcohol may be the most consumed psychoactive substance in the world (García-Marchena et al. 2018). Problems directly derived from its consumption may be associated with manifestations of other psychiatric disorders in ways not always easy to understand. Alcohol use disorders appear as comorbidities or components of multimorbidities in diseases such as schizophrenia, bipolar mood disorder, major depressive disorder, personality disorders, and anxiety disorders, to name a few. Both of these disorders seem to function as a vulnerability factor for problematic alcohol use, and the disorders arising from substance use may be a risk for triggering or exacerbating pre-existing diseases, including other substance use disorders (Nielsen et al. 2017; Yang et al. 2018). Although the determinants of the association between mental pathologies linked to the ingestion of alcoholic beverages and other mental illnesses are not yet sufficiently known, there is still a consensus that multiple factors (biological, psychological, and environmental) with different weights and natures of the etiological combinations in each individual case contribute to this. It is always important to take into account the heterogeneity of individuals and populations, both in terms of causes and modes of evolution and responses to treatments.

When dealing with the consumption of other drugs, conjugated (term used here to indicate concomitant ingestion during intoxication of two or more substances, otherwise we could talk about subsequent administrations) or not the use of alcohol, it is noted that it is relatively common for both conditions to occur.

According to one study, up to 33.7% of people diagnosed with some type of schizophrenia may have concomitant diagnosis of alcohol use disorder (Yang et al. 2018). However, it is possible that the living conditions of people living with schizophrenia, including appropriate treatments, have a high impact on the risk of alcohol problems, as there are also studies presenting lower rates for this association (Kumar et al. 2015). Certain characteristics of people diagnosed with schizophrenia can predict problems with alcoholic beverages: severity of negative symptoms (low pathological will and impoverishment of affections), male gender, low schooling, depressive symptoms, and history of substance use among other family members; additionally, problem drinking can predict the worst course of schizophrenia, with worsening of its symptoms (Smith et al. 2011; Yang et al. 2018). Although more evidence is needed for safe claims, it is possible that excessive use of alcohol in people with schizophrenia leads to longer lasting deleterious consequences at the neurobiological level, with increased functional damage to the hippocampus and subcortical areas (Smith et al. 2011). The coexistence of the two pathologies may imply further deregulation of executive function, with cognitive impoverishment; problems in the prefrontal cortex seem to be key processes in these situations (Yang et al. 2018).

Major depression is related to increased risk for alcohol use disorders (Boden and Fergusson 2011). Also, people who drink excessively often report depressive symptoms and it is often difficult to determine in initial clinical evaluations what started first and whether depressive symptoms are predominantly caused by the pattern of drinking or whether harmful drinking has been stimulated by the affective state. It is worth remembering that both conditions are prevalent in populations around the planet. People with depressive syndromes have an increased risk for pathological drinking by 2–3 times compared to the general population (Yang et al. 2018). When both types of mental disorders are diagnosable in an individual, it is even possible to think that there is an overlapping of genetic vulnerabilities regarding the etiological factors (Polimanti et al. 2019). This does not exclude the need to take into account the possible occurrence of other events that may also be involved in the etiology of both, such as stress, trauma (especially in childhood), difficulties in interpersonal relationships, loneliness, material deprivation, among others.

Although there is still insufficient data, several studies point to anxiety in childhood and adolescence as a causal element of alcohol use disorders in adulthood (Dyer et al. 2019). In general, the multimorbidity related presence of anxiety and alcohol use disorders seems epidemiologically and clinically significant (Smith and Randall 2012). Several models to explain the coexistence of the two types of disorders have been proposed: interactive or common biological factors, self-medication, triggering of one problem by the other (Smith and Randall 2012). Data in the literature suggest that women are more susceptible to this form of multimorbidity than men and that its treatment may also offer specific gender challenges (Smith and Randall 2012). Social anxiety has particular relevance (up to 50% of those diagnosed with social anxiety make problematic use of alcohol) and there are studies highlighting the likely precedence of anxiety symptoms (especially phobic ones) over alcohol abuse; there is apparently an attempt at self-medication for psychic discomfort and improved behavioral performance (Miloyan et al. 2017; Koyuncu et al. 2019). Furthermore, it is important to remember that generalized anxiety, panic, and post-traumatic stress disorders have an important relationship with alcohol use disorders; the spectrum of obsessive-compulsive disorders has a less robust association in studies (Brady et al. 2013).

Insomnia is an important symptom that can result from the excessive use of alcohol, and also lead to complications from the consumption of the substance. The investigation of sleep difficulties should never be neglected. It is often impossible to determine whether insomnia is only a secondary occurrence and, especially when it does not disappear after a reasonable period of abstention from drinking, it should be considered an independent problem and treated as such (Brower 2015).

In addition to recurrent depressions that occur without episodes of mania or hypomania, it is essential to contemplate multimorbidity including alcohol consumption disorders and bipolar mood disorders. The causes of such multimorbidities are still little known, but it is possible that the stress caused by mood instability, as well as irritability, often difficult to tolerate and dysfunctional in interpersonal relationships could explain this at least partially (Azorin et al. 2017). What has been shown is that alcohol abuse, as well as the use of other drugs, implies a worse evolution of bipolar disorder, with poorer response to treatment and higher risk of associated suicide; apparently men are more affected than women and there is also a more frequent connection of episodes of mania (Messer et al. 2017; Carrà et al. 2014).

Personality disorders should also be taken into account when investigating multimorbidity with respect to alcohol. Research to date has shown that antisocial personality disorder and "borderline" personality disorder are the most prominent in this case (Yang et al. 2018). As in other mental health problems, personality disorders can have varying levels of severity. Confirming the logical deductions, research shows that cases of multimorbidity are more common in more severe cases (Cavicchioli et al. 2019). It is important to consider that outcomes are unfavorable when estimating results of interventions to treat alcohol use disorders in people who also have a personality disorder and, even if there are not enough studies, it seems important that treatments should be designed specifically for such cases (Newton-Howes and Foulds 2018). It can be quite difficult to diagnose personality problems (when these are not prominent) in patients with severe alcohol problems, because the long evolution of alcoholism can contribute to lasting changes in personality traits that define their identity; on the other hand, some behaviors can be primarily characteristic of a personality that was relatively pathological before the onset of drinking or other drugs.

Marijuana and Other Cannabinoids

The consequences of marijuana use, still considered an illicit drug in most countries and one of the most widely used illicit substances in the world, have sparked much controversy among users, health professionals, and public policy managers. It is worth highlighting the questions regarding how harmful it can be to health, its therapeutic potential, use objectives, whether its use should be decriminalized, whether it should be commercialized legally (as it already is in some places) and perhaps more. One fact that must be addressed is that the marijuana consumed in the second decade of the twenty-first century is quite different from that which circulated in the last decades of the twentieth century (even considering that there have always been variations between plants or samples of the drug and its effects on humans, depending on the place and mode of cultivation and use, especially taking into account the age at which the user began consumption and the quantities and frequencies throughout life). *Cannabis sativa* contains more than 100 different cannabinoids, including delta-9-tetrahydrocannabinol and cannabidiol, the first known to promote the effects sought by users who want to experience changes in the psychic state, as well as likely to cause potential health damage and the second associated with therapeutic actions for some diseases (Lafaye et al. 2017). There are also synthetic cannabinoids whose consumption has become increasingly common since their emergence in the 1970s with possible accentuation of the magnitude of risks (Lafaye et al. 2017). Delta-9-tetrahydrocannabinol levels have been found in increasing amounts (in the 1970s they were detected in concentrations of approximately 3%, but during the second decade of the 2000s they were between 16 and 20% and some samples of new preparation and cultivation techniques rose to 40%), while cannabidiol appears in almost negligible concentrations in "street" marijuana samples (Curran et al. 2016; Lafaye et al. 2017). Cannabidiol, in addition to acting beneficially in some human diseases, seems to mitigate the harmful effects of delta-9-tetrahydrocannabinol; falls in concentrations of the former and increases in the latter have made marijuana (herbal), hashishe, and oily derivatives potentially more harmful than they were in the past (Lafaye et al. 2017). Thus, when discussing the therapeutic effects provided by *Cannabis sativa,* one should bear in mind the changes described above and especially that such beneficial effects would be linked to certain cannabinoids (such as cannabidiol) and not to the whole plant. It is important to remember that when the scientific literature talks about damages caused by the ingestion of marijuana and natural or similar synthetic derivatives, it considers the drugs with their set of many cannabinoids and does not disqualify the possibility of therapeutic potentials of specific extractions, made under controlled conditions, as in the case of cannabidiol. It is possible that the increase in the delta-9-tetrahydrocannabinol to cannabidiol ratio is related to the appearance of long-lasting psychotic syndromes after long periods of consumption (Lafaye et al. 2017). Similarly, the ingestion of synthetic cannabinoids whose formulations may contain high proportions of delta-9-tetrahydrocanabinol also poses a threat to health, the proportions of which are still insufficiently known.

The human being has an endogenous cannabinoid system with production of body substances of this category active in several neurotransmitter systems and whose functions have been increasingly researched, in addition to the receptors that are also targets for endogenous and exogenous cannabinoids (Leweke and Koethe 2008). There is evidence from studies in basic, clinical, and epidemiological areas that the disruption of the endocannabinoid system may be related to the onset of diseases such as schizophrenia, mood disorders such as bipolar disorder and major depression and anxiety disorders (Leweke and Koethe 2008). The use of marijuana and its derivatives and also synthetic cannabinoids for "recreational" use could play a significant role in such an imbalance of the natural functions of the endocannabinoid system and thus in the emergence of mental illnesses; perinatal and adolescent periods seem to be more at risk (Leweke and Koethe 2008). The onset of transient psychotic symptoms and symptomatic worsening of pre-existing psychotic disorders may also occur due to acute actions of marijuana and its derivatives (Leweke and Koethe 2008). There are studies indicating that synthetic cannabinoids produce more symptoms of mental impairment than herbal marijuana, but it is a subject that still lacks more evidence to make claims with greater accuracy (Mensen et al. 2019). The specific use of cannabidiol alone appears to be therapeutic in controlling schizophrenia (Leweke et al. 2018).

People with mental illness such as schizophrenia, mood disorders, anxiety disorders, and some personality disorders seem to be more vulnerable to exposure to marijuana and related disorders (Leweke and Koethe 2008; Merikangas et al. 2008; Shalit et al. 2019; Wittchen et al. 2007). It is reasonable to assume that people with important changes in mental functioning may feel distressed and seek relief for this. Still in this line of thought it is not uncommon for mental illnesses in their acute periods or when they leave after-effects that imply decreased critical capacity would also make people living with them more susceptible to consuming substances and have greater difficulty in controlling possible consumption. Evidence is accumulating suggesting that there is a two-fold greater risk of long-term psychotic states among marijuana users and other forms of cannabinoids than in the general population, in addition to possible worsening of symptoms in pre-existing psychotic diseases (Castle 2013; Leweke and Koethe 2008). However, research on causality in studies in this area still lacks clarification and the association between the consumption of certain cannabinoids and the emergence, exacerbation of symptomatic manifestations or interference in responses to treatment needs to continue to be evaluated for better understanding (Radhakrishnan et al. 2014). Limitations for stronger conclusions also apply to bipolar disorder and anxiety disorders, but similar concerns seem to be reasonable about the harm caused by the consumption of marijuana,

marijuana derivatives, and other cannabinoids both as risk factors for the onset of such diseases, such as worsening outcomes in people who already have them and use these drugs; they have been associated with the onset of manic symptoms in vulnerable populations (Leweke and Koethe 2008). The rates of more severe marijuana use problems (which are eventually identified as abuse and also addiction) seem to be high among people who have already had the bipolar disorder diagnosed. There are findings that point to numbers around 30%; there is also the suggestion that those with biological vulnerability to bipolar mood disorder have their first episode of mania earlier and have episodes of both mania and depression more often than people who do not consume cannabis (Bally et al. 2014). Another relevant aspect is the possibility that a cannabinoid-induced psychosis may turn into schizophrenia or bipolar disorder; otherwise the psychotic condition would disappear within weeks or a few months after cessation of consumption. There are data in the medical literature that draw attention to this type of unfolding of a psychosis primarily induced by cannabinoids (Starzer et al. 2018).

Individuals with reduced cognitive abilities may be more at risk of use and complications with psychoactive substances. However, what seems to be more common is that people without cognitive problems may develop cognitive problems after prolonged use of cannabinoids (even more synthetic ones) encompassing work memory, decision-making skills, behavioral flexibility, inhibitory control, and planning ability (Cohen et al. 2017; Mizrahi et al. 2017; Pattij et al. 2008). The continued activation of CB1 receptors seems to be related to the emergence of such deficiencies in executive function (Mizrahi et al. 2017). Thus, people who are diagnosed with problematic use of long-lasting cannabinoids may present losses of cognition skills and it is not yet known how reversible such damage could be in case of consumption interruption. When a person starts the consumption during adolescence of marijuana and its correlates seems to increase the intellectual disadvantage in the future when compared to the later start (Pattij et al. 2008). Adolescence is a crucial period for brain "organization," a period in which neural circuits acquire greater specificity and potential for acuity; drug use (marijuana may be the most used in this phase of life) can compromise the natural development of brain tissue making it less functional (Meruelo et al. 2017).

Cocaine/Crack

Even if epidemiological data show a lower frequency of cocaine and crack use among people with psychiatric diagnoses compared to alcohol and tobacco, these substances also represent important risks of worse evolution of diseases, which should always be considered by health professionals. Psychiatric illnesses increase the chances of cocaine/crack use, as well as of other substances. The first condition of increased morbidity would be concomitant problems with other substances such as alcohol, marijuana, hallucinogens, and various drugs (Castro Neto et al. 2016; García-Marchena et al. 2018). Regarding multimorbidities, among people who have concomitant diagnoses of substance use disorder and some other psychiatric disorder, problems with cocaine appear as the third highest prevalence, considering alcohol and other drugs (Rodríguez-Jiménez et al. 2008). Possibly attention deficit disorder, with or without hyperactivity, (whose acronym is ADHD) detectable in childhood or adolescence and without adequate treatment increases the probability of cocaine use, as a Mexican study with these populations points out (Tejeda-Romero et al. 2018). ADHD also appeared as a significant vulnerability factor for problems with the use of alcohol, tobacco, and illicit substances among young Austrian males (17–18 years), in a study with a sample of 3280 individuals, and should be the focus of attention in the research of multimorbidities among adolescents (Riegler et al. 2017). There is no yet sufficient data for more consistent statements, but the hypothesis has been raised that ADHD without effective treatment is a risk factor for cocaine/crack use disorder among adolescents and young adults, perhaps as self-medication; additionally, it is considered that the use of other substances such as alcohol and marijuana before cocaine/crack may occur in the search for relief from the psychic discomfort caused by ADHD (Levin et al. 2018). Possibly people with ADHD and cocaine/crack use in addition to difficulties in the cognitive sphere also have deregulation of affective control with greater impairment of functioning in interpersonal relationships (Miguel et al. 2016). In this multimorbidity responses to treatments for both conditions seem to be interrelated (Levin et al. 2018). It is expected that individuals with single episode depression or recurrent episodes, bipolar mood disorder, anxiety and schizophrenia have increased morbidity with more complicated evolution of acute episodes and long-term illness and consequently worse quality of life as cocaine/crack use disorders as well as other drugs are more severe (Lozano et al. 2017). Vulnerability to diagnosis of cocaine use disorder, as well as alcohol use disorder is higher in people who are also diagnosed with bipolar mood disorder, as studies in different places in the Western world point out (Arias et al. 2017; Grant et al. 2015; Toftdahl et al. 2016). Some of the negative aspects of this association are lower adherence to treatment, greater damage to cognitive function, and higher risk of suicide (Fagan et al. 2015; Passos et al. 2016). Personality disorders are also important in multimorbidities with cocaine use disorders; some of the dysfunctional behaviors in interpersonal relationships in this situation may be due to the damage in capacities needed to make decisions appropriate to social demands, which apparently are based on neurobiological functioning (Verdejo-Garcia et al. 2017).

Nicotine

Nicotine cannot be forgotten when talking about substance use and multimorbidity with psychiatric disorders. When tobacco use is detected it is almost impossible that there is no nicotine addiction due to the very high addictive power of this drug. People with mental illness are more vulnerable to tobacco use than the general population (Prochaska et al. 2017). Nicotine addiction is also associated with anxiety disorders, depression, and attention deficit disorder and its effects are thought to bring some relief from the symptoms of these diseases; however, nicotine withdrawal syndrome aggravates them (Kutlu et al. 2015). Schizophrenia also has a strong relationship with tobacco dependence and there is evidence to suggest a common genetic vulnerability to this multimorbidity (Quigley and MacCabe 2019). It is possible that individuals with schizophrenia use tobacco as self-medication to alleviate extra pyramidal symptoms and to achieve some compensation for negative symptoms, including seeking to expand cognitive capabilities, but the evidence suggests that few or no benefits are achieved with this resource and the risks of negative outcomes increase with smoking among these patients (Sagud et al. 2019).

Final Considerations

In general the existence of psychiatric multimorbidity in individuals who may be diagnosed with a substance use disorder may be closer to the rule than to the exception. A relatively recent study in the USA (already cited in this chapter) points to the plurality of substances used (although with variations as to what is more common or rare) and to diagnoses of mental illness (Grant et al. 2015). This study performed with samples extracted from the general population (not hospitalized or selected from some treatment center) using DSM-5 criteria, detected problems with substances such as cocaine, amphetamines, cannabinoids, opioids, hallucinogens, club-drugs, sedatives, and solvents/inhalants in addition to alcohol; mental illnesses such as major depression, dysthymia, bipolar disorder, post-traumatic stress disorder, antisocial, borderline and schizotypic personality disorders, various anxiety disorders such as generalized anxiety, panic disorder, and social phobia appeared with significant prevalences, both considering the most recent year and life (Grant et al. 2015). In addition to the substances included here it is pertinent to consider that other drug use disorders may also have increased prevalence among people living with psychiatric disorders. Thus, opioids, benzodiazepines, inhalants, "club drugs" such as ecstasy and methamphetamine, in addition to new drugs that appear and take time to be recognized by the scientific community, deserve appropriate research in this context. As in many health areas, studies conducted to answer relevant and well-articulated questions prepared with appropriate methods and with good analysis of data obtained are still a shortcoming when talking about multimorbidity involving substance use disorders and other mental disorders. Research in the area of epidemiology has produced more expressive data. The knowledge in the field of neurobiology and consequently of therapy is essential for necessary advances and depends on a lot of investment in good quality studies. It is also important that interventions that depend on good political practices are not petrified by ideological rigidity or by strange fidelities to the first commitment to good practices in health and to the well-being of individuals and societies.

References

Arias, F., Szerman, N., Vega, P., Mesías, B., Basurte, I., & Rentero, D. (2017). Bipolar disorder and substance use disorder. *Adicciones, 29*(3), 186–194. https://doi.org/10.20882/adicciones.782.

Azorin, J. M., Perret, L. C., Fakra, E., Tassy, S., Simon, N., Adida, M., & Belzeaux, R. (2017). Alcohol use and bipolar disorders: Risk factors associated with their co-occurrence and sequence of onsets. *Drug and Alcohol Dependence, 179*, 205–212. https://doi.org/10.1016/j.drugalcdep.2017.07.005.

Bally, N., Zullino, D., & Aubry, J. M. (2014). Cannabis use and first manic episode. *Journal of Affective Disorders, 165*, 103–108. https://doi.org/10.1016/j.jad.2014.04.038.

Boden, J. M., & Fergusson, D. M. (2011). Alcohol and depression. *Addiction (Abingdon, England), 106*(5), 906–914. https://doi.org/10.1111/j.1360-0443.2010.03351.x.

Brady, K. T., Haynes, L. F., Hartwell, K. J., & Killeen, T. K. (2013). Substance use disorders and anxiety: A treatment challenge for social workers. *Social Work in Public Health, 28*(3–4), 407–423. https://doi.org/10.1080/19371918.2013.774675.

Brower, K. J. (2015). Assessment and treatment of insomnia in adult patients with alcohol use disorders. *Alcohol (Fayetteville, NY), 49*(4), 417–427. https://doi.org/10.1016/j.alcohol.2014.12.003.

Carrà, G., Bartoli, F., Crocamo, C., Brady, K. T., & Clerici, M. (2014). Attempted suicide in people with co-occurring bipolar and substance use disorders: Systematic review and meta-analysis. *Journal of Affective Disorders, 167*, 125–135. https://doi.org/10.1016/j.jad.2014.05.066.

Castle, D. J. (2013). Cannabis and psychosis: What causes what? *F1000 Medicine Reports, 5*, 1. https://doi.org/10.3410/M5-1.

Castro Neto, A., Silva, D., & Figueiroa, M. (2016). Main mental disorders in crack-cocaine users treated at psychosocial care centers for alcohol and drugs in the city of Recife, Brazil. *Trends in Psychiatry and Psychotherapy, 38*(4), 227–233. https://doi.org/10.1590/2237-6089-2016-0002.

Catalá-López, F., Alonso-Arroyo, A., Page, M. J., Hutton, B., Tabarés-Seisdedos, R., & Aleixandre-Benavent, R. (2018). Mapping of global scientific research in comorbidity and multimorbidity: A cross-sectional analysis. *PLoS One, 13*(1), e0189091. https://doi.org/10.1371/journal.pone.0189091.

Cavicchioli, M., Prudenziati, F., Movalli, M., Ramella, P., & Maffei, C. (2019). The severity of personality pathology: A risk factor for concurrent substance use disorders in alcohol use disorder. *Journal of Dual Diagnosis, 15*(3), 159–171. https://doi.org/10.1080/15504263.2019.1612131.

Cohen, K., Kapitány-Fövény, M., Mama, Y., Arieli, M., Rosca, P., Demetrovics, Z., & Weinstein, A. (2017). The effects of synthetic cannabinoids on executive function. *Psychopharmacology, 234*(7), 1121–1134. https://doi.org/10.1007/s00213-017-4546-4.

Curran, H. V., Freeman, T. P., Mokrysz, C., Lewis, D. A., Morgan, C. J., & Parsons, L. H. (2016). Keep off the grass? Cannabis, cognition and addiction. *Nature Reviews. Neuroscience, 17*(5), 293–306. https://doi.org/10.1038/nrn.2016.28.

De Micheli, D., Andrade, A., & Galduróz, J. C. (2020). Limitations of DSM-5 diagnostic criteria for substance use disorder in adolescents: what have we learned after using these criteria for several years? *Brazilian Journal of Psychiatry*, in press. https://doi.org/10.1590/1516-4446-2020-1151.

Dyer, M. L., Easey, K. E., Heron, J., Hickman, M., & Munafò, M. R. (2019). Associations of child and adolescent anxiety with later alcohol use and disorders: A systematic review and meta-analysis of prospective cohort studies. *Addiction (Abingdon, England), 114*(6), 968–982. https://doi.org/10.1111/add.14575.

Fagan, C. S., Carmody, T. J., McClintock, S. M., Suris, A., Nakamura, A., Jeon-Slaughter, H., et al. (2015). The effect of cognitive functioning on treatment attendance and adherence in comorbid bipolar disorder and cocaine dependence. *Journal of Substance Abuse Treatment, 49*, 15–20. https://doi.org/10.1016/j.jsat.2014.06.008.

García-Marchena, N., Ladrón de Guevara-Miranda, D., Pedraz, M., Araos, P. F., Rubio, G., Ruiz, J. J., et al. (2018). Higher impulsivity as a distinctive trait of severe cocaine addiction among individuals treated for cocaine or alcohol use disorders. *Frontiers in Psychiatry, 9*, 26. https://doi.org/10.3389/fpsyt.2018.00026.

Grant, B. F., Goldstein, R. B., Saha, T. D., Chou, S. P., Jung, J., Zhang, H., et al. (2015). Epidemiology of DSM-5 alcohol use disorder: Results from the national epidemiologic survey on alcohol and related conditions III. *JAMA Psychiatry, 72*(8), 757–766. https://doi.org/10.1001/jamapsychiatry.2015.0584.

Jakovljevic, M., & Borovecki, F. (2018). Epigenetics, resilience, comorbidity and treatment outcome. *Psychiatria Danubina, 30*(3), 242–253. https://doi.org/10.24869/psyd.2018.242.

Koyuncu, A., İnce, E., Ertekin, E., & Tükel, R. (2019). Comorbidity in social anxiety disorder: Diagnostic and therapeutic challenges. *Drugs in Context, 8*, 212573. https://doi.org/10.7573/dic.212573.

Kumar, C. N., Thirthalli, J., Suresha, K. K., Arunachala, U., & Gangadhar, B. N. (2015). Alcohol use disorders in patients with schizophrenia: Comparative study with general population controls. *Addictive Behaviors, 45*, 22–25. https://doi.org/10.1016/j.addbeh.2015.01.009.

Kutlu, M. G., Parikh, V., & Gould, T. J. (2015). Nicotine addiction and psychiatric disorders. *International Review of Neurobiology, 124*, 171–208. https://doi.org/10.1016/bs.irn.2015.08.004.

Lafaye, G., Karila, L., Blecha, L., & Benyamina, A. (2017). Cannabis, cannabinoids, and health. *Dialogues in Clinical Neuroscience, 19*(3), 309–316.

Leal-Galícia, P., Betancourt Ocampo, D., González González, A., & Romo Parra, H. (2018). Breve historia sobre la marihuana en Occidente. *Revista De Neurología, 67*(04), 133. https://doi.org/10.33588/rn.6704.2017522.

Levin, F. R., Choi, C. J., Pavlicova, M., Mariani, J. J., Mahony, A., Brooks, D. J., Nunes, E. V., & Grabowski, J. (2018). How treatment improvement in ADHD and cocaine dependence are related to one another: A secondary analysis. *Drug and Alcohol Dependence, 188*, 135–140. https://doi.org/10.1016/j.drugalcdep.2018.03.043.

Leweke, F. M., & Koethe, D. (2008). Cannabis and psychiatric disorders: It is not only addiction. *Addiction Biology, 13*(2), 264–275. https://doi.org/10.1111/j.1369-1600.2008.00106.x.

Leweke, F. M., Mueller, J. K., Lange, B., Fritze, S., Topor, C. E., Koethe, D., & Rohleder, C. (2018). Role of the endocannabinoid system in the pathophysiology of schizophrenia: Implications for pharmacological intervention. *CNS Drugs, 32*(7), 605–619. https://doi.org/10.1007/s40263-018-0539-z.

Lozano, Ó. M., Rojas, A. J., & Fernández Calderón, F. (2017). Psychiatric comorbidity and severity of dependence on substance users: How it impacts on their health-related quality of life? *Journal of Mental Health (Abingdon, England), 26*(2), 119–126. https://doi.org/10.1080/09638237.2016.1177771.

Mensen, V. T., Vreeker, A., Nordgren, J., Atkinson, A., de la Torre, R., Farré, M., et al. (2019). Psychopathological symptoms associated with synthetic cannabinoid use: A comparison with natural cannabis. *Psychopharmacology, 236*(9), 2677–2685. https://doi.org/10.1007/s00213-019-05238-8.

Merikangas, K. R., Herrell, R., Swendsen, J., Rössler, W., Ajdacic-Gross, V., & Angst, J. (2008). Specificity of bipolar spectrum conditions in the comorbidity of mood and substance use disorders: Results from the Zurich cohort study. *Archives of General Psychiatry, 65*(1), 47–52. https://doi.org/10.1001/archgenpsychiatry.2007.18.

Meruelo, A. D., Castro, N., Cota, C. I., & Tapert, S. F. (2017). Cannabis and alcohol use, and the developing brain. *Behavioural Brain Research, 325*(Pt A), 44–50. https://doi.org/10.1016/j.bbr.2017.02.025.

Messer, T., Lammers, G., Müller-Siecheneder, F., Schmidt, R. F., & Latifi, S. (2017). Substance abuse in patients with bipolar disorder: A systematic review and meta-analysis. *Psychiatry Research, 253*, 338–350. https://doi.org/10.1016/j.psychres.2017.02.067.

Miguel, C. S., Martins, P. A., Moleda, N., Klein, M., Chaim-Avancini, T., Gobbo, M. A., et al. (2016). Cognition and impulsivity in adults with attention deficit hyperactivity disorder with and without cocaine and/or crack dependence. *Drug and Alcohol Dependence, 160*, 97–104. https://doi.org/10.1016/j.drugalcdep.2015.12.040.

Miloyan, B., Bulley, A., Brilot, B., & Suddendorf, T. (2017). The association of social anxiety disorder, alcohol use disorder and reproduction: Results from four nationally representative samples of adults in the USA. *PLoS One, 12*(11), e0188436. https://doi.org/10.1371/journal.pone.0188436.

Mizrahi, R., Watts, J. J., & Tseng, K. Y. (2017). Mechanisms contributing to cognitive deficits in cannabis users. *Neuropharmacology, 124*, 84–88. https://doi.org/10.1016/j.neuropharm.2017.04.018.

Newton-Howes, G., & Foulds, J. (2018). Personality disorder and treatment outcome in alcohol use disorder. *Current Opinion in Psychiatry, 31*(1), 50–56. https://doi.org/10.1097/YCO.0000000000000375.

Nielsen, S. M., Toftdahl, N. G., Nordentoft, M., & Hjorthøj, C. (2017). Association between alcohol, cannabis, and other illicit substance abuse and risk of developing schizophrenia: A nationwide population based register study. *Psychological Medicine, 47*(9), 1668–1677. https://doi.org/10.1017/S0033291717000162.

Passos, I. C., Mwangi, B., Cao, B., Hamilton, J. E., Wu, M. J., Zhang, X. Y., et al. (2016). Identifying a clinical signature of suicidality among patients with mood disorders: A pilot study using a machine learning approach. *Journal of Affective Disorders, 193*, 109–116. https://doi.org/10.1016/j.jad.2015.12.066.

Pattij, T., Wiskerke, J., & Schoffelmeer, A. N. (2008). Cannabinoid modulation of executive functions. *European Journal of Pharmacology, 585*(2–3), 458–463. https://doi.org/10.1016/j.ejphar.2008.02.099.

Polimanti, R., Peterson, R. E., Ong, J. S., MacGregor, S., Edwards, A. C., Clarke, T. K., et al. (2019). Evidence of causal effect of major depression on alcohol dependence: Findings from the psychiatric genomics consortium. *Psychological Medicine, 49*(7), 1218–1226. https://doi.org/10.1017/S0033291719000667.

Prochaska, J. J., Das, S., & Young-Wolff, K. C. (2017). Smoking, mental illness, and public health. *Annual Review of Public Health, 38*, 165–185. https://doi.org/10.1146/annurev-publhealth-031816-044618.

Quigley, H., & MacCabe, J. H. (2019). The relationship between nicotine and psychosis. *Therapeutic Advances in Psychopharmacology, 9*, 2045125319859969. https://doi.org/10.1177/2045125319859969.

Radhakrishnan, R., Wilkinson, S. T., & D'Souza, D. C. (2014). Gone to pot - a review of the association between cannabis and psychosis. *Frontiers in Psychiatry, 5*, 54. https://doi.org/10.3389/fpsyt.2014.00054.

Riegler, A., Völkl-Kernstock, S., Lesch, O., Walter, H., & Skala, K. (2017). Attention deficit hyperactivity disorder and substance abuse: An investigation in young Austrian males. *Journal of Affective Disorders, 217*, 60–65. https://doi.org/10.1016/j.jad.2017.03.072.

Rodríguez-Jiménez, R., Aragüés, M., Jiménez-Arriero, M. A., Ponce, G., Muñoz, A., Bagney, A., et al. (2008). Patología dual en pacientes psiquiátricos hospitalizados: prevalencia y características generales [Dual diagnosis in psychiatric inpatients: Prevalence and general characteristics]. *Investigacion Clinica, 49*(2), 195–205.

Sagud, M., Mihaljevic Peles, A., & Pivac, N. (2019). Smoking in schizophrenia: Recent findings about an old problem. *Current Opinion in Psychiatry, 32*(5), 402–408. https://doi.org/10.1097/YCO.0000000000000529.

Shalit, N., Rehm, J., & Lev-Ran, S. (2019). The association between cannabis use and psychiatric comorbidity in people with personality disorders: A population-based longitudinal study. *Psychiatry Research, 278*, 70–77. https://doi.org/10.1016/j.psychres.2019.05.041.

Smith, J. P., & Randall, C. L. (2012). Anxiety and alcohol use disorders: Comorbidity and treatment considerations. *Alcohol Research: Current Reviews, 34*(4), 414–431.

Smith, M. J., Wang, L., Cronenwett, W., Goldman, M. B., Mamah, D., Barch, D. M., & Csernansky, J. G. (2011). Alcohol use disorders contribute to hippocampal and subcortical shape differences in schizophrenia. *Schizophrenia Research, 131*(1–3), 174–183. https://doi.org/10.1016/j.schres.2011.05.014.

Smith, S., Soubhi, H., Fortin, M., Hudon, C., & O'Dowd, T. (2012). Managing patients with multimorbidity: Systematic review of interventions in primary care and community settings. *BMJ, 345*(sep03 1), e5205–e5205. https://doi.org/10.1136/bmj.e5205.

Starzer, M., Nordentoft, M., & Hjorthøj, C. (2018). Rates and predictors of conversion to schizophrenia or bipolar disorder following substance-induced psychosis. *The American Journal of Psychiatry, 175*(4), 343–350. https://doi.org/10.1176/appi.ajp.2017.17020223.

Tejeda-Romero, C., Kobashi-Margáin, R., Alvarez-Arellano, L., Corona, J., & González-García, N. (2018). Differences in substance use, psychiatric disorders and social factors between Mexican adolescents and young adults. *The American Journal on Addictions, 27*(8), 625–631. https://doi.org/10.1111/ajad.12808.

Toftdahl, N. G., Nordentoft, M., & Hjorthøj, C. (2016). Prevalence of substance use disorders in psychiatric patients: A nationwide Danish population-based study. *Social Psychiatry and Psychiatric Epidemiology, 51*(1), 129–140. https://doi.org/10.1007/s00127-015-1104-4.

Verdejo-Garcia, A., Verdejo-Román, J., Albein-Urios, N., Martínez-González, J. M., & Soriano-Mas, C. (2017). Brain substrates of social decision-making in dual diagnosis: Cocaine dependence and personality disorders. *Addiction Biology, 22*(2), 457–467. https://doi.org/10.1111/adb.12318.

Wittchen, H. U., Fröhlich, C., Behrendt, S., Günther, A., Rehm, J., Zimmermann, P., et al. (2007). Cannabis use and cannabis use disorders and their relationship to mental disorders: A 10-year prospective-longitudinal community study in adolescents. *Drug and Alcohol Dependence, 88*(Suppl 1), S60–S70. https://doi.org/10.1016/j.drugalcdep.2006.12.013.

Xavier da Silveira, D., & Doering Silveira, E. B. (2017). *Padrões de uso de drogas*. Retrived from http://www.aberta.senad.gov.br/medias/original/201704/20170424-094251-001.pdf

Xu, X., Mishra, G. D., & Jones, M. (2017). Evidence on multimorbidity from definition to intervention: An overview of systematic reviews. *Ageing Research Reviews, 37*, 53–68. https://doi.org/10.1016/j.arr.2017.05.003.

Yang, P., Tao, R., He, C., Liu, S., Wang, Y., & Zhang, X. (2018). The risk factors of the alcohol use disorders-through review of its comorbidities. *Frontiers in Neuroscience, 12*, 303. https://doi.org/10.3389/fnins.2018.00303.

Chapter 15
Behavioral Pharmacology: Contributions to Understanding Substance-Related and Addictive Disorders

Drielle Feitosa Silva and André Amaral Bravin

Introduction

Historically, drugs self-administration has always been present in the time line of human beings, being a drug defined as any "exogenous chemical substance, not necessary for the normal functioning of the cell, that significantly alters the functions of certain cells in the body when ingested at relatively low doses" (Carlson 2002, p. 97). Written accounts of *Homo sapiens* ancestors indicate that the species has been using substances since antiquity. The use of these and their effects on human behavior have already been mentioned in books such as the Bible, the Koran, and even in Homer's writings. Although drug self-administration by humans is a long-standing practice, the scientific study of the mechanisms and effects provoked by these chemical agents is just over a century old (Poling 1986a).

In the early 1950s, interest in the behavioral effects of drugs evolved greatly due to the insertion and prescription of chlorpromazine (an antipsychotic) for the psychiatric treatment of schizophrenia (Poling 2000). After proving the efficacy of this class of drugs, interest arose in investigating the effects of other drugs to treat mental illnesses, such as antidepressants, anxiolytics, among others, enabling the discovery of new drugs for clinical use. This paradigm provided the context for the emergence of more studies on the mechanisms of drug action (Branch 1991; Bravin et al. 2008).

Initially, the main hypothesis explaining the action and effectiveness of the drugs was that they acted on the emotional states that were behind the behavioral manifestations issued by the body. For example, there was a belief that anxiolytics promoted the decrease or "break down" of anxiety (an underlying "mental" event), resulting consequently in the decrease of overt (public) behaviors labeled as "anxious." According to Bravin et al. (2008):

D. F. Silva · A. A. Bravin (✉)
Universidade Federal de Jataí, Jataí, GO, Brazil

D. De Micheli et al. (eds.), *Drugs and Human Behavior*,
https://doi.org/10.1007/978-3-030-62855-0_15

> The fact that some drugs affected in a certain way the response rate of animals kept in positive reinforcement schedules, and the fact that the same drug acted in the opposite way in animals kept in negative reinforcement schedules, opened the interpretive possibility that the underlying emotional states of the behaviors kept by positive reinforcement were distinct from the underlying emotional states of the behaviors kept by negative reinforcement. From this (emotional states) would derive the difference in the pharmacological response of the animals (p. 124).

However, this also opened up the possibility of another interpretation, that the behavioral context (i.e., the contingencies of reinforcement) could be investigated. Since these "emotional states" were derived from the environmental aspects induced by the contingencies, studying them directly was a revolutionary possibility, since one could then manipulate tangible aspects of the organism–environment relationship, without resorting to underlying variables (i.e., intervening variables) such as these so-called emotional states. This possibility had been exemplified by Skinner and Heron's own work in 1937 (Skinner and Heron 1937), but it was the work of Dews (1955) that inaugurated a new tradition in the field.

Dews (1955) conducted an experiment in which he used pigeons deprived of food as experimental subjects, and trained them to peck a key that worked in a 50 Fixed-Ratio schedule—FR 50—in which after 50 pecks on the key, food was presented; or 15-min Fixed-Interval schedule—FI 15′—in which the first peck occurred after the 15-min interval was reinforced with food. These schedules generated high and low response rates, respectively. After behavior stabilization, saline or pentobarbital injections were administered in different doses. The results showed that, under the effect of this drug, the response in the FI schedule had its rate reduced, while in the FR schedule the response rate had increased. Considering that the effect of the same dose of the same drug on the same animal was different in those different schedules, it was clear that the environmental variables could modify how the drug influenced the behavior. Thus, this study by Dews is commonly recognized as the historical landmark of the discipline focused on investigating the behavioral effects of drugs, which would come to be known as Behavioral Pharmacology (Bravin et al. 2008; Dews 1955).

In *Behavioral Pharmacology*, Thompson and Schuster (1968) define behavioral pharmacology as "a branch of the biological sciences that uses the tools and concepts of experimental psychology and pharmacology to explore the behavioral actions of drugs" (p. 1). Therefore, this science is dedicated to the use of behavior control techniques to delineate the effect of the drug on the organism and/or uses the drug to analyze behavioral processes.

From this, the rationale and the level of interpretation used for understanding the behavioral mechanisms of drug action arise, that is, the identification of the independent variables (antecedent and consequent) that control behavior, and how they are affected when using drugs. According to Thomspon (1984a), to specify the behavioral mechanism responsible for the effect of a drug it is necessary (a) to identify the environmental variables that regulate the studied behavior and (b) to characterize how the influence of these variables is altered by the drug.

In some functional analyses, the emphasis may be on the elicitation function of the drug (i.e., the drug as an unconditioned stimulus—US), for example, when some antipsychotics elicit aversive respondents in a person diagnosed with schizophrenia (Oliveira and Furegato 2012). However, the most common functional analysis is the respondent–operant relationship, where the drug, in some instance, will modulate the control exerted by an existing environmental variable. These environmental variables that control behavior and can be modulated by the action of drugs are those variables antecedent or consequent to an operant response. In addition, since other variables also control the frequency of responses (e.g., motivating operations; reinforcement history), the drug can also affect them. Thus, the objective of Behavioral Pharmacology would be to describe how the drug would alter the behavioral variables involved, such as deprivation, discrimination of stimuli, reinforcements (whether positive or negative) and their properties, or even changes directly made in the organism, to cite some possible examples (Branch 1991; Bravin et al. 2008). Therefore, it is assumed that the drug can take place of US (unconditioned stimulus), Sd (discriminatory stimulus), R+ (positive reinforcement stimulus), R– (negative reinforcement stimulus), or even, alter the establishment of certain stimuli, such as reinforcements (i.e., acting as a motivating operation), for example.

Generally, research in Behavioral Pharmacology uses animal models to investigate the effects of substances on behavior, since the drug self-administration in animals is very similar to self-administration in humans (Spanagel 2017). Consequently, animal models are useful to uncover behavioral mechanisms related to drug use and to create intervention strategies for substance use in humans. One of the behavioral models for the study of drug addiction is called *drug-seeking behavior*, pointed out by some authors (Spanagel 2017) as the standard animal model to understand some properties of substance abuse and to test potential anti-craving and anti-relapse components.

Drug-seeking behavior is conceptualized as the behavior in which the responses issued generate drug infusions in the body (Self 2004). In this paradigm, an animal is trained to self-inject a drug and, after this training, the behavior is submitted to extinction. When the self-administration behavior is extinguished, other stimuli are presented. A stimulus recovers the *drug-seeking behavior* if, to some extent, it causes a further increase in the response rate, when you withhold the presentation of the drug as a reinforcement. At least three events can cause the new response: (a) injection of a small dose of the drug (reinstatement); (b) stressors; and (c) reacquisition (for more details on nomenclature or other processes, see Bouton 2002). It is important to note that after the presentation of (a) the drug, (b) the stressor stimulus, or (c) the conditioned stimulus, the drug demand responses are measured when the animal is in extinction (i.e., if a new lever press occurs, it will not generate drugs as reinforcement). From this, it can be inferred that the subject, whose behavior was previously extinct and currently "detoxified" from the *drug*, has its *drug-seeking behavior* increased.

The recovery reinstatement of *drug-seeking behavior* response can be useful to study the physiological basis of drug *craving*, and the behavioral aspects of reactions to environmental stimuli. Since it is possible to make an analogy between the events that induce *drug-seeking behavior* in laboratory animals and those events that provoke *craving* in humans, this has been a promising alternative in experimental research. Nevertheless, the predictive validity criterion of this model still needs to be better attested in studies of anti-craving properties. Other limitations on the use of the model as an analogy for aspects of substance use fall on the fact that (a) the experimental protocols include an extinction phase (recovery is only tested after the extinction of the behavior), and it is not necessarily true that dependent humans will necessarily go through this process; (b) in the model, the operant response is reinstated, but once the test is done in extinction, the subjects do not "relapse" because there is no new drug self-administration (which is why the model is called *drug-seeking behavior*). Therefore, experiments in *drug-seeking behavior* may provide some useful data on *craving* and triggers in humans, but they still lack data on predictive validity and analogy regarding relapse (Spanagel 2017).

Whereas *craving* in humans includes an intense desire to seek the drug, another suitable model for studying fissure responses in animals is incubation, developed by Shaham and colleagues (Grimm et al. 2001). In this model, rats were shaped to press a lever to obtain drug infusion, and were subjected to two experimental conditions of extinction, in which the presentation of cocaine was interrupted. The acquisition of the operant behavior occurred with the lever pressure being reinforced by cocaine infusion. In this condition, the light of the box (*house light*—HL) was on, and lever press was reinforced with the infusion of the drug (drug as R+) which was paired with a light + sound compound stimulus (conditioned reinforcement). After acquisition and maintenance of self-administration behavior, cocaine was withdrawn, which occurred for different periods of time: 1, 2, 4, 7, 15, 29, or 60 days. During the period of withdrawal of the drug, the animals were re-exposed to the same box, however, during re-exposure, the light from the box and the lever were absent.

The first extinction resistance test occurred with the return of the box light (HL) and the lever. In this condition, 1 h sessions (HL + lever) were succeeded by intervals of 5 min. (without HL and without lever), which occurred over 6–8 sessions, until the criterion of <15 responses/session was reached (operational definition of extinction in this experiment). The researchers observed that deprived animals for 1 day showed less resistance to extinction when compared to those deprived animals for 60 days.

The second resistance to extinction test occurred after the last extinction session of the previous test. However, in this condition, 1 h sessions (HL + lever) were succeeded by intervals of 5 min. (with HL and lever). Moreover, when starting the test, for 5 s, the conditioned reinforcement (light + sound) was released non-contingent to the response. During the whole test, each lever press generated light + sound as a consequence of the response (but not drug infusion). Again, the researchers observed that the number of lever pressures was lower in rats that were deprived of cocaine for a single day and higher in animals that were deprived for 60 days, i.e. resistance to extinction increased the greater the deprivation of the animal was. But it is important to note that resistance to extinction in the second test, when conditioned reinforcements are presented (i.e., reacquisition), is even greater when compared to the first test where only contextual stimuli (HL + lever) are present. Finally, the researchers discuss that their findings make analogy to the clinical issue with humans, where a delayed-onset craving syndrome develops (or "incubates") in the first 2 months of cocaine abstinence (Grimm et al. 2001).

By analogy, the study of Grimm et al. (2001) helps to interpret circumstances where a person stops using drugs during a hospitalization (the equivalent of removing the HL and lever from the environment). However, when the individual returns to their natural environment (the equivalent of reinserting the HL and lever from the environment), where their user friends or parties are present, the probability of relapse increases. Furthermore, the study suggests that the resumption of activities that generated as a consequence conditioned reinforcements associated with the use of the substance, such as conversation with user friends, dance, music, and/or lights at a party (the equivalent of light + sound) increases the frequency of pre-current responses to drug use, potentiating the chance of a relapse. Added to these factors is the "incubation" itself, which is consistent with clinical findings in which prolonged periods of abstinence also favor relapses (resistance to extinction).

The Reflex Conditioning (The Drug as US): Functional Alternatives for Understanding Abstinence, Tolerance, and Overdose

From the point of view of respondent behavior, the drug takes on the function of unconditioned stimulus (US) that elicits responses in the body, that is, it elicits unconditioned responses (UR). One of these effects is the metabolization responses of the drug itself, which from another perspective would be "compensatory responses" (UR). In order to maintain the dynamic balance of the body (i.e., homeostasis), organic cascades occur when a substance is administered, regulating the organism with other respondents opposed to those initiated by the drug (Benvenuti 2007; Leonardi and Bravin 2011). Thus, procedures performed before the administration of the drug (for example, seeing someone preparing a heroin injection), since they have been conditioned with the consumption of the drug, may begin to elicit compensatory responses, generating a desire for its consumption (i.e., abstinence/craving by the drug). Abstinence encompasses a set of variable grouping and severity symptoms, both in the absolute or relative absence of a substance, after repeated and prolonged use and/or administration in high doses of that substance (Benvenuti 2007; WHO 2019). Abstinence becomes conditioned when other stimuli are reliably related to the use of the substance (e.g., friends, places, subjects, etc.), so that these may have the same eliciting property of the drug compensatory responses, generating conditioned abstinence, which may be described by the user as desire or craving for the consumption of the drug, depending on the severity of the elicited respondents (which in part has to do with the biochemical properties of the substance).

The interpretation of conditioned abstinence occurs when the organism has not yet made use of the substance, but is being exposed to eliciting stimuli that have been conditioned with its use (CS). If, for some reason, the person self-administers the drug at that moment, it will have a minor physiological effect in relation to what it was previously accustomed to. This decrease in effect as a function of the compensatory responses of the drug is called behavioral tolerance (Siegel 2001; Thomspon 1984b). Tolerance (decrease in the initial effects of the drug along its chronic administration) generates as an effect the need to use increasing quantities of the drug for its effects to occur again. Once this cycle is established, the quantities of the drug are larger and larger, as the organism begins to elicit ever greater compensatory responses, too. A class of drug well known for its tolerance effects are opioids (e.g., morphine, heroin, codeine). Morphine administration, for example, initially results in analgesia (inhibits pain response). After repeated doses of morphine, the analgesic effect is gradually reduced compared to the initial effects produced by the drug. An example described in the literature is that heroin-tolerant users may consume up to a 100 times greater amounts of the drug in order to obtain the same effects as their initial use (Benvenuti 2007; Leonardi and Bravin 2011; Thomspon 1984b).

A related effect to the development of tolerance concerns the use of the substance in a different environment than usual, that is, without the presence of conditioned stimuli that elicit compensatory responses. If this occurs, the compensatory responses are not elicited and do not "prepare" the body to receive that high dose of the drug to which the body was already used. As an effect, the body collapses because without the compensatory responses, the person may overdose (in this case, called contextual overdose) (Siegel 2001).

The Operant Conditioning (The Drug as Sd, R+ and R−): Functional Alternatives for Understanding Drug Self-Administration

In the operant paradigm, the drug can act as a discriminative stimulus (Sd), in the presence of which a certain response is reinforced and in its absence (SΔ), such a response is not. Consider, for example, a group of marijuana users. When smoking, they are likely to verbalize being hungry. This may reflect marijuana's role as a discriminative stimulus, in which responses related to obtaining food (or social reinforcement among peers) were more successful in the presence of the drug than in its absence (Poling 1986b).

Another property of the drug, within the operant behavior, is to act as a positive or negative reinforcement stimulus. Reinforcing stimuli are changes in the environment that strengthen behaviors that precede them in time. Positive reinforcement refers to the addition of a stimulus in the environment; negative reinforcement involves the withdrawal of some stimulus, both with a view to increasing the frequency of the behavior.

The drug as positive reinforcement is common in both humans and non-human animals and it is the target of successive studies within behavioral pharmacology (Leonardi and Bravin 2011). According to Poling (1986c), Shirley Spragg observed that morphine-dependent chimpanzees would learn to select one of two boxes if the experimenter injected the substance into the animal with a syringe that was hidden under the box. Other researchers such as Headlee, Nichols, and Coppock showed that morphine injections acted as positive reinforcement for dependent rats. In the case of humans, it is believed that drugs that are self-administered (i.e., the use of which is not otherwise induced) can occupy the function of positive reinforcer stimuli (Poling 1986c). Although there is dispute over the view that the drug is a reinforcement in itself (an intrinsic reinforcement), it is undeniable that the reinforcing value of the positive consequences produced by the drug can be modified according to environmental variables and the individual's learning history (Silva et al. 2001).

A drug is acting as a negative reinforcement stimulus when the response of an organism occurs in such a way as to avoid or escape the substance, or to decrease the aversive stimulation of the immediate environment. Laboratory findings suggest that monkeys often emit responses that prevent exposure to LSD. Human beings also regularly avoid contact with certain types of drugs, especially prescription drugs. For example, a child with type 1 diabetes may spend much of his or her time away from home to avoid the injection of insulin by his or her parents (Poling 1986c). People diagnosed with schizophrenia may often vomit to avoid exposure to the antipsychotic drug administered, or start smoking cigarettes to reduce the side effects (Oliveira and Furegato 2012). Also, a drug addicted individual may use the substance to escape the symptoms generated by abstinence (Poling 1986c; Garcia-Mijares and Silva 2006).

Since the drug can assume the function of a positive reinforcement, its use can also be understood under the paradigm of choice behavior, competing with other reinforcements. According to Garcia-Mijares and Silva (2006), a situation of choice encompasses an environmental condition in which there are two or more response options towards which the behavior may vary. According to the matching law, in a given choice situation, the responses in each of the alternatives will be proportional to the reinforcement contingent on each one. Matching is obtained as a product of "melioration," which refers to the tendency of organisms to devote more time and/or effort to the alternatives that produce the highest rate of local reinforcement. The response rate of an organism will be higher in the alternative whose local reinforcement value of the consequence is higher. It is unlikely that in the presence of two alternatives, the response producing the lowest reinforcing consequence will be issued.

Another possible model of choice behavior is "maximization," which suggests that subjects will choose the most cost-effective alternative in the long run. The value of this cost-benefit refers to the future consequences of this decision and the cost of response, which is measured from the effort made and time spent in issuing it. Therefore, the choice is not made about one alternative over the other, but about the best combination among them (Garcia-Mijares and Silva 2006; Heyman 1996; Silva et al. 2001).

From this perspective, according to Garcia-Mijares and Silva (2006), drug addiction is considered a process in which the chronic consumption of the substance culminates in the reduction of the reinforcing value of other activities, such as spending time with the family, working, studying, among others, in favor of activities associated with drug consumption. Thus, the behavior of addicts is controlled by local and immediate reinforcements related to drug use, since its reinforcing value is greater than the local reinforcing value of other activities. Thus, the strategy of addicts is melioration. In contrast, non-dependent users maximize because their behavior is controlled by the combined reinforcing value of drugs and competing activities, both local and future.

An important factor in understanding drug use as a behavior of choice refers to the perspective of self-control and impulsiveness. It is known that delaying the consequence of responding diminishes its reinforcing power. In typical experiments using delayed discount reinforcement procedures, humans and non-human animals can choose between a small immediate reinforcer and a greater delayed reinforcer. We call impulsiveness the choice that produces the small and immediate reinforcement. In the case of drug use behavior, self-control would mean choosing the late benefits of abstinence rather than immediate reinforcement of drug use. Dependent users, however, engage in impulsive behavioral patterns, as they tend to behave in a way that produces local and immediate reinforcement of drug use (Kurti and Dallery 2012).

This evidence suggests that the view of chemical dependency as purely neurochemical controlled behavior or as a nosological entity is mistaken. Since it is an organism that behaves according to previous and consequent stimuli, drug abuse is governed by the same principles of so-called normal behavior and, therefore, is susceptible to modification (Silva et al. 2001). Some strategies can be useful in the treatment of substance use disorder.

Behavioral Alternatives for Substance Dependence Intervention

As mentioned above, the drug can act as a negative reinforcement when the individual presents withdrawal symptoms. The person, deprived of the drug, re-administers the substance to escape the aversive stimulation. It can therefore be said that abstinence syndrome leads to drug use (Benvenuti 2007). Because the symptoms of abstinence syndrome are caused by conditioned environmental stimuli, an important task would be to identify these variables and their eliciting intensity. Examples of stimuli that elicit abstinence symptoms are: places, companies, period of the day, time, use of other drugs, among others. In addition, the sight of another person using the drug, talking about drugs, seeing someone using the drug in anti-drug campaigns are frequent eliciting stimuli for emotional states characteristic of the abstinence syndrome. However, identifying these eliciting variables is a difficult task, due to the traditional clinical model of obtaining data only with verbal reports. To get around this problem, one possibility would be the mode of care called Therapeutic Accompaniment, whose intervention takes place in the user's natural environment. Nevertheless, even if the "cues" or "triggers" that precede the use of the drug in the natural environment are identified, keeping the individual away from that environment is not always possible (Benvenuti 2007).

Other forms of intervention, whose focus is on the operant level, are dedicated to promoting self-control in dependent users. These strategies may include: decreasing the value of immediate reinforcement of drug use, for example, by contingent more aversive consequences to the drug use response; decreasing the delay of alternative reinforcement, such as allowing the user to watch a movie at the end of a drug-free week; increasing the salience of late reinforcement, from reflection on the long-term benefits of abstinence; or manipulating variables that contribute to impulsive choice, for example, when the user commits at the beginning of the week to making weekend plans that exclude drug use (Kurti and Dallery 2012).

In this sense, possible approaches involving increasing the reinforcing value of a competing response to drug use or simply increasing the reinforcing value of other responses are: *Community Reinforcement Approach* and Contingency Management (Kurti and Dallery 2012; Miguel et al. 2015).

The Community Reinforcement Approach (CRA) initially focused on the treatment of alcoholism and was later extended to other forms of dependency (Miguel et al. 2015). According to his theoretical perspective, what maintains dependence is the presence of drug-related reinforcers and the lack of alternative reinforcers to drug use. CRA privileges social contingencies, with the participation of family and friends, promoting recreational and occupational activities, since it is believed that these variables influence the user to change his consumption behavior (Schenker and Minayo 2004). Thus, this approach proposes to create a social environment to compete with the reinforcers produced by the drug and seeks to reduce or eliminate conditional reinforcements (usually social reinforcements) associated with substance use, also offering coping strategies, social skills training, and behavioral therapy for couples (Miguel et al. 2015).

In Contingency Management (CM), the maintenance of addiction is defined as the product of unconditioned and conditioned reinforcements associated with drug use and the lack of alternative reinforcements to it. Thus, the unequal competition between reinforcements related to substance use and reinforcements not related to it makes it difficult to modify behavior. The MC proposes that problem behaviors can be modified through punishment or other powerful reinforcers contingent upon responses incompatible with substance use, such as verified abstinence from the drug and adherence to drug and behavioral treatments. Although punishment may eventually be effective, its use is questionable because it has several disadvantages, such as high rates of withdrawal from treatment, aversive emotional states, and losses in interpersonal relationships between users and team members, to name a few. The use of positive reinforcement in contingency management has more advantageous results than the use of punishment (Miguel et al. 2015).

The following components are necessary for effective contingency management: (a) employ a powerful concurrent reinforcer as an alternative to drug use; (b) develop an effective reinforcement schedule; (c) list appropriate target behavior; (d) objectively and systematically check acquisition of target behavior; (e) immediately reinforce components of target behaviors. Generally, the target behavior chosen is a measurable form of drug abstinence. However, treatment based on contingency management can also reinforce adherence behaviors (in cases of alcoholism and heroin addiction), treatment assiduity, and goal achievement.

One of the most common interventions in CM employs incentives through vouchers. For example, patients receive vouchers contingent upon checking for drug abstinence. These vouchers can be exchanged for products. The value of the voucher can be increased as a function of continuous maintenance of abstinence, as in the case of vouchers whose value increases with each urine sample with a negative result for drug presence. This method has proven effective in promoting long periods of abstinence from various substances (Miguel et al. 2015).

A meta-analysis conducted by Prendergast et al. (2006) demonstrates that the CM is effective in the treatment of several types of addition, especially in opiates and cocaine. This study also suggests that CM is among the most effective approaches in promoting abstinence during the treatment of substance dependence. Another study, conducted by Alessi et al. (2008), indicates that CM intervention using prizes was effective in promoting smoking reduction in tobacco users.

While there is criticism of the cost of voucher and prize-based interventions in CM, it is possible to decrease spending on requesting donations of products and services from private and public funds and use them to reinforce behavior modification. The survey conducted by García-Rodríguez et al. (2008) within the *Proyecto Hombre* program indicates that this intervention model generated a lower cost than the value of the donations: of the 15,670 euros collected, the expenses with the program corresponded to 3734 euros. These same funds were later used in another phase of the program. From this, it can be seen that the cost-benefit of this strategy is economically viable, in view of the effectiveness of CM-based interventions (García-Rodríguez et al. 2008).

Also, according to Miguel et al. (2015) it is possible to mix CRA and CM interventions. Some studies suggest that combining the two approaches generates abstinence more quickly, a higher rate of maintenance of abstinence after follow-up, greater adherence to treatment, less alcohol intoxication, fewer depressive symptoms, and less frequency of hospitalization than Contingency Management alone.

Final Considerations

In short, the studies in Behavioral Pharmacology have shed light on the behavioral mechanism of drug action, whose functioning goes beyond the biochemical factors produced by the drug. By evidencing the influence on the effects of the drug exercised by the environment, Behavioral Pharmacology has contributed to the deconstruction of the view of substance use and abuse as a psychopathology or as a deviation disorder (Silva et al. 2001). Considering chemical dependence as "normal" operant behavior, resulting from the relations of the organism with its environment, it is possible to trace prevention and intervention strategies that take place outside the individual.

In this way, the contributions of Behavior Analysis can be verified from the effectiveness of the intervention programs based on the Community Reinforcement Approach and Contingency Management, which have proved powerful alternatives in the treatment of substance use disorders. It is expected that in the future, data from these interventions will inspire political leadership in the use of these contingency management interventions for large-scale interventions rather than treating the issue of drug addiction as a moral or mental disorder.

Acknowledgements The authors thank Fundação de Amparo à Pesquisa do Estado de Goiás (FAPEG) for funding the research from which this product came (edital 03/2015, process n° 201610267001035).

References

Alessi, S. M., Petry, N. M., & Urso, J. (2008). Contingency management promotes smoking reductions in residential substance abuse patients. *Journal of Applied Behavior Analysis, 41*(4), 617–622. https://doi.org/10.1901/jaba.2008.41-617.

Benvenuti, M. F. (2007). Uso de drogas, recaída e o papel do condicionamento respondente: Possibilidades do trabalho do psicólogo em ambiente natural. In D. Zamignani, R. Kovac, & J. S. Vermes (Eds.), *A Clínica de Portas Abertas* (pp. 307–327). São Paulo, Brazil: ESETec – Paradigma.

Bouton, M. E. (2002). Context, ambiguity, and unlearning: Sources of relapse after behavioral extinction. *Biological Psychiatry, 52*(10), 976–986. https://doi.org/10.1016/s0006-3223(02)01546-9.

Branch, M. N. (1991). Behavioral pharmacology. In I. H. Iversen & K. A. Lattal (Eds.), *Experimental analysis of behavior* (pp. 21–78). New York, NY: Elsevier Science.

Bravin, A. A., Pandossio, J. E., & Albuquerque, A. R. (2008). O que é Farmacologia Comportamental? In W. C. M. P. Silva (Ed.), *Sobre Comportamento e Cognição: Reflexões Teórico-Conceituais e Implicações para Pesquisa* (Vol. 20, pp. 123–136). Santo André, Brazil: ESETec.

Carlson, N. C. (2002). *Fisiologia do Comportamento.* Barueri, Brazil: Manole.

Dews, P. B. (1955). Studies on behavior. I. Differential sensitivity to pentobarbital of pecking performance in pigeons depending on the schedule of reward. *The Journal of Pharmacology and Experimental Therapeutics, 113*(4), 393–401.

Garcia-Mijares, M., & Silva, M. (2006). Dependência de drogas. *Psicologia USP, 17*(4), 213–240. https://doi.org/10.1590/s0103-65642006000400012.

García-Rodríguez, O., Secades-Villa, R., Higgins, S. T., Fernández-Hermida, J. R., & Carballo, J. L. (2008). Financing a voucher program for cocaine abusers through community donations in Spain. *Journal of Applied Behavior Analysis, 41*(4), 623–628. https://doi.org/10.1901/jaba.2008.41-623.

Grimm, J. W., Hope, B. T., Wise, R. A., & Shaham, Y. (2001). Neuroadaptation. Incubation of cocaine craving after withdrawal. *Nature, 412*(6843), 141–142. https://doi.org/10.1038/35084134.

Heyman, G. (1996). Resolving the contradictions of addiction. *Behavioral and Brain Sciences, 19*(4), 561–574. https://doi.org/10.1017/s0140525x00042990.

Kurti, A. N., & Dallery, J. (2012). Review of Heyman's addiction: a disorder of choice. *Journal of Applied Behavior Analysis, 45*(1), 229–240. https://doi.org/10.1901/jaba.2012.45-229.

Leonardi, J. L., & Bravin, A. A. (2011). Uma introdução à farmacologia comportamental. *Interação em Psicolologia, 15*(2), 193–201. https://doi.org/10.5380/psi.v15i2.20514.

Miguel, A. Q. C., Yamauchi, R., Simões, V., Silva, C. J., & Laranjeira, R. R. (2015). From theory to treatment: Understanding addiction from an operant behavioral perspective. *Journal of Modern Education Review, 5*(8), 778–787. https://doi.org/10.15341/jmer(2155-7993)/08.05.2015/006.

Oliveira, M. R., & Furegato, F. A. R. (2012). Esquizofrenia e dependência de tabaco: Uma revisão integrativa. *Enfermería Global, 25*, 404–425.

Poling, A. (1986a). Historical origins of behavioral pharmacology. In *A primer of human behavioral pharmacology* (pp. 1–20). New York, NY and London, UK: Plenum Press.

Poling, A. (1986b). Stimulus properties of drugs. In *A primer of human behavioral pharmacology* (pp. 81–102). New York, NY and London, UK: Plenum Press.

Poling, A. (1986c). Drug abuse. In *A primer of human behavioral pharmacology* (pp. 177–208). New York, NY and London, UK: Plenum Press.

Poling, A. (2000). Introduction. In A. Poling & T. Byrne (Eds.), *Introduction to behavioral pharmacology* (pp. 9–25). Reno, NV: New Harbinger Publications.

Prendergast, M., Podus, D., Finney, J., Greenwell, L., & Roll, J. (2006). Contingency management for treatment of substance use disorders: A meta-analysis. *Addiction, 101*(11), 1546–1560. https://doi.org/10.1111/j.1360-0443.2006.01581.x.

Schenker, M., & Minayo, M. (2004). A importância da família no tratamento do uso abusivo de drogas: uma revisão da literatura. *Cadernos de Saúde Pública, 20*(3), 649–659. https://doi.org/10.1590/s0102-311x2004000300002.

Self, D. W. (2004). Regulation of drug-taking and -seeking behaviors by neuroadaptations in the mesolimbic dopamine system. *Neuropharmacology, 47*(1), 242–255.

Siegel, S. (2001). Pavlovian conditioning and drug overdose: When tolerance fails. *Addiction Research & Theory, 9*(5), 503–513. https://doi.org/10.3109/16066350109141767.

Silva, M. T. A., Guerra, L. G. G. C., Gonçalves, F. L., & Garcia-Mijares, M. (2001). Análise funcional das dependências de drogas. In H. J. Guilhardi (Ed.), *Sobre Comportamento e Cognição: Expondo a Variabilidade* (Vol. 7, pp. 422–442). São Paulo, Brazil: ESETec.

Skinner, B. F., & Heron, W. T. (1937). Effects of caffeine and benzedrine upon conditioning and extinction. *The Psychological Record, 1*, 340–346.

Spanagel, R. (2017). Animal models of addiction. *Dialogues in Clinical Neuroscience, 19*(3), 247–258.

Thompson, T., & Schuster, C. R. (1968). Behavioral pharmacology as a basic science. In T. Thompson & C. R. Schuster (Eds.), *Behavioral pharmacology* (pp. 1–7). Eaglewood Cliffs, NJ: Prentice Hall.

Thomspon, T. (1984a). Introduction. In T. Thompson, P. B. Dews, & J. E. Barret (Eds.), *Advances in behavioral pharmacology* (Vol. 4, pp. 2–5). Gainesville, FL: Academic Press.

Thomspon, T. (1984b). Drugs may alter the way antecedent factor modulate current behavior. In T. Thompson, P. B. Dews, & J. E. Barret (Eds.), *Advances in behavioral pharmacology* (Vol. 4, pp. 6–14). Gainesville, FL: Academic Press.

World Health Organization (WHO). (2019). *International statistical classification of diseases and related health problems, eleventh revision*. Retrieved from https://icd.who.int/browse10/2019/en

Chapter 16
Disorders Due to Substance Use in Clinical Behavior Analysis: Theory and Practice Observed in a Clinical Case

Fernanda Calixto

Introduction

The consumption of psychoactive substances is a constant habit in several civilizations since ancient times. Since the Greco-Roman civilizations, references to opium are found and the consumption of coca leaf is represented in the sculptures of the Andean peoples of the early third century BC. In relation to alcoholic beverages, it is possible to find descriptions of the consumption of the most diverse types of wines and beers in practically all prehistoric and contemporary civilizations. The use of psychoactive substances, as it is today, occurred for various reasons, whether religious, for medicinal purposes or merely for pleasure (Escohotado, 1998).

But what factors make the consumption of psychoactive substances so constant in many individual lives? It is important to point out that these substances cause changes in the central nervous system. Because of such changes, an individual, when consuming the substance, may present changes in mood and consciousness as well as in the way of acting (Robbins & Everitt, 1996). A common effect of cocaine, for example, is the increase of feelings of confidence, animation, and disinhibition. In addition, even though illegal drugs are usually cited, several legal substances present in our daily lives—such as alcohol and tobacco—also cause psychoactive effects.

The use of psychoactive substances becomes a factor of social concern, since excessive consumption and dependence can lead to various health damages, risk of death, in addition to negatively affecting the social coexistence and productivity of its users (Andrade et al. 2017; Bedendo et al. 2017; Fiore, 2008). Health can be affected by the constant use of the substance itself (e.g. permanent damage to the blood vessels of the heart and brain caused by cocaine), consumption habits (e.g.

F. Calixto (✉)
Paradigma Centre, Sciences and Behavioral Technology, São Paulo, SP, Brazil

D. De Micheli et al. (eds.), *Drugs and Human Behavior*,
https://doi.org/10.1007/978-3-030-62855-0_16

hepatitis caused by sharing syringes), and behavioral changes caused by the use (e.g. having sex without prevention or drunken driving). Social coexistence is harmed, since the user constantly moves away from friends and family who are against the use and starts to relate only with other users (Yamauchi et al. 2019).

In relation to the risk of morbidity and mortality, the 2018 World Drug Report released worrying information. Worldwide, deaths directly caused by drug use increased by 60% between 2000 and 2019. In the Brazilian context, the rate of violent deaths from homicides related to the use and abuse of alcohol, marijuana, and cocaine ranges from 29.7% to 69.6%. An additional concern is the constant increase in the supply of psychoactive substances. In relation to cocaine, for example, global manufacturing reached its highest level in history in 2016, with an estimated production of 1410 tons (United Nations Office on Drugs and Crime (UNODC), 2018).

The excessive consumption of substances with social and health damages is framed in DSM-5 as the substance use disorder and covers distinct categories of drugs, among which: alcohol, caffeine, marijuana, hallucinogens, inhalants, opioids, sedatives, anxiolytics, stimulants, tobacco and other substances. Among the diagnostic criteria are (a) the substance consumption in increasing amounts or for a longer period of time than originally intended; (b) the persistent desire to reduce the use of the substance and a history of failure to decrease or discontinue use; (c) large amount of time spent to obtain and consume the substance; (d) intense desire to consume the drug in the environment where the drug was previously used; (e) socioeconomic losses related to the pattern of consumption; (f) continuity of consumption even when it entails risks to its physical integrity; and (g) presence of withdrawal symptoms in the absence of the substance in the body (American Psychiatric Association (APA), 2013).

Due to its deleterious effects on health, productivity, and social relations of the individual diagnosed with substance use disorder, the reduction in consumption has become a source of extreme social, scientific, and therapeutic concern. For these reasons, dependence on psychoactive substances is the target of analysis and intervention in analytical-behavioral therapy, with the purpose of promoting effective evidence-based interventions.

According to analytical-behavioral principles, the behavioral pattern that we understand by chemical dependency is learned and governed by the same principles and laws of any behavior (Rachlin, 2000). The challenge of the therapist at CT is to identify in the history of the client how that complex pattern of consumption was constructed and what are the variables responsible for its maintenance. In the following topic, the behavioral analytical perspective of factors related to the acquisition and maintenance of psychoactive substances excessive consumption will be addressed. Later, a clinical case of an individual diagnosed with alcohol use disorder will be presented.

Analytical-Behavioral View of Substance Use Disorder

As mentioned, excessive consumption of psychoactive substances produces numerous health hazards, even increasing the risk of mortality. Information about the negative effects is constantly linked in the media and by the medical community and, therefore, it is likely that a large part of the population has knowledge about them. A basic therapeutic challenge is to understand why individuals continue to engage in behavioral patterns that clearly cause harm to their health and life.

In behavioral sciences, it is considered, based on extensive scientific evidence, that the consequences of what we do effect on our own actions, strengthening or weakening them (Schneider, 2012), and the closer the consequences are to action in time, the greater are its effects (Rachlin, 2000). As mentioned above, the consumption of psychoactive substances immediately causes changes in the body of the consumer and these changes often act as immediate reinforcing consequences of the act of consuming. The physiological changes that the substance causes in the body, with the activation of the reward mechanism and release of dopamine, may be sufficient to strengthen various classes of responses involved in consumption. In comparison, the deleterious effects of the same act tend to occur only in the long term after a long period of use. As an example of the negative delayed effects of consumption, we damage to the health, social, and professional life. In other words, if on the one hand we have the immediate pleasure of using, on the other hand, contact with the aversive consequences tends to occur only after a few months or years (such as the loss of a job and the removal of family and friends).

In addition, other reinforcing consequences, also immediate, may participate in the strengthening of the substance consumption behavior (Avery, 2011; Silverman, Roll, & Higgins, 2008). We consider that social reinforcing consequences act on strengthening, for example, when consuming the substance tends to occur in social contexts and the attention of relevant people is a participating factor in the addiction picture. In this case, we can think of user who increases his consumption at parties and always consumes with his group of friends. For some users, the consumption of the substance also acts as a facilitator for sexual encounters, since by feeling uninhibited and relaxed, initiatives would tend to happen more frequently. Borloti, Haydu, and Machado (2015), for example, described a clinical case in which crack use was functionally related to obtaining sexual boosters.

We consider that negative reinforcing consequences also relate functionally to consumption when substance use often eliminates or delays contact with aversive events. For example, it is extremely common to report that drinking decreases states of anxiety and stress (Anthenelli & Grandison, 2012). An increase in the consumption of psychoactive substances commonly occurs in situations considered problematic, such as difficulties at work or in the family. Often the consumption occurs to avoid the negative effects of the body in the absence of the substance. In this case, we have the use to alleviate the symptoms of fissure of which several states of physical malaise are part, such as nausea, body aches, trembling, among others in periods of abstinence. For the individual within the framework of substance use disorder, states of cleftness are placated by substance consumption, thus maintaining a contingency of constant negative reinforcement. In summary, for all consumers of psychoactive substances, potential positive and negative reinforcements act to maintain consumption.

After specifying the consequences related to the pattern of consumption, it is important to detail (1) how the learning of consumption patterns occurs and (2) why consumption occurs in specific contexts. As all behavior is determined by its consequences, the act of abusive consumption of psychoactive substances has determination in the three levels of selection (Borloti et al., 2015).

In the first level of selection, the phylogenetic, we consider the characteristics of the organism that make it sensitive to the effects of the substance consumed. In this case, we can cite the unconditional reflexes elicited by the presence of the substance possible by the activation of neurotransmitters in the reward brain circuit that guarantees the intensification of pleasure sensations (Laranjeira, 2010). In this way, the organism is prepared by a long selection process to react differently to the presence of the psychoactive substance and the organism's own differential reaction can be reinforcing enough to participate in the maintenance of consumption.

Regarding the ontogenetic level, our analysis is focused on the specific learning history of substance use throughout the user's life. In this case, all contexts in which consumption occurs—through a process of pairing and modeling—may begin to elicit the intense desire to consume the substance again and evoke consumption responses (Banaco & Montan, 2018). Often, we are not talking about physical contexts (such as the place of consumption), but about people (friends usually present) or even private events (such as states of anxiety and stress) that are functionally related to consumption and begin to elicit fissure sensations and evoke the entire behavioral chain of substance consumption.

In relation to the third level of selection, we consider the customs passed down between generations and maintained by cultural contingencies. For example, it is possible that, in a family context, consumption practices of alcoholic beverages or other substances are passed down between generations and act to strengthen abusive use.

By analyzing the acquisition of behaviors related to the consumption of substances we can realize that a gradual learning process occurs. Usually, in the beginning, the amount consumed is less and the consumption occurs less frequently. Gradually, a process of tolerance is common, in which the responses before elicited occur in a smaller magnitude in the presence of the same amount used before and, in this case, increasing amounts are necessary to produce the same effect (Higgins, Heil, & Sigmon, 2007). It is also common that, through modeling processes, consumption becomes part of a more complex behavioral chain. In the beginning, for example, it is possible that the use of cocaine occurs only in the presence of a friend who supplies the substance and, with time, the user learns to seek and buy on his own and the consumption starts to happen even in the friend absence.

When we consider a picture of substance use disorder, we are referring to a user who no longer makes use only for the pleasure of consuming, i.e. their behavior is no longer controlled solely by immediate positive reinforcing consequences. The excess consumption starts to flow into an aversive contingency in which "reducing the crack in all its aversive states" becomes the main control variable. In general terms, consumption that was previously controlled by powerful positive reinforcement gradually becomes functionally related to their negative reinforcement.

In relation to social and professional damages, the main cause is the fact that most of the user's behaviors tend to occur due to producing contact with the substance. For example, throughout the day there can be all the planning of how to get the money to buy the substance (which often occurs through non-licit ways), how to get to the place to consume, and how to "get rid" of personal demands and people who act hindering or preventing consumption. In this process, we often have a total distance from the work context and from all people who do not approve of consumption. Additionally, due to the very effects of the substance use (for example, drowsiness, delusions, sudden changes in mood), responses that impede social and professional coexistence are now presented, making it even more difficult for the user to engage socially and professionally. As time goes by, the user starts to present a life of impoverished social and professional relationships, making the substance (and the contexts related to its consumption) its only source of reinforces, whether positive or negative (Rachlin, 2000).

The role of the analytic-behavioral therapist in acting with individuals within the framework of substance use disorder must necessarily involve the identification of all consequences they have selected and act on the maintenance of consumption, as well as the identification of both the contexts that evoke the use and the pairings that have occurred that now act as triggers increasing the reinforcing value in the substance. Only after this analysis it is possible to act aiming at reducing the consumption of the substance. A safe path is to act in the management of previous conditions (eliminating triggers in this way) and in the strengthening of alternative abilities that allow the access to the social reinforcers produced by the substance use and of additional reinforcers that may be scarce in the individual's life. In the following, a clinical case will be presented to facilitate the understanding and analysis of concepts presented above.

Clinical Case

Participant and Therapeutic Procedure

Bruno (fictitious name), male, was 25 years old (at the beginning of the therapeutic process), single, and a professional in a large company. He lived with his mother only. His three older brothers lived outside the country for work and study reasons. The father was absent in his life since early childhood when he left home and moved to another state. Bruno sought therapy with the initial complaint in his words of "*feeling depressed and having more and more difficulties to deal with his mother and people from work.*" In the first session, Bruno reported on the consumption of alcoholic beverages. The beer consumption was daily and, according to Bruno, the perception of his drinking problem came about when he noticed the garbage full of cans and his mother started complaining about it. He claimed that he did not know the exact daily amount of consumption, but he believed it was around six cans.

The relationship with the mother was involved in conflict. Mother constantly compared him to her siblings and used negative adjectives to refer to his professional life, his scarce social life, and even his appearance. According to Bruno, his mother's aggressive lines also occurred in the past with her siblings and that was the main reason they left home. When asked the reasons for staying with his mother, he reports that it is purely for financial reasons. Regarding the fact that he did not go to university, Bruno reports again that he always preferred work to study and that the company in which he works would provide opportunities for growth if he started some university training in the area in which he performs his duties.

Regarding social life, Bruno reports "*being of few friends*." Two friends from the neighborhood who studied with him in high school rarely go home on weekends, a situation in which they usually drink and play (*online*) until late at night. In the absence of friends, Bruno reports that he often plays all night while consuming beer. I ask if there are situations where he attends his friends' house or goes out together and he reports that rarely "a *couple of months ago we went on André's birthday* (fictitious name of one of his friends)."

In the work context, Bruno reports that he has had great difficulties in arriving on time "*I feel sleepy all the time*" and the constant delays of up to 4 hours would be jeopardizing his continuity in employment. Bruno reports that, in order to make up for his delays, he usually stays late at the company. In some situations he worked all night (the company works 24 h), but he would have "*felt destroyed in the following days.*" I ask about the social coexistence with my co-workers and Bruno reports that he coexists friendly with everyone, but "*feels abused*" because, in his words "*every problem that happens they ask me to solve, as I am a god person, I end up realizing it.*" He also reports that the head of the sector constantly asks him to take on duty from other employees who are missing for various reasons, which he ends up doing at least twice a week. For this fact, Bruno reports that he considers unfair the company's complaint about his delays "*there are days that I leave after 10 pm, as they expect me to arrive the next day at 9 am.*"

Still on his social relations, Bruno says he recently had a conflict situation with a new employee. She posted in her social network a comment in favor of the death of racist people. On seeing the post, Bruno began to argue with her personally at lunchtime about the fact that violence generates more violence. According to Bruno, she understood his speech as a defense of racism, a fact he vehemently denies in the session. Bruno is afraid that other people in the sector were taking him for a racist, but he reported that he does not get very close to people at work, remaining isolated most of the time.

The first sessions with Bruno focused on establishing the therapeutic relationship, gathering information, mapping functional hypotheses, and establishing complaints and therapeutic goals. The intervention itself involved: (a) self-monitoring; (b) functional analysis of alcohol consumption; (c) training in social skills; (d) management of previous situations that culminated in consumption coupled with instruction for gradual reduction of consumption; (e) training of alternative and competing responses for access to other enforcers. Additionally, because of the potential long-term reinforcing consequences, the planning of an agenda that allowed free time to attend a university course was the focus of intervention. The intervention lasted 14 sessions that occurred weekly.

Results

Self-monitoring

We defined in session that Bruno's drinking behavior would be measured in two ways: an application would be used to record at the time of consumption the exact time and amount of beer cans consumed; additionally, daily Bruno would count the cans in the trash can. Both forms of recording were trained over a week and the client together with the therapist decided that the measures chosen were adequate due to the low cost of response.

Before the monitoring period, Bruno claimed to consume between 3 and 6 cans a day (maximum). However, the results obtained in the monitoring showed that the daily consumption varied between 6 and 8, reaching peaks of 15 beers over a Saturday that remained at home all day playing. The monitoring was initiated in the third session and maintained throughout the 14 weeks of intervention.

Functional Analysis of Alcohol Consumption

In the fourth intervention session, based on the records of the self-monitoring of alcohol consumption, we started the functional analysis in order to relate the drinking behavior with its environmental variables. The objective of the fourth session was to analyze the self-monitoring records obtained so far, identifying with Bruno the times at which beer consumption occurred, the contexts in which the behavior would occur (i.e., motivational operations and previous stimuli), and the reinforcing, positive and negative, and aversive consequences of its consumption.

To assist in the functional analysis, a table, of contexts, feelings, situations, and common consequences in Bruno's drinking behavior, was presented in session and he should score each item from 0 to 3. Regarding the previous situations, 0 referred to "I never drink"; 1 "I rarely drink"; 2 "I often drink"; and 3 "I always drink." Regarding the consequences of drinking, 0 referred to "never happen," 1 "rarely happen," 2 "frequently happen," and 3 "always happen."

Bruno's score results in the session revealed that score 3 was scored in the following previous situations: (a) I always drink alone, (b) While playing *online*, (c) After a stressful day, (d) After arguments at work, (e) After arguments at home, (f)

When I feel anxious. Regarding the potential reinforcing consequences, the highest score was regarding the following aspects: (a) I feel relaxed, (b) I feel "light" in the head. Regarding the potential aversive consequences we had: (a) Delay, (b) Hangover the next day, (c) Mood swings.

At the end of the fourth session Bruno was instructed to continue his self-monitoring, now recording the contexts and consequences related to drinking behavior in order to verify whether the functional hypotheses raised in session were correct. In the fifth and sixth session Bruno's records were analyzed and the conclusion was that his drinking behavior occurred primarily when he was drinking: (a) he was alone at home, (b) after discussions (at home and at work), (c) when he felt stressed, (d) anxious about not attending college, and (e) with the possibility of losing his job due to his constant delays. Throughout the following sessions, interventions were conducted with the objective of managing the conditions identified as precedents of beer consumption, coupled with the procedure of gradual reduction of consumption, and of training social skills.

Social Skills Training

During the sessions, Bruno described a series of situations in his home in which his mother verbally assaulted him. According to him, that was "*his mother's way of being and he would have to hold on to it until he had money to move in.*" Asked how Bruno reacts in these situations, he reports that "he *ends up being quiet so as not to make the situation worse.*" He tells of a day when he was helping his mother to file her income tax return and verbal assaults occurred. Bruno was collecting all the documentation and inserting it in the system that he "frequently" stopped. At those moments, the mother started complaining and saying that his brother would probably know how to solve everything faster and that "*he wasn't even good enough for that.*" He reports that he felt a lot of anger throughout the execution of the task, but that he said nothing and continued. After finishing, he locked himself in his room and drank late into the night.

Regarding the work, Bruno described the countless requests he receives to stay until later and every time he gives in even if staying at work has been accompanied by aversive consequences. Bruno reports a pre-holiday situation in which he had bought a bus ticket, but was unable to board because he stayed up to three hours after the end of his shift. According to Bruno, saying this is not something that makes him extremely anxious and that always ends up doing the will of others to avoid further problems.

According to the functional analysis of Bruno's drinking behavior, it is possible to verify that the boss's abusive requests and the mother's aggressions are variables that increased alcohol consumption. In general, drinking, for Bruno, was a strategy to avoid the related aversive private events that were products of maternal abuse and the difficulty to say no in the work environment. Because such situations were repeated, one focus of the intervention was social skills training. Specifically, assertive social coping skills (see Del Prette & Del Prette, 1999) such as expressing anger adequately and asking for behavior change; interacting with authorities (i.e., mother and boss); and dealing with criticism were trained through *role playing* in which aversive situations experienced with the mother and boss were acted on with the therapist and appropriate responses involving addressing the situation were trained. The components of the training were self-observation to identify factors that hinder coping behavior, modeling, and behavioral testing. The appropriate expression of negative feelings as well as the defense of one's own rights in the relationship with the mother and her superiors was listed as a therapeutic goal throughout the sessions.

Background Management and Gradual Reduction

Bruno's records, as well as his report in session, revealed that the beer was bought in brass format in an amount always higher than two bales, usually with 12 cans in the amount of 473 ml each. The beer was allocated in the refrigerator and in the freezer in the total amount. We defined in session the gradual reduction of beer consumption by stipulating that over 3 weeks consumption would drop from eight to two beers per day. The planned reduction was 10% after three days of consumption. For example, during the first 3 days Bruno would consume the 8 beers (average quantity identified in the self-monitoring phase), in the following three days he would consume 6 beers, then 4 beers until he reached the total of 2 beers per day. The gradual reduction in the consumption of psychoactive substances is recommended as an intervention because it reduces the probability of fissure responses produced by the absence of the substance. Experimental results support the effectiveness of the gradual reduction compared to the abrupt reduction in maintaining a reduced consumption of psychoactive substances (Foxx & Brown, 1979).

To facilitate the consumption of the agreed quantity in the period, the purchase of beer should take place on a daily basis and only in the agreed quantity to be consumed. The objective of the daily purchase was to increase the response cost of the purchase and consumption of beer as well as to facilitate self-observation of the consumption itself throughout the therapeutic process.

Training of Alternative and Competing Responses for Access to Other Boosters

During the sessions it became clear that Bruno had difficulties in engaging in a routine that would privilege the emission of behaviors that produced social reinforcement and backward reinforcements of great magnitude. Much of Bruno's free time was spent playing alone. Staying in his room was also an escape behavior and avoidance of contact with his mother, since meeting his mother was a context for potential verbal aggressions. With regard to backward reinforcements, Bruno listed entering a university as it would increase his chances of growing in his career and ultimately allow his financial independence and the possibility of paying rent in a republic or even in a single apartment.

Consuming beer in high quantity was established in session as a behavior incompatible with those that would produce reinforcements in the future, since drinking decreases the probability of quality social contact and increases delays at work, as well as, working until later as a strategy to compensate for their delays. Staying late at work is incompatible with entering a university, since the courses that Bruno hoped for were all nocturnal, starting classes around 7 pm. As Bruno reported, "*I get home and go to my room, I know it's easier to stay there alone, I stop thinking about what bothers me, the beer ends up being part of i., I wake up broken, it's hard to wake up, I end up staying late to take care of everything.*"

After the functional analysis of excessive drinking behavior, the gradual reduction, and training of social skills, the final part of the intervention was focused on programming Bruno's routine so as to allow social engagement, arrival, and departure at work at the stipulated time.

Specifically in relation to social interaction, we listed in session friends/knowwho Bruno could invite to alternative programs when playing *online,* since playing was context for the consumption of alcohol in excess. Bruno decided that he would like to meet again with a friend who lived "around" but had not seen him in a while. The social programs defined were the following: going to the cinema, to a restaurant and riding a bike in some public park. Even in his friend's absence, Bruno defined that he would engage in such activities to avoid staying at home alone playing and drinking. Increasing the possibilities of activities in which Bruno could engage is a way to increase his reinforcement potential and, in this way, increase the frequency of alternative repertoires to excessive consumption. Such intervention has a strong experimental basis and demonstrates that the best way to reduce compulsions is to strengthen competing/alternative responses that enable contact with various reinforces (Bernardes, 2008).

By the end of the therapeutic period, Bruno had reached the goal of drinking a maximum of two cans a day, demonstrating a reduction of at least 75% in beer consumption. In several sessions, Bruno reported that he remained days without consuming beer or any alcoholic beverage. Throughout the therapeutic period, Bruno reported several situations in which he acted with confrontation and in an appropriate manner to the verbal aggressions of his mother. Instead of going to his room to play (and consequently drink), Bruno reports that he tried to engage in the activities defined as competitors in the company of his friend or even alone. In the penultimate session, Bruno reported that a few days ago he was not late to get to work and left later only when everyone in the sector had to stay after hours.

Final Considerations

The excessive consumption of psychoactive substances is a behavioral pattern that causes various social, professional, and health damages. As a long-term result, being within the substance use disorder picture greatly decreases the probability of contact with backward enhancers of high magnitude related to a healthy mental life (such as being productive, healthy, and maintaining quality relationships).

The role of the behavior analyst acting in cases of this type of disorder is to identify, throughout the therapeutic process, how the pattern of excessive consumption was selected and maintained in the life history of his client. Additionally, the focus of analysis is on enriching the individual's repertoire so that his or her abilities allow access to multiple reinforces that compete with his or her pattern of excessive consumption. Bruno's case is an example that, without the identification of the variables that evoke and elicit his behavior of consuming alcohol, as well as the accurate analysis of all the effects of consumption in his life, it will be difficult to intervene in a contextual and effective manner. The analysis of behavior is thus presented as an effective model in establishing interventions that, in addition to reducing the picture of dependence, guarantee the promotion of quality of life through the expansion of the client's behavioral repertoire.

References

American Psychiatric Association (APA). (2013). *Diagnostic and statistical manual of mental disorders* (5th ed.). Washington, DC: APA.

Anthenelli, R., & Grandison, L. (2012). Effects of stress on alcohol consumption. *Alcohol Research: Current Reviews, 34*(4), 381–382.

Andrade, A. L. M., Teixeira, L. R. D. S., Zoner, C. C., Niro, N. N., Scatena, A., & Amaral, R. A. D. (2017). Factors associated with postpartum depression in social vulnerability women. SMAD. *Revista eletrônica saúde mental álcool e drogas, 13*(4), 196–204. http://dx.doi.org/10.11606/issn.1806-6976.v13i4p196-204.

Avery, M. (2011). *Behavior analysis and addictive behavior: A chance for change*. Retrieved from http://opensiuc.lib.siu.edu/gs_rp/48

Banaco, R., & Montan, R. N. M. (2018). Teoria analítico-comportamental. In N. A. Zanelatto & R. Laranjeira (Eds.), *O tratamento da dependência química e as terapias cognitivo-comportamentais: um guia para terapeutas* (2nd ed., pp. 115–132). Porto Alegre, Brazil: Artmed.

Bedendo, A., Andrade, A. L. M., Opaleye, E. S., & Noto, A. R. (2017). Binge drinking: a pattern associated with a risk of problems of alcohol use among university students. *Revista latino-americana de enfermagem, 25*. e2925–e2933. http://dx.doi.org/10.1590/1518-8345.1891.2925.

Bernardes, A. M. T. (2008). Efeito de enriquecimento ambiental na auto-administração oral de álcool em ratos (Master's thesis, Universidade de São Paulo, São Paulo, Brasil). https://doi.org/10.11606/D.47.2008.tde-05062008-172705

Borloti, E. B., Haydu, V. B., & Machado, A. R. (2015). Crack: Análise comportamental e exemplos das funções da dependência. *Acta Comportamentalia, 23*(3), 323–338.

Del Prette, Z. A. P., & Del Prette, A. (1999). *Psicologia das habilidades sociais: terapia e educação*. Petrópolis, Brazil: Vozes.

Escohotado, A. (1998). *Historia general de las drogas*. Madrid, Spain: Alianza Editorial.

Fiore, M. (2008). Prazer e risco: uma discussão a respeito dos saberes médicos sobre o uso de drogas. In B. C. Labate, S. L. Goulart, M. Fiore, E. MacRae, & H. Carneiro (Eds.), *Drogas e cultura: novas perspectivas* (pp. 141–153). Salvador, Brazil: EDUFBA.

Foxx, R. M., & Brown, R. A. (1979). Nicotine fading and self-monitoring for cigarette abstinence or controlled smoking. *Journal of Applied Behavior Analysis, 12*(1), 111–125. https://doi.org/10.1901/jaba.1979.12-111.

Higgins, S. T., Heil, S. H., & Sigmon, S. C. (2007). A behavioral approach to the treatment of substance use disorders. In P. Sturmey (Ed.), *Functional analysis in clinical treatment* (pp. 261–282). Burlington, VT: Elsevier.

Laranjeira, R. (2010). Tratamento da dependência do crack – as bases e os mitos. In M. Ribeiro & R. Laranjeira (Eds.), *O tratamento do usuário de crack: avaliação clínica, psicossocial, neuropsicológica e de risco, terapias psicológicas, farmacologia e reabilitação, ambientes de tratamento* (pp. 13–42). São Paulo, Brazil: Leitura Médica.

Rachlin, H. (2000). *The science of self-control.* Cambridge, UK: Harvard University Press.

Robbins, T. W., & Everitt, B. J. (1996). Neurobehavioural mechanisms of reward and motivation. *Current Opinion in Neurobiology, 6*(2), 228–236. https://doi.org/10.1016/s0959-4388(96)80077-8.

Schneider, M. S. (2012). *The science of consequences: How they affect genes, change the brain, and impact our world.* New York, NY: Prometheus Books.

Silverman, K., Roll, J. M., & Higgins, S. T. (2008). Introduction to the special issue on the behavior analysis and treatment of drug addiction. *Journal of Applied Behavior Analysis, 41*(4), 471–480. https://doi.org/10.1901/jaba.2008.41-471.

United Nations Office on Drugs and Crime (UNODC). (2018). *World drug report 2018.* Vienna: UNODC.

Yamauchi, L. M., Andrade, A. L. M., Pinheiro, B. O., Enumo, S. R. F., & De Micheli, D. (2019). Evaluation of the social representation of the use of alcoholic beverages by adolescents. *Estudos de Psicologia (Campinas), 36*, e180098. http://dx.doi.org/10.1590/1982-0275201936e180098.

Chapter 17
Psychological Trauma: Biological and Psychosocial Aspects of Substance Use Disorders

Richard Alecsander Reichert, Fernanda Machado Lopes, Eroy Aparecida da Silva, Adriana Scatena, André Luiz Monezi Andrade, and Denise De Micheli

Introduction

The evolution of the etiological concept of addiction has been transformed from the *syndrome* concept proposed by Edwards and Gross (1976), going through the various genetic and neuroimaging studies, which has brought significant contributions to this field of studies. However, many questions are still to be answered (De Micheli et al. 2020).

In recent decades, scientific knowledge has undergone several transformations, changing the way human behavior and mental disorders are understood. Genetics, for example, has progressed rapidly with the mapping of the entire human genome. This effort, however, was not enough to understand why there are psychopathologies, because, as Maté (2010) states, far from being autonomous dictators of people's destinies, genes are controlled by the environment in which they are inserted and, without environmental stimuli, would not function in such a way. In other words, despite the advances, many questions remained unanswered, demanding broader approaches. The integration of neuroscientific approaches to psychological and behavioral theories has made possible the emergence of new perspectives that consider the effects of the environment on the brain, i.e. the influence of

R. A. Reichert (✉)
Universidade do Vale do Itajaí, Itajaí, SC, Brazil

F. M. Lopes
Universidade Federal de Santa Catarina, Florianópolis, SC, Brazil

E. A. da Silva · A. Scatena · D. De Micheli
Universidade Federal de São Paulo, São Paulo, SP, Brazil

A. L. M. Andrade
Pontifícia Universidade Católica de Campinas, Campinas, SP, Brazil

D. De Micheli et al. (eds.), *Drugs and Human Behavior*,
https://doi.org/10.1007/978-3-030-62855-0_17

environmental events on the process of cognitive, emotional, and social development (Andrade and Micheli 2017; Brietzke et al. 2012).

Among the various misconceptions present in the discussions about drugs and which are consistently reinforced in the media, the belief that use undoubtedly leads to addiction stands out, considering the action of substances in the body the only determining factor (Souza et al. 2015). It is an undeniable fact that some people can become addicted after making frequent use of substances, with possible adverse consequences in many areas of their lives. However, it is important to comprehend what makes these individuals more vulnerable (Bedendo et al. 2015). Currently, scientific evidence shows that substance dependence is a complex and multidetermined disorder, influenced by genetic, socio-environmental, and psychological factors (Brown and Feng 2017; Enoch and Albaugh 2017; De Micheli et al. 2016; Francke et al. 2013; Magnusson et al. 2011).

Heroin, for example, is considered a drug of high potential addiction, but only for a minority of people, also depending on contextual factors, as demonstrated by Norman Zinberg's (1984) study on American soldiers in the Vietnam War. This study suggested that addiction is not caused by the drug itself, but by the needs of the individuals who used the substance and demonstrated the importance of social context in maintaining drug use patterns. If the addiction were caused solely by heroin and its action on the brain, most soldiers would continue to use it upon returning from the war. This vulnerability, however, encompasses factors other than genetic and biological variables, including family, community, social, cultural, economic, and political circumstances (Andrade and Micheli 2016).

Many addictions symptoms have a biological dimension. However, the belief that these behaviors can be reduced to biochemical processes in the brain to the functioning of nerve circuits or any other neurobiological, psychological, or social aspects acting in isolation is equivocal. To define the so-called addictions (a term popularly misused to refer to addiction) as an inherited or acquired disease is to limit the concept to an exclusively medical condition, disregarding its multifactorial nature and its variations. Although many cases present symptoms and diagnostic criteria that characterize a disorder, the biomedical model of disease alone is not sufficient to explain the issue. Therefore, over time, different perspectives and alternative definitions of "addiction" have emerged, considering it a multifaceted phenomenon, a complex and dynamic relationship between human beings and their environment. Therefore, a multi-level analysis, from different angles, is necessary, considering the interaction of several variables (Bedendo et al. 2013).

The etiology of problems related to the use of alcohol and other drugs is multifactorial, that is, influenced by several biogenetic and psychosocial factors. Adversity in childhood, such as physical and emotional abuse and neglect, is associated with the development of mental disorders in adults, including substance abuse. However, the mechanisms by which these environmental factors interact and predispose to the use and dependence of these substances are still poorly understood, mainly due to the limited knowledge about the genetic and biological aspects that mediate this process (Abrahao et al. 2012; Andrade et al. 2011; Fite et al. 2019; Rambau et al. 2018; Salokangas et al. 2019).

Exposure to stressful events and traumatic experiences can lead to changes in neurophysiological and behavioral development, increasing the risk of disorders due to the use of substances and related psychopathologies. Several studies show that there is a strong correlation between exposure to aversive environments/traumatic experiences and the development of psychological disorders such as anxiety, depression, and substance use disorders (Andrade et al., 2011; Campbell et al. 2009; Cerezo and Pérez-García 2019; Frade et al. 2013; Mingione et al. 2012; Meyers et al. 2019; Polimanti et al. 2017; Shin et al. 2018; Ten Have et al. 2019; Wolitzky-Taylor et al. 2016).

This chapter aims to elucidate the relationships between exposure to stressful events and traumatic experiences throughout life, especially in childhood, with the development of substance use disorders.

The Concept of Psychological Trauma

Psychological trauma can be defined as something generally catastrophic or aversive that causes emotional or cognitive damage, generating damage to the adaptive functioning of the individual (APA 2014; Santos 2017). It can result from some unique, unexpected traumatic situation, such as accident, death or threat of death, rape, natural disaster or assault; or from recurring traumatic experiences (Viola et al. 2011).

Continuous and prolonged exposure to traumatic experiences, especially those occurring since childhood, can produce negative impacts that are difficult to repair (Viola et al. 2011). Regardless of the event, trauma commonly generates physical and psychological suffering, a feeling of helplessness, helplessness, or fear, and stress. However, the subjective experience of the subject concerning the trauma, i.e. the way he or she experiences, means, and interprets the event, will determine whether the consequences of the event will be harmful and potentially disruptive. Thus, the consequences of the trauma will depend on factors such as the individual's history, his internal psychological resources (*coping* mechanisms), his support network, his resilience, among others (Bonanno and Diminich 2013; Santos 2017; Torres Bernal and Mille 2011).

The Relationships between Trauma and Use and Dependency on Substances: What Do the Researches Show?

Child neglect represents a global problem recognized as serious public health and human rights issues, covering physical and emotional abuse, sexual abuse, neglect, commercial sexual exploitation, child trafficking, and other forms of violence. These traumatic experiences have repercussions on physical and emotional health, resulting in immediate and long-term damage to dignity and socio-emotional cognitive development, such as increasing the likelihood of a range of health problems in adult life, including substance use disorders (Diehl et al. 2019; Hunt et al. 2017; Naal et al. 2018; Ngo et al. 2018; Silva et al. 2018; Sivolap and Portnova 2016; Wolitzky-Taylor et al. 2016).

These adversities increase the risk and severity of symptoms of psychopathologies in adult life. Patients with a history of childhood trauma have worse outcomes and higher rates of clinical disorders compared to individuals who did not experience trauma earlier in life. Although not a sufficient or necessary factor, evidence indicates that childhood stress is a risk factor for the development of mental disorders, influencing the expression of symptoms and the results of the therapeutic process (Brietzke et al. 2012; Heinonen et al. 2018).

Longitudinal research indicates that mistreatment in early life is related to the higher likelihood of developing psychopathologies in adulthood, including addiction to alcohol and other drugs (Enoch 2011; Kaplow and Widom 2007; Schilling et al. 2007). A literature review of the past 25 years of studies on childhood maltreatment and its impact on individuals' lifetime mental health has shown that child abuse increases the risk of developing many mental disorders, including anxiety disorders, depression, and harmful use of alcohol and other drugs (Sivolap and Portnova 2016).

Tractenberg et al. (2012) analyzed the occurrence of trauma and posttraumatic stress disorder (PTSD) among crack-dependent women and found a trauma exposure rate equivalent to 86.9% and PTSD corresponding to 15.1%. The most frequently reported types of events were aggression/physical abuse and witnessing violence to other people. The study also found that women who had experienced traumatic experiences during childhood and adolescence started using substances at an earlier age.

Because of this, it is a consensus in the scientific community that the early exposure to stress can affect developmental neuroimmune aspects and trigger psychopathologies in the future (Viola et al. 2011; Park et al. 2019). Hari (2018) states that a large number of substance dependence cases result from trauma experienced, especially in the early stages of life, is a correlation of magnitude rarely seen in epidemiology or public health.

Posttraumatic Stress Disorder and Substance Use Disorders

Posttraumatic stress disorder (PTSD) and substance use disorder (SUD) are conditions that often co-occur. PTSD–SUD comorbidity is associated with a more complex and costly clinical course when compared to any single disorder, including physical health problems, social harm, low treatment compliance, and worse prognosis (Hruska and Delahanty 2014; McCauley et al. 2012).

Studies on neurobiological and psychological mechanisms responsible for the PTSD–SUD correlation have resulted in explanatory models for the development of comorbidities, which differ in the order in which the comorbidity developed: (a) *hypothesis of the use of substances secondary to the psychiatric disorder*, which assumes that the use of substances is a strategy of self-medication to attenuate or alleviate sufferings arising from the psychiatric condition; (b) the psychiatric *disorder secondary to substance use hypothesis*, in which substance use may generate or intensify symptoms of psychiatric disorders; and (c) the *two-way hypothesis* or *shared vulnerability hypothesis*, which assumes that both disorders were mutually influenced (Cordeiro et al. 2019; Hruska and Delahanty 2014; Stewart and Conrod 2008).

In order to develop strategies to prevent and treat disorders associated with the use of substances and related psychopathologies, such as PTSD, it is necessary to identify the individual, family, community, social and political vulnerabilities to which individuals and communities are exposed (Andrade et al. 2016; Schaub et al. 2018). In this way, it becomes possible to formulate effective interventions and public policies that meet the real individual and collective needs. Some of these vulnerabilities that may predispose to physical and emotional health problems and generate or intensify social harm will be discussed below.

Exposure to Natural Disasters and the Use of Substances

Schiff and Fang (2016) analyzed the relationships between exposure to natural or human-made disasters and substance use by adolescents. The results of the review suggest a strong correlation between exposure to natural disasters and adolescent drug use. Vulnerable groups include adolescents who have been exposed to traumatic events and who live in regions with frequent disasters.

In the same direction, Maclean et al. (2016) investigated the impact of the experience of a natural disaster (fire, tornado, earthquake, hurricane) at the age of five on the mental health of adults and the disorders associated with substance use. The researchers used data from the *National Epidemiologic Survey of Alcohol and Related Conditions* from 2004 to 2005, including 27,129 individuals between the ages of 21 and 64. The results indicated that experiencing one or more natural disasters at age five increases the risk of psychological disorders in adult life, especially anxiety disorders.

Armed Conflicts: Physical and Emotional Health Impacts and Substance Use Relationships

Armed conflicts and forced displacement of people can last for years and even decades, impacting the physical and emotional health of the population often subjected to daily stressors and traumatic events. This context demands the formulation and execution of research, programs, and policies for humanitarian aid and recovery in the short, medium, and long term, which include the treatment of unhealthy behaviors (Makhashvili et al. 2014; Porter and Haslam 2005; Roberts et al. 2014).

The Republic of Georgia, for example, has gone through two main phases of conflict. The first occurred in the early 1990s, with fighting leading to the internal displacement of 300,000 people. The second took place in August 2008, due to a conflict between Georgia and Russia (Russian-Georgian War), leading to some 128,000 people being internally displaced. Considering this reality, a survey was conducted with a sample of 3600 internally displaced persons and former IDPs, measuring two outcomes of alcohol use disorders: (a) harmful alcohol use, with a score in the *Alcohol Use Disorders Identification Test* (AUDIT) corresponding to ≥8; and (b) excessive episodic consumption, equivalent to >60 g of alcohol each consumption at least once a week. Also, individual characteristics and demographic and socioeconomic aspects were recorded. The results showed that 71% of men and 16% of women were currently drinking, with 28% of men and 1% of women exhibiting risk drinking, and 12% of men and 2% of women exhibiting oppressive episodic drinking behavior. Characteristics such as age, the occurrence of severe injury, experiences of traumatic events, and symptoms of depression were associated with hazardous alcohol use (Roberts et al. 2014).

In line with this, studies indicate a high prevalence of mental disorders in populations affected by armed conflict, especially PTSD, anxiety, and depression. There are also concerns about alcohol and other drug use disorders among these populations. In these contexts of conflict, precarious living conditions, impoverishment, loss of family and friends, without means of subsistence and social support, the behavior of exacerbated alcohol use is interpreted as a form of self-medication in the face of stressors, to relieve the symptoms of stress, anxiety, and depression. In other words, the consumption of alcohol can exercise the function of facing adversity. However, exacerbated use can have implications at the individual level (e.g., non-communicable diseases, cardiovascular problems, cirrhosis, alcohol hepatitis) and at the collective level (e.g., exacerbation of gender-based violence), which is a significant public health concern (Ezard 2011; Roberts et al. 2014; Scherrer et al. 2008; Steel et al. 2009).

Consumption of Alcohol, Tobacco, and Other Drugs Among Immigrants

González-López et al. (2012) analyzed the prevalence of alcohol, tobacco, and other drug use among Latin American immigrants. The study showed that 61.4% of immigrants consumed alcohol in the month before the survey, 13.2% of participants were at risk for alcohol dependence, 30% were smokers, and 5.3% had used illicit substances (marijuana, hashish, and cocaine).

Part of this population is exposed to several risk factors, such as distance from family, social isolation, homelessness, exposure to constant hazards, discrimination, and social exclusion (Garcia 2008). Navarro-Lashayas and Eiroa-Orosa (2017) and Ramos et al. (2016) also found interrelations between stressful events, psychological suffering, and consumption of alcohol and other drugs among immigrants. As an aggravating factor, most individuals at high risk for substance use disorders do not have access to treatment because they encounter barriers such as limited language proficiency, financial difficulties, and lack of documentation, in addition to barriers at the system level, such as insufficient treatment services prepared to assist foreigners (Pagano et al. 2016). According to the authors, this information could help to overcome barriers that prevent the full citizenship and social participation of these individuals in society, in order to alleviate the stress resulting from the vulnerabilities to which they are exposed.

Traumas and Alcohol Use Among American Indians and Alaskan Natives

Enoch and Albaugh (2017) raised risk factors for alcohol use disorders in American Indians and Alaska natives. The authors identified environmental risk factors found in all societies, such as childhood trauma (neglect, physical and emotional abuse, etc.), geographical isolation, lack of economic opportunities, among others. Also, unique stressors were identified for indigenous populations, which include emotional and psychological trauma resulting from a denial of rights, loss of life, land, and cultural identity, which represent vulnerabilities to alcohol dependency in this population. According to the authors, the evaluation of these social determinants of health, such as socioeconomic status, education levels, and trauma, can lead to essential variables on which prevention efforts should focus.

Gender Vulnerabilities and Human Rights: Violence, Trauma, and Substance Dependence during Pregnancy and Early Motherhood

Torchalla et al. (2015) surveyed women living in poor and vulnerable neighborhoods such as Downtown Eastside, Vancouver—Canada. The objective was to explore personal issues related to traumatic experiences and gender-based violence among women substance users during pregnancy and early motherhood. The study participants' narratives highlighted the presence of multiple and ongoing adversity and trauma, from childhood to adulthood. The researchers found social problems such as homelessness, gender-based violence, and the sex trade, so psychological trauma is a collective experience for these women. Given this, the authors signaled that harm reduction services for poor and marginalized women should integrate an understanding of trauma and its relationships with substance use and dependence. These programs should include environmental, social, economic, and political interventions, addressing issues such as gender vulnerabilities and human rights, and providing positive environments and more integrative care to these people.

"Life at the River Is a Living Hell": The Case of Fishing Women in Zambia

Michalopoulos et al. (2017) conducted a survey of women fish traders from Zambia. The researchers found a relationship between the history of trauma, PTSD, substance use, and HIV risk behaviors. Most participants reported poor living and working conditions and described their work and quality of life as "suffering" due to the lack of essential elements for survival such as food, clothing, shelter, and access to education, and said they prefer another occupation but have no alternative employment, with the fish trade being the only viable option for women with a minimum level of schooling. The women interviewed also reported various approaches by fishers requesting sex in exchange for money, and punishment for denying blackmail. Also, the Government of Zambia implemented a fishing ban in the country for some months of the year to ensure the replenishment of depleted natural resources of lakes and rivers, which causes suffering to fisherwomen for lack of food for their families.

These women face risks of gender-based violence, such as intimate partner violence and sexual assault in rivers and at home, increasing exposure and risks of HIV and traumatic symptoms. The conceptual framework (Fig. 17.1) shows some of the vulnerabilities to which women fish traders in Zambia are exposed.

In this context, according to researchers, the use of substances (alcohol, cocaine, heroin, marijuana, and local synthetic drugs) emerges as a frequently reported strategy to deal with the stressors above.

Neurobiological and Behavioral Aspects Related to Traumatic Experiences and Their Relationship to Substance Use Disorders

When people are born, the brain is one of the most immature organs. The development of the fetal and neonatal brain, a process influenced by genetic and environmental factors, is fundamental to its functioning, including cognitive, emotional, and social performance (Andrade et al. 2014; Brietzke et al. 2012; Gressens et al. 2001). Since the brain—in constant related with the environment—controls mood, emotional self-control, and social behavior, neurological consequences from

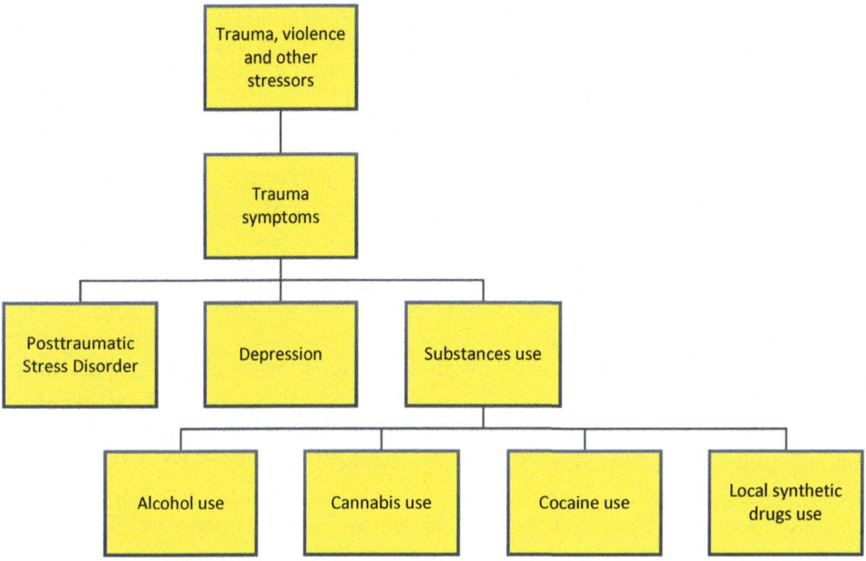

Fig. 17.1 Vulnerabilities associated with risky behavior among female fish traders in Zambia. Source: Adapted from Michalopoulos et al. (2017)

adverse experiences can lead to deficits in individuals' personal and social lives. There are three environmental conditions essential to the development of the human brain: nutrition, physical safety, and affective-emotional bond. In the industrialized world, except in cases of gross neglect or extreme poverty, children's nutritional and shelter needs are generally met. The third need, on the other hand, is more likely to be neglected (Maté 2010).

Emotional nutrition is an essential condition for neurobiological development and is decisive for the maturation of circuits essential to human life, which are involved in the processing of emotions and control of behavior, with implications for behavioral dependencies (Andrade et al. 2018). The lack of emotional nutrition can be represented by neglect and physical and emotional abuse. Individuals exposed to these stressors, especially in childhood, may suffer many lifelong impairments if they are subjected to such adversities and lack access to the protective resources necessary for their healthy development.

After traumatic events, animals and humans present physiological, behavioral, and emotional symptoms of distress. Studies have shown that laboratory animals exposed to aversive stimuli, such as shocks, had higher fear response rates and became more passive when submitted to new situations. This behavior was called "learned helplessness," which has significant repercussions on the individual's performance, adaptation, and survival (Maier and Seligman 1976).

Another study, performed by Caldji et al. (1998), showed, using an animal model study, that differences in the frequency of licking and breastfeeding of puppies contribute to the development of individual differences in stress responses.

In comparison with the children of mothers who exhibited low lick levels, the children who received more lickings had: reduced fear; increased density of the central benzodiazepine receptor (natural brain tranquilizer) in the central, lateral, and basolateral tonsil nuclei and the locus coeruleus; and decreased density of the corticotropin-releasing hormone receptor (which plays a role in the stress response) in the locus coeruleus. These results suggest that maternal care during childhood regulates behavioral responses to stress in the offspring, shaping the development of neural systems that measure fear.

In humans, children continuously exposed to adverse situations experience intense emotions of anger, fear, shame, among others. Therefore, some behavior patterns are developed in order to avoid the recurrence of these emotional responses (Viola et al. 2011). Maternal deprivation and other types of adversity early in life can result in high levels of cortisol (stress hormone) in the body. Chronically high levels of cortisol can damage important brain mechanisms associated with memory and the processing of emotions, with repercussions for the entire life of individuals. Also, neglect and physical and emotional abuse early in life can compromise the development of bonding systems and the ability to reward interpersonal relationships and commitment to social and cultural values. Children depend physically and emotionally on their parents, and their loving response releases endorphins in the brain, relieving the discomfort caused by separation. If they do not respond or respond inadequately, endorphins are not released. Later in life, those children who have not received the attentive presence of their parents are at higher risk of seeking satisfaction from external sources. Individuals who have gone through these experiences may seek other ways to stimulate reward pathways in the brain, such as drugs, sex, and aggression (Andrade et al. 2017a, b, 2018).

Prenatal stress also produces disorders in the structural and functional development of the nervous system, resulting in behavioral changes such as hyper responsiveness to stressors and new strengthening stimuli, increased anxiety, damage to memory and learning, altered circadian rhythm (biological cycle), and more significant response to the strengthening properties of psychoactive substances. In a review conducted by Campbell et al. (2009), experimental studies with animals have shown that those exposed to prenatal stress present changes in limbic structures and neurotransmitter systems, such as dopamine and glutamate. These changes may contribute to a higher propensity for self-administration of large amounts of drugs or relapses after periods of abstinence. In humans, children of mothers who have suffered stress during pregnancy or have experienced adversity early in life, there are changes in motor development, differences in brain morphology, and increased risk for the development of neuropsychiatric disorders such as sleep disorders, anxiety, depression, attention deficit and hyperactivity disorders, substance use disorders, among others.

Veer et al. (2015) observed lower volumes of right tonsils in patients with PTSD compared to controls. Although the results are not conclusive, the study provides more evidence on how adverse experiences in childhood can impact brain development and affect areas such as the amygdala, a region involved in processing emotional responses, which can make an individual more vulnerable to the development of psychological disorders.

Magnetic resonance studies show that exposure to traumatic events in the early stages of life can result in structural and functional changes in the brain, such as a reduction in the hippocampus and the corpus callosum, and thus damage to the functioning and cognitive performance. Differences have also been observed in the volume of the tonsil, a region involved in the processing of emotional responses. The result of alterations (reduction in size, interruption in functioning) in the corpus callosum, a structure that promotes communication between the two cerebral hemispheres, maybe a "split" in the processing of emotions: both parts may not work together, especially when the individual is under stress. These changes in essential regions of emotional processing and brain communication can make an individual more vulnerable to the development of psychological disorders (Brietzke et al. 2012; Maté 2010; Veer et al. 2015).

Meyers et al. (2019) examined the association of adverse experiences before 10 years of age concerning neurocognitive development, using data from the *Collaborative Study of the Genetics of Alcoholism* (COGA), with a sample composed of individuals aged 12–22 years. The researchers also analyzed other predictors, such as substance use, impulsivity, and alcohol use disorders by parents. They found that those exposed to traumas of sexual aggression in childhood presented atypical frontal neurophysiological development, which may reflect changes in frontal lobe development, synaptic pruning, and cortical maturation involving circuits related to inhibitory control. These areas may be associated with an increased probability of internalizing psychopathologies and disorders due to the use of alcohol and other drugs. These findings reinforce the evidence that early exposure to traumatic experiences, such as sexual assault, may increase the risks of mental health problems and substance use in adult life.

Kaag et al. (2018) found a significant increase in neural activation in several brain regions in cocaine users during the presentation of the substance to the user, including the frontostriatal circuit and the amygdala, which may contribute to worse cognitive control and increased recurrence of behavior. The relationship between childhood trauma, anxiety, and increased reactivity to drug-related clues was also observed. The severity of cocaine use was positively associated with the level of anxiety of users. Furthermore, results indicated a negative correlation between anxiety and functional connectivity between the dorsomedial prefrontal cortex and the ventromedial prefrontal cortex and the dorsal and ventral striated. The impairment of functional connectivity between the amygdala and prefrontal cortex may result in impaired emotional regulation. Although this study does not allow conclusions on causality, it provides essential information on how trauma in childhood can contribute to the installation and maintenance of substance use disorders, based on evidence that traumatic experiences induce changes in neurological development, especially in regions such as prefrontal cortex, striated, and amygdala.

Changes in the hypothalamic–pituitary–adrenal axis (HPA) and the stress response circuit are also related to the appearance of psychiatric disorders. Stress induces secretion of glucocorticoid hormones cortisol in human and non-human primates and corticosterone (glucocorticoid class hormone) in rodents. Activation of the HPA axis, corticotrophin-releasing hormone, and peripheral catecholamine systems in response to acute stress is essential for survival. Chronic activation of these systems, however, may increase the risk of various physiological problems and increase vulnerability to the development of psychopathologies such as anxiety, depression, and substance use disorders (Enoch 2011; Sapolsky et al. 2000).

There is also the participation of Monoamine Oxidase (MAO)—an enzyme that degrades serotonin, noradrenalin, and dopamine in the brain—in moderating the effects of stress throughout life and its relationship with the beginning of substance use. Research shows that alleles of MAO type A play a role in the pathogenesis of problems related to the use of alcohol and other drugs, through gene–environment interactions with psychosocial stress in the early stages of life. Some neuroimaging studies have shown the influence of MAO-A on the definition of anterior cingulate cortex function, brain circuitry region related to the control of executive functions, impulse control, and reward-related behavior. These findings suggest that gene and environment interactions with early maltreatment can result in inhibitory control deficits and facilitate substance use in adolescence (Fite et al. 2019).

After exposure to traumatic situations, there is an increase in the level of endorphins in the brain, which remains high during the period to help ease physical and emotional pain from the trauma. Then, however, endorphin levels gradually decrease, which can lead to a period of abstinence that can last for hours or days. For this reason, after experiencing a traumatic event, people usually report the use of alcohol to relieve symptoms of anxiety, irritability, and depression. Alcohol has the potential to alleviate these symptoms to the extent that it compensates for deficits in endorphin activity after adverse experiences. Therefore, chronic exposure to this cycle can lead to dependence on this drug (Jacobsen et al. 2001; Volpicelli et al. 1999). For this reason, the self-medication hypothesis postulates that individuals exposed to traumatic experiences are at higher risk of using substances to control emotional suffering resulting from exposure to adversity (Ramos et al. 2016).

Prevention of Use and Dependence and Substances and Other Disorders

Is there any way to reduce the impacts of traumatic experiences and decrease the likelihood of developing psychological disorders, such as substance use disorders? Rowe et al. (2010) examined the influence of Hurricane Katrina's impact on individual and family risk factors and their relationship to PTSD symptoms and substance use behavior among American adolescents. The results indicated that the impact of the hurricane was more strongly related to the development of PTSD, while the interaction with other risk factors, such as low family cohesion and parental monitoring, was associated with teenage substance use. These observations support Enoch's (2011) statement that mediating factors, such as gene–environment interactions and family and peer relationships, are essential for resilience and prevention of psychopathologies.

Concerning harmful substance consumption, current studies have called attention to the importance of understanding the development of both individual and family resilience, i.e. the ability to deal with diversity and adversity of life in the face of suffering and its overcoming, as well as risk and protection factors (Santos 2017; Silva et al. 2015; Yamauchi et al. 2019). Preventive programs must pay attention to the individual, family, social and programmatic vulnerabilities to which individuals and communities are exposed. The understanding that behavior is multidetermined and influenced by a complex interaction of biological and environmental factors is of paramount importance for the formulation of public policies and practical interventions committed to the needs of the suffering population (Bedendo et al. 2018). Understanding the biopsychosocial basis of substance use disorders is critical to the development of new, comprehensive, integrative, and effective personalized preventive strategies (Almeida et al, 2018; Andrade et al. 2017a; Bedendo et al. 2019; Enoch 2011; Fite et al. 2019; Rose et al. 2019).

Therefore, prevention should focus on early intervention in families to prevent mistreatment in the early stages of life, reducing the impacts of early stress on the socio-emotional cognitive development of children and adolescents (Silva et al. 2015). Especially in adolescence, a critically vulnerable time for the development of harmful substance use habits, it is essential to have programs for the development of positive parental practices, peer-to-peer mediation, among other interventions (Schaub et al. 2018). The manipulation of the environment in which individuals live may decrease the risk of substance use disorders (Enoch 2011; Enoch and Albaugh 2017; Schilling et al. 2007).

Final Considerations

Despite the vast body of evidence already available, more research, especially longitudinal studies, is needed to elucidate the mechanisms that measure this relationship. Given its complexity, substance abuse has to be analyzed from a critical scientific perspective, in a broad spectrum considering the individual about the social context. Thus, a biopsychosocial analysis is fundamental for the recognition and understanding of the multiplicity of factors that interact and influence human actions and decisions, and above all, for the formulation of public policies and more effective human and bioethical interventions.

References

Abrahao, K. P., Quadros, I. M. H., Andrade, A. L. M., & Souza-Formigoni, M. L. O. (2012). Accumbal dopamine D2 receptor function is associated with individual variability in ethanol behavioral sensitization. *Neuropharmacology, 62*(2), 882–889. https://doi.org/10.1016/j.neuropharm.2011.09.017.

Almeida, D. E. R. G., Andrade, A. L. M., Cruz, F. D., & Micheli, D. D. (2018). Perception of freedom in leisure among substance users and nonusers. *Psico-USF, 23*(1), 13–24. https://doi.org/10.1590/1413-82712018230102.

American Psychiatric Association (APA). (2014). *Manual diagnóstico e estatístico de transtornos mentais* (5th ed.). Porto Alegre, Brazil: Artmed Editora.
Andrade, A. L. M., Abrahao, K. P., Goeldner, F. O., & Souza-Formigoni, M. L. O. (2011). Administration of the 5-HT2C receptor antagonist SB-242084 into the nucleus accumbens blocks the expression of ethanol-induced behavioral sensitization in albino Swiss mice. *Neuroscience, 189*, 178–186. https://doi.org/10.1016/j.neuroscience.2011.05.028.
Andrade, A. L. M., Bedendo, A., Enumo, S. R. F., & Micheli, D. (2018). Brain development in adolescence: General aspects and update. *Adolescência e Saude, 15*(Supl. 1), 62–67. Retrieved from https://www.adolescenciaesaude.com/detalhe_artigo.asp?id=759#.
Andrade, A. L. M., De Micheli, D., & Fisberg, M. (2014). Cognitive aspects of fetal alcohol syndrome in young adults: Two case studies. *Interação em Psicologia, 17*(2), 217–223. https://doi.org/10.5380/psi.v17i2.27359.
Andrade, A. L. M., Lacerda, R. B., Gomide, H. P., Ronzani, T. M., Sartes, L. M. A., Martins, L. F., et al. (2016). Web-based self-help intervention reduces alcohol consumption in both heavy-drinking and dependent alcohol users: A pilot study. *Addictive Behaviors, 63*, 63–71. https://doi.org/10.1016/j.addbeh.2016.06.027.
Andrade, A. L. M., & De Micheli, D. (2016). *Innovations in the treatment of substance addiction* (1st ed.). New York, NY: Springer. https://doi.org/10.1007/978-3-319-43172-7.
Andrade, A. L. M., & De Micheli, D. (2017). *Inovações no Tratamento de Dependência de Drogas* (1st ed.). Rio de Janeiro, Brazil: Atheneu.
Andrade, A. L. M., Scatena, A., & De Micheli, D. (2017a). Evaluation of a preventive intervention in alcoholic and non-alcoholic drivers – A pilot study. *SMAD Revista eletrônica saúde mental álcool e drogas, 13*(4), 205–212. https://doi.org/10.11606/issn.1806-6976.v13i4p205-212.
Andrade, A. L. M., Teixeira, L. R. D. S., Zoner, C. C., Niro, N. N., Scatena, A., & Amaral, R. A. D. (2017b). Factors associated with postpartum depression in social vulnerability women. *SMAD. Revista eletrônica saúde mental álcool e drogas, 13*(4), 196–204. https://doi.org/10.11606/issn.1806-6976.v13i4p196-204.
Bedendo, A., Andrade, A. L. M., & Noto, A. R. (2015). Sports and substance use in high school students different perspectives of this relationship. *SMAD Revista Eletrônica Saúde Mental Álcool e Drogas, 11*(2), 85–96. https://doi.org/10.11606/issn.1806-6976.v11i2p85-96.
Bedendo, A., Andrade, A. L. M., & Noto, A. R. (2018). Internet-based alcohol interventions for college students: Systematic review. *Revista Panamericana de Salud Pública, 42*, e54. https://doi.org/10.26633/RPSP.2018.54.
Bedendo, A., Ferri, C. P., Souza, A. A. L., Andrade, A. L. M., & Noto, A. R. (2019). Pragmatic randomized controlled trial of a web-based intervention for alcohol use among Brazilian college students: Motivation as a moderating effect. *Drug and Alcohol Dependence, 199*, 92–100. https://doi.org/10.1016/j.drugalcdep.2019.02.021.
Bedendo, A., Opaleye, E. S., Andrade, A. L. M., & Noto, A. R. (2013). Heavy episodic drinking and soccer practice among high school students in Brazil: The contextual aspects of this relationship. *BMC Public Health, 13*(1), 247. https://doi.org/10.1186/1471-2458-13-247.
Bonanno, G. A., & Diminich, E. D. (2013). Annual research review: Positive adjustment to adversity - trajectories of minimal-impact resilience and emergent resilience. *Journal of Child Psychology and Psychiatry, 54*(4), 378–401. https://doi.org/10.1111/jcpp.12021.
Brietzke, E., Sant'Anna, M., Jackowski, A., Grassi-Oliveira, R., Bucker, J., Zugman, A., et al. (2012). Impact of childhood stress on psychopathology. *Revista Brasileira de Psiquiatria, 34*(4), 480–488. https://doi.org/10.1016/j.rbp.2012.04.009.
Brown, A., & Feng, J. (2017). Drug addiction and DNA modifications. *Advances in Experimental Medicine and Biology, 978*, 105–125. https://doi.org/10.1007/978-3-319-53889-1_6.
Caldji, C., Tannenbaum, B., Sharma, S., Francis, D., Plotsky, P., & Meaney, M. (1998). Maternal care during infancy regulates the development of neural systems mediating the expression of fearfulness in the rat. *Proceedings of the National Academy of Sciences, 95*(9), 5335–5340. https://doi.org/10.1073/pnas.95.9.5335.
Campbell, J., Szumlinski, K., & Kippin, T. (2009). Contribution of early environmental stress to alcoholism vulnerability. *Alcohol, 43*(7), 547–554. https://doi.org/10.1016/j.alcohol.2009.09.029.

Cerezo, M., & Pérez-García, E. (2019). Childhood victimization by adults and peers and health-risk behaviors in adulthood. *The Spanish Journal of Psychology, 22*, e20. https://doi.org/10.1017/sjp.2019.24.
Cordeiro, D., Diehl, A., & Mari, J. (2019). Comorbidades psiquiátricas. In A. Diehl, D. Cordeiro, & R. Laranjeira (Eds.), *Dependência química: prevenção, tratamento e políticas públicas* (2nd ed., pp. 75–89). Porto Alegre, Brazil: Artmed.
De Micheli, D., Andrade, A. L. M., Silva, E. A., & Souza-Formigoni, M. L. O. (2016). *Drug abuse in adolescence* (1st ed.). New York, NY: Springer. https://doi.org/10.1007/978-3-319-17795-3.
De Micheli, D., Andrade, A., & Galduróz, J. C. (2020). Limitations of DSM-5 diagnostic criteria for substance use disorder in adolescents: what have we learned after using these criteria for several years? *Brazilian Journal of Psychiatry*, in press. https://doi.org/10.1590/1516-4446-2020-1151.
Diehl, A., Clemente, J., Pillon, S., Santana, P., da Silva, C., & Mari, J. (2019). Early childhood maltreatment experience and later sexual behavior in Brazilian adults undergoing treatment for substance dependence. *Brazilian Journal of Psychiatry, 41*(3), 199–207. https://doi.org/10.1590/1516-4446-2017-0020.
Edwards, G., & Gross, M. (1976). Alcohol dependence: Provisional description of a clinical syndrome. *BMJ, 1*(6017), 1058–1061. https://doi.org/10.1136/bmj.1.6017.1058.
Enoch, M. (2011). The role of early life stress as a predictor for alcohol and drug dependence. *Psychopharmacology, 214*(1), 17–31. https://doi.org/10.1007/s00213-010-1916-6.
Enoch, M., & Albaugh, B. (2017). Review: Genetic and environmental risk factors for alcohol use disorders in American Indians and Alaskan natives. *The American Journal on Addictions, 26*(5), 461–468.
Ezard, N. (2011). Substance use among populations displaced by conflict: A literature review. *Disasters, 36*(3), 533–557. https://doi.org/10.1111/j.1467-7717.2011.01261.x.
Fite, P., Brown, S., Hossain, W., Manzardo, A., Butler, M., & Bortolato, M. (2019). Tobacco and cannabis use in college students are predicted by sex-dimorphic interactions between MAOA genotype and child abuse. *CNS Neuroscience & Therapeutics, 25*(1), 101–111. https://doi.org/10.1111/cns.13002.
Frade, I. F., De Micheli, D., Andrade, A. L. M., & de Souza-Formigoni, M. L. O. (2013). Relationship between stress symptoms and drug use among secondary students. *The Spanish Journal of Psychology, 16*, e4. https://doi.org/10.1017/sjp.2013.5.
Francke, I., Viola, T., Tractenberg, S., & Grassi-Oliveira, R. (2013). Childhood neglect and increased withdrawal and depressive severity in crack cocaine users during early abstinence. *Child Abuse & Neglect, 37*(10), 883–889. https://doi.org/10.1016/j.chiabu.2013.04.008.
Garcia, V. (2008). Problem drinking among transnational Mexican migrants: Exploring migrant status and situational factors. *Human Organization, 67*(1), 12–24.
González-López, J., Rodríguez-Gázquez, M., & Lomas-Campos, M. (2012). Prevalence of alcohol, tobacco and street drugs consumption in adult Latin American immigrants. *Revista Latino-Americana de Enfermagem, 20*(3), 528–535. https://doi.org/10.1590/S0104-11692012000300014.
Gressens, P., Mesples, B., Sahir, N., Marret, S., & Sola, A. (2001). Environmental factors and disturbances of brain development. *Seminars in Neonatology, 6*(2), 185–194. https://doi.org/10.1053/siny.2001.0048.
Hari, J. (2018). *Na fissura: uma história do fracasso no combate às drogas*. São Paulo, Brazil: Companhia das Letras.
Heinonen, E., Knekt, P., Härkänen, T., Virtala, E., & Lindfors, O. (2018). Associations of early childhood adversities with mental disorders, psychological functioning, and suitability for psychotherapy in adulthood. *Psychiatry Research, 264*, 366–373. https://doi.org/10.1016/j.psychres.2018.04.011.
Hruska, B., & Delahanty, D. L. (2014). PTSD-SUD biological mechanisms: Self-medication and beyond. In P. Ouimette & J. P. Read (Eds.), *Trauma and substance abuse: Causes, consequences, and treatment of comorbid disorders* (pp. 35–52). Washington, DC: American Psychological Association.

Hunt, T., Slack, K., & Berger, L. (2017). Adverse childhood experiences and behavioral problems in middle childhood. *Child Abuse & Neglect, 67*, 391–402. https://doi.org/10.1016/j.chiabu.2016.11.005.

Jacobsen, L., Southwick, S., & Kosten, T. (2001). Substance use disorders in patients with post-traumatic stress disorder: A review of the literature. *American Journal of Psychiatry, 158*(8), 1184–1190. https://doi.org/10.1176/appi.ajp.158.8.1184.

Kaag, A., Reneman, L., Homberg, J., van den Brink, W., & van Wingen, G. (2018). Enhanced amygdala-striatal functional connectivity during the processing of cocaine cues in male cocaine users with a history of childhood trauma. *Frontiers in Psychiatry, 9*, 70. https://doi.org/10.3389/fpsyt.2018.00070.

Kaplow, J., & Widom, C. (2007). Age of onset of child maltreatment predicts long-term mental health outcomes. *Journal of Abnormal Psychology, 116*(1), 176–187. https://doi.org/10.1037/0021-843X.116.1.176.

Maclean, J., Popovici, I., & French, M. (2016). Are natural disasters in early childhood associated with mental health and substance use disorders as an adult? *Social Science & Medicine, 151*, 78–91. https://doi.org/10.1016/j.socscimed.2016.01.006.

Magnusson, Å., Lundholm, C., Göransson, M., Copeland, W., Heilig, M., & Pedersen, N. (2011). Familial influence and childhood trauma in female alcoholism. *Psychological Medicine, 42*(2), 381–389. https://doi.org/10.1017/S0033291711001310.

Maier, S., & Seligman, M. (1976). Learned helplessness: Theory and evidence. *Journal of Experimental Psychology: General, 105*(1), 3–46. https://doi.org/10.1037/0096-3445.105.1.3.

Makhashvili, N., Chikovani, I., McKee, M., Bisson, J., Patel, V., & Roberts, B. (2014). Mental disorders and their association with disability among internally displaced persons and returnees in Georgia. *Journal of Traumatic Stress, 27*(5), 509–518. https://doi.org/10.1002/jts.21949.

Maté, G. (2010). *In the realm of hungry ghosts: Close encounters with addiction*. Berkeley, CA: North Atlantic.

McCauley, J., Killeen, T., Gros, D., Brady, K., & Back, S. (2012). Posttraumatic stress disorder and co-occurring substance use disorders: Advances in assessment and treatment. *Clinical Psychology: Science and Practice, 19*(3), 283–304. https://doi.org/10.1111/cpsp.12006.

Meyers, J., McCutcheon, V., Pandey, A., Kamarajan, C., Subbie, S., Chorlian, D., et al. (2019). Early sexual trauma exposure and neural response inhibition in adolescence and young adults: Trajectories of frontal theta oscillations during a go/no-go task. *Journal of the American Academy of Child and Adolescent Psychiatry, 58*(2), 242–255. https://doi.org/10.1016/j.jaac.2018.07.905.

Michalopoulos, L., Baca-Atlas, S., Simona, S., Jiwatram-Negrón, T., Ncube, A., & Chery, M. (2017). "Life at the river is a living hell:" a qualitative study of trauma, mental health, substance use and HIV risk behavior among female fish traders from the Kafue flatlands in Zambia. *BMC Women's Health, 17*(1), 15. https://doi.org/10.1186/s12905-017-0369-z.

Mingione, C., Heffner, J., Blom, T., & Anthenelli, R. (2012). Childhood adversity, serotonin transporter (5-HTTLPR) genotype, and risk for cigarette smoking and nicotine dependence in alcohol dependent adults. *Drug and Alcohol Dependence, 123*(1–3), 201–206. https://doi.org/10.1016/j.drugalcdep.2011.11.013.

Naal, H., El Jalkh, T., & Haddad, R. (2018). Adverse childhood experiences in substance use disorder outpatients of a Lebanese addiction center. *Psychology, Health & Medicine, 23*(9), 1137–1144. https://doi.org/10.1080/13548506.2018.1469781.

Navarro-Lashayas, M., & Eiroa-Orosa, F. (2017). Substance use and psychological distress is related with accommodation status among homeless immigrants. *American Journal of Orthopsychiatry, 87*(1), 23–33. https://doi.org/10.1037/ort0000213.

Ngo, Q., Veliz, P., Kusunoki, Y., Stein, S., & Boyd, C. (2018). Adolescent sexual violence: Prevalence, adolescent risks, and violence characteristics. *Preventive Medicine, 116*, 68–74. https://doi.org/10.1016/j.ypmed.2018.08.032.

Pagano, A., García, V., Recarte, C., & Lee, J. (2016). Sociopolitical contexts for addiction recovery: Anexos in U.S. Latino communities. *International Journal of Drug Policy, 37*, 52–59. https://doi.org/10.1016/j.drugpo.2016.08.002.

Park, C., Rosenblat, J., Brietzke, E., Pan, Z., Lee, Y., Cao, B., et al. (2019). Stress, epigenetics and depression: A systematic review. *Neuroscience & Biobehavioral Reviews, 102*, 139–152. https://doi.org/10.1016/j.neubiorev.2019.04.010.

Polimanti, R., Kaufman, J., Zhao, H., Kranzler, H., Ursano, R., Kessler, R., et al. (2017). A genome-wide gene-by-trauma interaction study of alcohol misuse in two independent cohorts identifies PRKG1 as a risk locus. *Molecular Psychiatry, 23*(1), 154–160. https://doi.org/10.1038/mp.2017.24.

Porter, M., & Haslam, N. (2005). Predisplacement and Postdisplacement factors associated with mental health of refugees and internally displaced persons. *JAMA, 294*(5), 602. https://doi.org/10.1001/jama.294.5.602.

Rambau, S., Forstner, A., Wegener, I., Mücke, M., Wissussek, C., Staufenbiel, S., et al. (2018). Childhood adversities, bonding, and personality in social anxiety disorder with alcohol use disorder. *Psychiatry Research, 262*, 295–302. https://doi.org/10.1016/j.psychres.2018.02.006.

Ramos, Z., Fortuna, L., Porche, M., Wang, Y., Shrout, P., Loder, S., et al. (2016). Posttraumatic stress symptoms and their relationship to drug and alcohol use in an international sample of Latino immigrants. *Journal of Immigrant and Minority Health, 19*(3), 552–561. https://doi.org/10.1007/s10903-016-0426-y.

Roberts, B., Murphy, A., Chikovani, I., Makhashvili, N., Patel, V., & McKee, M. (2014). Individual and community level risk-factors for alcohol use disorder among conflict-affected persons in Georgia. *PLoS One, 9*(5), e98299. https://doi.org/10.1371/journal.pone.0098299.

Rose, E., Picci, G., & Fishbein, D. (2019). Neurocognitive precursors of substance misuse corresponding to risk, resistance, and resilience pathways: Implications for prevention science. *Frontiers in Psychiatry, 10*, 399. https://doi.org/10.3389/fpsyt.2019.00399.

Rowe, C., La Greca, A., & Alexandersson, A. (2010). Family and individual factors associated with substance involvement and PTS symptoms among adolescents in greater New Orleans after Hurricane Katrina. *Journal of Consulting and Clinical Psychology, 78*(6), 806–817. https://doi.org/10.1037/a0020808.

Salokangas, R., Schultze-Lutter, F., Schmidt, S., Pesonen, H., Luutonen, S., Patterson, P., et al. (2019). Childhood physical abuse and emotional neglect are specifically associated with adult mental disorders. *Journal of Mental Health, 29*, 1–9. https://doi.org/10.1080/09638237.2018.1521940.

Santos, M. (2017). Trauma psicológico e resiliência: relação com o tipo de evento potencialmente traumático e o crescimento pós-traumático (Masters's thesis), Universidade de Lisboa, Portugal.

Sapolsky, R., Romero, L., & Munck, A. (2000). How do glucocorticoids influence stress responses? Integrating permissive, suppressive, stimulatory, and preparative actions. *Endocrine Reviews, 21*(1), 55–89. https://doi.org/10.1210/edrv.21.1.0389.

Schaub, M. P., Tiburcio, M., Martinez, N., Ambekar, A., Balhara, Y. P. S., Wenger, A., Poznyak, V., et al. (2018). Alcohol e-help: Study protocol for a web-based self-help program to reduce alcohol use in adults with drinking patterns considered harmful, hazardous or suggestive of dependence in middle-income countries. *Addiction, 113*(2), 346–352. https://doi.org/10.1111/add.14034.

Scherrer, J., Xian, H., Lyons, M., Goldberg, J., Eisen, S., True, W., et al. (2008). Posttraumatic stress disorder; combat exposure; and nicotine dependence, alcohol dependence, and major depression in male twins. *Comprehensive Psychiatry, 49*(3), 297–304. https://doi.org/10.1016/j.comppsych.2007.11.001.

Schiff, M., & Fang, L. (2016). Adolescents' exposure to disasters and substance use. *Current Psychiatry Reports, 18*(6), 57. https://doi.org/10.1007/s11920-016-0693-2.

Schilling, E., Aseltine, R., & Gore, S. (2007). Adverse childhood experiences and mental health in young adults: A longitudinal survey. *BMC Public Health, 7*, 30. https://doi.org/10.1186/1471-2458-7-30.

Shin, S., McDonald, S., & Conley, D. (2018). Patterns of adverse childhood experiences and substance use among young adults: A latent class analysis. *Addictive Behaviors, 78*, 187–192. https://doi.org/10.1016/j.addbeh.2017.11.020.

Silva, E. A., Rodrigues, T. P., de Micheli, D., & Andrade, A. L. M. (2015). Strategies for treating families affected by substance abuse users. *Revista Psicologia em Pesquisa, 9*(2), 198–204. https://doi.org/10.5327/Z1982-1247201500020010.

Silva, M. A. A., Andrade, A. L. M., & De Micheli, D. (2018). Evaluation of the implementation of brief interventions to substance abuse in a Socieducative context. *Revista Psicologia em Pesquisa, 12*(1), 9. https://doi.org/10.24879/2018001200100125.

Sivolap, Y., & Portnova, A. (2016). Childhood maltreatment and its impact on the mental health. *Zhurnal Nevrologii I Psikhiatrii Im. S.S. Korsakova, 116*(7), 108. https://doi.org/10.3389/fpsyt.2019.00415.

Souza, F. B., Andrade, A. L. M., Rodrigues, T. P., Nascimento, M. O., & De Micheli, D. (2015). Evaluation of teachers' conceptions about substance misuse in public and private schools: An exploratory. *Estudos e Pesquisas em Psicologia, 15*(3), 1081–1095. https://doi.org/10.12957/epp.2015.19429.

Steel, Z., Chey, T., Silove, D., Marnane, C., Bryant, R., & van Ommeren, M. (2009). Association of torture and other potentially traumatic events with mental health outcomes among populations exposed to mass conflict and displacement. *JAMA, 302*(5), 537–549. https://doi.org/10.1001/jama.2009.1132.

Stewart, S., & Conrod, P. (2008). *Anxiety and substance use disorders*. New York, NY: Springer.

Ten Have, M., de Graaf, R., van Dorsselaer, S., Tuithof, M., Kleinjan, M., & Penninx, B. (2019). Childhood maltreatment, vulnerability characteristics and adult incident common mental disorders: 3-year longitudinal data among >10,000 adults in the general population. *Journal of Psychiatric Research, 113*, 199–207.

Torchalla, I., Linden, I., Strehlau, V., Neilson, E., & Krausz, M. (2015). "Like a lots happened with my whole childhood": Violence, trauma, and addiction in pregnant and postpartum women from Vancouver's downtown eastside. *Harm Reduction Journal, 12*(1), 199–207. https://doi.org/10.1016/j.jpsychires.2019.03.029.

Torres Bernal, A., & Mille, D. (2011). Healing from trauma: Utilizing effective assessment strategies to develop accessible and inclusive goals. *Kairos – Slovenian Journal of Psychotherapy, 5*(1/2), 28–42.

Tractenberg, S., Viola, T., Rosa, C., Donati, J., Francke, I., Pezzi, J., & Grassi-Oliveira, R. (2012). Exposição a trauma e transtorno de estresse pós-traumático em usuárias de crack. *Jornal Brasileiro de Psiquiatria, 61*(4), 206–213. https://doi.org/10.1590/S0047-20852012000400003.

Veer, I., Oei, N., van Buchem, M., Spinhoven, P., Elzinga, B., & Rombouts, S. (2015). Evidence for smaller right amygdala volumes in posttraumatic stress disorder following childhood trauma. *Psychiatry Research: Neuroimaging, 233*(3), 436–442. https://doi.org/10.1016/j.pscychresns.2015.07.016.

Viola, T., Schiavon, B., Renner, A., & Grassi-Oliveira, R. (2011). Trauma complexo e suas implicações diagnósticas. *Revista de Psiquiatria do Rio Grande do Sul, 33*(1), 55–62. https://doi.org/10.1590/S0101-81082011000100010.

Volpicelli, J., Balaraman, G., Hahn, J., Wallace, H., & Bux, D. (1999). The role of uncontrollable trauma in the development of PTSD and alcohol addiction. *Alcohol Research & Health, 23*(4), 256–262.

Wolitzky-Taylor, K., Sewart, A., Vrshek-Schallhorn, S., Zinbarg, R., Mineka, S., Hammen, C., et al. (2016). The effects of childhood and adolescent adversity on substance use disorders and poor health in early adulthood. *Journal of Youth and Adolescence, 46*(1), 15–27. https://doi.org/10.1007/s10964-016-0566-3.

Yamauchi, L. M., Andrade, A. L. M., Pinheiro, B. O., Enumo, S. R. F., & De Micheli, D. (2019). Evaluation of the social representation of the use of alcoholic beverages by adolescents. *Estudos de Psicologia (Campinas), 36*, e180098. https://doi.org/10.1590/1982-0275201936e180098.

Zinberg, N. (1984). *Drug, set, and setting: The basis for controlled intoxicant use*. New Haven, CT: Yale University.

Chapter 18
Motivational Interviewing in the Treatment of Substance Dependents: Clinical Fundamentals for Increased Adherence to Treatment

Neliana Buzi Figlie and Janaina Luisi Turisco Caverni

Introduction

The Motivational Interviewing initially aimed to motivate changes people with problems related to the consumption of alcohol and other drugs. In this context, it was found that these individuals had great difficulties in changing their behavior, even with their lives in ruins, being seen as resistant to change. In the 1980s, the Motivational Interviewing in the health environment emerged, acting especially in alcohol dependence, being concerned, above all, with adherence to treatment (Rollnick, Miller, & Butler, 2009).

The authors William Miller and Stephen Rollnick believed in the possibility of offering a new, more dignified approach, taking into account mainly the motivation and ambivalence within the process of change. On the other hand, at that time when treatments were mainly guided by the principle of confrontation: they believed that people with problems related to the use of alcohol or drugs had very rigid defenses, which prevented them from recognizing their situation and, consequently, treating them would only be through confrontation (Miller & Rollnick, 2013; Rollnick et al., 2009).

Historical Overview

Initially, in its first edition, the Motivational Interviewing focused on people with problems related to alcohol and other drugs. However, soon after its first publication, several studies were conducted and it is now possible to find the Motivational

N. B. Figlie (✉) · J. L. T. Caverni
Universidade Federal de São Paulo, São Paulo, SP, Brazil
e-mail: neliana@nelianafiglie.com.br

D. De Micheli et al. (eds.), *Drugs and Human Behavior*,
https://doi.org/10.1007/978-3-030-62855-0_18

Interviewing in other fields of intervention, with emphasis on family and justice (Simmons et al., 2016), sexual risk behaviors (Pettifor et al., 2015), nutrition in young diabetics (Nansel et al., 2015), pregnant and obese women (Lindhardt et al., 2015), oral health prevention (Masoe, Blinkhorn, Taylor, & Blinkhorn, 2015), and even the use of Motivational Interviewing to reduce threats in conversations about risky environmental behaviors (Klonek, Güntner, Lehmann-Willenbrock, & Kauffeld, 2015).

In its first publication, in 1983, the Motivational Interviewing drew attention to its principles, strategies, and pitfalls (Rollnick & Miller, 1995). In its second edition, the authors emphasized the importance of professionals developing some essential skills during the conversation and the PARR (English OARS) concept emerged (Miller & Rollnick, 2002). In 2008, Miller and Rollnick dared in their proposal and published "Motivational Interviewing in Health Care," broadening the target audience that could benefit from the approach. However, after so many adaptations, through findings of clinical trials, the authors concluded that more changes would be necessary for the real understanding and effectiveness of the Motivational Interviewing and made a new publication in 2013, in which they proposed significant paradigmatic changes and included the concept of the "Spirit" of the Motivational Interviewing which is described as collaborative, evocative and with respect for the autonomy of the client (Figlie, Guimarães, Selma, & Laranjeira, 2015; Miller, Moyers, Arciniega, Ernst, & Forcehimes, 2005; Miller & Rollnick, 2013; Miller, Yahne, Moyers, Martinez, & Pirritano, 2004). The Motivational Interviewing is currently considered a counseling approach and has been gaining space, besides health, in the areas of Education (Snape & Atkinson, 2016), Justice (Coulton et al., 2017), and Social Assistance (Hohman, 2012) and recently in Sports (2019).

Current Surveys

One of the important aspects observed in current research is how much behavior change remains after an intervention based on the Motivational Interviewing. A study of 461 patients who met the criteria for DSM-IV for substance use dependence compared four weeks of structured intervention in the Motivational Interviewing with traditional counseling, and the results showed that there was no difference between groups in the percentage of substance positive urine samples. However, the Motivational Interviewing led to changes in substance use patterns that were maintained over 12 weeks (Ball et al., 2007).

A meta-analysis with 59 randomized studies making a total of 13,342 adult participants diagnosed as substance-dependent according to DSM-IV found that, compared to no treatment, Motivational Interviewing resulted in a significant reduction in the use of substances after intervention (standardized difference of means [SMD] = 0.79, 95% CI 0.48–1.09), as well as in the 12-month follow-up (SMD = 0.15, 95% CI 0.04–0.25). No difference in substance use was observed when the Motivational Interviewing was compared with traditional treatment for substance use disorders (TUSs), other types of treatment, evaluation, and feedback (Smedslund et al., 2011).

Some tests were performed comparing the combination of Motivational Interviewing and treatment intervention for TUSs with a traditional intervention with promising initial results. Another randomized trial of 105 cocaine dependence patients (DSM-IV) compared a detoxification intervention with a Motivational Interviewing intervention. Patients who received the Motivational Interviewing-based detoxification increased their use of *coping* strategies and were less frequent in cocaine positive urine samples (Stotts, Schmitz, Rhoades, & Grabowski, 2001). Other systematic reviews and meta-analyses have reported that the Motivational Interviewing showed effectiveness in treating substance abuse in adolescents (Tait & Hulse, 2003) and college students (Carey, Scott-Sheldon, Carey, & DeMartini, 2007) and in smoking cessation (Lai, Cahill, Qin, & Tang, 2010).

A differential of the Motivational Interviewing is that with training, it can be effectively performed by doctors, counselors, and other professionals, indicating that the profession seems not to affect the effectiveness of the Motivational Interviewing. Effects are observed in one to four sessions, with a "dose" minimum of about 20 min. It is worth noting that more sessions have been associated more effectively (Rubak, Sandbaek, Lauritzen, & Christensen, 2005).

A review article analyzed the association between professional, patient, and post-intervention behavior in 19 controlled clinical trials using the Motivational Interviewing. Three constructs associated with the outcome of the studies were found, namely the appearance of change statements in patients was associated with better outcomes; the perception of discrepancy by clients was associated with better outcomes; behaviors inconsistent with the Motivational Interviewing by the professional as offering information and advice without permission were associated with worse outcomes (Apodaca & Longabaugh, 2009).

What Is a Motivational Interviewing?

The Motivational Interviewing is a collaborative conversation style aimed at strengthening motivation and commitment to change. Table 18.1 shows the different definitions of the Motivational Interviewing, according to the perception of a layperson, practitioner, and a technical definition (Miller & Rollnick, 2013).

Table 18.1 Definitions of the motivational interviewing

Law	Practicant	Technical
Collaborative conversation style to reinforce one's own motivation and commitment to change	Person-centered style of counseling to address questions about ambivalence for change	A style of collaborative communication oriented towards a specific goal, which is to encourage change, has as its purpose to strengthen personal motivation for commitment to change, gathering and exploring one's own reasons, within an atmosphere of acceptance and compassion

Source: Miller and Rollnick (2013)

A very important aspect to take into account is how motivated a person is or not to any kind of behavior change, because in general there is something in human nature that resists change by feeling coerced and forced to do so. Ironically, sometimes the recognition of the other's right and freedom not to change is what makes change possible. The Motivational Interviewing considers that motivation can be activated, stimulated, and constructed, unlike some approaches that believe that motivation is innate. It was then observed that motivation is a state and not a personality trait, and can thus fluctuate depending on the situation or even be evoked and stimulated at any time by a professional in training (Miller & Rollnick, 2013; Rollnick et al., 2009).

Until today many approaches or treatments believed that they could only help the client if they wanted to, but the Motivational Interviewing has proven otherwise. Because it is an approach that has a specific goal: to solve ambivalence, it is understood as a brief intervention that can be used by a wide range of professionals in different services (Moyers, Houck, Glynn, Hallgren, & Manuel, 2017).

The Motivational Interviewing involves more listening than speaking: the client is expected to speak for most of the intervention (approximately 75% of the time). The idea is for the client to change speaking (from English "*Change talking*")· replacing the premise: "I have what you need" X "You have what I need and together we will get it" (Miller & Rollnick, 2013). This conversation provides the client with a learning opportunity, with full and free acceptance, without fear of the feelings, values and thoughts that the professional may have. Therefore, the role of the professional is of paramount importance, and he should follow some basic premises that will help him during the Motivational Interviewing practice, presented in Box 18.1.

Box 18.1 Basic Assumptions that will Help the Professional During the Motivational Interviewing Practice

1. Empathy, congruence, collaborative spirit in increasing motivation for change;
2. Adoption of a calm and eliciting style;
3. Consider natural ambivalence. The motivation for change should be elicited in the client and not imposed;
4. Resistance can be reduced or increased through interpersonal interactions. The professional is directive in helping the client to examine and solve the ambivalence;
5. The *client-professional* relationship must be collaborative and friendly; clients are responsible for their progress. The professional acts as a facilitator in the process, stimulating and supporting the client's self-efficacy;
6. Abstinence is the safest goal, but not always the best choice, especially with customers in pre-contemplation or contemplation.

The following are presented and described four fundamental concepts for the Motivational Interviewing Clinic.

Ambivalence

The Motivational Interviewing always begins his work with the prospecting of ambivalence, which is defined by the person and not by the professional. Example: a marijuana addict who does not visualize problems with the use of the substance, but accepts to work on his family relationship problems. The interviewer's posture is to start with the possibilities that the person allows and develops a collaborative conversation, where both build in partnership, the focus of the intervention.

In this context, ambivalence is a mental state in which a person has coexisting and conflicting feelings about something. The difficulties with ambivalence in relation to change are not specific to the use of substances. It is a characteristic of the human condition and taking this condition into account is a fundamental step towards behavior change (Miller & Rollnick, 2013).

We can observe the existence of ambivalence mainly in people who present problems with the use of substances in the search for treatment, because they arrive with fluctuating and conflicting motivations, at the same time they want and do not want to change. This conflict seems to have a special potential to keep people imprisoned, creating great stress, procrastination, and illness (Rollnick et al., 2009).

A professional who listens to a common manifestation of ambivalence such as "I want to stop drinking, but I can't stop having a beer with my friends," instead of judging as something wrong, abnormal, unacceptable, and as a sign of little motivation will be able to take this ambivalence into account as expected, acceptable, and understandable and, from then on, raise significant information to be used in the process of change (Arkowitz, Westra, Miller, & Rollnick, 2011).

It is important to stress that working with ambivalence is working with the essence of the problem, with the real motivations that will lead you to maintain or change your behavior (Miller & Rollnick, 2001). Taking into account that motivation is perceived as a state of readiness that can oscillate with time and suffer the influence of interpersonal relationships, it is up to the professional to evoke, extract, or even elicit the motives, the reasons, the desires of the person to change, thus helping to resignify the change itself.

The Motivational Interviewing Process

There is a flow to follow within the Motivational Interviewing, represented by processes that can be viewed in Fig. 18.1.

The processes are recursive: one does not end when the next begins. They can flow into each other, overlap, and appeal. This is the confluence of these four

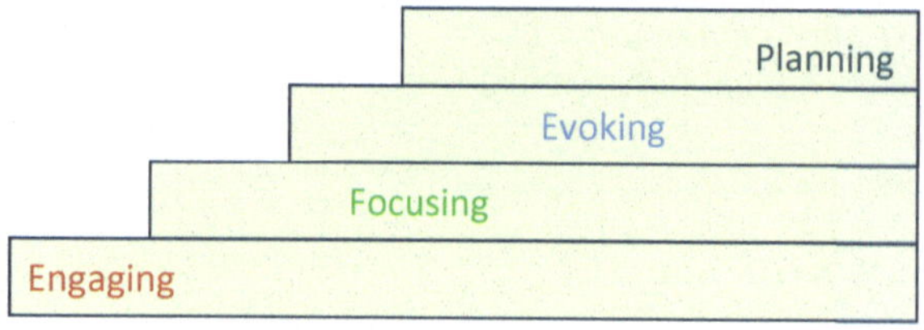

Fig. 18.1 Four processes in motivational interviewing (Miller & Rollnick, 2013)

processes that best describe the Motivational Interviewing. Since the four processes are sequential and recursive, they are represented as steps on the ladder (Fig. 18.1). Each subsequent process is based on those that were placed before and continue in progression from the previous one, as a foundation. In the course of a conversation, one can also walk up and down the ladder, returning to a previous step that requires renewed attention (Miller & Rollnick, 2013).

Engaging

The initial process takes place with Engagement: if the professional does not engage or even gets involved with a client, the next meetings are unlikely to happen.

Engagement consists in building a therapeutic alliance. When the professional manages to establish a good therapeutic alliance with the client, there is more engagement in the treatment, enabling greater adherence to it. Here, engagement is defined as a process of building a helping relationship, which seeks a solution to the problem pointed out. This relationship is based on mutual respect and trust. The engaged client is not passive to his own change process, he is extremely active within his skills and resources (Miller & Rollnick, 2013).

Focusing

The focus is on developing and maintaining the specific direction of the conversation for change. The client, during the service, may often be involved in a series of events and his tendency may be to focus on the symptoms or the most recent facts that led him there, undervaluing or even ignoring the "cause" factor. It is up to the professional to worry about keeping the focus during the care, so that the conversation is not lost halfway (Miller & Rollnick, 2013). Here it is expected that the ambivalence is defined, because it will be the focus of the intervention.

Evoking

Evoking is the movement of the professional to extract from the person his own feelings concerning the purpose of change. This is the essence of the Motivational Interviewing. All the conclusions or paths to be taken should be a conclusion that the client reaches alone, with the help of the professional and not with his induction. Here, it is up to the professional to take advantage of the client's own ideas, values, skills, and reasons so that the client discovers how and why he intends to act in a certain way and be truly active in his own process (Miller & Rollnick, 2013).

Planning

Planning is in building the movement of "when" and "how" to change. Taking as a basis the readiness for change, there is a moment when the client lessens his questions and begins to prepare himself for an attitude. At this time, planning is fundamental, as it develops the formulation of a specific action plan and can encourage the client to increase his commitment to change. It is worth pointing out that the planning should not be prescribed but evoked from the client; likewise, it should not be punctual and should always be reviewed—this is why it is the final process (Miller & Rollnick, 2013).

Essential Skills in The Motivational Interviewing

For the conversation to happen in a collaborative way, some skills must be trained and cultivated. Some strategies have been created to facilitate and reinforce this conversation, such as using reflective listening, affirming, summarizing and open-ended questions (PARR) in a ratio of at least 2:1, i.e. with each open-ended question asked it would be interesting to use reflections, affirming reinforcement or even a summary. In this context, the questions are used to a lower proportion as it is expected that all the other strategies can generate more speech in the client, so that the client speaks more than the professional and has a greater openness to be heard, by facilitating communication. In this way, more material emerges for the professional to work and thus strengthen the client as the protagonist of his/her own life. *See below the acronym of PARR (in English OARS): Q: open questions. A: affirm—positive reinforcement. A: reflect. A: summary (Figlie & Payá, 2004; Miller et al., 2004; Miller & Rollnick, 2013).

Asking Open Questions

A good way to start a conversation is to ask questions in a way that encourages the client to talk as much as possible. Open questions are those that cannot be answered easily with a simple word or phrase. Here are some examples of initial questions: Could you talk a little more about this behavior? What did you do to stay abstinent for a week? What has happened since we last met? The main purpose of an open-ended question is to open communication, strengthening and encouraging client autonomy.

Reflective Listening

The Reflective Listening is the main strategy in the Motivational Interviewing and should constitute a substantial proportion during the initial phase of the conversation. The crucial element in reflective listening is how the professional responds to what the client says. Thomas Gordon outlined the model of reflective thinking that connects what the client said with what the professional heard, with the professional's thinking about what the client wanted to say to finally connect what the client wanted to say with what he actually said (Gordon, 1970). By reflecting, the professional puts himself in the relationship, but at the same time he must be faithful to what the client said. For this reason, the Motivational Interviewing does not work with interpretation and demands from the professional the neutrality to faithfully reflect what the person said.

Offering reflective listening requires training and practice to think reflexively. The process of active listening requires: (a) Careful attention to what the client says; (b) Clear visualization of what has been said; (c) Formulation of the hypothesis concerning the problem, without assumptions or interpretations; (d) Articulating the hypothesis through a non-defensive approach. To evaluate if the reflection made was effective, it is enough to analyze the client's reaction. If it expresses agreement, it does not present a defensive posture, it opens space for the client to speak more and presents a more relaxed or motivated verbal posture, these are signs that the reflection was effective. On the other hand, if the client begins to warn or threaten, persuade, argue, disagree, judge, criticize or blame, retract, distract, be indulgent or change subjects, these are clear indications that the reflection was not effective and it is up to the professional to reformulate. It is also essential to evaluate the non-verbal communication by receiving the reflection.

There are two types of reflection: simple and complex. The simple reflections are a repetition of what the client said, without adding much information. They have the function of establishing the connection, linking the client to the intervention so that he feels understood. It also serves as a possibility for the professional to better elaborate his listening, before making the complex reflections, or in moments of tension in the conversation.

Example: Customer: I want to stop drinking, but I have a lot of free time lately.

Professional: You're telling me you want to stop drinking, but you have plenty of free time.

Complex reflections, as the name says, add information to the client's listening and there are different types of complex reflections (Figlie, 2013; Miller & Rollnick, 2013), described below:

- Amplified reflection: A very useful approach is to reflect something that the client has said in an exaggerated or amplified way. If the strategy is successful, it will encourage the client to step back and elicit the other side of ambivalence. But beware: an overblown or sarcastic statement may elicit even more resistance.
- Example: Client: I have no problem with marijuana, all my friends smoke. I'll stop at whatever time I want!

- Professional: So, you mean that you have no problems with marijuana and that your parents' concern for you is not necessary.
- Double Reflection: Implies in recognizing what the client said and adding the other side of ambivalence. This can be done by using material that the client has previously offered, even in another session.
- Example: Customer: I am very frustrated.
- Professional: It seems that you are frustrated, but we also know that the fact that you are frustrated makes you seek a relief in the drink.
- Reflection of feelings: It is the deepest form of reflection, in which emotional elements are incorporated so that the client is aware of his feelings. It is important to point out that this type of reflection is only used when the client's history is known or when he or she clearly demonstrates their feelings.
- Example: Client: I can't stop drinking.
- Professional: I understand that this situation discourages you and makes you feel powerless over drinking.
- Metaphor or paraphrasing: Moves far beyond content to provide a model for understanding, using image figures, popular sayings and metaphors.
- Example: Customer: I can't stop drinking. I've tried everything! Nothing works. Professional: I have the impression that you feel like a dead end.

Affirmation: Positive Reinforcement

The positive reinforcement also has its place in the Motivational Interviewing, being one of its peculiarities. It can be accomplished through appreciation, positive reinforcement, and understanding on the part of the professional, who endorses the person's qualities, values, skills, and positive strengths. Here are some examples:

- Your strength of will and determination made you attend the consultation today. Thank you for coming!
- You're determined to try and be a better father and recover from this disease.
- You've been under enormous pressure this week. It shows how important your health is to you!

Positive reinforcement is a form of genuine support, encouragement, and true recognition of what is of value in every human being—and not offering mere praise. Positive reinforcement must be genuine.

Summary

Summaries are sets of reflections and statements and can be used to connect the issues that were discussed, demonstrating that you listened to the client, as well as working as a didactic strategy for the client to organize their ideas. Abstracts provide links between the content present and those discussed previously. In the

Motivational Interviewing, the summaries can be used at various times during the session: when the client placed several ideas simultaneously and the professional tries to connect them and reflect them to the client for a better understanding; or in transition phases in the processes during the intervention, for an educational purpose. It works as a strong indication for the client that it is being listened to attentively by the professional, generating less resistance and increasing the therapeutic bond.

The Spirit of Motivational Interviewing

The underlying set of mind and heart within which the Motivational Interviewing is practiced is understood as the "Spirit of the Motivational Interviewing" and includes some attitudes of the professional towards his client, such as partnership, acceptance, evocation, and compassion, described in Fig. 18.2 (Figlie et al., 2015; Miller & Rollnick, 2013).

Partnership

The first of the four vital aspects of the spirit involves partnership. It is not something done by an expert to a passive recipient, a teacher to a student, a master to a disciple. In fact, it is not done "for" or "in" someone absolutely. Motivational Interviewing is done "with" a person. It is an active collaboration between

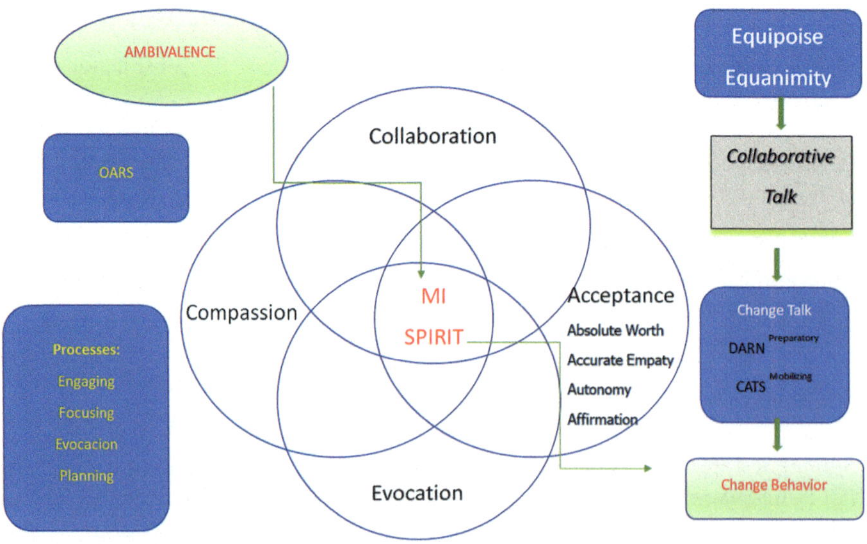

Fig. 18.2 The underlying spirit of MI (Adapted by Figlie from Miller & Rollnick, 2013)

specialists. People are the undisputed experts in themselves. No one has been with them longer, or knows them better than themselves. The method involves exploration, interest, and support instead of persuasion or argument, and curiosity on the part of the professional enters into the field of constructive curiosity. Professionals try to create a positive interpersonal atmosphere favorable to change, but not coercive.

Acceptance

For the understanding of MI, acceptance has a strong influence on the works of Carl Rogers and proposes that the professional be interested and value the potential of each individual. Accepting the person does not necessarily mean that the professional approves or endorses the client's actions, that is, whether the professional approves or disapproves is irrelevant (posture of neutrality). Acceptance consists of the recognition of the absolute worth that the client gives to his/her arguments and reasons, accurate empathy, support for the client's autonomy, affirmation of speech, and postures in favor of the client's health and integrity of life. The idea of acceptance is to know how to live with differences, where the professional and client can talk collaboratively, each with their own point of view.

Paradoxically, when the professional accepts the client in the way he presents himself (it is worth remembering that accepting does not imply agreeing), he feels accepted and, therefore, freer and more willing to experience movements of change naturally.

Evocation

Evoke the forces that motivate the person, rather than persuade. Evoking means to remember. Motivation comes from desire, reasons and needs, which means what can make move, engine that causes or determines something. Motivation is an internal resource. Evoking brings the proposal of helping the client to remember his or her own unique elements that can become reasons for a change in behavior.

The professional here tries to evoke the lines of change: any speech of the client that favors the movement towards a specific goal of change, by evoking the desires, reasons, capacities, and abilities of the change, in order to finally make it a necessity for the person.

Compassion

Compassion can be understood as a means of trying to get the professional closer to the person and not to the person's problem. Observe that there is suffering and a motivation to help. Once the professional is able to have access to the uniqueness of each one, it becomes possible to better understand the individual complexities that hinder behavioral changes. It is an act of getting closer in order to truly help. The authors reinforce the invitation to "put your hand in the mass" WITH the person and not FOR THE person, in order to empower them and count on the active help of the professional.

The concept of compassion, for the Motivational Interviewing, is not in a personal feeling that the professional should develop for his client. For the authors, the compassionate professional is the one who actively promotes the well-being of the other, placing it as a priority before himself. In the most different segments and types of services, the compassionate professional is identified as one who does not see in the client another number, another case, or as a source of income: he sees in the client a unique person, a priority, and full of possibilities, but with some suffering. The final target of each meeting is the client and should not be addressed at any time to satisfy the professional's own interests.

Final Considerations

The Motivational Interviewing is simple, but it's not easy. The processes of change involved are natural and, in an intuitive sense, we all know and recognize. Perhaps this is one of the reasons why the Motivational Interviewing was born. However, its practice requires the integration of some quite complex skills that can be improved with practice. Reflective listening alone is a challenge. For someone who is good at this, it may seem easy, as natural as breathing, until you try to do it.

Motivational Interviewing is an approach that has a theoretical basis and is not merely a set of techniques (Lundahl & Burke, 2009). It is a counseling approach with a practical and objective methodology, which can be conducted by any professional, as long as he or she is trained to do so. Faced with this, through tests and adaptations with scientific rigor, the Motivational Interviewing aims, in addition to changing behavior, to add a humanist and constructivist view on changes in risk behaviors.

References

Apodaca, T., & Longabaugh, R. (2009). Mechanisms of change in motivational interviewing: A review and preliminary evaluation of the evidence. *Addiction, 104*(5), 705–715. https://doi.org/10.1111/j.1360-0443.2009.02527.x.

Arkowitz, H., Westra, H., Miller, W., & Rollnick, S. (2011). *Entrevista Motivacional no Tratamento de Problemas Psicológicos*. São Paulo, Brazil: Roca.

Ball, S., Martino, S., Nich, C., Frankforter, T., Van Horn, D., Crits-Christoph, P., & Carroll, K. (2007). Site matters: Multisite randomized trial of motivational enhancement therapy in community drug abuse clinics. *Journal of Consulting and Clinical Psychology, 75*(4), 556–567. https://doi.org/10.1037/0022-006x.75.4.556.

Carey, K., Scott-Sheldon, L., Carey, M., & DeMartini, K. (2007). Individual-level interventions to reduce college student drinking: A meta-analytic review. *Addictive Behaviors, 32*(11), 2469–2494. https://doi.org/10.1016/j.addbeh.2007.05.004.

Coulton, S., Stockdale, K., Marchand, C., Hendrie, N., Billings, J., Boniface, S., & Wilson, E. (2017). Pragmatic randomised controlled trial to evaluate the effectiveness and cost effectiveness of a multi-component intervention to reduce substance use and risk-taking behaviour in adolescents involved in the criminal justice system: A trial protocol (RISKIT-CJS). *BMC Public Health, 17*(1), 6. https://doi.org/10.1186/s12889-017-4170-6.

Figlie, N. B., Guimarães, L. P., Selma, B., & Laranjeira, R. (2015). Entrevista motivacional. In N. B. Figlie, R. Laranjeira, & S. Bordin (Eds.), *Aconselhamento em dependência química* (3rd ed.). São Paulo, Brazil: Grupo Gen.

Gordon, T. (1970). *Parent effectiveness training*. New York, NY: Wyden.

Hohman, M. (2012). *Motivational interviewing in social work practice*. New York, NY: The Guilford Press.

Klonek, F., Güntner, A., Lehmann-Willenbrock, N., & Kauffeld, S. (2015). Using motivational interviewing to reduce threats in conversations about environmental behavior. *Frontiers in Psychology, 6*, e01015. https://doi.org/10.3389/fpsyg.2015.01015.

Lai, D., Cahill, K., Qin, Y., & Tang, J. (2010). Motivational interviewing for smoking cessation. *Cochrane Database of Systematic Reviews, 1*, CD006936. https://doi.org/10.1002/14651858.cd006936.pub2.

Lindhardt, C., Rubak, S., Mogensen, O., Hansen, H., Goldstein, H., Lamont, R., & Joergensen, J. (2015). Healthcare professionals experience with motivational interviewing in their encounter with obese pregnant women. *Midwifery, 31*(7), 678–684. https://doi.org/10.1016/j.midw.2015.03.010.

Lundahl, B., & Burke, B. (2009). The effectiveness and applicability of motivational interviewing: a practice-friendly review of four meta-analyses. *Journal of Clinical Psychology, 65*(11), 1232–1245. https://doi.org/10.1002/jclp.20638.

Masoe, A., Blinkhorn, A., Taylor, J., & Blinkhorn, F. (2015). An assessment of preventive care offered to orthodontic patients by oral health therapists in NSW Australia. *International Dental Journal, 65*(4), 196–202. https://doi.org/10.1111/idj.12169.

Miller, W., Moyers, T., Arciniega, L., Ernst, D., & Forcehimes, A. (2005). Training, supervision and quality monitoring of the COMBINE Study behavioral interventions. *Journal of Studies on Alcohol, 15*, 188–195. https://doi.org/10.15288/jsas.2005.s15.188.

Miller, W., Yahne, C., Moyers, T., Martinez, J., & Pirritano, M. (2004). A randomized trial of methods to help clinicians learn motivational interviewing. *Journal of Consulting and Clinical Psychology, 72*(6), 1050–1062. https://doi.org/10.1037/0022-006x.72.6.1050.

Miller, W. R., & Rollnick, S. (2001). *Entrevista motivacional – preparando as pessoas para a mudança de comportamentos aditivos*. Porto Alegre, Brazil: Artmed.

Miller, W. R., & Rollnick, S. (2002). *Motivational interviewing – Preparing people for change* (2nd ed.). New York, NY: The Guilford Press.

Miller, W. R., & Rollnick, S. (2013). *Motivational interview – Helping people change* (3rd ed.). New York, NY: The Guilford Press.

Moyers, T., Houck, J., Glynn, L., Hallgren, K., & Manuel, J. (2017). A randomized controlled trial to influence client language in substance use disorder treatment. *Drug and Alcohol Dependence, 172*, 43–50. https://doi.org/10.1016/j.drugalcdep.2016.11.036.

Nansel, T., Laffel, L., Haynie, D., Mehta, S., Lipsky, L., Volkening, L., & Liu, A. (2015). Improving dietary quality in youth with type 1 diabetes: Randomized clinical trial of a family-based behavioral intervention. *International Journal of Behavioral Nutrition and Physical Activity, 12*(1), 58. https://doi.org/10.1186/s12966-015-0214-4.

Pettifor, A., Corneli, A., Kamanga, G., McKenna, K., Rosenberg, N., Yu, X., & Hoffman, I. (2015). HPTN 062: A pilot randomized controlled trial exploring the effect of a motivational-interviewing intervention on sexual behavior among individuals with acute HIV infection in Lilongwe, Malawi. *PLoS ONE, 10*(5), e0124452. https://doi.org/10.1371/journal.pone.0124452.

Rollnick, S., & Miller, W. (1995). What is Motivational Interviewing? *Behavioural and Cognitive Psychotherapy, 23*(4), 325–334. https://doi.org/10.1017/s135246580001643x.

Rollnick, S., Miller, W. R., & Butler, C. C. (2009). *Entrevista Motivacional no cuidado da saúde: ajudando pacientes a mudar o comportamento*. Porto Alegre: Artmed.

Rubak, S., Sandbaek, A., Lauritzen, T., & Christensen, B. (2005). Motivational interviewing: A systematic review and meta-analysis. *The British Journal of General Practice: The Journal of the Royal College of General Practitioners, 55*(513), 305–312.

Rollnick, S., Fader, J., Breckon, J., Moyers, T.B. (2019). Coaching Athletes to Be Their Best: Motivational Interviewing in Sports. New Yourk: NY, The Guilford Press.

Simmons, C., Howell, K., Duke, M., & Beck, J. (2016). Enhancing the impact of family justice centers via motivational interviewing. *Trauma, Violence & Abuse, 17*(5), 532–541. https://doi.org/10.1177/1524838015585312.

Smedslund, G., Berg, R., Hammerstrøm, K., Steiro, A., Leiknes, K., Dahl, H., & Karlsen, K. (2011). Motivational interviewing for substance abuse. *Cochrane Database of Systematic Reviews, 5*, CD008063. https://doi.org/10.1002/14651858.cd008063.pub2.

Snape, L., & Atkinson, C. (2016). The evidence for student-focused motivational interviewing in educational settings: a review of the literature. *Advances in School Mental Health Promotion, 9*(2), 119–139. https://doi.org/10.1080/1754730x.2016.1157027.

Stotts, A. L., Schmitz, J. M., Rhoades, H. M., & Grabowski, J. (2001). Motivational interviewing with cocaine-dependent patients: A pilot study. *Journal of Consulting and Clinical Psychology, 69*(5), 858–862. https://doi.org/10.1037//0022-006x.69.5.858.

Tait, R. J., & Hulse, G. K. (2003). A systematic review of the effectiveness of brief interventions with substance using adolescents by type of drug. *Drug and Alcohol Review, 22*(3), 337–346. https://doi.org/10.1080/0959523031000154481.

Chapter 19
Assessment and Intervention in Social and Coping Skills for Alcohol and Drug Users

Lucas Guimarães Cardoso de Sá

Introduction

Substance use disorder (SUD) can be characterized by a set of cognitive, behavioral, and physiological symptoms, indicating constant self-administration of psychoactive substances, even if this results in significant problems for the individual and loss of voluntary control of consumption, tolerance to the effects of the drug, and specific symptoms when abstinence is performed (American Psychiatric Association, 2014). Studies indicate that, historically, alcohol seems to have been the drug that generated the most search for treatment for SUD in Brazil (Carlini, 2006; Noto & Galduróz, 1999), but in recent decades, cocaine, in the form of crack cocaine, divides space in the search for interventions (Borini, Guimarães, & Borini, 2003; Dias, Araújo, & Laranjeira, 2011; Duailibi, Ribeiro, & Laranjeira, 2008; Kessler & Pechansky, 2008).

SUD is a complex disorder only explained by biological, social, environmental, and psychological factors integrated. Thus, a multidimensional and integrative model is the best way to understand it (Donovan, 2009). Very diverse variables make up a multifactorial explanatory model for abusive or substance-dependent consumption. Studying them is relevant to understand the role of each one and how they can be integrated.

Part of the psychological variables, coping skills are defined as a set of adaptive cognitive and behavioral strategies available in the individual's repertoire to be used in specific moments of abstinence protection (Donovan, 2009). The assumption is that, among the factors that contribute to the maintenance of SUD is the maladaptive way of dealing with daily stress situations, whether in family, at work, with friends, or even in brief interactions with unfamiliar people. Stress, in this case, should be understood as an imbalance between the demands of the environment and the

L. G. C. de Sá (✉)
Universidade Federal do Maranhão, São Luis, MA, Brazil

D. De Micheli et al. (eds.), *Drugs and Human Behavior*,
https://doi.org/10.1007/978-3-030-62855-0_19

resources of the individual, and may lead those with poorly developed repertoires of coping skills to use the substance in an attempt to re-establish balance (Monti, Kadden, Rohsenow, Cooney, & Abrams, 2005). For example, it would be the case of a person who drinks to deal with unpleasant feelings caused by not being able to express feelings of discontent in an interpersonal relationship, or of one who uses crack cocaine to alleviate the unease generated by an argument. When the environment continuously demands the use of behavioral repertoires that the individual does not possess, substance consumption can become constant, characterizing abuse or dependence. Some studies show the relationship between previous stressors and substance consumption (Brown et al., 1990; Hassanbeigi et al. 2013; Saha, 2013).

In view of this, for the promotion and maintenance of abstinence, it would be important to evaluate and teach the individual to discriminate which stress situations offer a risk of using psychoactive substances and which alternative behaviors could be used to prevent or deal with such adverse situations, thus increasing the probability of avoiding a lapse or a relapse (Frade et al., 2013; Marlatt & Donovan, 2009). Successfully coping with increasingly difficult situations of a high risk of psychoactive substance use would lead the individual to establish a realistic sense of confidence in his or her own ability to deal with adverse moments, facilitating the process of maintaining abstinence. This model, known as relapse prevention, is described in detail in Marlatt and Donovan (2009).

Relapse prevention, based on a cognitive-behavioral model, is centered on the development of cognitive and behavioral strategies to avoid the occurrence of a lapse or, if this is not possible, that it becomes a relapse (Marlatt & Witkiewitz, 2009). Such a rationale is in accordance with one of the most popular definitions of coping, described as "the constantly changing cognitive and behavioral efforts to manage specific external and internal demands that are appraised as taxing or exceeding the resources of the person" (Lazarus & Folkman, 1984, p. 141). In this definition, coping is not seen as a stable profile, but as a changeable process linked to specific contexts.

The definition, although part of a broader coping theory, applies to the specific context of substance dependence. As previously mentioned, dependence on alcohol or other drugs would be, among other variables, the result of inadequate coping, a maladaptive response in the management of demands inflicted on the individual. According to Donovan (2009), the most common demands imposed on people who wish to maintain abstinence from alcohol or other drugs are: (a) pressure to use, which includes frequenting old places where the substance was consumed and maintaining contact with former fellow users; (b) desire to obtain the benefits that the consumption provided, such as belonging to a social group; (c) experience of unpleasant feelings, such as sadness, loneliness, and boredom; and (d) experience of anger and resentment resulting from interpersonal conflicts.

As cited in Monti et al. (2005) the repertoire of coping skills is one of the variables that help determine the use or non-use of the substance. However, several others, classified within specific factors, also contribute to this. Donovan (2009) explains that, following a time *continuum* related to the moment of lapse, there is (1) the distal personal factor, which involves variables of the individual himself, such as his life history and heredity; (2) the background intermediary factor, composed of variables related to the lifestyle, the daily life of a person, such as daily pressures, social support, sense of effectiveness, expectations, and motivations in relation to the process of change; (3) the proximal precipitating factor, which includes variables linked to situations of high risk of substance consumption, such as cravings and commitment to maintain abstinence; and, finally, (4) the transitional factor, which includes variables linked to the break-in abstinence, such as the commitment to return to a state of sobriety. Each of the factors, with the exception of the distal, implies the use of distinct types of coping skills, requiring coping skills that can be anticipatory, immediate, or restorative.

Still according to Donovan (2009), in the anticipatory coping, linked to the intermediary factor of background, thoughts and behaviors are directed towards the construction of an environment less susceptible to stressful situations, or to its rapid and effective solution before it can cause cravings. If there are no cravings, the chance of a lapse or relapse decreases considerably. Thus, in a metaphorical way, the use of anticipatory skills, such as properly criticizing, praising, or expressing pleasure, would work as the primary prevention of relapse. In the immediate coping, which can be a consequence of the low performance of anticipatory skills, thoughts and behaviors are used as a way of dealing with a craving already installed, at a moment when there is a high risk of substance use. It is linked to the proximal precipitating factor and an important skill would be, for example, to think about the negative consequences of the use and positive of not using the substance (Rohsenow, Martin, & Monti, 2005). In the metaphor initiated earlier, it would be the equivalent of secondary relapse prevention. Finally, restorative skills, linked to transitional factors, aim to minimize the affective and cognitive consequences generated by the consumption of the substance, reducing the chance of a more intense and prolonged relapse and leading the individual back to the previous state of abstinence. Asking for help and remembering the benefits that had been achieved with sobriety are examples of restorative abilities. In the metaphor adopted, they would be like the tertiary prevention of relapse.

For Marlatt and Witkiewitz (2009), the coping skills have at least two other important categories. As for the psychological characteristic, they can be cognitive, if mental processes are used to control behavior, or else behavioral, if they involve some form of action. As for the context, they can be of the interpersonal types, when used to deal with a problem situation in which other people constitute an important factor, or else intrapersonal, when used for a problem situation in which only the individual himself constitutes the relevant factor.

In this way, each coping skill has at least three distinct qualities: the moment, the psychological characteristic, and the context. There are several skills that could contribute to the maintenance of abstinence, whether they are anticipatory, immediate, or restorative; cognitive or behavioral; interpersonal or intrapersonal. Examples would be conversational skills, making and receiving praise, making constructive criticism, refusing to drink or do drugs, solving relationship problems, controlling anger and negative thoughts, identifying, avoiding, and dodging risky situations, asking for help, thinking about negative consequences of using and positive consequences of not using the drug, among others (Monti et al., 2005; Rangé & Marlatt, 2008; Rohsenow et al., 2005).

In examining the various coping skills cited above, it can be seen that many of them are social skills. Although they are not synonymous, since coping is a broader construct that includes intrapersonal skills, it is undeniable that coping in substance dependence necessarily includes the performance of social skills. They are an important part of coping skills, since they enable the structuring of responsible, stable, and secure bonds, which generates social insertion and prevents the emergence of cravings, lapses, and relapses (Sakiyama, Ribeiro, & Padin, 2012).

A performance based on a poor repertoire of social skills could generate a set of negative situations and feelings that maintain consumption and lead to less efficiency in facing adverse situations, making it difficult to maintain abstinence (Longabaugh and Morgenstern 1999). Rangé and Marlatt (2008, p. 92) highlight that "the development of skills for effective coping has to involve basic social skills, assertive behaviors and confrontation skills, which include an ability to identify risk situations, to handle emotions and to provide cognitive restructuring." Therefore, some subclasses of social skills end up working for immediate coping, such as expressing feelings to another person at the moment of compulsive desire, but mainly in anticipatory coping, as they commonly prevent a neutral social situation from becoming a situation of risk for the use of psychoactive substances.

For Del Prette and Del Prette (2017), social skills are a descriptive construct and represent the classes of social behaviors that a person must use to successfully complete a given social task. It is important to highlight its descriptive character, as having a good repertoire of social skills is a necessary, although not sufficient, condition for a behavior to be performed adequately. An individual may, for example, be hampered by anxiety and not complete the social task successfully. Thus, social skills need to lead to socially competent behavior.

Social competence is an evaluative construct of the person's performance in a particular social task and the consequences obtained from that performance. According to Del Prette and Del Prette (2005, p. 33), it is the "ability to articulate thoughts, feelings and actions according to personal objectives and the demands of the situation and culture, generating positive consequences for the individual and his relationship with other people." The criteria that characterize the functionality of social competence and that serve as a basis for the evaluation of social performance are highlighted: the achievement of the objectives of an interpersonal situation, maintenance or improvement in the relationship with other people, maintenance or improvement in self-esteem, maintenance or extension of socially recognized human rights, and social approval of the verbal community (related to the form and occasion of the performance). According to these criteria, social skills contribute to the strengthening, both positive (e.g., making a request and being met) and negative (e.g., interrupting unfair criticism) of an individual's performance (Del Prette & Del Prette, 2008; Del Prette & Del Prette, 2010).

Therefore, in the process of maintaining abstinence, social skills, by allowing socially competent behaviors, increase the probability of achieving goals which, in this case, would include identifying and moving away from risky situations and maintaining self-control, as well as improving self-esteem and the quality of their relationships with other people (Villalba, 1995). This could produce comfortable interpersonal relationships for the individual, protecting him or her from relapse, since the likelihood or intensity of cravings would be reduced. Since these aspects are related to important social and psychological components of addiction, they can help to strengthen abstinence from alcohol and other drugs.

Historical Overview and Current Researches

The statement that the repertoire of coping skills is related to abstinence from psychoactive substances has been found in the literature since the 1970s. As examples, Van Hasselt, Hersen, and Milliones (1978) reviewed the various studies that had employed social skills training as an intervention technique until then, suggesting its usefulness for the treatment of alcohol and other drug addicts. Oei and Jackson (1982) showed a strong relationship between increased social skills repertoire and decreased alcohol consumption. Monti et al. (1990) found that in the months following a communication skills training in a treatment program for alcoholism, there was a significant decrease in the rate of alcohol use when compared to that registered in a treatment in which there was not the same training. In another study, Monti et al. (1997) taught cocaine users how to deal with situations of frustration, anger, negative feelings, social pressure to use the drug, and other skills. The results showed that in the following 3 months these patients used the drug less and had shorter periods of relapse when compared to those in a control group. Scheier, Botvin, Diaz, and Griffin (1999) found that measures of low social competence and poor ability to refuse are related to alcohol consumption.

Ames and Roitzsch (2000) found that the frequency and strength of minor stressors predict the appearance of cravings, and that social support moderates the relationship between the number of stressors and the cravings in substance abuse. Barkin, Smith, and DuRant (2002) presented results indicating that decision-making skills and drug resistance abilities are among the significant predictors of adolescent substance use. Gossop, Stewart, Browne, and Marsden (2002) described that heroin addicts who remained abstinent after intervention reported increased use of coping skills in post-treatment compared to pretreatment. Those who relapsed reported no change in this direction. The use of coping responses was associated with a reduction in the chances of returning to drug use and the risk of lapses leading to a relapse.

Rohsenow et al. (2005) report that less cocaine use is related to 13 different strategies in the immediate coping. Epstein, Zhou, Bang, and Botvin (2007) found that the use of refusal skills and resistance to media influence are related to the lower probability of students consuming alcohol at present and in the future. For those with high perceptions of the benefits of drinking, less frequent use of refusal skills increases the likelihood of drinking in the future. A study by Forys, McKellar, and Moos (2007) indicated that the greater the general and specific coping repertoire for drinking, the lower the consumption, drinking problems, and frequency of other drug use. Hasking and Oei (2007) showed results indicating that immediate coping skills are predictors of frequency, though not the volume of alcohol consumption. Thus, training these skills could be a strategy to delay relapse and prevent the frequency of drinking episodes, but does not seem to limit excessive drinking on a single occasion. Mattoo, Chakrabarti, and Anjaiah (2009) report that alcohol-dependent or opioid-users who relapsed in the past 6 months of treatment had lower mean scores for adaptive coping strategies when compared to a group without relapse episodes in the same period. Wagner and Oliveira (2009) compared the social skills repertoire of adolescent abusers or marijuana addicts with other non-users, and found that the first group had a lower repertoire of self-exposure skills to strangers and new situations and of self-control of aggressiveness.

Wagner, Silva, Zanettelo, and Oliveira (2010) found that adolescent marijuana users had a significantly lower repertoire of self-control of aggressiveness in aversive situations than non-users. The results of Ritchie, Weldon, Freeman, MacPherson, and Davies (2011) showed that the greatest risk situations requiring coping in a relapse prevention program with mentally disturbed offenders were, in the decreasing order of importance, dealing with: pleasant moments, negative emotions, physical discomfort, cravings, social pressure, conflict with others, positive feelings, and with ideas of testing control. Felicissimo et al. (2013) presented in a 20-year literature review a series of studies on the relationship between social skills and alcohol abuse and dependence. Sá and Del Prette (2014) indicate that conversational and social disinhibition skills and self-exposure to strangers and new situations skills seem to be relevant for alcohol users, since they have a significant negative correlation with alcohol involvement. For cocaine users, the ability to control their own aggressiveness would deserve attention, also because they have a negative correlation with the level of involvement with the substance. The authors call attention to possible differences in the skills required according to the type of substance preferably used.

Horta et al. (2016) presented variables that are related to low scores in social skills in crack cocaine users, such as early motivational stages, higher scores of depression, child mourning, and having committed theft or assault to obtain the substance. Felicissimo et al. (2016) indicated that alcoholics have a lower repertoire of self-control skills of aggressiveness compared to non-alcoholics. Andretta et al. (2016) compared the repertoire of social skills between women and men crack users and showed that women have a significantly larger repertoire than men in conversation and expression of positive feelings skills. Also, they indicated that deficits in women are more frequent in conversation and social resourcefulness, self-exposure to strangers, and self-control of aggressiveness, while in men they are more frequent in conversation and social resourcefulness and self-control of aggressiveness skills. Limberger and Andretta (2018) highlighted that the repertoire of communication skills and assertiveness in childhood and adolescence were a relevant factor for crack consumption in the lives of three adult women interviewed. Schneider and Andretta (2017) presented that the more elaborated repertoire of risky confrontation skills and a lower repertoire of conversation and social resourcefulness skills increase the probability of involvement with crack cocaine. Rocha (2017) identified that assertiveness for refusal was the class of skills that presented the worst rating in a study with patients with alcoholic liver disease. Albuquerque and Nappo (2018) pointed out that the difficulty in dealing with emotions, especially frustration generated by problems in interpersonal relationships, is the main cause of relapse of crack cocaine consumers. Silva, Hatanaka, Rondina, and Silva (2018), in a study with multiple substance users, found that almost half of the sample had a below-average repertoire of social skills, especially in risky self-assertion and in conversation and social disinhibition.

All this historical journey to the present day leaves no doubt as to the relationship that exists between social and coping skills and the consumption of alcohol, cocaine, crack cocaine, heroin, or marijuana. Therefore, assessing and proposing interventions based on these skills seem to be relevant for the treatment of substance use disorders.

Coping Skills-Based Evaluation and Intervention

The assessment of coping skills as part of a comprehensive evaluation in the context of SUD should consider a variety of techniques and methods that allow for complete and reliable information. Interviews with the individual and other informants, observations, documents, role-plays are examples of techniques that can be used in this context (Argimon & Oliveira, 2009; Lopes, Andrade et al., 2017; Andretta, & Oliveira, 2019; Shaub et al., 2018)

Nevertheless, the greatest attention in the evaluation process has still been given to testing. One of the most popular tools for assessing coping in substance users is the *Coping Response Inventory* (CRI) of Moos (1992), which assesses general coping but is used in researches in SUD. Based on CRI, Marijuana Treatment Project Research Group (2004) developed the *Coping Strategy Scale* (CSS) for *marijuana* users. This test has a translation into Portuguese, without a description of its psychometric properties, in Jungerman and Zanelatto (2007).

The *Coping Behaviors Inventory* (CBI), by Litman, Stapleton, Oppenheim, and Peleg (1983), has 36 items to measure the immediate coping to alcoholism. There are studies of translation and cross-cultural adaptation (Constant et al., 2014) and measurement of psychometric properties (Constant et al., 2018) for Brazil. The *Urge Specific Strategies Questionnaire* (USS) was developed by Rohsenow et al. (2001) from a group of questions used by Monti et al. (1993). Initially, it contained 11 questions about the coping of drinking cravings, and then it had 16 questions. In Monti et al. (2005), there is a version of the instrument with 11 questions translated into Portuguese, but without any description of its psychometric properties, named *Questionário de Estratégias Específicas às Fissuras*. An adaptation of this instrument for *cocaine* addicts was named by Rohsenow et al. (2005) as *Urge Specific Strategies Questionnaire-Cocaine* (USS-C) and contains 21 questions. In Brazil, pilot studies are being conducted with this instrument (Sousa, Martins, Haidar, &

Sá, 2020). Also developed by Rohsenow et al. (2005), the *General Change Strategies-Cocaine* (GCS-C) investigates the frequency with which 21 life-style changing skills are used to maintain cocaine abstinence. Finally, Humke and Radnitz (2005) made an adaptation for alcoholism of *Coping With Temptations Inventory* (CWTI), an instrument originally used for nicotine addiction, and produced *The Alcohol Abuse Coping Response Inventory* (AACRI), which contains 51 items to address high-risk drinking situations. No reports of research involving these instruments have been found in Brazil.

In Brazil, the most widely used instrument for assessing the repertoire of social and coping skills was the social skills inventory (Del Prette & Del Prette, 2001). As it is a general instrument, not directed to the context of SUD, the *Inventory of Anticipatory Coping Skills for Abstinence from Alcohol and other Drugs* (Sá & Del Prette, 2016; Sá, Olaz & Del Prette, 2017) was developed. This test has 30 items, divided into three factors that assess (1) Assertiveness and planning for high-risk situations of substance use; (2) Emotional expression of positive feelings for maintaining abstinence; and (3) Emotional self-control in adverse situations.

Studies on coping skills-based interventions indicate that they can be developed through different methods, leading to important results in reducing cravings, consumption, and substance use, abuse, or dependence problems. Duncan, Duncan, Beauchamp, Wells, and Ary (2000), after using a multimedia program to teach adolescents skills to refuse marijuana, found greater effectiveness and intention to refuse the drug, and a greater belief that refusal would be effective in stopping people offering drugs, compared to pre-intervention data. Litt, Kadden, Cooney, and Kabela (2003) identified growth in the general repertoire of coping skills after cognitive-behavioral therapy, although this was not significantly different from the repertoire observed in a group undergoing other modality of therapy. The authors suggest that the number of coping skills used matters more than the type that is employed. An investigation conducted by Rohsenow et al. (2004) compared a group of cocaine addicts who underwent training in coping skills to a control group that did not undergo this intervention. Participants of the former reported less craving for cocaine use than those of the latter. A secondary result of the intervention was a 24% reduction in the number of people using alcohol in the following 3 months. Women in the intervention group benefited more than those in the control group. They were less likely to use cocaine and alcohol in the first three months and to use alcohol 7–9 months after the intervention. Women also benefited more than men from relapses with cocaine after 6 months, and from the frequency of alcohol and cocaine use after 1 year.

Zywiak et al. (2006) suggested that active ingredients of cognitive-behavioral therapy such as risk assessment and refusal training offer protection against relapse and social pressure for alcohol use. Litt, Kadden, Kabela-Cormier, and Petry (2008) found that motivational interview and cognitive-behavioral therapy coupled with contingency management provided a greater increase in coping skills than other combinations of therapies in marijuana addicts, and also that there was a drop in coping skills scores over the follow-up period, suggesting that with longer abstinence time the use of these skills is less necessary. Litt, Kadden, and

Kabela-Cormier (2009) noted that individualized treatment, compared to a standardized treatment, generates a greater likelihood of coping responses, greater avoidance responses, distraction, refusing to drink, escaping the situation in cravings or waiting for the craving to go away, as well as a greater variety of coping skills used. When coping responses were used there was 30% less likelihood of drinking.

Mares and Torres (2010) evaluated a substance refusal training and reported that the percentage of abstinence achieved after the intervention reaffirms the importance of this skill as it favors the extinction of invitations to drink or use drugs. Conrod, Castellanos-Ryan, and Strang (2010) state that shorter and targeted interventions based on coping skills appear to be effective in reducing the use of alcohol and illicit substances in addicts and in reducing the amount of drinking, drinking frequency, and drinking-related problems in elementary and middle school students. Witkiewitz et al. (2011) investigated the hypothesis that training to refuse and to deal with social pressure to drink lead to different outcomes in different racial groups. The training was found to be associated with significantly lower levels of heavy drinking days and a lower likelihood of alcohol-related problems among African Americans when compared to non-Hispanic white clients and the group of African Americans who did not receive the intervention. Araújo et al. (2011) described a single case intervention based on immediate coping skills training for cravings in a crack cocaine addict. They presented the evaluation procedures and the skills training sessions to face the cravings, such as waiting to pass, using a positive image, using a negative image, respiratory relaxation, substitution, and distraction. In re-evaluation after 135 days, the patient was abstinent, with high motivation and low cravings. Dolan et al. (2013) indicated a significantly greater difference in the repertoire of immediate coping skills of abstinent people compared to those who had lapsed, both 6 and 12 months after a treatment in which such skills were taught. There was also a significant negative correlation between coping skills and drinking days.

McGillicuddy, Rychtarik, and Papandonatos (2015) compared a coping skills training for parents of teenage drug users to a 12-step group and a control group. The group that underwent resistance skills training acquired a greater repertoire of skills than the other groups, but obtained superior results only when compared to the control group, in this case equaling the 12-step group. Kiluk et al. (2017) compared a computerized cognitive-behavioral therapy program, based on coping skills, to a traditional treatment with individual and group therapy sessions, and found that there was an improvement in the quality of skills of cocaine users who were initially evaluated as having inadequate performances. Mellentin et al. (2017) point out that interventions for alcohol users that include immediate coping skills to deal with the cravings, along with stimulus exposure therapy, can be better than just the latter alone. Witkiewitz, Roos, Tofighi, and Van Horn (2018) sought to fill methodological gaps in the evaluation of the effectiveness of interventions and found that a broad repertoire of coping skills, in the number of strategies used, may be key to the effectiveness of an intervention for alcoholics. Chen (2019) presented results of an intervention protocol for heroin users that includes 12 skills training sessions and found that, compared to a control group, this protocol provided higher abstinence rates in 36 months of follow-up and lower treatment dropout rates. For Gorgulu (2019), the best predictor of motivation for the treatment of various psychoactive substances addiction is the level of coping skills. Sudhir (2018) presented social skills training, especially assertiveness, as one of the components of an intervention for SUD.

Although investigations on these models still require greater methodological systematization, the results found so far do not allow us to rule out the coping skills training at any level of substance abuse and dependence assessment and treatment. Studies suggest its relevance both as a complement to cognitive-behavioral therapy and as a specific therapy, equivalent to other approaches.

Final Considerations

Theory and research on social and coping skills in Substance Use Disorders are not exactly deficient, there is a reasonable amount of interest in the topic, but there are several questions that need to be answered in the coming years. It is known that there are several relationships between classes and subclasses of coping with substance involvement, but what are the strongest, what are the weakest relationships? Assertiveness, communication, conversation, and social disinhibition, and self-control of aggressiveness are some of the examples that appear frequently, but are they enough for an effective intervention? Which others should make up an intervention program? Which have anticipatory functions, which can be effective for immediate coping? What types should be taught in an intervention program? What is important is the quality of the skills, is it the type of skills or is it the number of skills in the repertoire to be used? Do standardized programs, with a predefined number of sessions in 8, 12, or 20 meetings, actually promote behavior change? Are customized programs better than standardized ones? What would be a good measure of behavior change: days of abstinence, reduction of consumption, change of related variables as motivation for treatment? Are group interventions equally effective than individual interventions? Are there differences between the skills affected and required for alcohol, crack cocaine, marijuana, and multiple substance users? As you can see, there are many questions for a long way to go.

Such responses are essential for a more accurate assessment that enables targeted and effective interventions. In order for them to occur, it is fundamental to bring theory and research closer to the practices adopted in the public centers of psychosocial attention, therapeutic communities, hospitals, and other treatment systems, including private practices. Today the distance is great and harmful for both sides. Theory and research do not advance as much as they could, since they do not find a fertile field of practical application that could give parameters on what works more and what works less. On the other hand, professional practice does not benefit from reliable empirical data to generate higher-quality evaluations and interventions, forcing psychologists and other professionals to work often on the basis of trial and error.

There is a need to define more standardized research methodologies, which allow results to be compared and progress to be targeted. Currently, there does not seem to be a clear direction followed by Brazilian and foreign researchers. Each one proposes an investigation that is not necessarily a later stage in relation to something already studied. Several lines are opened in a diffuse way, knowledge advances in many directions, but it does not deepen in any of them.

The academic, theoretical, and empirical relationships between social and coping skills and substance use disorder have long been reported. However, the use of assessment and treatment in coping skills in professional practice still seems to be a novelty, at least in Brazil. There is still a long way to go, paths that cross at many points. Challenge for the next decades of theory, research, and practice.

References

Albuquerque, R. C., & Nappo, S. A. (2018). Reasons to crack consumption relapse. Users' perspective. *Jornal Brasileiro de Psiquiatria, 67*(3), 194–200. https://doi.org/10.1590/0047-2085000000197.

Andrade, A. L. M., Scatena, A., & De Micheli, D. (2017). Evaluation of a preventive intervention in alcoholic and non-alcoholic drivers – a pilot study. SMAD. Revista eletrônica saúde mental álcool e drogas, 13(4), 205-212. https://doi.org/10.11606/issn.1806-6976.v13i4p205-212.

American Psychiatric Association. (2014). *Manual diagnóstico e estatístico de transtornos mentais* (5th ed.). Porto Alegre: Artmed.

Ames, S. C., & Roitzsch, J. C. (2000). The impact of minor stressful life events and social support on cravings: A study of inpatients receiving treatment for substance dependence. *Addictive Behaviors, 25*(4), 539–547. https://doi.org/10.1016/s0306-4603(00)00069-1.

Andretta, I., Limberger, J., & Schneider, J. A. (2016). Social skills in crack users: Differences between men and women. *Psicologia: Reflexão e Crítica, 29*(1), 4. https://doi.org/10.1186/s41155-016-0054-4.

Araújo, R. B., Balbinot, A. D., Castro, M. G. T., Rocha, M. R., Miguel, S. R. P. S., Cohen, M., & Pedroso, R. S. (2011). Tratamento de exposição a estímulos e treinamento de habilidades como coadjuvantes no manejo do craving em um dependente de crack. *Trends in Psychiatry and Psychotherapy, 33*(3), 181–188. https://doi.org/10.1590/S2237-60892011000300008.

Argimon, I. I. L., & Oliveira, M. S. (2009). Avaliação psicológica do dependente de substâncias psicoativas. In C. S. Hutz (Ed.), *Avanços e polêmicas em avaliação psicológica* (pp. 199–216). São Paulo: Casa do Psicólogo.

Barkin, S. L., Smith, K. S., & DuRant, R. H. (2002). Social skills and attitudes associated with substance use behaviors among young adolescents. *The Journal of Adolescent Health, 30*(6), 448–454. https://doi.org/10.1016/s1054-139x(01)00405-0.

Borini, P., Guimarães, R. C., & Borini, S. B. (2003). Usuários de drogas ilícitas internados em hospital psiquiátrico: Padrões de uso e aspectos demográficos e epidemiológicos. *Jornal Brasileiro de Psiquiatria, 52*(3), 171–179.

Brown, S. A., Vik, P. W., McQuaid, J. R., Patterson, T. L., Irwin, M. R., & Grant, I. (1990). Severity of psychosocial stress and outcome of alcoholism treatment. *Journal of Abnormal Psychology, 99*(4), 344–348. https://doi.org/10.1037//0021-843x.99.4.344.

Carlini, E. A. (2006). Epidemiologia do uso de álcool no Brasil. *Arquivos Médicos ABC, Suplemento, 2*, 4–7.

Chen, J., Yu, J., Cao, J., Xiao, Y., Gu, H., Zhong, R., & Wang, Z. (2019). Abstinence following a motivation-skill-desensitization-mental energy intervention for heroin dependence: A three-year follow-up result of a randomized controlled trial. *Current Medical Science, 39*(3), 472–482. https://doi.org/10.1007/s11596-019-2062-y.

Conrod, P. J., Castellanos-Ryan, N., & Strang, J. (2010). Brief, personality-targeted coping skills interventions and survival as a non-drug user over a 2-year period during adolescence. *Archives of General Psychiatry, 67*(1), 85–93. https://doi.org/10.1001/archgenpsychiatry.2009.173.

Constant, H. M. R. M., Figueiró, L. R., Signor, L., Bisch, N. K., Barros, H. M. T., & Ferigolo, M. (2014). Tradução, adaptação transcultural e validação de conteúdo da versão em português do coping behaviours inventory (CBI) para a população brasileira. *Cadernos de Saúde Pública, 30*(10), 2049–2056. https://doi.org/10.1590/0102-311X00176513.

Constant, H. M. R. M., Moret-Tatay, C., Benchaya, M. C., Oliveira, M., Barros, H. M. T., & Ferigolo, M. (2018). CBI-20: Psychometric properties for the coping behaviors inventory for alcohol abuse in Brazil. *Frontiers in Psychiatry, 9*, 1–8. https://doi.org/10.3389/fpsyt.2018.00585.

Del Prette, A., & Del Prette, Z. A. P. (2017). *Competência social e habilidades sociais: Manual teórico-prático*. Petrópolis: Vozes.

Del Prette, Z. A. P., & Del Prette, A. (2001). *Inventário de habilidades sociais (IHS-Del Prette): Manual de aplicação, apuração e interpretação*. São Paulo: Casa do Psicólogo.

Del Prette, Z. A. P., & Del Prette, A. (2005). *Psicologia das habilidades sociais na infância: Teoria e prática*. Petrópolis: Vozes.

Del Prette, Z. A. P., & Del Prette, A. (2008). Psicologia das habilidades sociais: Terapia. In *educação e trabalho* (5th ed.). Vozes: Petrópolis.

Del Prette, Z. A. P., & Del Prette, A. (2010). Habilidades Sociais e Análise do Comportamento: Proximidade histórica e atualidades. *Perspectivas em Análise do Comportamento, 1*(2), 104–115.

Dias, A. C., Araújo, M. R., & Laranjeira, R. (2011). Evolução do consumo de crack em coorte com histórico de tratamento. *Revista de Saúde Pública, 45*(5), 938–948. https://doi.org/10.1590/S0034-89102011005000049.

Dolan, S. L., Rohsenow, D. J., Martin, R. A., & Monti, P. M. (2013). Urge-specific and lifestyle coping strategies of alcoholics: Relationships of specific strategies to treatment outcome. *Drug and Alcohol Dependence, 128*(1-2), 8–14. https://doi.org/10.1016/j.drugalcdep.2012.07.010.

Donovan, D. M. (2009). Avaliação dos comportamentos dependentes na prevenção da recaída. In D. Donovan & A. Marlatt (Eds.), *Avaliação dos comportamentos dependentes* (pp. 1–50). São Paulo: Roca.

Duailibi, L. B., Ribeiro, M., & Laranjeira, R. (2008). Profile of cocaine and crack users in Brazil. *Cadernos de Saúde Pública, 24*(suppl. 4), 545–557. https://doi.org/10.1590/S0102-311X2008001600007.

Duncan, T. E., Duncan, S. C., Beauchamp, N., Wells, J., & Ary, D. V. (2000). Development and evaluation of an interactive CD-ROM refusal skills program to prevent youth substance use: "Refuse to use". *Journal of Behavioral Medicine, 23*(1), 59–72. https://doi.org/10.1023/a:1005420304147.

Epstein, J. A., Zhou, X. K., Bang, H., & Botvin, G. J. (2007). Do competence skills moderate the impact of social influences to drink and perceived social benefits of drinking on alcohol use among inner-city adolescents? *Prevention Science, 8*(1), 65–73. https://doi.org/10.1007/s11121-006-0054-1.

Felicissimo, F. B., Casela, A. L. M., & Ronzani, T. M. (2013). Habilidades sociais e alcoolismo: Uma revisão da literatura. *Psicologia Em Estudo, 18*(1), 137–145. https://doi.org/10.1590/S1413-73722013000100014.

Felicissimo, F. B., Santos, J. A., Fontoura, L. O., & Ronzani, T. M. (2016). Habilidades sociais em alcoolistas: um estudo comparativo. *Psicologia: Teoria e Pesquisa, 32*(2), 1–6. https://doi.org/10.1590/0102-3772e322212.

Forys, K., McKellar, J., & Moos, R. (2007). Participation in specific treatment components predicts alcohol-specific and general coping skills. *Addictive Behaviors, 32*, 1669–1680. https://doi.org/10.1016/j.addbeh.2006.11.023.

Frade, I. F., De Micheli, D., Andrade, A. L. M., & de Souza-Formigoni, M. L. O. (2013). Relationship between stress symptoms and drug use among secondary students. The Spanish journal of psychology, 16, e4. https://doi.org/10.1017/sjp.2013.5.

Gorgulu, T. (2019). The effect of self-efficacy and coping strategies on treatment motivation of individuals in the substance addiction group work process. *Dusunen Adam: The Journal of Psychiatry and Neurological Sciences*, 33–42. https://doi.org/10.14744/dajpns.2019.00005.

Gossop, M., Stewart, D., Browne, N., & Marsden, J. (2002). Factors associated with abstinence, lapse or relapse to heroin use after residential treatment: Protective effect of coping responses. *Addiction, 97*(10), 1259–1267. https://doi.org/10.1046/j.1360-0443.2002.00227.x.

Hasking, P. A., & Oei, T. P. (2007). Alcohol expectancies, self-efficacy and coping in an alcohol-dependent sample. *Addictive Behaviors, 32*(1), 99–113. https://doi.org/10.1016/j.addbeh.2006.03.024.

Hassanbeigi, A., Askari, J., Hassanbeigi, D., & Pourmovahed (2013). The relationship between stress and addiction. Procedia-Social and Behavioral Sciences, 84, 1333-1340. Doi: https://doi.org/10.1016/j.sbspro.2013.06.752

Horta, R. L., Schäfer, J. L., Coelho, L. R. M., Rodrigues, V. S., Oliveira, M. S., & Teixeira, V. A. (2016). Condições associadas a prejuízo de desempenho em habilidades sociais em uma amostra de conveniência de usuários de crack. *Cadernos de Saúde Pública, 32*(4), e00010715. https://doi.org/10.1590/0102-311X00010715.

Humke, C., & Radnitz, C. L. (2005). An instrument for assessing coping with temptation: Psychometric properties of the alcohol abuse coping response inventory. *Substance Use & Misuse, 40*(1), 37–62. https://doi.org/10.1081/ja-200030493.

Jungerman, F. S., & Zanelatto, N. A. (2007). *Tratamento psicológico do usuário de maconha e seus familiares: Um manual para terapeutas*. São Paulo: Roca.

Kessler, F., & Pechansky, F. (2008). Uma visão psiquiátrica sobre o fenômeno do crack na atualidade. *Revista de Psiquiatria do RS, 30*(2), 96–98.

Kiluk, B. D., DeVito, E. E., Buck, M. B., Hunkele, K., Nich, C., & Carroll, K. M. (2017). Effect of computerized cognitive behavioral therapy on acquisition of coping skills among cocaine-dependent individuals enrolled in methadone maintenance. *Journal of Substance Abuse Treatment, 82*, 87–92. https://doi.org/10.1016/j.jsat.2017.09.011.

Lazarus, R. S., & Folkman, S. (1984). *Stress, appraisal and coping*. New York: Springer Publishing Company.

Limberger, J., & Andretta, I. (2018). Desenvolvimento das habilidades sociais na vida de mulheres usuárias de crack: estudo de casos múltiplos. *Temas Em Psicologia, 25*(4), 1709–1724. https://doi.org/10.9788/tp2017.4-11pt.

Litman, G. K., Stapleton, J., Oppenheim, A. N., & Peleg, M. (1983). An instrument for measuring coping behaviours in hospitalized alcoholics: Implications for relapse prevention treatment. *British Journal of Addiction, 78*(3), 269–276. https://doi.org/10.1111/j.1360-0443.1983.tb02511.x.

Litt, M. D., Kadden, R. M., Cooney, N. L., & Kabela, E. (2003). Coping skills and treatment outcomes in cognitive-behavioral and interactional group therapy for alcoholism. *Journal of Consulting and Clinical Psychology, 71*(1), 118–128. https://doi.org/10.1037//0022-006x.71.1.118.

Litt, M. D., Kadden, R. M., & Kabela-Cormier, E. (2009). Individualized assessment and treatment program for alcohol dependence: Results of an initial study to train coping skills. *Addiction, 104*(11), 1837–1838. https://doi.org/10.1111/j.1360-0443.2009.02693.x.

Litt, M. D., Kadden, R. M., Kabela-Cormier, E., & Petry, N. M. (2008). Coping skills training and contingency management treatments for marijuana dependence: Exploring mechanisms of behavior change. *Addiction, 103*(4), 638–648.

Longabaugh, R., & Morgenstern, J. (1999). Cognitive-behavioral coping-skills therapy for alcohol dependence. Current status and future directions. *Alcohol Research & Health, 23*(2), 78–85.

Lopes, F. M., Andretta, I., & Oliveira, M. S. (2019). Avaliação psicológica dos transtornos relacionados a substâncias psicoativas. In M. N. Baptista et al. (Eds.), *Compêndio de avaliação psicológica* (pp. 692–702). São Paulo: Vozes.

Mares, M. F., & Torres, L. B. (2010). Mantenimiento de las habilidades de rehusarse al consumo em usuarios crônicos de alcohol y drogas: Un estudio de casos. *Salud Mental, 33*, 47–55.

Marijuana Treatment Project Research Group. (2004). Brief treatments for cannabis dependence: Findings from a randomized multisite trial. *Journal of Consulting and Clinical Psychology, 72*(3), 455–466. https://doi.org/10.1037/0022-006X.72.3.455.

Marlatt, G. A., & Donovan, D. M. (2009). *Prevenção da recaída: Estratégias de manutenção no tratamento de comportamentos adictivos* (2nd ed.). Porto Alegre: Artmed.

Marlatt, G. A., & Witkiewitz, K. (2009). Problemas com álcool e drogas. In A. Marlatt & D. Donovan (Eds.), *Prevenção da recaída: Estratégias de manutenção no tratamento de comportamentos adictivos* (2nd ed., pp. 15–50). Porto Alegre: Artmed.

Mattoo, S. K., Chakrabarti, S., & Anjaiah, M. (2009). Psychosocial factors associated with relapse in men with alcohol or opioid dependence. *The Indian Journal of Medical Research, 130*(6), 702–708.

McGillicuddy, N. B., Rychtarik, R. G., & Papandonatos, G. D. (2015). Skill training versus 12-step facilitation for parents of substance-abusing teens. *Journal of Substance Abuse Treatment, 50*, 11–17. https://doi.org/10.1016/j.jsat.2014.09.006.

Mellentin, A. I., Skøt, L., Nielsen, B., Schippers, G. M., Nielsen, A. S., Stenager, E., & Juhl, C. (2017). Cue exposure therapy for the treatment of alcohol use disorders: A meta-analytic review. *Clinical Psychology Review, 57*, 195–207. https://doi.org/10.1016/j.cpr.2017.07.006.

Monti, P. M., Abrams, D. B., Binkoff, J. A., Zwick, W. R., Liepman, M. R., Nirenberg, T. D., & Rohsenow, D. J. (1990). Communication skills training, communication skills training with family and cognitive behavioral mood management training for alcoholics. *Journal of Studies on Alcohol, 51*(3), 263–270. https://doi.org/10.15288/jsa.1990.51.263.

Monti, P. M., Kadden, R. M., Rohsenow, D. J., Cooney, N. L., & Abrams, D. B. (2005). *Tratando a dependência de álcool: Um guia de treinamento das habilidades de enfrentamento*. São Paulo: Roca.

Monti, P. M., Rohsenow, D. J., Michalec, E., Martin, R. A., & Abrams, D. B. (1997). Brief coping skills treatment for cocaine abuse: Substance use outcomes at three months. *Addiction, 92*(12), 1717–1728.

Monti, P. M., Rohsenow, D. J., Rubonis, A. V., Niaura, R. S., Sirota, A. D., & Abrams, D. B. (1993). Cue exposure with coping skills treatment for male alcoholics: A preliminary investigation. *Journal of Consulting and Clinical Psychology, 61*(6), 1011–1019. https://doi.org/10.1037//0022-006x.61.6.1011.

Moos, R. H. (1992). *Coping response inventory adult form*. Palo Alto: Center for Health Care Evaluation, Stanford University and Department of Veterans Affairs Medical Center.

Noto, A. R., & Galduróz, J. C. F. (1999). O uso de drogas psicotrópicas e a prevenção no Brasil. *Ciência e Saúde Coletiva, 4*(1), 145–151. https://doi.org/10.1590/S1413-81231999000100012.

Oei, T. P., & Jackson, P. R. (1982). Social skills and cognitive behavioral approaches to the treatment of problem drinking. *Journal of Studies on Alcohol, 43*(5), 532–547. https://doi.org/10.15288/jsa.1982.43.532.

Rangé, B., & Marlatt, G. A. (2008). Terapia cognitivo-comportamental de transtornos de abuso de álcool e drogas. *Revista Brasileira de Psiquiatria, 30*, 88–95. https://doi.org/10.1590/S1516-44462008000600006.

Ritchie, G., Weldon, S., Freeman, L., MacPherson, G., & Davies, K. (2011). Outcomes of a drug and alcohol relapse prevention programme in a population of mentally disordered offenders. *The British Journal of Forensic Practice, 13*, 32–43. https://doi.org/10.5042/bjfp.2011.0048.

Rocha, H. G. (2017). Fatores psicossocias relacionados à manutenção da abstinência alcoólica no pós-transplante hepático (Master's thesis, Universidade de Brasília, Brasília, Brasil). Retrieved from https://repositorio.unb.br/handle/10482/25180

Rohsenow, D. J., Martin, R. A., & Monti, P. M. (2005). Urge-specific and lifestyle coping strategies of cocaine abusers: Relationships to treatment outcomes. *Drug and Alcohol Dependence, 78*(2), 211–219. https://doi.org/10.1016/j.drugalcdep.2005.03.001.

Rohsenow, D. J., Monti, P. M., Martin, R. A., Colby, S. M., Myers, M. G., Gulliver, S. B., & Abrams, D. B. (2004). Motivational enhancement and coping skills training for cocaine abusers: Effects on substance use outcomes. *Addiction, 99*(7), 862–874. https://doi.org/10.1111/j.1360-0443.2004.00743.x.

Rohsenow, D. J., Monti, P. M., Rubonis, A. V., Gulliver, S. B., Colby, S. M., Binkoff, J. A., & Abrams, D. B. (2001). Cue exposure with coping skills training and communication skills training for alcohol dependence: 6- and 12-month outcomes. *Addiction, 96*(8), 1161–1174. https://doi.org/10.1046/j.1360-0443.2001.96811619.x.

Sá, L. G. C., & Del Prette, Z. A. P. (2014). Habilidades sociais como preditoras do envolvimento com álcool e outras drogas: Um estudo exploratório. *Interação em Psicologia, 18*(2), 30660. https://doi.org/10.5380/psi.v18i2.30660.

Sá, L. G. C., & Del Prette, Z. A. P. (2016). Habilidades de enfrentamento antecipatório para abstinência de substâncias: Construção de um novo instrumento de medida. *Avances En Psicologia Latinoamericana, 34*(2), 351–364. https://doi.org/10.12804/apl34.2.2016.09.

Sá, L. G. C., Olaz, F. O., & Del Prette, Z. A. P. (2017). Initial psychometric properties of the inventory of anticipatory coping skills for abstinence from alcohol and other drugs. *Avaliação Psicológica, 16*(2), 176–186. https://doi.org/10.15689/AP.2017.1602.08.

Saha, A. (2013). A study on relapse prevention in cases of alcohol dependence syndrome. *American Journal of Life Sciences, 1*(4), 184–188. https://doi.org/10.11648/j.ajls.20130104.17.

Sakiyama, H. M. T., Ribeiro, M., & Padin, M. F. R. (2012). Prevenção de recaída e habilidades sociais. In M. Ribeiro & R. Laranjeira (Eds.), *O tratamento do usuário de crack* (pp. 337–350). Porto Alegre: Artmed.

Schaub, M. P., Tiburcio, M., Martinez, N., Ambekar, A., Balhara, Y. P. S., Wenger, A., Poznyak, V, et al.. (2018). Alcohol e-Help: study protocol for a web-based self-help program to reduce alcohol use in adults with drinking patterns considered harmful, hazardous or suggestive of dependence in middle-income countries. Addiction, 113(2), 346-352. http://dx.doi.org/10.1111/add.14034.

Scheier, L. M., Botvin, G. J., Diaz, T., & Griffin, K. W. (1999). Social skills, competence, and drug refusal efficacy as predictors of adolescent alcohol use. *Journal of Drug Education, 29*(3), 251–278. https://doi.org/10.2190/M3CT-WWJM-5JAQ-WP15.

Schneider, J. A., & Andretta, I. (2017). Habilidades sociais de usuários de crack em tratamento nas comunidades terapêuticas: Relação com características sociodemográficas e de padrão de consumo. *Revista Colombiana de Psicologia, 26*(1), 83–98. https://doi.org/10.15446/rcp.v26n1.54032.

Silva, M. L., Hatanaka, Y. F., Rondina, R. C., & Silva, N. R. (2018). Avaliação do repertório de habilidades sociais de usuários de substâncias psicoativas em tratamento. *Cadernos Brasileiros de Terapia Ocupacional, 26*(4), 849–858. https://doi.org/10.4322/2526-8910.ctoao1633.

Sousa, J. M., Martins, V. M. S., Haidar, F. C., & Sá, L. G. C. (2020). Adaptação Brasileira do Questionário de Estratégias Específicas à Fissura (USSQ).

Sudhir, P. M. (2018). Cognitive behavioural interventions in addictive disorders. *Indian Journal of Psychiatry, 60*(Suppl. 4), S479–S484. https://doi.org/10.4103/psychiatry.IndianJPsychiatry_15_18.

Van Hasselt, V. B., Hersen, M., & Milliones, J. (1978). Social skills training in alcoholics and drug addicts: A review. *Addictive Behaviors, 3*, 221–233. https://doi.org/10.1016/0306-4603(78)90023-0.

Villalba, E. A. (1995). Proyecto de entrenamiento en habilidades socials com toxicómanos. In F. G. Rodríguez, J. M. L. Rubio, & L. J. Expósito (Eds.), *Habilidades sociales y salud* (pp. 127–132). Madri: Biblioteca Eudema.

Wagner, M. F., & Oliveira, M. S. (2009). Estudo das habilidades sociais em adolescentes usuários de maconha. *Psicologia em Estudo, 14*(1), 101–110.

Wagner, M. F., Silva, J. G., Zanettelo, L. B., & Oliveira, M. S. (2010). O uso da maconha associado ao déficit de habilidades sociais em adolescentes. *Revista Eletrônica Saúde Mental, Álcool e Drogas, 6*(2), 255273.

Witkiewitz, K., Roos, C. R., Tofighi, D., & Van Horn, M. L. (2018). Broad coping repertoire mediates the effect of the combined behavioral intervention on alcohol outcomes in the COMBINE study: An application of latent class mediation. *Journal of Studies on Alcohol and Drugs, 79*(2), 199–207. https://doi.org/10.15288/jsad.2018.79.199.

Witkiewitz, K., Villarroel, N. A., Hartzler, B., & Donovan, D. M. (2011). Drinking outcomes following drink refusal skills training: Differential effects for African American and non-Hispanic White clients. *Psychology of Addictive Behaviors, 25*(1), 162–167. https://doi.org/10.1037/a0022254.

Zywiak, W. H., Stout, R. L., Longabaugh, R., Dyck, I., Connors, G. J., & Maisto, S. A. (2006). Relapse-onset factors in project MATCH: The relapse questionnaire. *Journal of Substance Abuse Treatment, 31*(4), 341–345. https://doi.org/10.1016/j.jsat.2006.05.007.

Chapter 20
Psychoeducation in the Treatment of Smoking and Alcohol Use Disorder

Fernanda Machado Lopes, Weridiane Lehmkuhl da Luz, Joana Bender Remus, and Ilana Andretta

Introduction

Psychoeducation is a psychotherapeutic strategy that consists of transmitting relevant theoretical and technical information to patients and their families about symptoms and treatment, with the objective of making them aware of the pathology and/or problem in question and formulating effective methods of coping (Dobson & Dobson, 2011; Lemes & Ondere Neto, 2017; Marques, 2016; Zanelatto, 2013). It is assumed that the more informed patients are about their current physical and/or mental condition and the functioning of the treatment to be performed, the more they will be motivated and involved in their therapeutic process (Knijnik & Kunzler, 2014; Lukens & McFarlane, 2004).

The emergence of psychoeducation occurred timidly due to the prevailing biomedical paradigm of health, which considered patients and family members to be lay people and incapable of understanding and getting involved in the therapeutic process (Andrade, 1997, as cited by Marques, 2016). It began to be used in 1970 as a complementary form to pharmacological therapy and in opposition to treatments and interventions used at the time, such as those that only incited the expression of feelings. It involves different theories and disciplines that, if related, help as a therapeutic resource by promoting understanding on the part of patients regarding the various factors that involve the situation they are facing (Marques, 2016; Nogueira, Crisostomo, Souza, & Prado, 2017, as cited in Lemes & Ondere Neto, 2017).

F. M. Lopes (✉) · W. L. da Luz · J. B. Remus
Universidade Federal de Santa Catarina, Florianópolis, SC, Brazil

I. Andretta
Universidade do Vale do Rio dos Sinos, São Leopoldo, RS, Brazil

D. De Micheli et al. (eds.), *Drugs and Human Behavior*,
https://doi.org/10.1007/978-3-030-62855-0_20

However, with the paradigm shift presented by the biopsychosocial model in the 1980s, psychoeducation began to gain new evidence. It presented itself as a way to help patients avoid relapses and prolonged hospitalizations in psychiatric treatments, a common practice at that time (Andrade, 1999, as cited by Marques, 2016). In this way, this practice began to consider the subject in the intervention center in order to clear up his doubts and welcome his worries through a structured intervention program that favors the patient's engagement in his treatment. Since by understanding his current situation, he felt more autonomous and responsible in decision-making (Carvalho, Malagris, & Rangé, 2019; Lemes & Ondere Neto, 2017; Lima & Mângia, 2015; Marques, 2016). Other benefits of psychoeducation include relief of symptoms, increased sense of control over symptoms, and increased confidence and motivation in treatment (Carvalho et al., 2019; Dobson & Dobson, 2011).

Lemes and Ondere Neto (2017) state that psychoeducation can be employed in different contexts such as hospital, organizational, educational institutions, among others. Its applicability in the context of health psychology stands out, where information on physical diseases, possible causes, and side effects of medication can help in treatment adherence. An example is the application of psychoeducation in the pre- and post-surgical moment, when patients may present restlessness and anxiety regarding the procedure to be performed and subsequent care. The follow-up, in these cases, aims to clarify doubts regarding the surgery, since understanding the functioning of the process as a whole tends to ease anxiogenic symptoms in these patients.

It is known that psychoeducation as a psychological technique contributes to the therapy, as knowledge is shared and treatment becomes meaningful to patients and to the therapist (Lemes & Ondere Neto, 2017; Marques, 2016). Thus, there is the possibility of a more horizontal and transparent therapeutic relationship, in which patients are also responsible for their treatment process, even helping in the planning of interventions (Carvalho et al., 2019).

Among the contexts in which psychoeducation is employed, the scope of psychotherapy is highlighted, especially under the cognitive-behavioral therapy (CBT) approach. CBT is a structured psychotherapy aimed at solving current problems and modifying dysfunctional (maladaptive) thoughts and behaviors, which are common to all psychological disorders (Beck, 2013). The treatment is based on a cognitive conceptualization, which is a schematic way of understanding the patient's beliefs and thought and behavior patterns. In addition, CBT is educational and emphasizes the active participation of patients in the therapeutic process, in order to teach them the theory that underlies the interventions performed, the techniques possibly used, and the symptomatic aspects of the disorder (if any) and/or the demands presented. Thus, patients develop a repertoire of effective strategies to their demands, and through psychoeducation, the psychotherapist teaches patients to be "their own therapists," emphasizing relapse prevention (Beck, 2013; Carvalho et al., 2019; Wright, Basco, & Thase, 2008).

In cognitive-behavioral psychotherapy, psychoeducation is one of the first steps, since it aims, among other things, to clarify patients about how the treatment works and adjust their expectations regarding psychotherapy (Dobson & Dobson, 2011).

However, this strategy is not restricted only to the beginning of therapy, but can be performed throughout the entire therapeutic process. One of its functions is to guide patients in terms of the construction of their beliefs and how they manifest themselves through thoughts, emotions, and daily behaviors, making them more aware of their functioning (Beck, 2013; Nogueira et al., 2017; Wright et al., 2008). Thus, the cognitive-behavioral psychotherapist is dedicated to teaching patients the monitoring of automatic thoughts, to test their validity and to modify those distorted, in addition to ways to identify and alter beliefs that contribute to distorted patterns of interpretation of reality (Beck, 2013; Carvalho et al., 2019). Thus, the understanding of the psychotherapeutic process is facilitated, playing a role of prevention, promotion, and health education (Lemes & Ondere Neto, 2017; Marques, 2016).

Methods and Modalities of Psychoeducation

There are several ways to perform psychoeducation and, therefore, the therapist should be sensitive to the needs that each patient presents, identifying situations that are likely to accomplish this strategy and considering how to do it in the most personalized way (Dobson & Dobson, 2011; Wright et al., 2008). For example, if patients' attention, awareness, or orientation abilities are impaired, the psychotherapist should be cautious and evaluate the feasibility and effectiveness of the application at this time. In addition, one should consider patients' desire for such information and the most indicated sources; there are patients who are more interested in more technical and scientific materials, and the recommendation of specific readings is advised, and may even instruct patients to conduct their own research (Dobson & Dobson, 2011).

In choosing psychoeducational methods, one should consider whether the language of the material is congruent with the level of patient literacy; the skills and resources available, such as Internet access; and the quality of the materials (Dobson & Dobson, 2011). It is not recommended that materials that have not been previously assessed by the psychotherapist be indicated (Dobson & Dobson, 2011; Wright et al., 2008). Also, as needed, it is suggested that materials be adapted to patients, such as the use of large print and audio recordings or videos (Wright et al., 2008).

Initially, it is essential to hear what patients already know about the subject, enabling possible mistakes to be clarified (Carvalho et al., 2019). During the sessions, mini-classes—brief and clear explanations of opportune subjects—and learning exercises of techniques such as, for example, the recording of automatic thoughts can be performed. CBT psychotherapy provides homework exercises to be performed between sessions, with psychoeducation being a resource allied to the therapy notebook. In addition to brief explanations on timely subjects, texts, films, videos, websites, mobile applications, and computer programs can also be used for this purpose (Beck, 2013; Carvalho et al., 2019; Wright et al., 2008). Attention is paid to the use of specific written materials that facilitate and contribute to the psychotherapeutic process, with concise information pertinent to patients (Dobson &

Dobson, 2011; Wright et al., 2008). It is essential to emphasize the importance of requesting feedback in order to verify patients' understanding about the information used in psychoeducation (Carvalho et al., 2019; Wright et al., 2008).

In terms of modality, psychoeducation can take place on an individual, intimate and private basis, or in groups. Group modality tends to provide more benefits when compared to individual care because they are configured as a protective space, free of prejudice and providing mutual trust (Menezes & Souza, 2012; Marques, 2016). The family can be inserted in the psychoeducation process; therefore, the groups can be formed only by patients, relatives/caregivers, or by all (Carvalho et al., 2019; Lemes & Ondere Neto, 2017; Zanelatto, 2013).

The groups integrated by family members/caregivers aim to share information, dispel myths, reduce prejudice, and develop skills to deal with the disease or disorder (Gonçalves-Pereira & Sampaio, 2011, as cited in Marques, 2016). In addition, they reduce the feeling of family isolation and provide experience exchange, enabling comfort to family members when developing a support network (Menezes & Souza, 2012; Ponce et al., 2011). Thus, the psychoeducation performed with the family provides a decrease in dysfunctional thoughts and behaviors, as well as intensifies the belief of self-efficacy by developing means that enable the confrontation of health-related aspects of the patients' family in a harmonious manner (Lemes & Ondere Neto, 2017; Lopes & Cachioni, 2012).

In groups with patients, psychoeducation provides dialogues, social learning, support, support network, and reinforcement in the face of positive changes (Carvalho et al., 2019). Patients are guided about the disorder or disease they have, their symptoms, and the different pathways through the exchange of experiences. By sharing and listening to experiences of similar situations, patients feel more motivated to help each other and to remain open to being helped (Nogueira et al., 2017).

Lemes and Ondere Neto (2017) conducted a systematic review on the application of psychoeducation in different contexts and problems. This study showed that the use of this strategy is applied to several physical and mental pathologies, such as cancer, phobias, bipolar affective disorder, anxiety disorder, post-traumatic stress disorder, among other psychiatric disorders, with positive results. The authors also mentioned the importance of using psychoeducation in substance use disorder (SUD), since they verified that it seems to contribute to the control of consumption behavior, collaborating in the confrontation of possible prejudices and social stigma and helping in the promotion of healthy habits (Lima and Mângia 2015; Nogueira et al., 2017).

Psychoeducation Applied to the Treatment of Smoking and Alcohol Use Disorder

The World Health Organization (WHO) defines drug dependence as a state characterized by the uncontrolled use of one or more psychoactive substances that end up causing harm in one or more areas of the subject's life, such as physical, social, and psychological problems. It consists of a chronic and recurrent disease (with relapses) that presents itself as one of the greatest challenges of the world's health systems, which can be effectively treated (Mathias & Abreu, 2019; Morandi & Guimarães, 2015).

The diagnosis of this disorder has evolved over time. The Diagnostic and Statistical Manual of Mental Disorders third edition (DSM III) gave rise to the classification of substance abuse, and in DSM IV it was identified as a distinct diagnosis with specific symptoms (Farina, Terroso, Lopes, & Argimon, 2013). Currently, DSM 5 describes that the essential quality to characterize a SUD is the presence of a grouping of cognitive, behavioral, and physiological symptoms that end up indicating continuous use by the individual, regardless of considerable substance-related problems (American Psychiatric Association - APA, 2014). The psychoactive substances present in drugs cause changes in the way people think and act, and each substance has a mechanism of action and provides a different effect, which can be agitation, euphoria, sleepiness, relaxation, hallucinations, among others.

In general, some characteristic of SUD are the basic changes in brain circuits that, even after the detoxification process, may persist in the case of patients with severe disorders, such as chronic alcohol use disorders. Through constant relapses and craving (intense desire for the drug), behavioral effects of these brain alterations can be observed (American Psychiatric Association - APA 2014). Thus, drugs are conceived as a problem when individuals have the belief that they will only find pleasure and relief by using the substance. A vicious circle forms when people use drugs to feel better; the use generates problems that drive people to use it again (Knapp & Luz, 2008; Mathias & Abreu, 2019).

The factors that lead to the use of the substances are diverse, such as family, genetic, and/or social. The diagnosis of SUD is based on a pathological pattern of behaviors associated with its use, under conditions related to low control, social deterioration, risky use, and pharmacological criteria (American Psychiatric Association - APA 2014; Mathias & Abreu, 2019). It is recurrent that, during the SUD treatment process, including alcohol and tobacco use, there are high rates of relapse, treatment abandonment, and lack of motivation (Foes, Ferreira, & Paludo, 2015; Gigliotti, Carneiro, & Ferreira, 2008). Therefore, specialists in this area recommend that the therapeutic strategy be broader and actively involve the user, which highlights the use of psychoeducation as one of the first techniques used in treatment (Foes et al., 2015; Moraes & Boschetti, 2013).

Through psychoeducation, myths and "false beliefs" on alcohol and tobacco, the effects of continued use, and withdrawal symptoms can be dispelled (Zanelatto, 2013). In the case of alcohol, for example, abrupt discontinuation after chronic consumption can lead to a severe withdrawal syndrome, including symptoms ranging from tremors to seizures and *Delirium Tremens* (a condition of generalized agitation and mental confusion, with high blood pressure, fever, and hallucinations). In this sense, psychoeducation is an important strategy, since it allows presenting the scenario in which an abusive use of these drugs is characterized, helping patients to understand what makes it so difficult to stop consuming the substance (Knijnik & Kunzler, 2014).

Some relevant themes for psychoeducation of alcohol and tobacco dependence are texts about mechanisms of action of each drug in the central nervous system and in the reward circuit, the concepts of tolerance, craving, abstinence syndrome, and the cognitive model of relapse itself (Foes et al., 2015; Knapp & Luz, 2008; Moraes & Boschetti, 2013; Zanelatto, 2013). In the cognitive model, there are specificities such as permissive beliefs for drug use and the identification of automatic thoughts in moments of craving (Knapp et al. 2008; Zanelatto, 2013). Through the identification of craving-stimulus situations, patient and therapist are able to debate when and why it occurs, duration, symptoms, and patient behaviors towards this moment (Câmara, 2019; Foes et al., 2015; Knapp & Luz, 2008; Rangé & Marlatt, 2008). Thus, the patient understands that the craving is momentary and the therapist should assist him in the repertoire of techniques for these situations, such as distraction, for example, decreasing the probability of drug use and, consequently, increasing adherence to treatment.

In a similar way, psychoeducation on the abstinence syndrome should be performed, because its effects can be anxiogenic to patients. The clarification that symptoms such as difficulty in concentration, changes in sleep and appetite, irritability, anxiety and depressive symptoms come from abstinence and start to diminish in a period of time from two to four weeks allows patients to know that this phase is part of the treatment and means that their body is recovering. At the same time, knowing that the withdrawal syndrome is temporary, as well as the craving, may increase their motivation to continue treatment and decrease the chance of relapse (Gigliotti et al., 2008; Rangé & Marlatt, 2008; Silva, Ferreira, & Zanelatto, 2013).

Thus, one of the goals of CBT, specifically psychoeducation in the treatment of alcohol and tobacco use disorder, is to teach patients to question their automatic thoughts and beliefs regarding these drugs, as well as to provide them with information for this purpose (Knapp & Luz, 2008). Another important issue to be addressed in psychoeducation is where to seek help and how the addiction treatment process occurs, in order to guide users also with regard to the public health network (Foes et al., 2015).

The themes of psychoeducation in the treatment of alcohol and tobacco use disorders can also be applied in group modalities and with patients' relatives (Farina et al., 2013; Foes et al., 2015; Knapp & Luz, 2008; Lima & Mângia, 2015). The treatment started to be carried out through psychosocial care, with the individuals inserted in their daily contexts, with the family having an important role as partner in the singular therapeutic project (Lima & Mângia, 2015).

When psychoeducation on alcohol and tobacco use disorders is performed in groups, the benefits presented above are widely perceived. It provides new knowledge to patients about their demands, facilitates understanding about the problems to be faced, as well as clarifying doubts, directly helping in the bond with therapists and adherence to treatment (Farina et al., 2013). Therapists seek to accept the collaborations of the group members, making them feel constructive in the psychoeducational process (Farina et al., 2013). This situation is clearer when patients' interactions occur after teaching about some concept related to the addiction process. Patients feel comfortable reporting their experiences in terms of what they have just learned, which demonstrates an integration between them and the therapeutic team, making them feel more understood and able to go through the process of change (Farina et al., 2013).

In relation to the family, the impacts can be financial, social, occupational, and even health, and it is fundamental to carry out psychoeducation on SUD with the families of alcohol and tobacco dependents (Lima and Mângia 2015). Thus, there is a greater understanding and demystification of the functioning of dependence on these drugs, which reduces anxiety and tension in the family environment (Foes et al., 2015; Lima and Mângia 2015). Moreover, by providing information on services and the health network, social isolation is reduced and support to users and family members is promoted (Lima and Mângia 2015). The family begins to identify itself as an important agent and assumes the role of partner in treatment (Foes et al., 2015).

An example of the application of psychoeducation in groups in the treatment of alcohol and other drug users and their families is reported by Foes et al. (2015). Through the *Caindo na Real* program, two stages of psychoeducational groups were carried out: the first, with users only, topics related to the effects of drug use, classification, dependence, action on the central nervous system and the reward circuit, treatment, and where to seek help in these cases were discussed. The second stage was carried out with family members, and topics regarding the different drugs such as cocaine, alcohol, and marijuana were discussed. At the end of the program, a handout was prepared with the main information discussed, which was given to users and their families.

Psychoeducation in the Treatment of Smoking

Although illicit drugs can cause high damage to the lives of individuals and their families, the protagonists in terms of large-scale harm in Brazil, especially in economic and health terms, are alcohol and tobacco (Laranjeira, 2014). Smoking, due to tobacco-related diseases, has been considered the largest avoidable cause of death in the world, generating high financial and social costs (Mendes et al., 2016; Pinto, Pichon-Riviere, & Bardach, 2015; Pressman & Gigliotti, 2011). To deal with this problem, the Brazilian Ministry of Health and the National Cancer Institute (INCA) have developed, among other actions that make up the Brazilian National Tobacco Control Program (such as the 100% smoke-free environment), a free treatment program for smokers who wish to quit smoking. This first-line treatment for smoking cessation is structured in four sessions of cognitive-behavioral approach, followed by monthly maintenance sessions, generally in group modality, although it can also be offered individually (Brasil, 2008; Portes, Machado, & Turci, 2018).

The characterization of the treatment of the smoker in group modality recommended by INCA is of a psychoeducation group, since its objective is to discuss scientifically regarding the aspects related to the nature of the problem, offer information on the treatment, and promote self-knowledge (Neufeld, Maltoni, Ivatiuk, &

Rangé, 2017). Each session has specific objectives to be discussed in terms of theme and participants receive a hornbook at the end of each meeting to read at home and make notes of more particular aspects. Homework assignments are also suggested so that they can continue the work between sessions (Brasil, 2008). The maximum number of participants is 15 smokers per group.

The first session, entitled *Understanding why you smoke and how it affects health,* has three main goals in terms of psychoeducation: to discuss ambivalence, the three types of addictions, and the methods of smoking cessation. In relation to ambivalence, understanding that every psychotropic drug has the potential to be abused because it generates a sense of pleasure (due to its action on the brain's reward circuit) helps to accept that quitting smoking is a difficult process in which there is an oscillation of motivation. Teaching patients to use decision-making techniques, as well as knowing the stages of motivation for change (details on the Transtheoretical model and stages of change can be accessed in Prochaska & DiClemente, 1992 and in Prochaska et al. 1997) can be useful for the decision to quit smoking (Brasil, 2008). The evaluation and understanding of the three types of addiction (physical, psychological, and behavioral) help patients to know themselves about the triggers and factors that maintain their smoking habit and serves as a basis for the therapist to direct the treatment in terms of technique choice (more cognitive or behavioral) and indication of whether or not to use drugs (nicotine replacement) as coadjuvants. Still in the first session, patients are taught two modes of cessation: abrupt stop, in which they choose the "D" day and from there, they do not smoke cigarettes anymore; or gradual stop, which can be carried out by reduction (systematically reduces the number of cigarettes each day until it ceases) or postponement (delays the time of the first cigarette each day until it ceases), so that each patient chooses what best fits his case (Brasil, 2008; Pinto et al., 2015; Portes et al., 2018; Silva et al., 2013).

The objectives of the second session, entitled *Living the first days without cigarettes,* involve psychoeducation actions on the abstinence syndrome and on relaxation techniques. As previously discussed, as patients understand that the discomfort of abstinence has an "expiration date," which tends to gradually reduce and disappear in up to 4 weeks, they feel encouraged to face it more confidently. On the other hand, learning about relaxation techniques can be useful both in times of craving and in other situations that require anxiety management, besides promoting a sense of self-control and self-efficacy in patients (Brasil, 2008; Silva et al., 2013).

In the third session, entitled *Overcoming obstacles to staying smoke-free,* the group's coordinator works on issues related to possible weight gain, making suggestions on low-calorie food intake and on the importance of not replacing cigarettes with sweets. The issue of concomitant use of alcohol and tobacco (including cases of cross-dependence) is also addressed, alerting to the fact that alcoholic beverages can serve as a trigger to craving and to reduce resistance to temptation, facilitating relapse. Besides food and alcohol, the third meeting discussed the physical benefits experienced when quitting smoking, such as improved breath and smell, stimulating the exchange of information between those who have already achieved abstinence and those who are still ambivalent (Brasil, 2008). Silva et al. (2013) add the importance of discussing short- and long-term risks of the drug and the benefits obtained after cessation, seeking to encourage and motivate those who have not yet made the attempt to quit.

The objectives of the fourth and last structured session, entitled *Benefits obtained after quitting smoking*, are fundamentally aimed to value the indirect benefits of quitting, such as improved self-esteem, a feeling of freedom and self-control, and to work on preventing relapse. The most frequent situations and reasons why former smokers return to smoking are presented and discussed. Participants are encouraged to plan, including coping strategies for craving situations. Finally, in the monthly maintenance meetings, the learning obtained during the structured sessions is resumed, valuing the gains of not smoking and seeking to motivate those who relapsed. In addition, the strategies for self-monitoring and confronting the situations predicted as eliciting relapse are reviewed and stimulated, with a view to maintaining abstinence in the long term (Brasil, 2008; Silva et al., 2013).

As verified in studies conducted in Brazil, psychoeducation is a useful strategy both for the treatment of smoking (Brasil, 2008; Polônio, Amaral, Ueda & Carvalho, 2018; Silva et al., 2013) and for alcohol and other drugs (Farina et al., 2013; Lima & Mângia, 2015; Morandi & Guimarães, 2015). The following is a brief case report in which the psychoeducation strategy, among other CBT techniques, was applied in the treatment of a patient with Alcohol Use Disorder.

Clinical Case

Rogério (fictitious name) is a patient who sought therapy on the advice of his mother because she thought her son was losing control over his use of alcohol. He is 46 years old and recently went through a complicated separation after 12 years of marriage. From this union, he has two children, with whom he reported having an ambivalent relationship. When stressed and irritated, he identifies himself as very rigid and intolerant with them, but soon after, he becomes guilty when he perceives himself as rude. He says that the marriage ended because he had no admiration for his wife and also because he was solely responsible for the family's support and, over time, the couple distanced themselves and fights became more and more frequent.

In relation to his professional life, he says that he did business administration and that he "was programmed" to take over the business of the family of origin. His family has a construction company that, according to him, has "excellent income." He started working in the company as a trainee and today has a director position. He says he does not feel as the "owner of the company" because his father is still the president, and the two are very different in the administration.

In the first sessions, Rogério reported episodes of excessive alcohol use in his life. From an early age he liked to drink a lot at parties, always proud to be the last one out. In several situations, he had a bad experience with excessive drinking and there was one episode, at the age of 22, when he suffered a serious accident for driving under the influence of alcohol. After leaving this party where he had drunk too much, he lost control in the direction of a car, which was in excessive speed, and hit a spotlight (the car had total loss). At this moment, psychoeducation on the neurobiological and behavioral effects of alcohol use was performed, explaining that it is a depressor of the central nervous system and, therefore, slows down the cognitive functions necessary to drive, such as attention, perception, and reaction time, among others. When asked about the reasons why he drank too much, he referred that he was always a person who overcharged himself. He needed to be the best student, the best professional, and stand out from his friends to feel better. He said that his father has never paid much attention to him and that he had only approached him to make collections.

He had several girlfriends, but one of them, with whom he dated for seven years, complained about his abusive use of alcohol. His ex-girlfriend did not like it when he drank, arguing that he was very different from the way he was without alcohol. There was even an episode where they argued and he pushed her, culminating in the end of the relationship. Psychoeducation was carried out emphasizing that executive functions such as impulsiveness control and the ability to think about consequences of actions are also abilities that are impaired under the effect of alcohol (and other drugs). Still on the subject of relationships, he mentioned that he met his wife through friends in common and stated that the relationship was good until the birth of his children. The couple loved to travel a lot, and for him, this was a period when he could escape the pressure of work. After the birth of the children, the frequency of travel was much reduced and Rogério became interested in other hobbies, such as poker. In recent times before the separation, he played three to four times a week with a group of friends, and on those evenings they went from dawn to dusk, they even drank more than 1/2 L of whiskey for each member of the table. He said that he lost a lot of money in this period and that his wife asked his family to help him to be in psychiatric treatment. He says that he never accepted the possibility of hospitalization, but that today he realizes that maybe it would have been better. His wife could not stand Rogério's rhythm and asked for a divorce. At this stage of psychotherapy, the issue of cross-dependence and the generalization of impulse uncontrol to other addictive behaviors, such as pathological gambling, was discussed.

Currently the couple shares the custody of their children, who stay in Rogério's apartment one night a week, and every 15 days the whole weekend. He said that he has already forgotten to pick up his children on some weekends and that because of this, his ex-wife is asking for a review of shared custody. He is aware that he likes to drink, especially when he is stressed with his work. He plays poker less often, but makes a daily use of alcohol. When he does not, he gets depressed and feels unproductive, with nausea and headache. He says he starts drinking and cannot stop. However, he has missed several important work meetings by not being able to wake up in the morning. He has not been exercising and is 10 kg over his ideal weight. Currently he has insomnia on average three times a week and is having financial problems because he has been very disorganized with expenses that he does not even know what they are.

Considering all these damages, psychoeducation was carried out regarding the withdrawal symptoms of alcohol and the beneficial factors of physical activity on mood and sleep, seeking to promote self-knowledge. In addition, problem-solving strategies are also being worked on with a view to broadening the repertoire of coping with complex situations and interpersonal skills. According to DSM-5 criteria, Rogério has a severe alcohol use disorder. This is characterized by the presence of an unsuccessful effort to control alcohol use (criterion A2); the need to use alcohol, and much time spent recovering from its effects (criteria A3 and A4); recurrent use resulting in the failure to play important roles (criterion A5); important professional and/or routine activities are abandoned due to alcohol use (criteria A6 and A7), and he presents withdrawal symptoms (criterion A11), for more than 12 months.

In the intermediate sessions, through guided discovery in the therapy, Rogério was able to relate the amount of damage in his live to his alcohol consumption pattern.

This technique allowed the patient to identify connections that seemed very threatening before the psychotherapeutic process. His therapist chose to start the treatment in this way because Rogério was very resistant to abandoning alcohol, as a compensatory strategy that alleviates important core beliefs. Alcohol was perceived as a form of relief from his automatic thoughts related to his disability and devaluation beliefs. Discussing with the patient about these aspects promoted self-knowledge about his way of functioning and reduced resistance.

When carrying out his records of dysfunctional thoughts, he identified that in each situation of difficulty, due to a high self-demand, he needed to resort to alcohol as a form of relief. By sharing his cognitive conceptualization and performing psychoeducation about his addictive beliefs (anticipatory, relief, and permissive), Rogério was able to observe that, since his adolescence, alcohol entered his life as a form of "relief" from the strong activation of his core beliefs and that he uses addictive beliefs to perpetuate its use. He realized how much alcohol was present in his life and gradually replaced it with other activities. Together with his therapist, he searched websites for information on the effects of alcohol use and identified that his disorder was serious. He started looking for physical activities and this provided him with new gratifications such as a change in his weight and physical appearance, as well as an improvement in his relationship with his children. At the academy, he made new friendships and is starting a new relationship. However, the work is still a risky situation because he feels pressured by his father. Currently, Rogério has been in abstinence for 45 days and has been working on how to deal with it, in prevention of relapse. The beliefs of devaluation and disability are partially relaxed and anxiety reduced; however, the need of a psychiatric evaluation for the use of some medication for the symptoms of anxiety and depression, still present in abstinence from alcohol, is not ruled out.

Final Considerations

This chapter presented and discussed how psychoeducation has proven to be a very potent and effective intervention in the therapeutic process, especially with individuals with problems regarding the use of tobacco and alcohol. The application of this strategy allows patients to have knowledge on their information processing and about the consequences of drug use, increasing their autonomy and motivation for the change process.

References

American Psychiatric Association - APA. (2014). *DSM-V: Manual de diagnóstico e estatístico dos transtornos mentais* (5th ed.). Porto Alegre: Artmed.

Beck, J. S. (2013). *Terapia cognitivo-comportamental: Teoria e prática* (2nd ed.). Porto Alegre: Artmed.

Brasil. (2008). *Deixando de Fumar sem mistérios: manual do coordenador. Ministério da Saúde. Secretaria de Atenção à Saúde. Instituto Nacional de Câncer. Coordenação de Prevenção e Vigilância*. Rio de Janeiro: INCA.

Câmara, U. (2019). Tabagismo. In M. R. Carvalho, L. E. N. Malagris, & B. Rangé (Eds.), *Psicoeducação em terapia cognitivo-comportamental* (pp. 177–185). Novo Hamburgo: Synopsys.

Carvalho, M. R., Malagris, L. E. N., & Rangé, B. (2019). Introdução: A psicoeducação na terapia cognitivo-comportamental. In M. R. Carvalho, L. E. N. Malagris, & B. Rangé (Eds.), *Psicoeducação em terapia cognitivo-comportamental* (pp. 15–28). Novo Hamburgo: Synopsys.

Dobson, D., & Dobson, K. S. (2011). Começando o tratamento: Habilidades básicas. In D. Dobson & K. S. Dobson (Eds.), *A terapia cognitivo-comportamental baseada em evidências* (pp. 69–75). Porto Alegre: Artmed.

Farina, M., Terroso, L. B., Lopes, R. M. F., & Argimon, I. I. L. (2013). Importância da psicoeducação em grupos de dependentes químicos: Relato de experiência. *Aletheia, 42*, 175–185.

Foes, V. F. L., Ferreira, L. S., & Paludo, S. S. (2015). Caindo na real: Relato de uma experiência de psicoeducação no tratamento da dependência química. *Revista Saúde e Desenvolvimento Humano, 3*(1), 61–70. https://doi.org/10.18316/2132.

Gigliotti, A., Carneiro, E., & Ferreira, M. (2008). Tratamento do tabagismo. In B. Rangé (Ed.), *Psicoterapias cognitivo-comportamentais: um diálogo com a psiquiatria* (pp. 351–371). Porto Alegre: Artmed.

Knapp, P., & Luz, E. (2008). Terapia cognitivo-comportamental dos comportamentos adictivos. In A. V. Cordioli (Ed.), *Psicoterapias: Abordagens atuais* (3rd ed., pp. 616–640). Porto Alegre: Artmed.

Knapp, P., Luz, E., & Baldisserotto, G. V. (2008). Terapia cognitiva no tratamento da dependência química. In B. Rangé (Ed.), *Psicoterapias cognitivo-comportamentais: um diálogo com a psiquiatria* (pp. 332–350). Porto Alegre: Artmed.

Knijnik, D. Z., & Kunzler, L. S. (2014). Psicoeducação e a reestruturação cognitiva. In W. V. Melo (Ed.), *Estratégias psicoterápicas e a terceira onda em terapia cognitiva* (pp. 24–56). Novo Hamburgo: Sinopsys.

Laranjeira, R. (2014). *II Levantamento Nacional de Álcool e Drogas (LENAD): Relatório 2012.* São Paulo: Instituto Nacional de Ciência e Tecnologia para Políticas Públicas de Álcool e Outras Drogas (INPAD), UNIFESP.

Lemes, C. B., & Ondere Neto, J. (2017). Aplicações da Psicoeducação no Contexto da Saúde. *Temas em Psicologia, 25*(1), 17–28.

Lima, H. A., & Mângia, E. F. (2015). Estratégias grupais voltadas aos familiares de pessoas com necessidades decorrentes do uso de substâncias psicoativas: uma revisão narrativa. *Revista de Terapia Ocupacional da Universidade de São Paulo, 26*(2), 294–300. https://doi.org/10.11606/issn.2238-6149.v26i2p294-300.

Lopes, L. O., & Cachioni, M. (2012). Intervenções psicoeducacionais para cuidadores de idosos com demência: uma revisão sistemática. *Jornal Brasileiro de Psiquiatria, 61*(4), 252–261. https://doi.org/10.1590/S0047-20852012000400009.

Lukens, E. P., & McFarlane, W. R. (2004). Psychoeducation as evidence-based practice: Considerations for practice, research and policy. *Brief Treatment and Crisis Intervention, 4*(3), 205–225. https://doi.org/10.1093/brief-treatment/mhh019.

Marques, M. F. (2016). *Cuidados de natureza psicoeducacional: de que falamos? VII Congresso Internacional ASPESM*. Disponível em https://dspace.uevora.pt/rdpc/handle/10174/23000

Mathias, A. C. R., & Abreu, M. A. (2019). Abuso de substâncias. In M. R. Carvalho, L. E. N. Malagris, & B. Rangé (Eds.), *Psicoeducação em terapia cognitivo-comportamental* (pp. 98–109). Novo Hamburgo: Synopsys.

Mendes, A. C. R., Toscano, C. M., Barcellos, R. M. S., Ribeiro, A. L. P., Ritzel, J. B., Cunha, V. S., & Duncan, B. B. (2016). Custos do programa de tratamento do tabagismo no Brasil. *Revista de Saúde Pública, 50*, 66. https://doi.org/10.1590/s1518-8787.2016050006303.

Menezes, S. L., & Souza, M. C. B. M. (2012). Implicações de um grupo de Psicoeducação no cotidiano de portadores de Transtorno Afetivo Bipolar. *Revista da Escola Enfermagem USP, 46*(1), 124–131. https://doi.org/10.1590/S0080-62342012000100017.

Moraes, P. B., & Boschetti, F. (2013). Técnicas cognitivas. In N. A. Zanelatto & R. Laranjeira (Eds.), *O Tratamento da dependência química e as terapias cognitivo-comportamentais: um guia para terapeutas* (pp. 293–310). Porto Alegre: Artmed.

Morandi, M., & Guimarães, L. P. (2015). Intervenções cognitivo-comportamentais no tratamento das dependências químicas. *Id Online Revista Multidisciplinar e de Psicologia, 9*(25), 203–216. https://doi.org/10.14295/idonline.v9i25.321.

Neufeld, C. B., Maltoni, J., Ivatiuk, A. L., & Rangé, B. (2017). Aspectos técnicos e o processo em TCCG. In C. B. Neufeld & B. P. Rangé (Eds.), *Terapia cognitivo-comportamental em grupos* (pp. 33–56). Porto Alegre: Artmed.

Nogueira, C. A., Crisostomo, K. N., Souza, R. S., & Prado, J. M. (2017). A importância da psicoeducação na terapia cognitivo-comportamental: uma revisão sistemática. *Revista das Ciências da Saúde do Oeste Baiano, 2*(1), 108–120.

Pinto, M. T., Pichon-Riviere, A., & Bardach, A. (2015). Estimativa da carga do tabagismo no Brasil: mortalidade, morbidade e custos. *Cadernos de Saúde Pública, 31*(6), 1283–1297. https://doi.org/10.1590/0102-311X00192013.

Polônio, I. B., Amaral, R. A., Ueda, I. G., & Carvalho, J. B. (2018). Uso da psicoeducação e da respiração profunda para tratamento do tabagismo. *Arquivos Médicos dos Hospitais e da Faculdade de Ciências Médicas da Santa Casa de São Paulo, 63*(3), 168–172. https://doi.org/10.26432/1809-3019.2018.63.3.168.

Ponce, C. C., Ordonez, T. N., Lima-Silva, T. B., dos Santos, G. D., Viola, L. F., Nunes, P. V., Forlenza, O. V., & Cachioni, M. (2011). Effects of a psychoeducational intervention in family caregivers of people with Alzheimer's disease. *Dementia & Neuropsychologia, 5*(3), 226–237. https://doi.org/10.1590/S1980-57642011DN05030011.

Portes, L. H., Machado, C. V., & Turci, S. R. B. (2018). Trajetória da política de controle do tabaco no Brasil de 1986 a 2016. *Cadernos de Saúde Pública, 34*(2). https://doi.org/10.1590/0102-311X00017317.

Pressman, S., & Gigliotti, A. (2011). Nicotina. In A. Diehl et al. (Eds.), *Dependência Química: Prevenção, tratamento e políticas públicas* (pp. 145–160). Porto Alegre: Artmed.

Prochaska, J. O., & DiClemente, C. (1992). Stages of change in the modification of problem behaviors. In M. Hersen, M. Eiser, & W. Miller (Eds.), *Progress in behavior modification* (pp. 184–214). Sycamore: Sycamore Press.

Prochaska, J. O., DiClemente, C., & Norcross, J. C. (1997). Search of how people change: Applications to addictive behavior. In G. A. Marlatt & G. Vandenbos (Eds.), *Addictive behaviors: Readings on etiology, prevention, and treatment* (pp. 671–696). Washington, DC, USA: American Psychological Association.

Rangé, B. P., & Marlatt, G. A. (2008). Terapia Cognitivo-Comportamental de transtornos de abuso de álcool e outras drogas. *Revista Brasileira de Psiquiatria, 30*, S88–S95. https://doi.org/10.1590/S1516-44462008000600006.

Silva, I. F., Ferreira, S. L., & Zanelatto, N. A. (2013). Terapia cognitivo-comportamental aplicada ao tratamento de dependentes de nicotina. In N. A. Zanelatto & R. Laranjeira (Eds.), *O tratamento da dependência química e as terapias cognitivo-comportamentais: um guia para terapeutas* (pp. 503–520). Porto Alegre: Artmed.

Wright, J. H., Basco, M. R., & Thase, M. E. (2008). *Aprendendo a Terapia Cognitivo-comportamental: Um guia ilustrado*. Porto Alegre: Artmed.

Zanelatto, N. A. (2013). Estrutura das sessões: temas centrais. In N. A. Zanelatto & R. Laranjeira (Eds.), *O Tratamento da dependência química e as terapias cognitivo-comportamentais: um guia para terapeutas* (pp. 356–418). Porto Alegre: Artmed.

Chapter 21
Mindfulness for the Treatment of Substance Use Disorders

Vívian Vargas de Barros, Emérita Sátiro Opaleye, Mayra Pires Alves Machado, and Ana Regina Noto

Introduction

The last decades have been marked with an increasing scientific interest from Western countries in an ancient technique of meditation called mindfulness. Curiosity is justified: there is evidence that this practice is associated with wellbeing and symptom relief outcomes in the treatment of a variety of clinical conditions, such as cancer, cardiovascular disease, chronic pain, depression, anxiety, and substance use disorder (SUD) (Gotink et al., 2015). Conceptualized as "paying attention to the present moment intentionally and without judgment" (Kabat-Zinn, 2009), the term mindfulness can be used both to denominate this metacognitive ability above, and the meditative practices used to train this ability (Sauer et al., 2013).

Jon Kabat-Zinn's pioneering work gave rise to the first mindfulness-based intervention (MBI) by systematizing these meditation practices in the mindfulness-based stress reduction (MBSR) program. MBI is characterized by integrating contemplative practices and conventional treatment techniques, preserving relevant elements in health contexts, such as program secularity and scientific evidence. The program must also be offered by a trained professional in the specific MBI. In addition to the technical knowledge required to deliver MBI to specific populations, the teacher must mainly have a sedimented personal mindfulness practice (Crane et al., 2017).

Usually, MBI is offered in groups in weekly meetings with an average of 2 h for 8 weeks. The sessions are structured with practices of mindfulness and psychoeducation directed to the specific population and discussions among participants to exchange experiences. This structured format of the programs, generally described in protocols, enhances the dissemination and implementation of MBI in different cultures and populations (Crane et al., 2017).

V. V. de Barros (✉) · E. S. Opaleye · M. P. A. Machado · A. R. Noto
Universidade Federal de São Paulo, São Paulo, SP, Brazil

D. De Micheli et al. (eds.), *Drugs and Human Behavior*,
https://doi.org/10.1007/978-3-030-62855-0_21

This chapter aims to present a broad, but not conclusive, view on how mindfulness has been useful as an adjunct to SUD treatment. Characteristics of existing MBI are described, especially of what has been worked on in Brazil (such as the mindfulness-based relapse prevention—MBRP), the theories that support the mechanisms by which mindfulness acts in the therapeutic process of SUD, and a brief presentation of the current scientific evidence on the topic, including studies conducted in Brazil.

Mindfulness in the Treatment of Substance Use Disorders

As research on MBI advanced, Bowen and colleagues sought to develop a new MBI to assist as an adjunct in the treatment of SUD, including elements of the Relapse Prevention program designed by Marlatt and Gordon in 1985, culminating with the Mindfulness-Based Relapse Prevention (MBRP) (Bowen, Chawla, & Marlatt, 2015). The MBRP maintained elements of Behavioral and Cognitive Psychology present in the Relapse Prevention program, with the main difference being the principle of acceptance and non-judgment. In contrast, traditional cognitive approaches seek to identify and restructure dysfunctional beliefs and thoughts. Mindfulness practices stimulate attention and acceptance of experiences (sensations, emotions, and thoughts) in challenging situations.

Studies in neurosciences have shown the potential for mindfulness in modifying brain functions involved in regulating attention, emotion, and self-consciousness (Tang, Hölzel, & Posner, 2015). This mechanism of self-regulation underpins the MBRP as mindfulness practices seek to stimulate full attention to triggers, the usual and automatic processes associated with the impulse for substance consumption, and, consequently, the relapse process of people recovering from SUD. The practices also stimulate the ability to pause, observe the present experience, and then understand the range of strategies that can be used to deal with challenging situations (Bowen et al., 2015). Another critical assumption of the program is to encourage a compassionate attitude and self-care, favoring the development of autonomy of individuals who are in the therapeutic process.

Each MBRP session has a specific theme and objective, pursuing to develop full attention skills in a gradual learning logic. The training begins with a practice that invites the participant to experience the usual trend of "autopilot" in contrast to the posture of "awareness" at each experience, moment by moment, without judgment. The first three sessions also aim at integrating mindfulness skills into daily life, stimulating awareness, especially to body sensations. Subsequent sessions deal with the recognition of emotions, thoughts, triggers, and impulses to react, emphasizing the acceptance of the present experience as well as the application of mindfulness practices to prevent relapses. The last two sessions highlight issues of self-care, support networks, and lifestyle balance. Compassionate attitudes, equanimity, empathy, acceptance, and conscious action towards the challenges of daily life and interpersonal relationships are also worked on over the program. The potential contribution of awareness to the treatment of SUD is discussed throughout the program, since the first session (Bowen et al., 2015).

Mindfulness Beyond Relapse Prevention

According to the experience of its creators, the MBRP was planned as an adjunct to the therapeutic process for relapse prevention (Bowen et al., 2015). More recent experiences, however, suggest the relevance of the program throughout the therapeutic process, improving the patient globally and not only in preventing post-treatment relapses (Machado, 2019).

SUD is characterized by the gradual loss of the ability to control substance consumption, associated with a series of comorbidities and vulnerabilities that vary from case to case, and is also accompanied by moral self-judgment and low self-esteem. In this context, mindfulness practices present themselves as a promising alternative to help the recovery process in general.

Within this perspective, Machado (2019), when evaluating the program in different secondary outpatient services named Centers of Psychosocial Attention—Alcohol and Drugs (CAPS-ad) in Brazil, confirmed benefits in several areas of the patients' lives under treatment for SUD, thus suggesting the potential for mindfulness far beyond the prevention of relapses. Such observations have broadened the range of possibilities of using the MBPR in the treatment of SUD.

How Mindfulness Promotes Change: Exploring Mechanisms of Action

To understand the mechanisms of change favored by MBI, it is necessary to return to the concept of mindfulness. Common sense considers the term mindfulness as an ability to pay attention to the present experience. However, this definition is insufficient and may lead to confusion, from a clinical point of view, since it is well known that *Self-Focused Attention* (SFA) is related to worse clinical outcomes, with increased emotional burden, psychological symptoms, and stress. This happens because, as people become aware that they are not doing well, the most common human pattern is to engage in mental rumination, to try to understand why they feel this way. Rumination comes with self-criticism, for there is a tendency to believe that this problem only happens to the person who experiences it and that they should be able to deal with it. Thus, a vicious circle of symptoms, rumination, and self-judgment occurs (Ingram, 1990). Therefore, attention alone is not enough, unless it is accompanied by an attitudinal component, which involves openness, curiosity, acceptance, and non-judgment of the present experience. This is where the most current definition of mindfulness comes in, from which the mechanisms of change will be explained:

> Mindfulness can be defined as a non-judgmental awareness, moment by moment, cultivated by paying attention in a specific way, that is, in the present moment, in a non-reactive way, without judging and with the most open heart as possible (Kabat-Zinn, 2005, p. 108).

Effectively, in the mindfulness approach as described above, when experiencing challenging emotional states, rather than engaging in ruminative or self-critical thoughts like "Why do I feel this way?" or "Why can't I handle it better?", the behavior would be to bring curious attention to how they experience these emotional states in the body; to allow thoughts to come and notice when they go, to observe and let emotions to be present, without rejecting or trying to resolve them. Therefore, both attention and the attitudinal component of non-judgment and non-reactivity are necessary for better clinical outcomes. Secondary analyses of a MBRP clinical trial have demonstrated the efficacy of participation in the program for craving reduction in people with SUD. The researchers evaluated that this association between involvement in the MBRP and craving reduction was mediated by changes in a latent mindfulness factor, defined as acceptance, non-judgment, and consciousness. These isolated components did not correlate with craving reduction (Witkiewitz, Bowen, Douglas, & Hsu, 2013).

Since SUD is complex by nature and requires multidisciplinary understanding and treatment, and since mindfulness involves diverse attentional and attitudinal skills, there are also several ways in which mindfulness can benefit people with SUD. Thus, these mechanisms are studied and described according to the respective theories that underpin the various approaches to this disorder. Therefore, some mechanisms of change from cognitive-behavioral theories will be described here because they are the theoretical basis of the MBRP program. Still, this description is not intended to be exhaustive.

According to the cognitive processing model, drug use is controlled by action plans that are stored in memory and are performed automatically. Thus, this theory suggests that intervention efforts should focus on (1) removing the stimuli that evoke the action plans, or (2) protecting or enhancing the processing resources needed to inhibit the execution of the action plans (Tiffany & Conklin, 2000). Participation in MBI can help individuals become aware of usually automated processes and behaviors. In the case of a person motivated to change their behavior concerning the use of substances, a greater ability to recognize what is present at the moment may favor them to identify more easily that they are about to consume the substance automatically, which in turn will allow them to inhibit the action of using, that is, to regulate automatic behaviors related to use (Tapper, 2018).

Another way to approach these mechanisms is through a radical behaviorism perspective. To review some[1] important concepts from this approach, one can use the example of a person who uses cocaine repeatedly with the same friend when

[1] To see more about the philosophical bases and basic concepts of behavior analysis, we suggest reading Baum (2018), Moreira and Medeiros (2018), Lombard-Platet, Watanabe, and Cassetari (2015), Skinner (2003, 2006), among others. To read more about the application of knowledge and analytical-behavioral technologies to Substance Use Disorders (SUDs), we suggest reading Banaco and Montan (2018) and Garcia-Mijares and Silva (2006).

they are at parties. The *classic* or *respondent conditioning* occurs by the repeated association between the external cue (friend, festive context) and the behavior of using the substance. *Operative conditioning* refers to positive (pleasurable sensations, social approval) and negative (relief of aversive sensations) reinforcements that increase the probability of the behavior occurring again. In SUD, other factors may act as cues (discriminatory stimuli) for the emission of behavior. Since negative affections are significant predictors of relapse, and people usually want to get rid of discomfort, conditioning can also be given by internal cues (private events), such as negative affects that predispose to the behavior of using cocaine. Relief from negative affects (negative reinforcement) explains the continuity of use even when it no longer provides the same level of pleasure due to the development of tolerance in addicts. However, together with the relief of discomfort, the Effect of Abstinence Violation (EVA) occurs, strengthening negative affects, favoring a complete cycle of relapse (Witkiewitz & Villarroel, 2009).

Considering the theoretical bases previously explained, one can understand how mindfulness contributes to this process of body and mind as the environment, following that, regardless of external situations, individuals repeat habitual patterns of thought and behavior. Thus, by understanding these internal patterns, people can extrapolate them to external circumstances. In this sense, the term *interoceptive conditioning* is used to describe the association between internal stimuli and responses (thoughts, emotions, and sensations) with another internal event (e.g., hyperventilation and panic attack) (Bouton, Mineka, & Barlow, 2001). If we consider exposure and desensitization as effective methods of response change, it is also possible to certify this process with internal stimuli (interoceptive exposure). An example of this would be to deliberately generate hyperventilation and observe if a panic attack occurs (Craske & Barlow, 2006). This strategy of interoceptive exposure may promote *decoupling* among the experiences, and it is possible either between two internal experiences, as in the example above, or between an internal experience (being sad) and an external behavior (using cocaine).

Mindfulness can foster this decoupling through curious awareness and non-judgment to the feelings or urges present, without the need to react automatically to this discomfort, allowing the choice of different behavior, which in turn can extinguish the conditioning between a trigger and substance use (Bowen & Marlatt, 2009; Curtiss et al. 2017; Levin, Luoma, & Haeger, 2015).

Still considering the body and mind as the environment, individuals can change their behavior patterns through internal reinforcements. Continuing with the example of the person with cocaine use disorder, imagine that they are sad. With mindfulness training, by recognizing the sadness, they may seek other internal elements that can work as reinforcements, such as noticing the sensations of breathing, allowing them to stay with the discomfort without having to run away from it, which on previous occasions was associated with the behavior of using cocaine to get rid of the sadness. Using systematic training, the very ability to explore discomfort (in this case, sadness) with curiosity can become a positive reinforcement in the sense of recognizing that we are capable of being with something unpleasant without having to run away, increasing the feeling of self-efficacy (Bowen, 2016).

It is a human being's pattern to avoid or escape from uncomfortable situations and stimuli, among them feelings. This process works as negative reinforcement because an aversive stimulus is removed, which in turn increases the probability of this behavior. Mindfulness favors interoceptive exposure, since it encourages the observation of experiences curiously and openly, collaborating to become aware of automatic behavior patterns, that is, of conditioned responses, which are also extrapolated to the external environment, daily life. As an example of this process, suppose that in the practice of mindfulness, an itch is observed in the body and a tendency to scratch it soon to get rid of this discomfort. By observing the experience, it is possible to perceive the urge to move and make a choice between scratching or not. This way, one learns to recognize the tendency to cling to the comfortable or avoid the uncomfortable, in addition to learning a new way to relate to and respond to these stimuli, for example, by creating a space for behavioral choice. With practice, these processes tend to reduce the suffering associated with avoiding discomfort and desire to seek or maintain comfort.

This last point goes back to a fundamental concept of mindfulness, known as acceptance. Acceptance does not refer to resignation or passivity, but a courageous recognition of what is present, so that strategies can be created that are appropriate to the reality that exists at that moment. Learning to deal with what is at stake, without the tendency to want to lock oneself in or get rid of experiences, learning that there are sufficient internal resources to deal with discomfort, which in turn promotes improved mental health. In analytic-behavioral terms, the practice of mindfulness (openly staying with discomfort, without reacting automatically to it) helps to replace the association between previous stimulus and response, through the desensitization that occurs, exposing the individual repeatedly to the interoceptive experience.

Thinking about the medium- and long-term changes provided by mindfulness, which favors a greater sustaining of favorable results in mental health, it is possible to understand what occurs from the point of view of radical behaviorism and behavior analysis. Initially, when people meet direct experiences (thoughts, feelings, and physical sensations), they tend to avoid them because they can be quite uncomfortable. So, the usual tendency for them is to focus on the interpretations, judgments, or ideas they have about these experiences, that is, the reality they create concerning what they live. As this process takes away contact with a potentially aversive initial experience, conditioning occurs to always avoid it (experiential avoidance), by negative reinforcement. As individuals train mindfulness, they recognize more quickly that they are avoiding and no longer want to, because they learn that it is possible to come into contact with discomfort with an attitude of approximation, curiosity, and kindness, allowing themselves actually to see what is annoying and accurately dimension it. Therefore, the behavior of avoidance is no longer reinforcing. When people notice that they are avoiding, they want to go back to what is actually happening because they know that by staying there, they have more chances to act appropriately to respond to the real needs of the moment. This way, this return to direct experience works as positive reinforcement, because they leave a "virtual" reality to a place of protagonist, where, although it may be uncomfortable, they have a chance to act. In conclusion, with the practice of mindfulness, we are reconditioning the behavior according to the Skinnerian principles described above.

Mindfulness for Substance Use Disorders: A Summary of Scientific Evidence

From a scientific point of view, MBI is still incipient in terms of results for SUD. In addition to the challenging research in the SUD field, with a large number of participant losses during follow-up and ethical issues involved, there are also several limitations regarding studies with mindfulness (Davidson & Kaszniak, 2015). There is great difficulty in measuring the quantity and quality of personal practice involved, with questions still open about the role formal or informal practices have on the results (Bowen & Kurtz, 2012). Equally, the very definition of mindfulness is not yet a consensus in many studies, some highlighting the attentional component, while others consider a more multifaceted construct, including elements of non-judgment and non-reactivity. Also, many mechanisms intermediate the relationship between the practice of mindfulness and the desired outcomes, and not all studies investigate this, leaving a gap in the functioning of mindfulness in this context. Although this is not a definitive list of limitations, they do present an idea of the challenges of science in reaching irrevocable conclusions.

The current literature on mindfulness for SUD is encouraging, considering the high rates of recurrence of SUD patients and the growing demand for new approaches in this area. In a 2014 systematic review, with 24 studies comparing different interventions with mindfulness training to control groups for various substances, MBI presented a reduction in the consumption of alcohol, cocaine, methamphetamine, marijuana, tobacco, and opiates to a significantly greater extent than control groups, both active (e.g., other interventions) and inactive (e.g., waiting list). Besides, MBI also showed improvements in psychological outcomes related to substance use, such as depressive symptoms and craving, and increased performance in cognitive tasks (memory, response inhibition, and decision-making) (Chiesa & Serretti, 2014).

The first meta-analysis on mindfulness and TUS was published in 2017 with 42 studies, only one with adolescents and the others with adults, among which 5 were exclusive with women and 4 with men (Li, Howard, Garland, McGovern, & Lazar, 2017). The positive effects of the MBI were consistent throughout the studies, even with different methodologies and modalities, for a diversity of populations, with significant results in reducing the frequency and severity of problematic substance use, craving intensity, and stress severity, when compared with the usual treatment.

Two more recent meta-analyses reinforce MBI's positive findings on SUD. Sancho et al. (2018) included only randomized and controlled clinical trials, but with extensive protocols for mindfulness training, including Yoga, and other addiction outcomes, such as pathological gambling. With 54 studies involving 4916 participants of all ages, the authors conclude that MBI is effective in reducing addiction, craving, and other addiction-related symptoms, as well as reducing symptoms of depression, anxiety, perceived stress, and emotional regulation difficulties. The most frequent interventions were MBRP, mindfulness training for smoking (MTS), mindfulness-oriented recovery enhancement (MORE), acceptance and commitment therapy (ACT), and its variations, as well as different types of Yoga. It should also be noted that the interventions combined with the usual treatments present better results than alone (Sancho et al., 2018). These results were quite similar to those found by Cavicchioli et al. (2018) in a meta-analysis of 37 studies and 3531 patients, who added in relation to the previous study, positive results for outcomes such as negative affects, post-traumatic symptoms, and avoidance-based coping strategies (Cavicchioli, Movalli, & Maffei, 2018).

When the MBRP was the specific analyzed intervention, Grant et al. (2017) through a meta-analysis of 9 studies aggregating 901 participants did not find significant results in favor of the intervention, when compared to control groups for relapses, frequency of use, abandonment of treatment, depressive and anxiety symptoms, and dispositional mindfulness. On the other hand, they found significant improvement in craving outcomes, withdrawal symptoms, and negative consequences of substance use for patients who received MBRP. The authors mention that the small number of research participants makes it difficult to identify a significant difference between the groups. It is also noteworthy that the only study included in this meta-analysis with at least 12-month follow-up was the study by Bowen et al. (2014), which found better results for MBRP compared to conventional relapse prevention only in this period, pointing out that the effects of the intervention may occur in the long term and, therefore, the studies designed so far have not been able to robustly identify these differences regarding the results on substance use, but rather, for a series of outcomes that intermediates the outcomes aspirated by MBRP.

According to current evidence, other factors for the adoption of MBRP in services should be considered if the objective is short-term responses, such as available resources, impact on the global health of participants at the expense of specific purposes of reduction or suppression of consumption, acceptability of the intervention by the patients, and feasibility of implementation (Grant et al., 2017).

Aware of the MBRP's potential, research in Brazil begins with the adaptation of the program and the creation of a research and professional training group in MBRP by the *Universidade Federal de São Paulo*. The first study conducted a pragmatic pilot trial to verify the effectiveness of MBRP as an adjunct to the standard treatment instituted for smoking (protocol of the Cancer Institute—INCA), with randomization of 86 patients. After 6 months of follow-up, the results found no difference between the groups, but in the analysis within each group, the intervention group relapsed less than the control group. The authors emphasize that the high number of dropouts in the study over time limited the analyses, having reached the end with only 19 participants. However, the unprecedented nature of the MBRP investigation into smoking was a high point of the study, in addition to being the first conducted in a Brazilian context (Souza, 2016).

A study evaluating the efficacy of MBRP in insomnia and in reducing the use of hypnotics among women was then carried out, with a follow-up of six months after intervention (Barros, 2017). Because it was the first study aimed at hypnotic dependence, which has characteristics slightly different from other dependencies, for example, the absence of cravings, it was of particular importance for the advancement of knowledge about the MBRP. In addition to preventing relapse, this study tested the efficacy of the program to assist in the process of substance withdrawal. The 70 participants received psychoeducation, after which they were randomized between the intervention group (IG) and the control group (CG), which received telephone follow-up. IG further reduced the dosage of hypnotics compared to CG shortly after the intervention but did not differentiate in other follow-ups. Even so, the reduction continued in the MBRP group until the last measurement, 6 months after the intervention, when there was also a significant improvement in the severity of insomnia and in the reduction of suffering in this group compared to the GC. These results indicate that despite the withdrawal of the drug, the quality of sleep remained more positive in the group that received the intervention, leading the authors to conclude that studies with longer follow-ups may be more sensitive in capturing significant differences between the two groups in terms of withdrawal of the drug.

Promising experiences with smoking and hypnotics excited the next stage of more challenging research in Brazil, with a feasibility study on the implementation of MBRP in reference services for the treatment of SUD, the CAPS-ad. The main results found are described in the section below.

Implementation of MBRP in Clinical Practice in CAPS-Ad and Inpatient Services

When MBRP was performed in outpatient treatment, several challenges were faced, starting with the profile of the very heterogeneous population (from homeless people with high dependency severity to people with upper schooling and less severe condition), and which impact in different ways on the development of the approach. These different profiles lead to different treatment demands and an impact on the regularity of outpatient attendance. Thus, the MBRP format with weekly meetings of two hours duration and structured content transmitted in each session ends up being more demanding for those who are unable to attend all the sessions, discouraging continuity when they miss one or another session (Fig. 21.1).

Still, concerning the structure of the MBRP, two other factors that configure higher demand are the amount of content in each session and the duration time. By bringing a new paradigm of approaching discomfort as opposed to the strategy of using substances to avoid it, there is a need to work on these contents more slowly and gradually, facilitating assimilation and consolidation of learning. Additionally, the two hours of each session exceed the usual duration of groups and activities in most outpatient settings, requiring efforts for concentration, tolerance, discipline, and organization of participants. Considering also the inherent challenges of the meditation process, such as drowsiness, physical and mental restlessness, difficulty

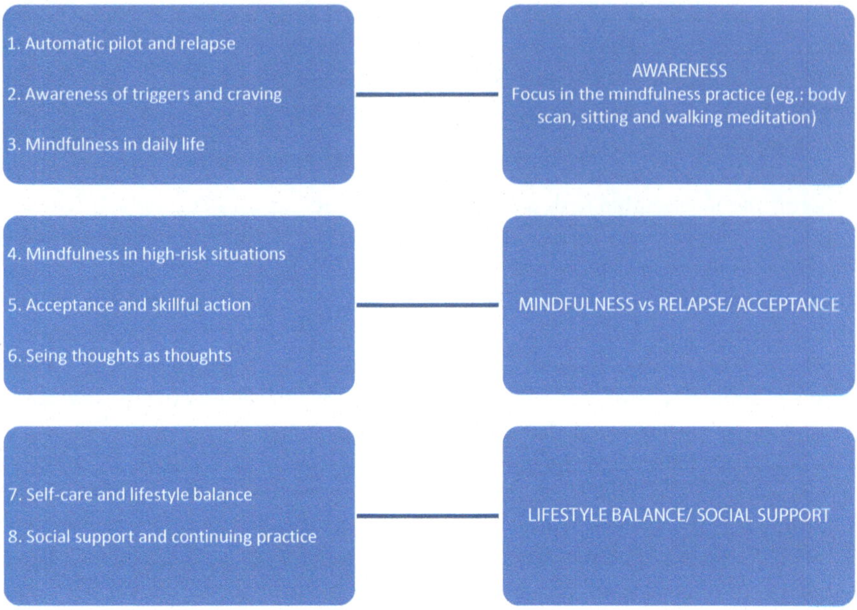

Fig. 21.1 Basic structure of the MBRP sessions

to connect with the body and mind openly and curiously, and resistance to uncomfortable experiences, shorter sessions may be more suitable for this population who, in general, are conditioned to impatience, immediacy, and intolerance to states such as mind-wandering and agitation.

Despite the challenges mentioned, when participants manage to engage in the proposed activities, they report several benefits, also perceived by the professionals who accompany them. Figure 21.2 summarizes the reports, both on aspects related to the development of mindfulness components (such as attention and attitudes) and related skills (such as self-compassion) and emotional and behavioral outcomes, including those related to substance use.

For these reasons, the adaptation of the program to a rolling and open format, in which participants can enter any session, is indicated, being more in line with other outpatient treatment interventions. It would favor that a more significant number of people participate in MBRP groups, also contributing to the development of autonomy for the execution of activities among sessions and continuity after treatment, ensuring long-term benefits. Currently, this format is being tested to happen in rolling cycles of 12 sessions with a length of an hour and a half, and participants can repeat them as many times as they wish.

However, rolling groups is not the case in long-term admission settings, since participants already remain at the treatment sites and do not face the logistical challenges related to treatment compliance. Provided that it is not offered to people in the initial detoxification phase, the original MBRP format seems to be quite adequate in this environment, favoring even adherence to treatment as a whole and interpersonal relationships within the institution.

Higher awareness of self and the present moment	Notice autopilot and have greater clarity of their actions	Acceptance of themselves and that the suffering they face is part of common shared humanity	Higher self-esteem, self-efficacy, and self-care
Cognitive defusion	Reduction in anxiety symptoms	Decrease and better control of irritation/aggression	Reduction in interpersonal conflicts
More calm and patience	An increased repertoire of significant and healthier activities	Sleep improvement	Greater awareness and management of triggers
	Ability to "stay with" the discomfort (non-reactivity)	Skillful actions related to their real needs	

Fig. 21.2 Perceptions of changes reported as benefits by people with SUD that received MBRP in CAPS-ad

Finally, there is still resistance in this population to different therapeutic approaches, in a culture quite "medicalocentric." This is a relevant barrier for people to initiate the MBRP, especially when there is a social representation that meditation is aimed at people of higher social class, calmer and "Zen" with healthy food, and practitioners of physical activity—that is, the opposite of the perception that people with SUD have of themselves. In this sense, the awareness of professionals for the application of the MBRP is fundamental, considering that many clients participate due to the encouragement of those responsible for their treatment, trusting their judgment.

However, the main barrier to the implementation and dissemination of the MBRP in public services is the professional training of MBRP. As with other IBMs, part of the professional training of the MBRP involves immersion retreats, which, despite favoring the personal practice of the instructors, makes the process more expensive and challenging to organize for the professionals. Generally, these services have already reduced staff in the face of the high demand for work. Therefore, it was also necessary to adapt the format of this training, so that it takes into consideration the challenges pointed out and guarantees its quality, especially related to the personal practice of the trainer.

Final Considerations

The MBRP is an intervention with sufficient scientific evidence to encourage its use as an adjunct to the treatment of SUD, and it has been identified that it can be implemented in different treatment contexts in Brazil, expanding the repertoire of therapeutic strategies. Applied in conjunction with other approaches, the MBRP can bring significant benefits to this population, especially concerning a recovering as a whole and not only focused on the drug relationship. The incentive to research in Brazil is of paramount importance to better adapt and disseminate this intervention.

References

Banaco, R., & Montan, R. (2018). Teoria analítico-comportamental. In N. Zanelatto & R. Laranjeira (Eds.), *O tratamento da dependência química e as terapias cognitivo-comportamentais: um guia para terapeutas* (2nd ed., pp. 115–132). Porto Alegre: Artmed.

Barros, V. V. (2017). Efeitos de Mindfulness no Padrão de Uso Crônico de Hipnóticos e na Insônia entre Mulheres Insones que Buscam por Tratamento (Doctoral dissertation, Universidade Federal de São Paulo, São Paulo, Brazil).

Baum, W. (2018). *Compreender o behaviorismo: Comportamento, cultura e evolução* (3rd ed.). Porto Alegre: Artmed.

Bouton, M. E., Mineka, S., & Barlow, D. H. (2001). A modern learning theory perspective on the etiology of panic disorder. *Psychological Review, 108*, 4–32. https://doi.org/10.1037/0033-295X.108.1.4.

Bowen, S. (2016, May). *Integrating contemporary behaviorist and traditional contemplative approaches: Towards an effective technology of behavior change*. In Oral communication presented at the International Symposium for Contemplative Studies of the Mind and Life Institute, San Diego.

Bowen, S., Chawla, N., & Marlatt, G. A. (2015). *Prevenção de Recaída Baseada em Mindfulness para comportamentos aditivos: um guia para o clínico*. Rio de Janeiro: Cognitiva.

Bowen, S., & Kurz, A. S. (2012). Between-session practice and therapeutic alliance as predictors of mindfulness after mindfulness-based relapse prevention. *Journal of Clinical Psychology, 68*(3), 236–245. https://doi.org/10.1002/jclp.20855.

Bowen, S., & Marlatt, A. (2009). Surfing the urge: Brief mindfulness-based intervention for college student smokers. *Psychology of Addictive Behaviors, 23*(4), 666–671. https://doi.org/10.1037/a0017127.

Bowen, S., Witkiewitz, K., Clifasefi, S. L., Grow, J., Chawla, N., Hsu, S. H., & Larimer, M. E. (2014). Relative efficacy of mindfulness-based relapse prevention, standard relapse prevention, and treatment as usual for substance use disorders: A randomized clinical trial. *JAMA Psychiatry, 71*(5), 547–556. https://doi.org/10.1001/jamapsychiatry.2013.4546.

Cavicchioli, M., Movalli, M., & Maffei, C. (2018). The clinical efficacy of mindfulness-based treatments for alcohol and drugs use disorders: A meta-analytic review of randomized and nonrandomized controlled trials. *European Addiction Research, 24*(3), 137–162. https://doi.org/10.1159/000490762.

Chiesa, A., & Serretti, A. (2014). Are mindfulness-based interventions effective for substance use disorders? A systematic review of the evidence. *Substance Use & Misuse, 49*(5), 492–512. https://doi.org/10.3109/10826084.2013.770027.

Crane, R. S., Brewer, J., Feldman, C., Kabat-Zinn, J., Santorelli, S., Williams, J. M. G., & Kuyken, W. (2017). What defines mindfulness-based programs? The warp and the weft. *Psychological Medicine, 47*(6), 990–999. https://doi.org/10.1017/S0033291716003317.

Craske, M., & Barlow, D. (2006). Transtorno de pânico e agorafobia. In D. Barlow (Ed.), *Manual clínico dos transtornos psicológicos – Tratamento passo a passo* (pp. 1–30). Porto Alegre: Artmed.

Curtiss, J., Klemanski, D. H., Andrews, L., Ito, M., & Hofmann, S. G. (2017). The conditional process model of mindfulness and emotion regulation: An empirical test. *Journal of Affective Disorders, 212*, 93–100. https://doi.org/10.1016/j.jad.2017.01.027.

Davidson, R. J., & Kaszniak, A. W. (2015). Conceptual and methodological issues in research on mindfulness and meditation. *American Psychologist, 70*(7), 581–592. https://doi.org/10.1037/a0039512.

Garcia-Mijares, M., & Silva, M. (2006). Dependência de drogas. *Psicologia USP, 17*(4), 213–240.

Gotink, R. A., Chu, P., Busschbach, J. J. V., Benson, H., Fricchione, G. L., & Hunink, M. G. M. (2015). Standardised mindfulness-based interventions in healthcare: An overview of systematic reviews and meta-analyses of RCTs. *PLoS ONE, 10*(4), e0124344. https://doi.org/10.1371/journal.pone.0124344.

Grant, S., Colaiaco, B., Motala, A., Shanman, R., Booth, M., Sorbero, M., & Hempel, S. (2017). Mindfulness-based relapse prevention for substance use disorders. *Journal of Addiction Medicine, 11*(5), 386–396. https://doi.org/10.1097/ADM.0000000000000338.

Ingram, R. E. (1990). Self-focused attention in clinical disorders: Review and a conceptual model. *Psychological Bulletin, 107*(2), 156–176. https://doi.org/10.1037/0033-2909.107.2.156.

Kabat-Zinn, J. (2005). *Coming to our senses: Healing ourselves and the world through mindfulness*. New York: Hyperion.

Kabat-Zinn, J. (2009). Full catastrophe living: How to cope with stress, pain and illness using mindfulness meditation. Delta.

Levin, M. E., Luoma, J. B., & Haeger, J. A. (2015). Decoupling as a mechanism of change in mindfulness and acceptance: A literature review. *Behavior Modification, 39*(6), 870–911. https://doi.org/10.1177/0145445515603707.

Li, W., Howard, M. O., Garland, E. L., McGovern, P., & Lazar, M. (2017). Mindfulness treatment for substance misuse: A systematic review and meta-analysis. *Journal of Substance Abuse Treatment, 75*, 62–96. https://doi.org/10.1016/j.jsat.2017.01.008.

Lombard-Platet, V., Watanabe, O., & Cassetari, L. (2015). *Psicologia experimental: manual teórico e prático de análise do comportamento*. São Paulo: Edicon.

Machado, M. P. A (2019). Mindfulness adjunto ao tratamento ambulatorial de transtornos por uso de substâncias (Doctoral dissertation, Universidade Federal de São Paulo, São Paulo, Brazil).

Moreira, M., & Medeiros, C. (2018). *Princípios básicos de análise do comportamento* (2nd ed.). Porto Alegre: Artmed.

Sancho, M., De Gracia, M., Rodríguez, R. C., Mallorquí-Bagué, N., Sánchez-González, J., Trujols, J., & Menchón, J. M. (2018). Mindfulness-based interventions for the treatment of substance and behavioral addictions: A systematic review. *Frontiers in Psychiatry, 9*, 95. https://doi.org/10.3389/fpsyt.2018.00095.

Sauer, S., Walach, H., Schmidt, S., Hinterberger, T., Lynch, S., Büssing, A., & Kohls, N. (2013). Assessment of mindfulness: Review on state of the art. *Mindfulness, 4*(1), 3–17. https://doi.org/10.1007/s12671-012-0122-5.

Skinner, B. F. (2003). *Ciência e comportamento humano*. São Paulo: Martins Fontes.

Skinner, B. F. (2006). *Sobre o behaviorismo*. São Paulo: Cultrix.

Souza, I. C. W. (2016). Avaliação da efetividade do programa de Mindfulness-Based Relapse Prevention (MBRP) como estratégia adjunta ao tratamento da dependência de tabaco (Doctoral dissertation, Universidade Federal de São Paulo, São Paulo, Brasil). Retrieved from https://www.repositorio.unifesp.br/handle/11600/47303

Tang, Y., Hölzel, B., & Posner, M. (2015). The neuroscience of mindfulness meditation. *Nature Reviews Neuroscience, 16*(4), 213–225.

Tapper, K. (2018). Mindfulness and craving: Effects and mechanisms. *Clinical Psychology Review, 59*, 101–117. https://doi.org/10.1016/j.cpr.2017.11.003.

Tiffany, S. T., & Conklin, C. A. (2000). A cognitive processing model of alcohol craving and compulsive alcohol use. *Addiction, 95*(8 Suppl 2), 145–153. https://doi.org/10.1080/09652140050111717.

Witkiewitz, K., Bowen, S., Douglas, H., & Hsu, S. H. (2013). Mindfulness-based relapse prevention for substance craving. *Addictive Behaviors, 38*(2), 1563–1571. https://doi.org/10.1016/j.addbeh.2012.04.001.

Witkiewitz, K., & Villarroel, N. A. (2009). Dynamic association between negative affect and alcohol lapses following alcohol treatment. *Journal of Consulting and Clinical Psychology, 77*(4), 633–644. https://doi.org/10.1037/a0015647.

Part IV
Public Policies Interventions

Chapter 22
Drug Use and Trafficking and the Criminal Liability of Court-Involved Youth

Marcelo Mayora Alves

Introduction

In this chapter we will deal with the relationships between the use and trade of drugs currently considered illegal in Brazil and the criminal responsibility of adolescents in conflict with the law. Before entering into the specific theme, it is necessary to make some introductory remarks which will be seen below.

The use of psychoactive substances is a historical invariant, in that it was present in all cultures known until today (Escohotado 2008). Drugs were used as religious, mystical, magical instruments, as medicines, as facilitators of interaction and communication, as recreational tools, as an escape from reality, as an aid to increase productivity, etc. Throughout history they have found multiple senses attributed to drug consumption, from the toxic practices of the artists of the *fin de siecle* (opium, hashish), to the "counter-culture" of the 1960s (LSD, marijuana), to the "crisis of counter-culture," which was accompanied by the consumption of heroin by the deviant *junkies of the* 1980s and cocaine by the *yuppies* of the financial bourgeoisie, reaching the consumption of *ecstasy* in the context of the youth festivals of the privileged classes and of crack in the scenes of extreme emotional misery; all of this without taking into account the abundant contemporary consumption of licit and as such socially accepted drugs, such as alcohol and other drugs, as well as without entering into the practices of substance use of traditional populations.

At a certain moment, recent in historical terms (a little over 100 years), numerous countries, due to geopolitical, economic, and moral factors, decided to ban some types of narcotic substances, thus producing crimes and criminalizations, starting the so-called war on drugs. This prohibitionist decision was concretized in United Nations Conventions, which guide and determine the policies on drugs that the member countries must adopt. The prohibitionist regime basically establishes that

M. M. Alves (✉)
Universidade Federal do Pampa (Unipampa), Santana do Livramento, RS, Brazil

D. De Micheli et al. (eds.), *Drugs and Human Behavior*,
https://doi.org/10.1007/978-3-030-62855-0_22

the drugs considered illicit must be fought by means of repressive measures. This strategy has been operationalized by police forces, in general militarized, that have real war apparatuses, used with the objective of seizing these products and arresting people who participate at some point in the network of production, circulation, and trade.

From this idea, some substances were made illegal, resulting in a clandestine market and a state apparatus (police, judiciary, and prison), supposedly designed to combat these drugs. Others, however, remained legal, such as alcohol and tobacco. The reasons for the differentiation between licit and illicit can be understood from a genealogy of prohibitions, since the decision regarding the legal fate of each substance is not necessarily based on scientific evidence, depending on numerous variables. It is also important to point out that the legal *status of* drugs—that is, their control regime—changes over time. Alcohol, for example, was banned in North American territory between 1919 and 1932; marijuana, prohibited and demonized during the twentieth century, has been undergoing a gradual legalization and regulation, a situation that is already a reality in countries like Canada and Uruguay. In short, the question that should guide rigorous reflection is the following: why are certain psychoactive substances with the potential to generate harm to the user's health considered licit or illicit?

Nowadays, the use of drugs, licit or illicit, is a phenomenon spread by society. The consumption of psychoactive substances reaches all social classes and all age groups. However, the senses and consequences of the practices vary according to the context in which the use occurs. According to Bourgois (2004, p. 95), "the pharmacological qualities of drugs are virtually insignificant outside their political-economic and sociocultural contexts". Therefore, an analysis that aims to deal generically with the use of a certain substance will suffer from relevant limitations, because the reflection on the subject requires contextualizing it.

One of the most important elements is class position. The trajectories of life and consumption tend to diversify according to the economic, cultural, and social capital of the subjects and their families, so that even if people use the same drug, in the same dose, the social effects will be different, since the social context is also different. Another important variable is the age group. Early onset of consumption is one of the factors that can contribute to the development of problematic consumption.[1] Furthermore, young people are more vulnerable to the seductions of drug advertising, whether expressed, as in the case of alcohol, or implicit, derived mainly from prohibition, which glamorizes—by making the use of psychoactive substances synonymous with rebellion.

> The almost childish attitude of the promoters of prohibition is really unacceptable because, ignoring the phenomena of collective psychology, they end up inducing in young people an

---

[1] Drug use can be unproblematic or problematic. The first are those controlled from self-management and that occupy a mere space in the sphere of the subject's other affective concerns, but that do not become the protagonists of his existence. The second are those who end up generating the breaking of the bonds of the consumer with his interpersonal network, disintegrating his affective bonds, and disturbing his other daily activities.

> attitude contrary to what they preach. Censorship, far from diminishing the consumer's desire, increases it. For it happens in open societies that the arguments of authority cause an undesirable change in the behavior of the public, setting in motion a mechanism of denial that leads to reinforcing precisely the option that official censorship puts under suspicion. Therefore, banning drug use and penalizing it is an effective mechanism to spread abuse behavior and reinforce the dynamics of compulsion. (Restrepo 2004, p. 109).

Knowing the number of drug users, licit or illicit, is a methodological challenge. This is because estimating this data requires information from the user himself, who is sometimes afraid to reveal his practice, especially when it is a criminal activity. The issue becomes even more complicated when we are dealing with data related to children and adolescents, due to ethical limitations regarding research. Therefore, statistics on this subject should be read and understood with caution. In fact, in this field, qualitative research is essential because it has a greater capacity to penetrate the universe of consumption and the consumer.

In any case, we can cite two reliable studies on the subject, which sought to estimate the number of drug users in Brazil, in different dimensions. The National Survey on Drug Use among Children and Adolescents in Brazil in Street Situations in the 27 Brazilian Capitals from the partnership of the then National Anti-Drug Secretariat with the Brazilian Center for Information on Psychotropic Drugs (2003) is the first to be cited. Based on a methodologically validated sample, the research demonstrated, among other data, that the substances most consumed by children and adolescents in street situation are tobacco (52.5%—use in the year), alcohol (62.4%—use in the year), and solvents (36.8%—use in the year). As for alcohol, beer is more consumed, and as for solvents, shoemaker's glue. Research also showed that the main form of acquisition of these substances was the personal purchase in commerce, which is forbidden to traders and configures the crime provided in art. 243 of the Statute of the Child and Adolescent ([ECA], Law No. 8.069 1990). Regarding illicit drugs, marijuana is the most consumed substance (32.1%—use in the year), followed by cocaine in the aspirated form (9.5%—use in the year) and crack (8.6%—use in the year). Finally, it is worth mentioning that the data inform that 44% of children and adolescents reported attempts to stop or reduce their use and, in these cases, 24.8% tried alone, without any kind of help.

The VI National Survey on the Consumption of Psychotropic Drugs among Primary and High School Students in the Public and Private Education Networks in the 27 Brazilian Capitals investigated the same topic, but based on research conducted among students from public and private schools in Brazilian capitals. In summary, the study concluded that "alcohol and tobacco are the drugs with the highest prevalence of use in life, in all capitals, followed by inhalants" and that "crack is not a prominent drug among students" (Brazilian Center for Information on Psychotropic Drugs 2012). According to the study, alcohol was the most consumed substance by students (42.4% use per year), followed by tobacco (9.6% use per year), solvents (5.2% use per year), marijuana (3.7% use per year), anxiolytics (2.6% use per year), cocaine (1.8% use per year), and crack (0.4% use per year). In addition, the study showed that students in private schools had a higher prevalence of drug use (use in life and last year), but those in public schools had higher rates of heavy use, when compared to those in private schools. Finally, the study concluded that there was a decrease in consumption, from a comparison with an identical survey conducted in 2004, with the exception of cocaine consumption, which showed a slight increase. Another interesting conclusion concerns the fact found that Brazilian students are not among those who use drugs the most, when compared with students from South America, Europe, and North America.

Similarly, several studies show a high rate of drug use by adolescents who comply with socio-educational measures in a regime of deprivation of liberty. Silva (2010, p. 128) analyzed 2691 cases and found the following results regarding drug use, 76.9% reported alcohol use, 64.8% cigarette use, 63.2% marijuana use, 30.1% cocaine use, 28.8% solvent use, 6.2% crack, and 2.2% used other psychoactive drugs. Of the 2691 interviewed, only 7.2% said they do not use drugs and 8.2% claimed they had already done some anti-drug treatment. Nardi et al. (2014) survey, which had a sample of 143 adolescents deprived of their liberty in Porto Alegre/RS, showed similar data.

It is important to emphasize that this type of investigation lacks methodological limitation, since the sample is made up of adolescents already selected by the socio-educational system, which occurs according to color and class variables. Thus, the data indicate only that the rate of drug use is higher among imprisoned adolescents than among adolescents in school situation, but it is not possible to conclude that drug use is a "cause" of infraction acts.

Therefore, poor teenagers are the most vulnerable to drug risks. In the first place, because of the chances of developing a problematic consumption and because of the difficulties they will encounter when seeking treatment. Secondly, and mainly, because of the chance of involvement in drug trafficking, which will tend to lead to incarceration or lethal victimization, as we will see.

Illicit Drugs and Court-Involved Youth

Brazil's current criminal drug policy is based on the so-called ideology of differentiation, which consists of establishing distinct punitive responses to drug possession (carrying drugs for personal use) and drug trafficking. The Brazilian legal system is one of the few that still criminalizes possession for personal use. In this case, the law establishes non-carceral penalties—verbal warning, community service, and therapeutic measures. For drug-trafficking cases, the Drug Act (Law No. 11.343 2006) establishes higher penalties, from 5 to 15 years of imprisonment.

In Brazil, teenagers between 12 and 18 years old are not held criminally responsible. They are, however, held accountable when they violate criminal law. The ECA (1990) establishes that when an adolescent engages in a conduct prescribed by adult law as a crime, they are considered to commit an infraction (*ato infracional*), and their punishment is called a Socio-Educational Measure (*Medida Socioeducativa*, MSE).

Article 112 of the ECA (1990) lists the following MSEs: verbal warning; damage compensation; community service; probation; "semi-liberty" custody; full custody (imprisonment); protection measures. When choosing an MSE, judges shall analyze the adolescent's compatibility with the measure, as well as the circumstances and seriousness of the infraction committed. In addition, judges should consider some principles, such as " [the adolescent's] full protection and best interests," as well as "proportionality [between offense and punishment], and minimum intervention." When making a decision, judges also may "take into account the [pre-sentence] report about the adolescent produced by a qualified professional" (Cornelius 2018, p. 71).

These MSEs may be imposed at the end of the procedure, after a trial, or at its beginning, as a diversion measure (remissão) (Law No. 8069 1990). In the latter case, however, only non-custodial MSEs may be imposed. This diversion measure is a form of conditional pardon granted by the Public Prosecutor's Office, according to the circumstances and consequences of the fact, as well as to the personality of the adolescent and his/her greater or lesser participation in the infraction.

Drug Use and Adolescents in Conflict with the Law

One of the main problems of the normative framework currently adopted by Brazil is the differentiation between the hypotheses of trafficking and possession. This is because the law does not set objective criteria, but merely states that in order to determine whether possession is for personal consumption, the judge must take into account the nature and quantity of the substance, the place where the action took place, the social and personal circumstances, the conduct and background of the subject caught. This normative vacuum results in selectivity, since the tendency is for the decision to occur based on variables of color and social class. For example: a young black man, living in the periphery, caught with 10 g of cocaine will probably be considered a trafficker, while a young white man, of middle class, caught with the same substance, in the same amount, will probably be considered a user. This is the trend, abundantly demonstrated by criminological studies (Batista 2003; Carvalho 2016; Mayora 2009).

As has already been clarified, the system of accountability of adolescents does not establish determined sentences, but MSEs should be applied according to the judge's analysis, based on relatively open criteria. There is only one overriding limitation, namely the impossibility of applying the detention measure (deprivation of liberty) in cases in which there was no violence or serious threat, repeated commission of other serious infractions, or unjustified non-compliance with previously imposed measures (Law No. 8069 1990). Thus, accountability for an infraction equated with a drug use offense does not allow for deprivation of liberty of the adolescent.

> It is contrary to the legal system, for subverting the principle of full protection of the unaccountable minor, to impose on the adolescent - who eventually commits an infraction consistent with own consumption of drugs - the extraordinary measure of internment, because not even the person over eighteen years of age, imputable, can suffer the deprivation of liberty due to transgression of art. 28 of Law No. 11343/2006 (Habeas Corpus 124682/SP, Reporting Justice Celso de Melo, judged on 16/12/2014)

What socio-educational measures are usually applied in the case of an adolescent who has responded to a lawsuit for an infraction equivalent to drug use? There are no official data, but it can be said that in general remission is granted, sometimes without any MSE, other times with the application of a warning, community service, or assisted freedom. It has also been common in these cases to apply projects of the so-called Therapeutic Justice, which consists of imposing compulsory treatment on adolescent drug users, based on the application of a protective social-educational measure, which allows the inclusion of the young person in an official or community program of assistance, guidance, and treatment to alcoholics and drug addicts (Law No. 8069 1990). According to Carvalho, Therapeutic Justice

> It re-edits the sanitary perspective in which the drug user is invariably seen as sick, endowed with the attribute of 'dangerousness' and establishes moralizing and normalized guidelines of authoritarian penal models based on dangerousness. (2016, p. 370).

According to the author,

> Common practices of therapeutic interventions such as mandatory laboratory testing to verify drug use, requiring regular and punctual attendance at therapy sessions, satisfactory work or school performance and abstinence from drug use are offensive to individual rights and guarantees, especially the dimensions of intimacy and private life. (2016, p. 370).

Silva (2010), in a research already mentioned, provides some clues on the issue. Based on quantitative analysis in records of infraction acts that occurred in Belo Horizonte/MG showed that in cases of drug use infraction, the decisions taken at the preliminary hearing are the following: dismissal (4.1%); remission (18.5%); remission with warning (36.5%); remission with community service (8.1%); remission with assisted release (7.9%); provisional admission (4.9%); continuity of the process (11.5%); others (15.4%).

As can be seen, there is a great variety of responses and the reprimand will vary according to the political-criminal conceptions of the judge and the other judicial actors who act in a given juvenile court, as well as according to the profile of the adolescent offender.

Drug Trafficking and Adolescents in Conflict with the Law

The prohibition of some drugs and the existence of users of such products have generated a vigorous clandestine market, with a transnational character. This clandestine economy of prohibited drugs is formed by a network of agents that occupy different positions of power, from the tip of production, through exportation/import and circulation until the arrival to the retail trade, which makes it possible for the consumer to acquire them.

In Brazil and in Latin America in general, retailing is operated on the outskirts of cities (towns, favelas), in places whose names vary in the different regions of the country ("boca de fumo," "biqueira," etc.), and its main agent is vulnerability. In this context, adolescents belonging to the working classes, excluded from the labor market, become involved in the illicit drug trade.

The business of retailing illicit drugs flourished in the 1970s after the spread of marijuana and cocaine consumption among the middle classes. From then on, an organizational structure was formed that is similar throughout the country, composed of the "owner" or "boss" of the mouth, the "managers," the "vapors and airplanes" (direct sellers)," the "rocketmen," and the "soldiers" (Misse, 2006, p. 193). This entire structure is composed, in general, of young people in situations of social vulnerability, but adolescents, under 18 years of age, participate in this scenario in the position of *mere servants of narco-trafficking*, to remember the expression of Caetano Veloso, or as *shareholders of nothing* (Zaconne 2007), occupying subordinate and high-risk positions (informants, airplanes, vapores, soldiers). The risks involve both the possibility of lethal victimization, in the context of *wars* against rival groups and the *settling of scores* within the group itself, as well as prison/internity, since the current drug policy fundamentally incarcerates the subject at the weakest end of the illicit drug economy.

The involvement of adolescents in drug trafficking stems from several factors. Firstly, because of class position and the limited chances of access to the formal market, which has contributed significantly to this adolescent finding work and income in the illicit activity. Secondly, in the face of the search for social recognition, which is a very scarce asset in this context. A youth who suffers from prejudiced looks and attitudes of rejection throughout life finds in drug trafficking a chance to affirm their own identity based on the possibility of displaying symbols of consumption proper to the upper classes, as well as through the affirmation of a type of masculinity that has been called *etos guerreiro* (Zaluar 2012), based on the notions of courage and fearlessness, the cult of violence and weapons, and the construction of an "other" to be fought, the enemy, which produces relationships of trust within the group itself.

> Experience in trafficking structures 'work' routines from relationships of trust. The turnover is high and profit allows the more progress in the structure of the business, access to the goods most coveted by young people, for example, clothes 'branded' ('to walk tidy'), cars, motorcycles and fun. [...] "We inside the periphery don't have many examples, nobody likes study very much. Our reference is those people on the street corner selling drugs, because they're wearing brand-name sneakers, with the pretty T-shirt, they're so wearing the cap that we wanted to wear. They so much with the girls all around them, because they have money, so that's our reference". (Rolim 2016, p. 182).

It is essential to stress that the retailing of illicit substances is not the monopoly of poor youth. Even middle-class youth combine their uses with sales. It is quite common for an adolescent of a given group to be responsible for buying a certain amount in the peripheral retail and then share it with his friends and acquaintances, sometimes charging some kind of premium, conduct that also characterizes an infraction of drug trafficking.

The characteristics of the peripheral retail market, criminalized, are in the genesis of the high rate of homicides displayed by Brazil, whose agents and victims are mostly adolescents and young people in vulnerable situations. On the one hand, the establishment of points of sale has required the practice of dominating territories, which has led to the need to dispute and protect them, through the use of weapons, a factor that has triggered real wars and a high rate of lethal conflicts, both among the participants in the illegal market themselves and by the police, on the pretext of combating drug trafficking. On the other hand, the organization of sales occurs, in general, through the delivery of the product on consignment: after the sale, the seller must deliver the money collected to the hierarchical superior. When there is some kind of *vacillation* in this flow the punishment can be death. These structural elements combine with the existence of an agent willing to practice extreme violence, due to a specific type of socialization, characterized by coexistence from early childhood with abandonment and mistreatment (Rolim 2016).

According to the latest Atlas of Violence (Institute of Applied Economic Research, Brazilian Forum of Public Security 2019, p. 25), the premature death of young people (15–29 years old) by homicide is a phenomenon that has grown in Brazil since the 1980s. According to the aforementioned study, in 2017, 35,783 youths were murdered in Brazil. This number represents the equivalent of 69.9 homicides for every 100,000 young people in the country, a record rate in the last 10 years. Homicides were the cause of 51.8% of the deaths of youths aged 15–19. It is important to mention that the rate of 69.9 homicides for every 100,000 youths in the country is significantly higher than the general rate of 31.1 homicides for every 100,000 inhabitants.

Poor adolescents involved in the illicit drug trade are also very likely to end up deprived of their freedom. Article 122, I, of the ECA (1990) provides that a measure of confinement in an educational establishment (deprivation of liberty in a closed regime) can only be applied in the face of an infraction committed with serious threat or violence to the person. Therefore, in thesis it would not be possible to apply this measure to cases of infraction equivalent to drug trafficking. However, it is quite common for magistrates to apply the MSE of internment in this type of case. Faced with the controversy, the Superior Court of Justice edited the precedent 492, which states that the infraction act analogous to drug trafficking, by itself, does not necessarily lead to the imposition of a socio-educational measure of internment of the adolescent. In fact, the STJ has endorsed the interpretation against the law that has been used by magistrates, in that the expression "does not necessarily lead" indicates that "although internment is not obligatory in cases of trafficking, it is not prohibited," while the expression "on its own" seems to indicate that "there are other circumstances that, in addition to drug trafficking, allow internment" (Cornelius 2018, p. 223).

Below is an example of an argument that allows the detention of adolescents due to an infraction analogous to drug trafficking, extracted from a subject in trial at the Bahia Court of Justice, by Minahim and Sposato:

> Drug trafficking should be considered one of the most serious criminal acts, since it is a practice that has been spreading addiction among the most vulnerable population, that is, the youngest and most unprotected in society. Drug trafficking is an infraction that presupposes the use of violence against society as a whole. (2011, p. 284)

The precedent, therefore, has not altered the tendency to trivialize the detention measure, used despite the letter of the law as a reprimand for the act of drug trafficking in the context of the punitive turn of juvenile justice. This type of decision has contributed to the increase in the number of adolescents deprived of their liberty.

In the last Annual Survey of the National System of Socio-Educational Assistance (SINASE), it is stated that 26,868 adolescents are deprived of their liberty, complying with the MSE of internment or semi-liberty, or provisionally internees (that is, without definitive condemnation), which configures a rate of 79 adolescents deprived of liberty per 100,000 inhabitants between 12 and 21 years old. The number of adolescents subjected to socio-educational measures deprived of their liberty has increased over the past two decades. In 1996, there were 4245 young people submitted to the MSE deprived of their liberty, so the current number represents an increase of approximately 440%.

Among adolescents deprived of their liberty, 49% were responsible for criminal acts equated to property crimes (46% for robbery and 3% for theft) and 24% were deprived of their liberty due to criminal acts equated to drug trafficking. In addition, 10% were convicted of an infraction equated to homicide, 3% for attempted homicide, 2% for carrying a firearm, 2% for latrine, 1% for rape, and the remainder for other less relevant infractions. The SINASE Annual Survey also shows that 96% of adolescents deprived of their liberty are men; that 57% are between 16 and 17 years of age, 23% between 18 and 21, 17% between 14 and 15, and 2% between 12 and 13 years of age. Finally, it shows that 61% are black or brown, 23% white, 0.81% yellow, 0.28% indigenous, and that in 14% of cases the information was not included.

In other words, almost a quarter of the adolescents who serve MSE deprivation of liberty have responded to the criminal act of drug trafficking. The data is similar to that found for imprisoned adults. In this case, 29% of the men arrested and 64% of the women arrested responded for drug trafficking (Ministry of Justice and Public Security, National Penitentiary Department 2017).

Final Considerations

Research on the subject has already shown that the policy currently adopted for the control of illicit substances, prohibitionism or the war on drugs, has not produced satisfactory results. On the one hand, it has not been able to reduce supply and demand, so that prohibited psychoactive substances are being produced, marketed, and consumed on a large scale, in the context of an illegal market, with relative ease of access to users. On the other hand, criminal drug policy has generated perverse effects such as prison overcrowding (a substrate in which the so-called criminal factions have germinated and flourished), urban violence (especially lethal conflicts derived from the context of the clandestine drug economy), violence, and police corruption, as well as difficulties in satisfying treatment for cases of problematic users.

For cases of drug use, the system of adolescents' accountability does not offer effective solutions, mainly because it does not differentiate between problematic and unproblematic uses nor uses according to the type of substance, offering a standard treatment to all adolescents caught committing this infraction. In fact, very few countries still keep consumption criminalized, so much so in respect for the guarantees of citizen's freedom, so much so that reception policies, aimed at the care of problematic consumers, tend to work better in legal environments.

Likewise, the accumulation of violence around the illicit drug trade imposes reflection on alternatives to the policy currently adopted, based on prohibition and combat. The clandestine market created by prohibition is the environment in which the real *civil war* is currently taking place in the country, whose rates of lethal violence are unacceptable.

The trivialization of the detention measure for adolescents involved in drug trafficking is another worrying factor. As we have seen, a quarter of all adolescents in detention are due to this infraction. The early experience of deprivation of liberty deepens the breakdown of family and social ties and contributes to the consolidation of a deviant career, which generates a tendency for recidivism, a factor that will contribute to this same youth ending up in prison after turning 18. On the other hand, this policy of combat and imprisonment does not produce any satisfactory result from the point of view of the declared objectives of prohibitionism, since it does not affect the supply of illicit substances nor the organization of retail sales. Adolescents who are at the tip of the trade are usually seized with small quantities and the next day their function has already been occupied by another young person of the same social class. The arrest of thousands of adolescents and young people removes from the market a minute quantity of drugs, much smaller than the eventual discovery of a wholesale trader.

Against this background, why does the war on drugs still continue to produce its dead and its prisoners? One possible answer is that the criminalization of drugs enables punitive power and allows permanent vigilance in relation to the popular classes, instrumentalizing social control directed at such groups.

In any case, the fact is that we are seeing significant changes in this field. The global trend is to review the prohibitionist policy, both by decriminalizing consumption and by formulating control regimes that allow legal access to substances considered illegal today.

References

Batista, V. M. (2003). Difíceis ganhos fáceis. In *Drogas E Juventude Pobre No Rio De Janeiro*. Rio De Janeiro, Brazil: Revan.

Bourgois, P. (2004). Crack-cocaina Y economia politica del sufrimiento social. *Monografias Humanitas, 5*, 95–103.

Carvalho, S. (2016). *A política criminal de drogas no Brasil: Estudo criminológico e dogmático*. São Paulo, Brazil: Saraiva.
Centro Brasileiro De Informações Sobre Drogas Psicotrópicas. (2003). *Levantamento nacional sobre o uso de drogas entre crianças e adolescentes em situação de rua nas 27 capitais brasileiras*. Retrieved from https://www.cebrid.com.br/wp-content/uploads/2012/10/Levantamento-Nacional-sobre-o-Uso-de-Drogas-entre-Crianças-e-Adolescentes-em-Situação-de-Rua-nas-27-Capitais-Brasileiras-2003.pdf
Centro Brasileiro De Informações Sobre Drogas Psicotrópicas. (2012). *VI Levantamento nacional sobre o consumo de drogas psicotrópicas entre estudantes do ensino fundamental e médio das redes pública e privada de ensino nas 27 capitais brasileiras*. Retrieved from https://Www.Cebrid.Com.Br/Wp-Content/Uploads/2012/10/Vi-Levantamento-Nacional-Sobre-O-Consumo-De-Drogas-Psicotrópicas-Entre-Estudantes-Do-Ensino-Fundamental-E-Médio-Das-Redes-Pública-E-Privada-De-Ensino-Nas-27-Capitais-Brasileiras.Pdf
Cornelius, E. G. (2018). *O pior dos dois mundos? A construção legítima da punição de adolescentes no superior tribunal de justiça*. São Paulo, Brazil: Ibccrim.
Escohotado, A. (2008). *Historia general de las drogas*. Madrid, Spain: Espasa Calpe.
Instituto de Pesquisa Econômica Aplicada, Fórum Brasileiro de Segurança Pública. (2019). *Atlas da violência 2019*. Retrieved from https://www.ipea.gov.br/portal/images/stories/PDFs/relatorio_institucional/190605_atlas_da_violencia_2019.pdf
Lei No 11.343, de 23 de agosto de. (2006). *Institui o Sistema Nacional de Políticas Públicas sobre Drogas - Sisnad; prescreve medidas para prevenção do uso indevido, atenção e reinserção social de usuários e dependentes de drogas; estabelece normas para repressão à produção não autorizada e ao tráfico ilícito de drogas; define crimes e dá outras providências*. Retrieved from http://www.planalto.gov.br/ccivil_03/_ato2004-2006/2006/lei/l11343.htm
Lei No 8.069, de 13 de julho de. (1990). *Dispõe sobre o Estatuto da Criança e do Adolescente e dá outras providências*. Retrieved from http://www.planalto.gov.br/ccivil_03/leis/l8069.htm
Mayora, M. (2009). *Entre a cultura do controle e o controle cultural: um estudo sobre práticas tóxicas na cidade de porto alegre*. Rio De Janeiro, Brazil: Lumen Juris.
Minahim, M. A., & Sposato, K. B. (2011). A internação de adolescentes pela lente dos tribunais. *Revista Direito GV, 7*(1), 277–298. https://doi.org/10.1590/S1808-24322011000100014.
Ministério da Justiça e Segurança Pública, Departamento Penitenciário Nacional. (2017). *Levantamento Nacional De Informações Penitenciárias Atualização – Junho de 2017*. Retrieved from http://depen.gov.br/DEPEN/depen/sisdepen/infopen/relatorios-sinteticos/infopen-jun-2017-rev-12072019-0721.pdf
Misse, M. (2006). *Crime E Violência No Brasil Contemporâneo*. Rio De Janeiro, Brazil: Lumen Juris.
Nardi, F. L., Jahn, G. M., & Dell'Aglio, D. D. (2014). Perfil de adolescentes em privação de liberdade: eventos estressores, uso de drogas e expectativas de futuro. *Psicologia Em Revista, 20*(1), 116–137. https://doi.org/10.5752/P.1678-9523.2014v20n1p116.
Restrepo, L. C. (2004). *La fruta prohibida. la droga como espejo de la cultura*. Madrid, Spain: Ediciones Libertarias.
Rolim, M. (2016). *A formação de jovens violentos: Estudo sobre a etiologia da violência extrema* (Doctoral dissertation), Universidade Federal do Rio Grande do Sul, Curitiba, Brazil. Retrieved from http://hdl.handle.net/10183/102225
Silva, G. M. (2010). *Ato infracional: Fluxo do sistema de justiça juvenil em Belo Horizonte*. (Master's thesis), Universidade Federal De Minas Gerais, Belo Horizonte, Brazil. Retrieved from http://hdl.handle.net/1843/VCSA-8BNN93
Zaconne, O. (2007). *Acionistas do nada: Quem são os traficantes de drogas*. Rio De Janeiro, Brazil: Revan.
Zaluar, A. (2012). Juventude violenta: Processos, retrocessos e novos percursos. *Dados – Revista De Ciências Sociais, 55*, 327–365. https://doi.org/10.1590/S0011-52582012000200003.

Chapter 23
Gender, Alcohol Dependence, and Public Policies

Silvia Brasiliano, Fabio Carezzato, and Patricia Brunfentrinker Hochgraf

Introduction

Until about 30 years ago, women were not included in most clinical research. The argument was often based on beliefs (National Institute on Drug Abuse [NIDA] 2019) that women were biologically more complicated than men and that, being primarily responsible for housework and family and young children care, they did not have time to participate in research.

The situation was so absurd that U.S. Senator Barbara Mikulski declared in 2010:

> Remember the famous study, take an aspirin a day to keep the heart attack away? That study was done on 10.000 men. Not one woman was included. In a study of the aging process, they told me women weren't included because the wasn't ladies' room available for study participants. Yet the results of these studies were being applied to men and women. I vowed to fix that (NIDA 2018a).

In 1991, the U.S. Department of Health and Human Services established the Office of Women's Health to ensure that broader public health issues related to sex and gender were addressed (NIDA 2018a). But it was not until 2014 that the National Institute of Health announced a new policy requiring that research involving animal and cellular models should include both sexes to receive their funding (NIDA 2019).

For many years, as could not be otherwise, substance use disorders were also considered a male problem. Although already in the Hammurabi code, which is from 1762 BC, we find phrases like *a wife who drinks wine … may be abandoned at any time* (Lal et al. 2015), only in 1995 did NIDA formally establish the Women and Sex/Gender Disorders Research Program. This program aimed to understand

S. Brasiliano (✉) · F. Carezzato · P. B. Hochgraf
Universidade de São Paulo, São Paulo, SP, Brazil
e-mail: brasili@netway.com.br

D. De Micheli et al. (eds.), *Drugs and Human Behavior*,
https://doi.org/10.1007/978-3-030-62855-0_23

the underlying causes of these disorders and the best ways to prevent and treat them in both men and women (NIDA 2019).

In this scenario it is not difficult to imagine why for decades dependent women have been considered more serious than men and a number of myths have been created, such as that alcoholic women have lower retention rates, respond poorly, and have a worse prognosis than men (Hochgraf 1995).

Although the problem of drugs is more present and studied among men, women constitute a growing and vulnerable group, and many are involved in pregnancy and motherhood (Galera et al. 2005).

Prevalence

Epidemiological studies, both in the world and in Brazil, point to a male predominance in the abuse of most substances (Slade et al. 2016). Men are more likely to be drinkers and, among these, men drink more problematically than women (McCaul et al. 2019).

In the USA, a large study conducted between 2012 and 2013, the National Epidemiologic Survey on Alcohol and Related Conditions (NESARC III), reported a prevalence of alcohol use disorders of 17.6% among men and 10.4% among women (Grant et al. 2015).

In Brazil, the II National Survey of Alcohol and Drugs (Instituto Nacional de Ciências e Tecnologia para Políticas Públicas de Álcool e Outras Drogas [INPAD] 2014), which in 2012 interviewed 4607 individuals over the age of 14, found a prevalence of 10.5% male and 3.6% female alcohol-dependent (2.9 men for 1 woman).

We can observe that in Brazil, while male alcohol dependence decreased, female alcohol dependence increased, thus narrowing the gender gap (INPAD 2014). This result is different from that of other countries where, although there is also a decrease in the male-to-female ratio, there is an increase for both genders in alcohol use and alcohol use disorders (Grant et al. 2017; McCaul et al. 2019). Williams et al. (2018), referring to white and Hispanic women in the USA, suggest that the increase in problem drinking among them may reflect changes in social norms and roles, such as the verified transition from domestic to formal work and the postponement of marriage. In addition, the increase in the years of formal education between them and the later age of pregnancy may contribute.

Female Specificities in Alcohol Use Disorders

There are numerous differences between men and women in the emergence and development of substance use disorders. The importance of this understanding lies in the implications for the development of more effective treatment and prevention strategies.

Review studies show a high genetic influence for both men and women in relation to alcohol use disorders, reaching 49% of inheritability. In addition to genetic influence there is an important environmental influence on this inheritability (Munn-Chernoff and Baker 2016; Verhulst et al. 2015).

Considering the beginning of use, women mention specific reasons for the use of psychoactive substances: weight control, dealing with stress and exhaustion and self-medication for feelings and psychic problems (NIDA 2015), while men tend not to give a single reason. In general, women initiate the use with their partners, different from men who are introduced to alcohol by friends. Living together with a substance abuser not only introduces and reinforces women's consumption, but also plays an important role in maintaining their behavior (Lal et al. 2015).

Another characteristic is that women begin to use alcohol later than men, but report a faster progression in the development of the same number of symptoms as men and a shorter length of time between onset of abuse and addiction (Holdcraft and Iacono 2004). This phenomenon is often referred to in the literature as *telescoping effect*. In addition to having a faster progression of their disorder, women generally present themselves to treatment with a more severe picture (Choi et al. 2015).

Still in relation to the pattern of use, women usually drink less alcohol and less frequently than men (Bravo et al. 2013; Health Canada 2001).

Physical issues have a major impact on male and female differences in the evolution of substance use disorders. Since women have less body water than men, assuming both have the same body weight, when ingesting an equal amount of alcohol women achieve a higher blood alcohol content. Another factor for the greater absorption of alcohol among them is due to the gastric concentration of the enzyme ADH (alcohol dehydrogenase), responsible for the metabolization of alcohol, being lower among women compared to men (Hochgraf and Brasiliano 2012).

Besides the higher blood concentration, two factors need to be considered. The first is that women have a higher vulnerability of all organs. The other is the influence of female hormones in the reward system via different neurotransmitters, which would also contribute to gender differences in this pathology (Anker and Carrol 2010). These reasons help understand why the consequences of alcohol abuse are worse in women than among men, with morbidity in alcohol-dependent women being 1.5–2.0 times higher than in those without problem drinking (Brady et al. 1993; Thomasson 2002).

This information is corroborated by other evidence. A study of hospitalized patients showed that men with alcohol problems die three times more than the general population, while women with the same problem die five times more than the general population (Lindenberg and Agren 1988). Similarly, in a recent meta-analysis of 81 studies, Roerecke and Rehn (2014) found a higher mortality rate in women than in men with alcohol-related disorders.

Pregnancy

No doubt the biggest difference between men and dependent women is that women get pregnant. There are numerous issues regarding the use of drugs during pregnancy, both political-social and physical.

It is important to make it clear that of all the psychoactive substances, alcohol is the one that causes the greatest number and most serious problems for the fetus and the newborn, as well as serious consequences for the child's development. Fetal alcohol spectrum disorders (FASD) describe a series of conditions that affect babies who have had prenatal exposure to alcohol. These disorders can manifest themselves in several ways, the most severe of which is fetal alcohol syndrome (FAS). It is estimated that in the USA there are 0.2–1.5 cases of FAS in 1000 live births and that this is the third most frequent cause of mental retardation in newborns (Center for Disease Control and Prevention 2019). This syndrome consists of any combination of the following: low weight for gestational age, malformations in the facial structure (short palpebral fissures, low nasal bridge, and indistinct philtrum), defects in the cardiac ventricular septum, malformations of the hands and feet (especially, syndactyly), and mental retardation that varies from mild to moderate. Problems in behavior and learning can also persist at least during childhood (Howell et al. 1999).

When considering FASD, it is estimated that 1 in every 13 pregnant women who have consumed alcohol during pregnancy will have a child with these disorders. Globally, it is estimated that every day 1700 babies are born with FASD (Lange et al. 2017). There is evidence that drinking in the first trimester increases the risk of FASD by 12 times, drinking in the second and third trimesters increases this risk by 61 times and in all trimesters by 65 times. Conversely, drinking in the first trimester alone is 5 times less risky than drinking in all quarters (May et al. 2013).

It is interesting to mention that the chronic consumption of alcohol by men seems to lead to hypomethylation in some regions of the sperm DNA and the transmission of these epigenetic alterations in fertilization could alter the expression of genes critical to normal development, thus increasing the risk of FASD (Cernach 2017). Since the frequency of consumption and the amount of alcohol that would be involved in this syndrome are unknown, as well as the role of nutritional deficiencies secondary to alcoholism, women are recommended not to drink during pregnancy. It should be emphasized that already in the Old Testament in the Holy Bible there are references to the deleterious effects of alcohol during pregnancy: "but he assured me: you will become pregnant and give birth to a child. However, do not drink wine or any other fermented beverage" (Biblia 1969).

A study conducted in Canada in 2011, which found that 14% of women had used alcohol in pregnancy, proposed that in view of the high prevalence, all pregnant women should be evaluated for alcohol and other drug use. Recalling that this is a period with greater motivation for unhealthy or dangerous behavior changes, the authors suggest working with harm reduction: encouraging abstinence or reduction in use, safe use, treatment of withdrawal symptoms, counseling, and pharmacotherapy. Special attention should be given to the risk of sexually transmitted diseases (Wong et al. 2011).

Reinforcing how much the investment in pregnancy is worth, Forray (2016) found that 96% of heavy drinkers, 73% of cocaine addicts, and 32% of smokers were able to stay abstinent in pregnancy. After delivery only half of the alcoholics relapsed; a lower rate was found for cocaine addicts (27%) and a slightly higher rate for smokers (58%).

Characteristics and Specific Needs of Treatment Programs

There is almost consensus in the literature that stigma is one of the main barriers to access, retention, and success in treatment. Alcohol use disorders are among the most severely stigmatized psychiatric disorder. In general, alcoholics are seen as dangerous, unpredictable, and blamed for their own condition (Keyes et al. 2010; Weine et al. 2016). In addition, individuals who suffer from substance use disorders are considered less ill and provoke more negative emotions, rejection, and a desire for social distance (Schomerus et al. 2011).

Women also suffer from stigma, although there is no consensus in the literature about the difference with men. While some studies indicate that they are more stigmatized (Pretorius et al. 2009; United Nations Office on Drugs and Crime 2004), others go in the opposite direction (Keyes et al. 2010). In any case, stereotypes of greater aggressiveness and sexual promiscuity are more linked to the female gender (Hochgraf 1995). Special emphasis has been placed on pregnancy, as there is a strong stigma towards women who use alcohol in pregnancy (Corrigan et al. 2018).

Despite all the changes in the social roles of men and women, it is not difficult to observe that this prejudice continues to exist to this day, making it difficult for dependent women to access treatment. Thus, they are generally underrepresented in therapeutic centers. It is estimated that only 23% of men and 15% of women with alcohol use disorders seek treatment (Health Canada 2001; McCrady et al. 2009) and the ratio of male-to-female users in mixed services may reach 10:1 (Greenfield et al. 2007).

In a recent editorial published in an important journal of gynecology and obstetrics, Prasad and Metz (2019) states:

> "Substance use disorders is associated with more stigma than other chronic diseases. As such, some people with substance use disorders will not seek treatment and some doctors refuse to treat patients with addiction. Similarly, some pharmaceutical companies will not work to develop new treatments for addicts, which has limited options for women with this chronic disease. Overtime, it is our hope that as a result of public education and broader acceptance of addiction as a treatable disease, that stigma will become less of a barrier to those who need treatment for substance use disorders" (2019, p.111).

Further on, the authors reiterate "...we can begin to medicalize out approach, rather than stigmatize pregnant women with substance use disorder" and "...relapse should be considered part of the substance use disorder disease process, rather than a transgression" (Prasad and Metz 2019, p. 111).

This stigma is believed to be one of the most important variables responsible for the fact that most women with alcohol problems prefer to seek help in general health centers rather than specialized centers (Bold et al. 2017).

Regarding treatment, a particularly important fact is the motivation for them to seek treatment. A work by Grosso et al. (2013) showed that women have more internal motivations: concern about the progression of alcoholism (61.1%), physical health (43.4%), mental health (38.9%), and family relations (38.3%) compared to men, whose motivations are predominantly external. An interesting fact of this work is that the reason why women seek treatment is associated negatively with treatment outcome and retention.

We should remember that, compared to men, women face more barriers to enter treatment: more social opposition, less support from family and friends, higher unemployment, greater economic barriers, more family responsibility, increased stigma, and social disapproval (Grosso et al. 2013). It is worth noting that married alcoholic women with children suffer more guilt and shame than men in the same situation (Thurang et al. 2010). Besides these, Becker and Duffy (2002) point out as obstacles: the repercussion of stigma on child protection items, fragility of maternity support services, negative attitude of health professionals and, finally, ineffective interagency service. In relation to pregnant women, the authors indicate that stigma against women who use alcohol can influence public policies related to the withdrawal of custody, inhibiting the demand of mothers for treatment. Despite the fear of losing their children, the concern with the impact that alcohol use can have on the child's life is a great motivator for seeking treatment (Powis et al. 2000). Assuming that children should stay with their biological parents as far as possible improves the relationship of women with problematic use of alcohol and other drugs with social welfare departments and also breaks with the idea that the search for addiction-related care leads to immediate loss of custody (Henderson et al. 1995).

Another problem faced by pregnant women with alcohol-related problems is that when they report their disorder during prenatal care, they are referred to services of high complexity, often far from the region where they live. This decreases the retention of these pregnant women to prenatal care and causes them to deny their problem (Becker and Duffy 2002).

Despite all these difficulties and contrary to what was believed, Bravo et al. (2013) in a 20-year longitudinal follow-up study of men and women treated for alcoholism concluded that women have greater retention to treatment and better long-term evolution in alcohol consumption. This evolution is possible as long as the important differences between men and women alcoholics are considered in the development of treatment programs, especially for women who often report preferring exclusive programs for them (Sugarman et al. 2016). Numerous studies have pointed out that they obtain the greatest benefit when treated in these programs, since they are the ones that enable their full participation (Choi et al. 2015). The same would not occur in mixed gender treatments, which generally fail to respond to women's needs, since men's interests tend to predominate by making it difficult, or even preventing to address their particular issues (Greenfield et al. 2010). Building a personal identity, improving self-esteem, developing positive interpersonal relationships, mother–child interaction, and vocational training are usually key focuses in the recovery of dependent women, which are hardly worked in mixed groups, usually more focused on men's conflicts with abstinence and its maintenance (Greenfield et al. 2010).

Ideally, gender-sensitive programs should include other factors, which have been pointed out in the literature, such as: facilities the service can offer to overcome structural (e.g., childcare and legal aid), attitudinal (such as shame at discussing the problem, hopelessness about results), personal (such as lack of employment, family responsibilities), and social barriers (such as partner and family members' opposition to treatment) (Verissimo and Grella 2017). Also, there is a need for health team members to recognize, create empathy, and deal with the specific nature of alcohol use in women (Brasiliano and Hochgraf 2006).

Although there is still little research studying the effectiveness of gender-sensitive treatments, two review and meta-analysis studies are important: in the first, Orwin et al. (2001) conducted an extensive review of treatments offered to women and concluded that, compared to mixed gender services, women only programs achieve additional beneficial results and are more effective, particularly when their approaches are intensified and directed specifically to the needs of the population they serve. In the other review, Ashley et al. (2003) found similar findings examining components of therapeutic approaches from 38 evolution studies, 7 with randomized clinical samples and 31 with non-randomized samples. The authors observed significantly higher results, such as: increased retention rates; decreased substance use; reduced HIV risk behaviors; and improvements in self-esteem, depression, and pre- and neonatal care associated with: day care centers, prenatal care, exclusive admission of women, workshops on women's issues, mental health approaches, and intensified programs.

A study by Sugarman et al. (2016) showed that women only recovery groups for drug use disorders are significantly more cohesive and more frequented than mixed gender groups. Women feel more welcome and secure in these groups and verbal support seems to be key to keeping them in treatment.

In conclusion, according to the National Institute on Drug Abuse (2018b) effective treatment for alcohol-dependent women ideally should include approaches that recognize sexual and gender differences, understand the types of trauma they often face, offer support for childcare, and use evidence-based strategies for treatment of pregnant women.

Final Considerations

Prevention programs, as well as treatment programs, aimed at women should be designed specifically for them and not adapted from male models. One of the main issues is to provide women with scientifically based information about their increased vulnerability to alcohol and the consequences of its use for their bodies and for pregnancy and breastfeeding. On this account, we reaffirm the need for scientific production that studies this population and its specificities.

Considering that women's consumption in general is in *binge* pattern we can prevent harm by focusing on situations of risk of violence, through the creation of a support network to which women feeling vulnerable when ontoxicated by alcohol may ask for help in bars and other places they drink, encouraging the use of safe transportation, either by specific transportation applications for this population or by walking along someone else whenever possible.

Professionals should be alerted to problem use screening on women, focusing on combating stigma and prejudice. As the use of women also presents the characteristic of being domestic and hidden from the family, the approach of health professionals is of great importance.

It is important to focus on the use of alcohol in pregnancy. Although the recommendation is not to drink anything during this period, there is a hidden tolerance for alcohol consumption and excess is more common than one might think. Training basic care professionals for an empathetic and judgment-free approach can make it easier to obtain information and early diagnosis of abuse, which favors, if necessary, the woman's referral to a therapeutic program that can guarantee her health and that of the baby.

It is also worth noting that a significant number of women with alcohol-related problems report having been victims of physical or sexual abuse by close relatives during their childhood or adolescence (Cesar 2006), and it is therefore of great importance to promote policies to prevent violence against women.

Finally, in recent years we have seen a growth in alcoholic beverage advertising aimed at women. This reflects directly on the increase in consumption by this population. Combating alcohol advertising in general is one of the most effective ways to decrease consumption, a policy whose success can be illustrated by anti-smoking campaigns.

References

Anker, J. J., & Carroll, M. E. (2010). Females are more vulnerable to drug abuse than males: Evidence from preclinical studies and the role of ovarian hormones. In J. Neill & J. Kulkarni (Eds.), *Biological basis of sex differences in psychopharmacology*. Berlin: Springer. https://doi.org/10.1007/7854_2010_93.

Ashley, O. S., Marsden, M. E., & Brady, T. M. (2003). Effectiveness of substance abuse treatment programming for women: A review. *American Journal of Drug and Alcohol Abuse, 29*(1), 19–53. https://doi.org/10.1081/ada-120018838.

Becker, J., & Duffy, C. (2002). *Women drug users and drugs service provision: Service-level responses to engagement and retention*. London, United Kingdom: Home Office.

Biblia, P. (1969). A Biblia Sagrada: Antigo e Novo Testamento. Tradução de João Ferreira de Almeida. Edição rev. e atualizada no Brasil. Brasília: Sociedade Bíblia do Brasil.

Bold, K., Epstein, E., & McCrady, B. (2017). Baseline health status and quality of life after alcohol treatment for women with alcohol dependence. *Addictive Behaviors, 64*, 35–41. https://doi.org/10.1016/j.addbeh.2016.08.014.

Brady, K. T., Grice, D. E., Dustan, L., & Randall, C. (1993). Gender differences in substance use disorders. *American Journal of Psychiatry, 150*(11), 1707–1711. https://doi.org/10.1176/ajp.150.11.1707.

Brasiliano, S., & Hochgraf, P. B. (2006). Drogadicção feminina: a experiência de um percurso. In D. X. Silveira & F. G. Moreira (Eds.), *Panorama atual de drogas e dependências* (pp. 289–295). São Paulo, Brazil: Editora Atheneu.

Bravo, F., Gral, A., Lligoña, A., & Colom, J. (2013). Gender differences in the long-term outcome of alcohol dependence treatment: An analysis of twenty-years prospective follow up. *Drug and Alcohol Dependence, 32*(4), 3881–3388. https://doi.org/10.1111/dar.12023.

Center for Disease Control and Prevention. (2019). *Fetal alcohol spectrum disorders (FASDs)*. Data & Statistics. Retrieved from https://www.cdc.gov/ncbddd/fasd/data.html

Cernach, M. C. S. P. (2017). Fatores genéticos na síndrome alcoólica fetal. In C. A. M. Segre (Ed.), *Efeitos do álcool na gestante, no feto e no recém-nascido* (2nd ed., pp. 45–52). São Paulo, Brazil: Sociedade de Pediatria de São Paulo.

Cesar, B. A. L. (2006). Alcoolismo feminino: um estudo de suas peculiaridades. Resultados preliminares. *Jornal Brasileiro de Psiquiatria, 55*(3), 208–211. https://doi.org/10.1590/S0047-20852006000300006.

Choi, S., Adams, S. M., Morse, S. A., & MacMaster, S. (2015). Gender differences in treatment retention among individuals with co-occurring substance abuse and mental health disorders. *Substance Use and Misuse, 50*(5), 653–663. https://doi.org/10.3109/10826084.2014.997828.

Corrigan, P. W., Shah, B. B., Lara, J. L., Michell, K. T., Simmes, D., & Jones, K. L. (2018). Addressing the public health concerns of fetal alcohol spectrum disorders: Impact of stigma and health literacy. *Drug and Alcohol Dependence, 185*(1), 266–270. https://doi.org/10.1016/j.drugalcdep.2017.12.027.

Forray, A. (2016). Substance use during pregnancy. *F1000 Research, 5*(1), 887. https://doi.org/10.12688/f1000research.7645.1.

Galera, S. A. F., Roldan, M. C. B., & O'Brien, B. (2005). Women living in a drug (and violence) context—The maternal role. *Revista Latino-Americana de Enfermagem, 13*, 1142–1147. https://doi.org/10.1590/S0104-11692005000800007.

Grant, B. F., Chou, S. P., Saha, T. D., Pickering, R. P., Kerridge, B. T., Ruan, W. J., et al. (2017). Prevalence of 12-month alcohol use, high-risk drinking, and DSM-IV alcohol use disorder in the United States, 2001-2002 to 2012-2013. Results from the National Epidemiologic Survey on alcohol and related conditions. *Journal of the American Medical Association Psychiatry, 74*(9), 911–923. https://doi.org/10.1001/jamapsychiatry.2017.2161.

Grant, B. F., Goldstein, R. B., Saha, T. D., Chou, S. P., Jung, J., Zhang, H., et al. (2015). Epidemiology of DSM-5 alcohol use disorder: Results from the National Epidemiologic Survey on alcohol and related conditions III. *Journal of the American Medical Association Psychiatry, 72*, 757–766. https://doi.org/10.1001/jamapsychiatry.2015.0584.

Greenfield, S. F., Back, S. E., Lawson, K., & Brady, K. T. (2010). Substance abuse in women. *Psychiatry Clinics of North America, 33*, 339–355. https://doi.org/10.1016/j.psc.2010.01.004.

Greenfield, S. F., Brooks, A. J., Gordon, S. M., Green, C. A., Kropp, F., McHugh, R. K., et al. (2007). Substance abuse treatment entry, retention, and outcome in women: A review of the literature. *Drug and Alcohol Dependence, 86*(1), 1–21. https://doi.org/10.1016/j.drugalcdep.2006.05.012.

Grosso, J., Epstein, E., McCrady, B., Gaba, A., Cook, S., Backer-Fulghum, L., & Graff, F. (2013). Women's motivators for seeking treatment for alcohol use disorders. *Addictive Behaviors, 38*(6), 2236–2245. https://doi.org/10.1016/j.addbeh.2013.02.004.

Health Canada. (2001). *Best practices – Treatment and rehabilitation for women with substance use problems*. Ontario, Canada: Publications Health Canada.

Henderson, D. J., Boyd, C. J., & Whitmarsh, J. (1995). Women and illicit drugs: Sexuality and crack cocaine. *Health Care for Women International, 16*(2), 113–124. https://doi.org/10.1080/07399339509516163.

Hochgraf, P. B. (1995). *Alcoolismo feminino: comparação das características sociodemográficas e padrão de evolução entre homens e mulheres alcoolistas* (Doctoral dissertation), Universidade de São Paulo, São Paulo, Brazil.

Hochgraf, P. B., & Brasiliano, S. (2012). Diagnóstico e tratamento da dependência de álcool no gênero feminino. In J. Rennó Jr. & H. L. Ribeiro (Eds.), *Tratado de Saúde Mental da Mulher* (pp. 123–129). São Paulo, Brazil: Editora Atheneu.
Holdcraft, L. C., & Iacono, W. G. (2004). Cross-generational effects on gender differences in psychoactive drug abuse and dependence. *Drug and Alcohol Dependence, 74*, 147–158. https://doi.org/10.1016/j.drugalcdep.2003.11.016.
Howell, E. M., Heiser, N., & Harrington, M. (1999). A review of recent findings on substance abuse treatment for pregnant women. *Journal of Substance Abuse Treatment, 16*(3), 195–219. https://doi.org/10.1016/S0740-5472(98)00032-4.
Instituto Nacional de Ciências e Tecnologia para Políticas Públicas de Álcool e outras Drogas. (2014). *II Levantamento Nacional de Álcool e Drogas*. Retrieved from https://inpad.org.br/wp-content/uploads/2014/03/Lenad-II-Relatório.pdf
Keyes, K. M., Hatzenbuehler, M. L., McLaughlin, K. A., Link, B., Olfson, M., Grant, B. F., & Hasin, D. (2010). Stigma and treatment for alcohol use disorders in the United States. *American Journal of Epidemiology, 172*, 1364–1372. https://doi.org/10.1093/aje/kwq304.
Lal, R., Deb, K. S., & Kedia, S. (2015). Substance use in women: Current status and future directions. *Indian Journal of Psychiatry, 57*(6), S275–S285. https://doi.org/10.4103/0019-5545.161491.
Lange, S., Probst, C., Gmel, G., Rehm, J., Burd, L., & Popova, S. (2017). Global prevalence of fetal alcohol Spectrum disorder among children and youth: A systematic review and meta-analysis. *Journal of the American Medical Association Pediatrics, 171*(10), 948–956. https://doi.org/10.1001/jamapediatrics.2017.1919.
Lindenberg, S., & Agren, G. (1988). Mortality among male and female hospitalized alcoholics in Stockholm 1962-1983. *British Journal of Addiction, 83*(10), 1193–1200. https://doi.org/10.1111/j.1360-0443.1988.tb03026.x.
May, P. A., Blankenship, J., Marais, A. S., Gossage, J. P., Kalberg, W. O., Joubert, B., et al. (2013). Maternal alcohol consumption producing fetal spectrum disorders (FASD): Quantity, frequency and time of drinking. *Drug and Alcohol Dependence, 133*(2), 502–512. https://doi.org/10.1016/j.drugalcdep.2013.07.013.
McCaul, M. E., Roach, D., Hasin, D. S., Weisner, C., Chang, G., & Sinha, R. (2019). Alcohol and women: A brief overview. *Alcoholism: Clinical and Experimental Research, 43*(5), 774–779. https://doi.org/10.1111/acer.13985.
McCrady, B. S., Epstein, E. E., Cook, S., Jensen, N., & Hildebrant, T. (2009). A randomized trial of individual and couple behavioral alcohol treatment for women. *Journal of Consulting and Clinical Psychology, 77*(2), 243–256. https://doi.org/10.1037/a0014686.
Munn-Chernoff, M. A., & Baker, J. H. (2016). A primer on the genetics of comorbid eating disorders and substance use disorders. *European Eating Disorders Review, 24*(2), 91–100. https://doi.org/10.1002/erv.2424.
National Institute on Drug Abuse. (2015). *Sex and gender differences in substance use: Drug facts*. Retrieved from http://ww.drugabuse.goc/publications/drugfacts/substance-use-in-women
National Institute on Drug Abuse. (2018a). *The importance of including women in research*. Retrieved from https://www.drugabuse.gov/publications/research-reports/substance-use-in-women/importance-including-women-in-research
National Institute on Drug Abuse. (2018b). *Substance use in women*. Retrieved from https://www.drugabuse.gov/publications/research-reports/substance-use-inwomen/summary
National Institute on Drug Abuse. (2019). *Sex and gender differences in substance use: Drug facts*. Retrieved from http://www.drugabuse.gov/publications/drugfacts/substance-use-in-women
Orwin, R., Francisco, L., & Bernichon, T. (2001). *Effectiveness of women's substance abuse treatment programs: A meta-analysis national evaluation data services, center for substance abuse treatment*. Arlington, VA: SAMHSA.
Powis, B., Gossop, M., Bury, C., Payne, K., & Griffiths, P. (2000). Drug-using mothers: Social, psychological and substance use problems of women opiate users with children. *Drug and Alcohol Review, 19*(2), 171–180. https://doi.org/10.1080/713659321.
Prasad, M. R., & Metz, T. D. (2019). Foreword: Substance abuse in pregnancy. *Clinical Obstetrics and Gynecology, 62*(1), 110–111. https://doi.org/10.1097/GRF.0000000000000420.

Pretorius, L., Naidoo, A. V., & Reddy, S. P. (2009). "Kitchen cupboard drinking": A review of South Africa women's secretive alcohol addiction, treatment history, and barriers to accessing treatment. *Social Work on Public Health, 24*, 89–99. https://doi.org/10.1080/19371910802569575.

Roerecke, M., & Rehn, J. (2014). Cause-specific mortality risk in alcohol use disorder treatment patients: A systematic review and meta-analysis. *International Journal of Epidemiology, 43*(3), 906–919. https://doi.org/10.1093/ije/dyu018.

Schomerus, G., Lucht, M., Holzinger, A., Matschinger, H., Carta, M. G., & Angermeyer, M. C. (2011). The stigma of alcohol dependence compared with other mental disorders: A review of population studies. *Alcohol and Alcoholism, 46*(2), 105–112. https://doi.org/10.1093/alcalc/agq089.

Slade, T., Chapman, C., Swift, W., Keyes, K., Tonks, Z., & Teesson, M. (2016). Birth cohort trends in the global epidemiology of alcohol use and alcohol-related harms in men and women: Systematic review and metaregression. *British Medical Journal Open, 6*, e011827. https://doi.org/10.1136/bmjopen-2016-011827.

Sugarman, D. E., Wigderson, S. B., Iles, B. R., Kaufman, J. S., Garrett, M., Fitzmaurice, E., et al. (2016). Measuring affiliation in group therapy for substance use disorders in the Women's recovery group study: Does it matter whether the group is all-women or mixed gender? *American Journal of Addiction, 25*, 573–580. https://doi.org/10.1111/ajad.12443.

Thomasson, H. R. (2002). Gender differences in alcohol metabolism. In M. Galanter et al. (Eds.), *Recent developments in alcoholism* (Vol. 12, pp. 163–179). https://doi.org/10.1007/0-306-47138-8_9.

Thurang, G. A., Fagerberg, I., Palmstierna, T., & Tops, A. B. (2010). Women's experiences of caring when in treatment for alcohol dependency. *Scandinavian Journal of Caring Science, 24*, 700–706. https://doi.org/10.1111/j.1471-6712.2009.00766.x.

United Nations Office on Drugs and Crime. (2004). *Substance abuse treatment and care for women: Case studies and lessons learned.* Retrieved from https://www.unodc.org/pdf/report_2004-08-30_1.pdf

Verhulst, B., Neale, M. C., & Kendler, K. S. (2015). The heritability of alcohol use disorders: A meta-analysis of twin and adoption studies. *Psychological Medicine, 45*, 1061–1072. https://doi.org/10.1017/S0033291714002165.

Verissimo, A. D. O., & Grella, C. E. (2017). Influence of gender and race/ethnicity on perceived barriers to help-seeking for alcohol or drug problems. *Journal of Substance Abuse Treatment, 75*, 54–61. https://doi.org/10.1016/j.jsat.2016.12.013.

Weine, E. R., Kim, N. S., & Lincoln, A. K. (2016). Understanding lay assessments of alcohol use disorders: Need for treatment and associated stigma. *Alcohol and Alcoholism, 51*(1), 98–105. https://doi.org/10.1093/alcalc/agv069.

Williams, E., Mulia, N., Karriker-Jaffe, K. J., & Lui, C. K. (2018). Changing racial/ethnic disparities in heavy drinking trajectories through adulthood: A comparative cohort study. *Alcoholism: Clinical and Experimental Research, 42*(1), 135–143. https://doi.org/10.1111/acer.13541.

Wong, S., Ordean, A., & Kahan, M. (2011). Substance use in pregnancy. *Journal of Obstetrics and Gynaecology Canada, 33*(4), 367–384. https://doi.org/10.1016/S1701-2163(16)34855-1.

Chapter 24
The Psychosocial Care Network as Organizer of Public Policy in the Care of People in Harmful Use of Alcohol and Other Drugs

Priscilla dos Santos Peixoto Borelli Tavares, Rogério da Silva Ferreira, and Sarah Raphaella Fonseca Silva

Introduction

From food to medicine, illness to treatment, legality to illegality, luxury to misery, pleasure to suffering—regardless of the cut that is made to build the narrative on drugs in society, there is a relationship established that changes according to the time, the subject who uses and the socio-cultural conditions. It was no different in the past; because, first of all, the history of drugs is also the history of the medicalization and criminalization of certain substances. While the use of drugs for medical reasons or with the intent to extend life is stimulated, it is repressed for recreation purposes. The last make life feels more intense and may shorten it, being classified as harmful by medical authorities (Vargas, 1998).

Therefore, there is a historical background that presents itself in contemporary times disguised as a new model, but that is actually a (re)construction of the institutionalizing ones. For example, the so-called Therapeutic Communities, which are financed by the Federal Government since 2011, but, acting in improper ways, still commit a series of contraventions (Instituto de Pesquisa Econômica Aplicada, 2018; Ministério Público Federal, 2018).

In association with this, prohibitionist and anti-drugs logics exist in the media and in the daily lives of the population; those are supported by narratives that reduce the issue of drug abuse to requests of law/law enforcement or healthcare guardianship.

Thus, to overestimate the drug as a prohibited substance and to reduce their use to a taboo creates repulsion and stigma, also turning the drug into social merchandise of exclusion and inclusion, of identity, and of an illegality frontier through the criminalization of conducts (Carneiro, 2018).

Researches and activists have been demonstrating, supported by the logic above mentioned, that the War on Drugs has been the central narrative of the system that

Priscilla dos Santos Peixoto Borelli Tavares (✉) · R. da Silva Ferreira · S. R. F. Silva
CAPS AD III Antônio Carlos Mussum, Rio de Janeiro, RJ, Brazil

D. De Micheli et al. (eds.), *Drugs and Human Behavior*,
https://doi.org/10.1007/978-3-030-62855-0_24

has been marginalizing, imprisoning, and shortening black lives for centuries in Brazil. This is validated by Law No. 11,343 of 2006[1]—called the Drug Law—(Borges, 2019; Oliveira & Ribeiro, 2018) and by using the argument of what was a mistaken crack cocaine epidemic (Bastos & Bertoni, 2014).

It is noticeable that both logics—Prohibitionism and the War on Drugs—do not seem to take care of people with needs originated from the use of alcohol and other drugs, of their families, and of the support network with which each subject counts, not just because of the absence of the issue mentioned in the report of the first and second National Conference on Mental Health,[2] but also because of the punishment that is given to these people, which is given either by legal/penal means or even by institutionalizing them with the purpose of achieving abstinence, since the overlapping between poverty and crime is present in the social imaginary.

The research conducted by Silva and Delduque (2015) endorses this perception when by analyzing 147 Bills gathered using the descriptor "alcohol, tobacco, and other drugs" on the Legislative Health Observatory database, it identifies that the occupation of the Brazilian Federal Legislative Branch with drug-related issues encourages punishment and pathologization practices, rather than the formulation of policies that effectively create alternatives or treatments designed for the harmful use of psychoactive substances.

This is also explained by the fact that citizenship-oriented care for the user of harmful substances is recent. So, aiming to divert from punishment to an ethical stance of concern for the other, according to Silva, Frazão, and Linhares (2014), only in the beginning of the twenty-first century, with the III National Health Conference, is Mental Health capable of associate the substance abuse issue with the Psychiatric Reform and with the principles of the Unified Health System.

In this sense, the complexity of the matter here exposed, its paradoxes, specificities, and crossings creating a need for questioning not only the current politics but also clinical practices, understanding that these go together in order to strengthen bets that converse with real needs of alcohol/drug users, their families, and the community (De Micheli et al., 2016).

The production that happens during an encounter with the other creates politics, which when attentive to the needs of the people living with substance abuse problems, reflects in the clinical practice. This interface of what separates, but does not distinguish itself, creates vectors in the sense of Psychiatric Reform and Harm Reduction Policy, which are currently weakened in front of the biomedical and religious hegemony discourse.

In order to strengthen care in freedom, with autonomy and responsibility, it is necessary to amplify the focus on the subject, understanding he or she as a bio-psycho-socio-spiritual being, and to share actions, literally producing know-how which meets the clinical practice that we wish to reaffirm to people with needs

[1] Modified by Decreto No 9.761, de 11 de abril de (2019).

[2] Held in 1988, 1992 respectively.

arising from alcohol and other drugs. To do so, it is imperative to think of care based on an intersectoral network.

History of the Care of People with Needs Resulting from Drug Use in Brazil

The context of care for people with needs arising from drug use in Brazil is marked by the isolation of users in psychiatric hospitals and by the prevalence of the psychiatric knowledge about the disease process.[3] Only with the appearance of the re-democratization movement in the country—after the military dictatorship period—and with the rise of the Sanitary Reform Movement, it becomes possible to expand the concept of health and to criticize the modern medical thought.

This thought, according to Guedes, Nogueira, and Camargo Jr. (2006), focuses on the signs and symptoms of the disease, and the search for the etiology of pathologies and their cures the main goal of medicine. These reasons corrupted the other determinants involved in the disease process, erasing the subject and ignoring the complexities of this mechanism—which are essential to plan the care of people with needs arising from drug use, since the subject's relationship with it is more complex than just a diagnosis of chemical dependence.

The 8th National Conference of Health was the milestone for the amplification process of the health concept. It conceptualizes health as:

> In its broadest sense, health is that resulting from the conditions of food, housing, education, income, environment, work, transportation, employment, leisure, freedom, access, and ownership of land and access to health services. It is thus, above all, the result of the social organization of productive forces, which can generate inequalities in living standards (Ministério da Saúde, 1986, p. 4).

In line with the Sanitary Reform Movement, the Brazilian Psychiatric Reform ratifies the criticism of the hospital-centered model of care, which isolates madness, and the monopoly of the psychiatry knowledge that happens in the Mental Health field. This ratification was a change in the area of Mental Health that deals with the defense of freedom and democracy, providing participation of the subject in his or her family and community and territorial coexistence, in opposition to the movement of the subject's submission to asylum institutions.

Therefore, the movement began in the late 1970s, when mental health workers formed the Mental Health Workers Movement—MTSM—in 1978. The MTSM was organized during the 1980s for the I National Mental Health Conference, in 1987, and at the end of the same year, the II MTSM National Congress was held. It was

[3] From the work spread by Philippe Pinel (1745–1826). However, in this period several denunciations regarding the precarious conditions of psychiatric care are registered, such as isolation, its logic of exclusion and the terrible conditions in which users were kept, both in public and private institutions and the policy of privatization of the sector that occurred during the military dictatorship.

during this congress that the movement changed since it went from being a movement of health professionals only to one with the effective participation of patients and family members. During this Conference, the motto adopted was "for a society without insane asylums," aiming their gradual abolition and the determination of May 18th as the National Day of Struggle Against Asylums (Amarante & Nunes, 2018).

Although only in 2000 was the first regulatory framework approved—the Law 10,216 of April 6, 2001, which provides for the protection and rights of people with mental disorders and seeks to reorient the mental health care model (Lei No 10.216, de 6 de abril de, 2001), this model had been going through changes since the previous decade.

In the following year, Psychosocial Care Centers are regulated as territorial and community-based services, substitutes for hospitalization in insane asylums (Portaria No 336, de 19 de fevereiro de, 2002). In 2003, the Ministry of Health endorsed a policy affirming the care of patients based on an expanded health perspective, provided in the territory and through an intersectoral network, in order to reduce the harm caused by drug use (Portaria No 457, de 16 de abril de, 2003).

Despite the advances seen in the health field, subsequent regulatory[4] benchmarks demonstrate the dispute of the projects existent in the area of care of people who use alcohol and other harmful drugs, mainly based on society's concern with the consumption of crack cocaine, which on the one hand-built narrative by strengthening the care offered by SUS, valuing services of psychosocial nature, and on the other, the isolation of these people, diverting the focus from the social determinants involved in drug consumption. In this dispute of projects and, consequently, of the public fund, in 2011 the Psychosocial Care Network is created.

The Care for People with Needs Resulting from the Use of Alcohol and Other Drugs in the Psychosocial Care Network: RAPS

The Psychosocial Care Network (RAPS) is one of the Health Care Networks—RAS—is a component of the Integrated Health Care System. The last is organized through an organized set of health care segments created to provide continuous and comprehensive care, capable to attend the healthcare needs of people in acute and chronic conditions with efficiency, effectiveness, quality, safety, and equity, coordinated and oriented by the Primary Health Care—PHC.

[4] National Drug Policy (Resolução No 3 GSIPR/CH/CONAD, 2005); Integrated Plan to Combat Crack Cocaine (Decreto No 7.179, de 20 de maio de, 2010); Crack cocaine, it is possible to win (Ministério da Justiça, 2011), even though there is an expansion of services such as CAPS and of the number of beds in general hospitals, at the same time there is also an increase of the number of beds in therapeutics communities.

The RAPS was instituted by the Directive GM/MS n° 3.088, of December 23, 2011 (republished on May 21, 2013), following the guidelines of this new model of care. Its main goals are to expand access for the population to psychosocial care in its different levels of complexity; to promote access for people with mental disorders and with needs arising from the use of crack, alcohol, and other drugs and their families to healthcare segments; to ensure the articulation and integration of the healthcare segments existent in the health networks of the territory, qualifying care through user embracement, ongoing care, and attention to emergencies (Portaria No 3.088, de 23 de dezembro de, 2011). To achieve these goals and break with this paradigm that fragments people and seeks ultimate answers as way of treatment, psychosocial care needs to operate and to produce network care based on the following components and healthcare segments: primary healthcare (primary healthcare care unit, street outreach teams, supporting teams to therapeutic residential care services, community centers); specialized psychosocial care (Psychosocial Care Centers); urgent and emergency care (The Mobile Emergency Medical Service—SAMU 192, stabilization rooms, 24 h Emergency Care Units, emergency care hospitals, primary care units); residential care of a transitional nature (outreach units, residential care facilities—UAA and UAI); hospital care (specialized psychiatric ward in general hospitals and referral hospital service to care for people with mental suffering or disorder and with needs arising from the use of crack, alcohol and other drugs); deinstitutionalization strategies (Residential Therapeutic Services) and psychosocial rehabilitation.

Although Residential Therapeutic Services (SRT) and psychosocial rehabilitation are components of RAPS, for the purposes of this study, those aspects will not be approached deeply, since the theoretical and practical dimensions of deinstitutionalization and psychosocial rehabilitation need to be tackled in a cross-sectoral manner. These need to be associated with other network devices and seen as coordinators of the psychiatric reform, enduring the current challenges of the mental health policy within the scope of alcohol and other drugs.

Primary Health Care

One of the strategies used by the Ministry of Health when expanding the access for general population to the psychosocial care provided by the Unified Health System (SUS) is the organization of primary health care and its other network points.

In the field of mental health, among others, the Family Health Strategy (ESF), street outreach teams, community centers have, therefore, the strategic role of reorienting health practices and actions through the perspective of integrality (Silva et al. 2018).

In this sense, territory-based and primary care services are viewed as main fields of action, as they function not only on a territorial logic of care but also use it to create a connection with the community and understand its dynamics, seeing more than a spatial/geographic cutout.

The territory used for these units should also include the symbolic, affective, and relationship dimensions that each individual develops in their lives in order to produce other forms of existing, in a way they can improve self-care and, consequently, of the community.

In order to guarantee the first access to health, primary care services should be the entrance for people with needs arising from the use of alcohol and other drugs. These must act in the territory and bet on its disruptive potential to break and transform the asylum culture into the community culture.

Therefore, the existence of a strong network of primary care services constitutes a solid basis for the expansion and overcome of service capacity. However, the constant challenges only reinforce the existing gap in primary care work, due to network integration challenges and to the lack of human resources who are properly trained for working in community care.

Aiming to qualify the work processes and to create an opening for the development of other logics able to sustain care in primary care services, cases that require other sorts of knowledge, not existent on the people who integrate the mini teams, need the matrix support of Family Health Support Centers—NASF.[5]

According to Fortes et al. (2014) the matrix support carried out by NASF is consolidated as a proposition to expand the frontiers of Mental Health care by changing fragmented visits to longitudinal attention, pharmacological based treatment to a biopsychosocial approach, that is, changing from specialized work to collaborative work.

The pedagogical and inter-consultation strategies used with the mini-teams in the NASF meetings, to deal with situations of greater difficulty related to the use of psychoactive substances, ensure the continuity of care in primary care services, as well as the possibility to share serious matters with the CAPS. In addition, they (re) affirm the role of primary care in access to health and monitoring of pregnant women and people suffering from sexually transmitted infections (STIs), HIV, tuberculosis, and other non-transmissible clinical comorbidities that affect the lives of these patients.

Street Outreach Offices (CnaR)

The homeless population who use alcohol and other drugs undergo vulnerabilities that have as a characteristic a relationship with the drug use permeated by misery, hunger, violence, and wrongdoings, demanding actions capable not only of

[5] Created by Portaria No 154, de 24 de janeiro de (2008), republished on March 4 of the same year, is decisive to the operation of the Family Health Strategy in RAPS, therefore strengthening the processes of health territorialization and regionalization. The NASF teams can be constituted by the following professionals: social workers, physical educators, pharmacists, physiotherapists, speech therapists, gynecologists, acupuncturists, homeopathic doctors, nutritionists, pediatricians, psychiatrists, and occupational therapists.

developing strategies to overcome these issues but also of creating ways to develop health and to reduce damage using the available resources, even if these are precarious.

In this perspective, the assistance to the homeless population in Brazil took its first steps with experiences that occurred diffusely in several states; among these experiences, emerge the Street Outreach Offices (CnaR), that appeared in the decade of 1990 in the city of Salvador, located in the state of Bahia, with the intention of providing health assistance to the homeless population who abuse alcohol and other drugs by developing harm reduction actions, enabling access to other existent points of the health network.

Inspired by these projects, the Street Outreach Offices are composed by groups of professionals who work in an itinerant way and in partnership with teams located in other points of attention of the health network, such as Basic Health Units, Centers of Psychosocial Attention, First-aid centers, among others, offering actions and healthcare services to the homeless population in general and taking into account their different health needs (Portaria No 122, de 25 de janeiro de, 2011).

The CnaRs are oriented by a transversal look of healthcare. On the one hand, primary care posture of prevention, promotion, and health care closely linked to the territory is embraced by them; on the other, the main focus is to not forget the original objective, which is working with mental health, more specifically with the harmful use of alcohol and other drugs.

Having the street as its working place and lightweight technologies[6] as the main instruments of practice, the Street Outreach Offices develop a great potential for developing bonds by accessing—even in an experiential way—morally covert themes such as the use of drugs. In this way, it reaches people with whom other health services have little connection and acquaintance. This kind of work has been positively evaluated, as reported in Silva et al. (2014), as it provides access to a public whose health care demand is still historically repressed. Associated with this, the Street Outreach Offices have also been successful in the treatment of neglected diseases that most frequently affect harmful users of alcohol and other drugs, such as tuberculosis and sexually transmitted infections.

Community and Culture Centers

These are spaces of sociability, production, and intervention of culture in the city (Portaria No 3.088, de 23 de dezembro de, 2011). Ferreira (2014), when researching the impact of these centers on users, highlights that those are spaces in which the

[6] Merhy (2005) argues that healthcare production technologies can be classified into three categories: light technologies, identified in bond production, reception, and management of work processes; light-hard technologies, referring to knowledge that is already systematized and less flexible, such as theories, medical practice and epidemiology; and hard technologies, concerning technological equipment, regulations, and organizational structures.

community can freely meet, develop together work, culture, and leisure spaces and bring discussions and opinions on their problems. This enables the inclusion of subjects who would normally be excluded, such as people with mental disorders, the elderly, and people who abuse substances.

To care is also to invest in culture and to give people the possibility of enjoying moments of leisure; therefore, the expansion of these services is fundamental, but also the promotion by other services of the RAPS of the opportunity to access art by their patients.

Psychosocial Care Centers, in their Different Modalities

The Psychosocial Care Centers (CAPS) are services of the Psychosocial Care Network, that care for people with severe and persistent mental disorders and people with needs arising from the use of alcohol and other drugs.

Despite being services belonging to the RAPS, and one of its places of specialized attention operating in a substitutive nature to the logic of asylum, currently they have to be understood as strategic and essential devices for monitoring situations that require comprehensive mental health care in the context of SUS. These units are designed based on the population number, in increasing order of complexity (CAPS I: from 20,000 to 70,000 inhabitants; CAPS II and CAPS AD II: from 70,000 to 200,000 inhabitants; CAPS III and CAPS AD III: above 200,000 inhabitants; and CAPSi: over 150,000 inhabitants). For cities that only count with a CAPS I, all age groups must receive treatment at the place. The units known as CAPS AD II and III are responsible for the treatment of adults, children or adolescents with needs resulting from the use of crack, alcohol and other drugs, whereas CAPSi only treats children and adolescents suffering from mental disorders or who abuse drugs (Portaria No 3.088, de 23 de dezembro de, 2011). Some units open on weekdays from 8 a.m. to 6 p.m, with the possibility of extending opening hours until 9 p.m., for example, CAPS II, AD II and i (Portaria No 336, de 19 de fevereiro de, 2002). Some are open 24 h a day, all days of the week, including weekends and holidays, such as the CAPS III and AD III; these count with night beds designed for attending crisis 24 h a day. (Portaria No 3.088, de 23 de dezembro de, 2011).

Although only CAPS III and AD III, as redefined by ordinance no. 130 of 2012, have 24-h crisis services, it is the work of all CAPS units to take on and monitor crisis situations, either by accessing CAPS units or when people suffering from mental disorders resort to the main entrances of mental health crisis units. Thus, as described in (Portaria No 336, de 19 de fevereiro de, 2002), the CAPS takes on the function of providing clinical care on a daily basis, avoiding hospitalizations in psychiatric hospitals. They are then considered Health Network Facilitators, ordering units of the mental health care network, and must develop activities directed to the territory—this being the place of possibilities and articulations with other health and mental health services and also with other policies, in the search for intersectoriality, rescuing the potentialities of community resources and promoting psychosocial reintegration.

While progress has been made towards the effectiveness of these units, expansion of its coverage, increase of financial investments made in community services, and significant reduction of the number of psychiatric beds, major challenges are still present, as these services have been proved to be insufficient when facing epidemiological challenges, the complexity of the problem, and the significant reduction in financial investments (FIOCRUZ, 2015).

When talking about the CAPS AD, these challenges expose significant obstacles, facing neo-institutionalization trends arising from social welfare policies, religious therapeutic communities, from the socio-educational system and the penal system, being the latter an issue that requires better evaluation due to the components of security measures in custodial psychiatric hospitals or in alternative measures (FIOCRUZ, 2015).

This new technology and its approaches, which are contrary to actions such as prohibitionism, institutionalization, and pathologization, are the reference, of the community and of the territory, for the care of people with needs related to the consumption of alcohol and other drugs (and their families) in terms of access, intake, and comprehensive care. Therefore, the approach of the CAPS AD units is based on the principles of harm reduction, which, according to the International Harm Reduction Association (2010), aim to reduce health and socioeconomic adverse consequences caused by drug use, without necessarily reducing its consumption, leading to benefits for the substance users, their families, and the community.

The CAPS AD units, aligned with harm reduction principles, must operate in the territory as a place that can also produce care, offering health assistance where drugs are available. Such proximity to territory allows one to understand its dynamics and vivacity, as well as the support network that each subject possesses.

Being much more than a place or a locus, the CAPS has the ethical and political proposal of recognizing alterity and different ways of living, while having a collective commitment to empower protagonism and different creative manners present in relationships and encounters (Santos & Yasui, 2016).

In this sense, the territorial work, not only in the monitoring of cases already registered, but also in the intake of people present in drug use scenes or psychotropic territories gives place and visibility to these subjects, diverting from stigmas and stereotypes to life quality production, using strategies of promotion, prevention, and protection.

Furthermore, although it may seem redundant, it is essential to emphasize that the CAPS AD, as Health Network Facilitators aware to the principles of harm reduction, psychiatric reform and of the SUS need to question, on a daily basis, the development of the network, which does not occur only through service provision flows and protocols, but more from a situation and its singularities. Therefore, the singular therapeutic project designed, triggers an intra- and intersectoral assemblage, generating, for all network points, joint accountability, and co-management of healthcare.

Urgent and Emergency Care

The development of new forms to care for people in psychological suffering, mental illness sufferers, and people with needs arising from the use of alcohol and other drugs in crisis situations at Urgent and Emergency care units is a fundamental aspect of the RAPS aligned with the psychiatric reform, as it is decisive and strategic because mental health crisis is historically seen as the gateway to psychiatric hospital admissions, only possible to be managed using asylum practices.

The RAPS attention points of urgent and emergency care, such as the Mobile Emergency Assistance Service (SAMU), stabilization rooms, 24-h Emergency Care Units (UPAs), urgent/emergency care hospitals, primary care units, among others, need to improve the services of patient intake and risk classification and care in urgent and emergency situations, in an articulated manner with the psychosocial network (Portaria No 3.088, de 23 de dezembro de, 2011).

Seeing beyond the mental health crisis improves and qualifies healthcare, as it enables the construction of life stories, of the patients' trajectories for the search of treatment, their emotional bonds, affects, and their network, pointing out to a possible path of care in the territory.

In this way, the proposition is to break paradigms, looking beyond mental health crisis and pathological symptoms that generate medicalized or stereotyped responses which have an impact on moral actions, especially for drug users. It also ensures the individualization of the crisis experience, affirming that the place for biological and/or psychical exacerbations, as well as one protected for when in risk or vulnerable, is also the territory community-based healthcare service, either by accompanying the patient to one of the urgent and emergency points of care or by coordinating care, arranging spots in night beds at CAPS AD III and CAPS III to follow the management of the crisis.

In this layout, networking is essential for a new approach and qualified response, where the crisis attention system foundation in mental health are not the stations, the specialized units, and crisis-oriented services themselves, but the extended healthcare network and clinical practice sustain the therapeutic projects of each patient in their territory, including, mainly, primary health care, keeping the capacity of intervention, and the community's own resources stored (Campos, 2014).

Hospital Care

The Brazilian Psychiatric Reform seeks a society without insane asylums. However, those are available when all other resources have been exhausted, meaning that users with mental disorders can be hospitalized. However, this hospitalization should be carried out as rapidly as possible. And, from the understanding that this person must be reintegrated into society, the hospitalization should be carried out preferably in general hospitals, and no longer in psychiatric ones. Mental health units in general hospitals are spaces of care equipped with mental health staff, designed for short stays, that must articulate with the other points of the psychosocial network so that the patient can return to his or her territory to continue the treatment.

In the case of people with needs arising from the use of alcohol and other drugs, hospitalization, when necessary, will be performed at the Referral Hospital Service - SHR, in Portuguese, in urgent/emergency situations resulting from the consumption or abstinence of alcohol and other drugs, as well as psychiatric and/or clinical comorbidities (Portaria No 3.088, de 23 de dezembro de, 2011).

Therefore, the hospitalization should be based on clinical criteria and recommended by the patients' CAPS, respecting the singular therapeutic project of each person. This system, along with the CAPS AD III night beds, makes it possible to replace hospitalization in psychiatric hospitals and in long-term institutions.

Outreach Unit

The outreach units are part of the transitional residential care service, instituted by Ordinance No. 121 of January 25, 2012. These units, existing in the modalities of Outreach Units for Adults (UAA, in Portuguese) and Outreach Units for Children—(UAI, in Portuguese), are of a transitional nature and have as reference a health unit, for example, CAPS AD. They are destined to voluntarily shelter and to offer continuous care for people at risk, socially vulnerable and which require therapeutic and protective monitoring, with health needs resulting from the use of alcohol and other drugs at risk.

There is little research on the work of the UAA and the UAI. Almeida (2019), when researching a UAA points out that this is a device that goes against the hospitalization and confinement model by providing places where patients can live together, promoting (re)construction of bonds, since it is not closed upon itself. The UAA team, in partnership with the CAPS team, must plan, coordinate, and accompany users' relationships on community spaces, expanding the possibilities of creating a negotiation field with the territory, family, and community. The author continues to highlight that the UAA brings the need to create different strategies for issues related to the treatment of people with needs arising from the use of alcohol and other drugs, to address the "inhabiting" question by those who are affected by inequality and marginalization due to use, who should occupy not only the space of their houses but also that of the city.

The dispute that determines the care of people with needs arising from the use of alcohol and other drugs, especially regarding the public fund, leads to little investment in this device when compared to therapeutic communities, which are also part of the RAPS. The need for a temporary distancing caused by the vulnerability is one of the signs of referral to therapeutic communities. However, therapeutic communities, as mentioned above, are characterized by a series of violations of rights and by a logic of treatment guided by religion, while the outreach units have care marked by the psychosocial attention perspective, guaranteeing freedom and the user access to social rights.

Final Considerations

The harmful use of alcohol and other drugs, being a multicausal phenomenon, demands a multifaceted network, to collectively think and execute actions that are consistent with each subject's stories, its actors, and their outcomes. For this reason, even though the RAPS services are divided into multiple levels and are responsible for different aspects of healthcare, they still need to cooperate in order to achieve a common goal, not dividing the responsibilities, but integrating them.

So, with the need to develop an articulated health network emerges a challenge: the need for communication. Because, for example, if someone drinks alcohol to relieve the hunger associated with life on the streets, it is necessary that the health-care field, in communication with others, facilitates this population's living conditions, so that it won't be necessary to drink in order to relieve hunger. At the same time, it is necessary to take care of a body that undergoes physiological, psychological, and social aggressions of this situation, and all of these aspects, precisely because of their complexity, are not covered by only one point of the attention network. But to enable this type of construction, it is necessary to analyze the health system itself, which, being implemented in a prohibitionist society—where care is often replaced by discipline—it is crucial to see people who abuse alcohol and other drugs as citizens before they can be seen as, sometimes, inadequate or even offenders.

This is essential discrimination to make before one can renounce a moral—which little can do as a judgment- and adopt the ethical position of a universal public policy which objective is to develop healthier projects for life and society.

It is worth mentioning that the new drug policy, sanctioned by Decree No. 9.761 of April 11th, 2019, goes against the advances made until then, seen in actions that generate health based on the construction of citizenship, since it engraves a supporting position to the war on drugs, removing the harm reduction policy as a guideline for working with substance abusers, therefore also disrespecting the rights of people who seek healthcare, enforcing abstinence as the only possible strategic horizon for treatment.

The new policy creates barriers of access and would possibly generate more if it were not for the fact that health teams, although influenced by the widespread morality bias, also remain guided by the principle of universality[7] which, as a pillar of the Unified Health System—SUS, defines that health is a right of all and not only

[7] Universalization: health is a right of citizenship for all people and it is up to the State to ensure this right, and access to actions and services must be guaranteed to all people, regardless of gender, race, occupation, or other social or personal characteristics.

of those who are abstinent. It ethically guides the worker to build possibilities in healthcare, even if the user's choice is not the same as the policy under discussion.

Therefore, the many services of the network must continue to articulate care for people who abuse alcohol and other drugs, working on improving the living conditions of the population, its social determinants and building singular therapeutic projects that include not only access to health services, but also to culture and leisure establishments.

References

Almeida, A. L. M. (2019). *Cuidado no território aos usuários de álcool e outras drogas: estudo de caso exploratório de uma Unidade de Acolhimento Adulto, um serviço residencial transitório* (Master's thesis, Fundação Oswaldo Cruz, Rio de Janeiro, Brazil). Retrieved from https://www.arca.fiocruz.br/handle/icict/40171

Amarante, P., & Nunes, M. O. (2018). A reforma psiquiátrica no SUS e a luta por uma sociedade sem manicômios. *Ciência & Saúde Coletiva, 23*(6), 2067–2074. https://doi.org/10.1590/1413-81232018236.07082018.

Bastos, F. I. P. M., & Bertoni, N. (Eds.). (2014). *Pesquisa nacional sobre o uso de crack: quem são os usuários de crack e/ou similares do Brasil? Quantos são nas capitais brasileiras?* Retrieved from https://www.arca.fiocruz.br/handle/icict/10019

Borges, J. (2019). *Encarceramento em massa*. São Paulo, Brazil: Pólen.

Campos, P. (2014). Crise, Rede e Hospitalidade: uma abordagem para a reforma psiquiátrica. In J. M. A. Soares, M. C. A. Carvalho, & P. R. Fagundes (Eds.), *Políticas e cuidado em saúde mental: Contribuição para a prática profissional*. Rio de Janeiro, Brazil: FIOCRUZ.

Carneiro, H. (2018). *Drogas: a história do proibicionismo*. São Paulo, Brazil: Autonomia Literária.

Decreto No 7.179, de 20 de maio de. (2010). *Institui o Plano Integrado de Enfrentamento ao Crack e outras Drogas, cria o seu Comitê Gestor, e dá outras providências*. Retrieved from http://www.planalto.gov.br/ccivil_03/_Ato2007-2010/2010/Decreto/D7179.htm

Decreto No 9.761, de 11 de abril de. (2019). *Aprova a Política Nacional sobre Drogas - Pnad, revoga o Decreto n° 4.345, de 26 de agosto de 2002, e dá outras providências*. Retrieved from http://www.in.gov.br/materia/-/asset_publisher/Kujrw0TZC2Mb/content/id/71137357/do1e-2019-04-11-decreto-n-9-761-de-11-de-abril-de-2019-711373 16

De Micheli, D. Andrade, A. L. M., Silva, E. A. & Souza-Formigoni, M. L. O. (2016). Drug Abuse in Adolescence. 1. ed. New York: Springer International Publishing. https://doi.org/10.1007/978-3-319-17795–3

Ferreira, P. H. R. (2014). *Centro de convivência e cultura e suas repercussões na vida de usuários de um centro de atenção psicossocial* (Master's Thesis, Universidade Estadual de Campinas, Brazil). Retrieved from http://taurus.unicamp.br/bitstream/REPOSIP/310870/1/Ferreira_PriscilaHelenaRubin_M.pdf

Fortes, S., Menezes, A., Athié, K., Chazan, L. F., Rocha, H., Thiesen, J., Ragoni, C., Pithon, T., & Machado, A. (2014). *Psiquiatria no século XXI: Transformações a partir da integração com a Aaenção primária pelo matriciamento*. Rio de Janeiro, Brazil: Physis.

Guedes, C. R., Nogueira, M. I., & Camargo, K. R., Jr. (2006). A subjetividade como anomalia: Contribuições epistemológicas para a crítica do modelo biomédico. *Ciência & Saúde Coletiva, 11*(4), 1093–1103. https://doi.org/10.1590/S1413-81232006000400030.

Instituto de Pesquisa Econômica Aplicada. (2018). *Comunidades Terapêuticas: temas para reflexão*. Brasília, Brazil: Author.

Lei No 10.216, de 6 de abril de. (2001). *Dispõe sobre a proteção e os direitos das pessoas portadoras de transtornos mentais e redireciona o modelo assistencial em saúde mental.* Retrieved from http://www.planalto.gov.br/ccivil_03/Leis/LEIS_2001/L10216.htm

Merhy, E. E. (2005). *Saúde: a cartografia do trabalho vivo.* São Paulo, Brazil: Hucitec.

Ministério da Justiça. (2011). *Crack, é possível vencer.* Retrieved from https://www.justica.gov.br/programas-e-planos/crack

Ministério da Saúde. (1986). *Relatório Final da 8ª Conferência Nacional de Saúde.* Retrieved from http://bvsms.saude.gov.br/bvs/publicacoes/8_conferencia_nacional_saude_relatorio_final.pdf

Ministério Público Federal. (2018) *Relatório de Inspeção Nacional em Comunidades Terapêuticas – 2017.* Retrieved from https://site.cfp.org.br/wp-content/uploads/2018/06/Relat%C3%B3rio-da-Inspe%C3%A7%C3%A3o-Nacional-em-Comunidades-Terap%C3%AAuticas.pdf

Oliveira, N., & Ribeiro, E. (2018). O massacre negro brasileiro na guerra às drogas: Reflexões sobre raça, necropolítica e o controle de psicoativos a partir da construção de uma experiência negra. *Revista Internacional de Direitos Humanos, 15*(28), 35–44.

Portaria No 122, de 25 de janeiro de. (2011). *Define as diretrizes de organização e funcionamento das Equipes de Consultório na Rua.* Retrieved from http://bvsms.saude.gov.br/bvs/saudelegis/gm/2012/prt0122_25_01_2012.html

Portaria No 154, de 24 de janeiro de. (2008). *Cria os Núcleos de Apoio à Saúde da Família - NASF.* Retrieved from http://bvsms.saude.gov.br/bvs/saudelegis/gm/2008/prt0154_24_01_2008.html

Portaria No 3.088, de 23 de dezembro de. (2011). *Institui a Rede de Atenção Psicossocial para pessoas com sofrimento ou transtorno mental e com necessidades decorrentes do uso de crack, álcool e outras drogas, no âmbito do Sistema Único de Saúde (SUS).* Retrieved from http://bvsms.saude.gov.br/bvs/saudelegis/gm/2011/prt3088_23_12_2011_rep.html

Portaria No 336, de 19 de fevereiro de. (2002). Retrieved from http://portal.saude.gov.br/portalarquivos/pdf/Portaria% 20GM% 203362002.pdf

Portaria No 4.279, de 30 de dezembro de. (2010). *Estabelece diretrizes para a organização da Rede de Atenção à Saúde no âmbito do Sistema Único de Saúde (SUS).* Retrieved from http://bvsms.saude.gov.br/bvs/saudelegis/gm/2010/prt4279_30_12_2010.html

Portaria No 457, de 16 de abril de. (2003). *Afirma sobre o cuidado dos usuários realizado a partir da perspectiva ampliada de saúde.* Retrieved from http://bvsms.saude.gov.br/bvs/saudelegis/gm/2003/prt0457_16_04_2003.html

Resolução No 3 GSIPR/CH/CONAD. (2005). Retrieved from https://www.justica.gov.br/central-de-conteudo/politicas-sobre-drogas/cartilhas-politicas-sobre-drogas/2011legislacaopoliticaspublicas.pdf

Santos, C. E., & Yasui, S. (2016). Muito além do CAPS AD: O cuidado no território e na vida. In A. C. S. Souza (Ed.), *Entre pedras e fissuras.* São Paulo, Brazil: Hucitec.

Silva, F. P., Frazão, I. S., & Linhares, F. M. P. (2014). Práticas de saúde das equipes dos Consultórios de Rua. *Cadernos de Saúde Pública, 30*(4), 805–814. https://doi.org/10.1590/0102-311X00100513.

Silva, M. B., & Delduque, M. C. (2015). Patologização e penalização do uso de drogas: uma análise socioantropológica de proposições legislativas (2007-2010). *Physis: Revista de Saúde Coletiva, 25*(1), 231–250. https://doi.org/10.1590/S0103-73312015000100013.

Silva, M. A. A., Andrade, A. L. M., & De Micheli, D. (2018). Evaluation of the Implementation of Brief Interventions to Substance Abuse in a Socieducative Context. *Revista Psicologia em Pesquisa, 12*(1). http://dx.doi.org/10.24879/2018001200100125.

Vargas, E. (1998). Os corpos intensivos: Sobre o estatuto social do consumo de drogas legais e ilegais. In L. F. Duarte & O. Leal (Eds.), *Doença, sofrimento, perturbação: perspectivas etnográficas.* Rio de Janeiro, Brazil: FIOCRUZ.

Chapter 25
Health Services and the Care Network for People Who Have Problems Arising from Drug Use and the Role of Professionals in Health Care

Vitor Leite Ferreira, Pollyanna Santos da Silveira, Leonardo Fernandes Martins, and Telmo Mota Ronzani

Introduction

The way drugs are viewed today incorporates aspects that began to be designed a little over a century ago and which have contributed to the construction of a negative and repulsive view of the people who use these substances, especially those considered illicit. The use of drugs are a topic of great interest and have prompted wide discussions in various sectors of society, having acquired throughout history and in different places, meanings and varied uses, and are still used in large quantities and their abuse considered a public health problem (Prates et al. 2014; Vargas 2006).

In this sense, it is indispensable to think about the care and access to health that are proposed by the State to drug users and addicts, which historically has demonstrated a coercive and inelastic posture towards the contexts of consumption and that even today is involved in antagonistic and heated debates. In addition, the negative attitudes and beliefs towards these users by health professionals, highlighted in the literature, call attention to the role that professionals have been playing in the daily life of health services and in the assistance network, and how they stand before the laws and guidelines that govern their professional activity, as well as the endless discussions that are drawn up in the political and social fields regarding the treatment given to drugs and the path that the user must go through the health network (Alves 2009; Costa et al. 2013; Ronzani and Furtado 2010).

V. L. Ferreira (✉) · T. M. Ronzani
Universidade Federal de Juiz de Fora, Juiz de Fora, MG, Brazil

P. S. da Silveira
Universidade Católica de Petrópolis, Petrópolis, RJ, Brazil

L. F. Martins
Universidade Salgado de Oliveira, Niterói, RJ, Brazil

D. De Micheli et al. (eds.), *Drugs and Human Behavior*,
https://doi.org/10.1007/978-3-030-62855-0_25

Stipulation of Social and Arbitrary Control of Substance Use

The proposals and public policies that are developed in order to address the problem of drugs arise from the moment that there is an increase, in the nineteenth century, in the consumption of substances resulting from the process of industrialization. Through this process, scientists began to isolate the active principles of plants, making the substances more potent, while other drugs had their consumption encouraged by emerging industry, attracting those who wanted to ease their pain and those who, in a hedonistic pursuit of pleasure, maintained a use that could feed their subjective travels. The ordering of this consumption, until then regulated by sociocultural strategies, suffers a disarray, therefore, which forces the State to interfere (Alves 2009; MacRae 2001; Ronzani 2018).

Claims in favor of the prohibition of commercialization, especially of alcoholic beverages, gained strength in U.S. territory with the creation of the Prohibitionist Party in the second half of the nineteenth century, supported by the interests of other conservative groups and a science that gained space in the field of health and wanted to give voice to its researchers and doctors, who in turn had the knowledge about the damage caused by substances. Such positions remain in vogue during the twentieth century, strengthened worldwide by the economic power that had become the U.S., in some sequences of Conventions and Conferences, whose objective was to combat drugs that could lead to abuse (Alves 2009; MacRae 2001).

Due to political interests, the issue of drug use and the consequent actions on how to deal with the consumption and commercialization of these substances were accompanied by antagonistic positions that influenced the implementation of drug programs and policies. The so-called prohibitionist current is based on the idea that the strong criminal repression of the planting, production, commercialization, and consumption of some substances leads to the reduction of their availability and their consequent extinction in society, in the idea of the "drug-free world." On the other hand, we would have the so-called anti-prohibitionists who defend that the regularization of the production chain and consumption of substances could generate greater control over the harmful consequences of their use, and other effects generated by prohibition, such as violence, organized crime, and large imprisonment of specific populations, thus reducing the social vulnerability associated with the consumption and commercialization of Karam (2017).

Prohibitionist strategies, implemented and led by the United States of America (USA), gained great strength in the world during the course of the twentieth century, consolidating and spreading hegemonically, without, however, demonstrating satisfactory results. It can be said that it failed consubstantially, if observed its main explicit objective, which was to promote abstinence from illicit drugs and to eradicate international drug trafficking (Costa et al. 2015). However, it can be affirmed that it was very efficient from the point of view of ideological and geopolitical control, criminalization, genocide, and mass imprisonment of a specific public (Ronzani 2018).

It seems simple at first to think that relegating some drugs to the category of illegal makes them inaccessible, but the history that followed shows us with strong evidence that this is not possible (Karam 2017). A clear example is the so-called Prohibition Act, instituted in the USA from 1920 to 1932, which prohibited the consumption of alcohol, something completely unimaginable to anyone in today's society, and which resulted in a vertiginous growth of the illegal market, violence, and the fortune of families involved in trafficking (Carneiro 2002). These consequences are also found around the trade of any other drug that has remained illicit, with strong illegal trade and high demand for consumption, feeding an immense network of trafficking that produces new and more powerful substances each year, which easily contradicts the initial pretensions of prohibition laws and observes an increasingly early onset of drug use by adolescents (Alves 2009; Franco and Rodrigues 2014; Karam 2017).

The popularization of this perspective of abstinence was present in the formulation of the whole political and social apparatus regarding illicit drugs in much of the world in the last century, including Brazil. The country was one of those responsible for the inclusion of marijuana in the illicit drugs panorama (Carlini 2006) and had the development of its policies focused on the repression and prohibition of some substances, following deliberations of international institutions like the United Nations (UN).

In this context, the *anti-drug* policy and actions towards users in Brazil are supported and justified by medical/pseudoscientific, legal/criminal, and moral/religious discourses (Ronzani 2018). Institutionalized medicine focused on a market practice excludes social and cultural interference from the health-disease process, taking the individual as a purely biological organism and decontextualized from its history and social environment, considering the disease as a physical mark on the body and a simple health counterpoint (Prates et al. 2014).

Thus, led by a still young Psychiatry and imbued with biomedical practices, the number of psychiatric hospitals began to grow, whose social function was to remove from the eyes of society all unacceptable behavior, which were summed up in some groups such as those of drug addicts, beggars, people with mental illnesses, and carriers of venereal diseases. That is, the institutionalization of a discourse, which defined a closed place and which isolated, in some cases for the rest of their lives, undesirable groups in the eyes of the good society. In the area of drugs, religious/moral and medical/pseudoscientific treatment is incorporated by health professionals and the developed treatments are organized, therefore, in a conception of total abstinence of the individual who profoundly transgressed his individuality, with the intention of correcting him before what would be considered correct (Prates et al. 2014).

The hegemony of the biomedical model and the prohibitionist view began to be questioned more intensely in the 1970s and 1980s. Psychiatric hospitals are the targets of accusations of neglect and insults suffered by their inmates, which gains the media and draws the attention of public and political opinion. The so-called Psychiatric Reform that starts from then on begins to evolve progressively with the support of professionals, families, and the community and to question the way these hospitals work, projecting alternative forms of treatment for the patients hospitalized there (Maciel 2012).

At the same time, there are social movements and user and professional groups that apply and advocate the inclusion of Harm Reduction as an alternative to the zero tolerance model regarding the use of substances. Viewed as a rational and pragmatic option to care for people with drug use problems and more in line with an action based on human rights, Harm Reduction is applied in accordance with the fact that drug use has always existed and that there will be no society without it, so one must care for the user in order to reduce the negative consequences, usually with intermediate goals and an expanded care of these people (Alves 2009).

Gaining strength with the political movements in favor of the redemocratization of the country, the Psychiatric Reform is then constituted in defense of the deinstitutionalization, of the guarantee of rights and in a better access to health, topics that were taken to discussion in the VIII National Health Conference of 1986. This event and the period in question are considered important for the establishment of different thinking about the field of health, which is now understood also as a social and psychological product and in congruence with the quality of life, in addition to opening paths for the creation of the Unified Health System (SUS), whose main guiding point is health as a citizen's right and duty of the State (Fertonani et al. 2015; Maciel 2012).

Enlargement and Establishment of Ideas

The expanded conceptions of health, the organization of hierarchical and networked services are implemented throughout the 1990s and during the 2000s, from the Health Reform Movement and the implementation of SUS (Costa et al. 2013). Among the main public policies are the Family Health Program of 1994, later called Family Health Strategy (Ministry of Health 1997), the National Drug Policy (PNAD), previously called National Anti-Drug Policy and reformulated in 2005, from the National Secretariat of Drug Policy (SENAD) (Resolution No. 3 GSIPR/CH/CONAD, 2005), the Policy of Integral Attention to Alcohol Users and Other Drugs of 2003 (PAIUAD), from the Ministry of Health (2003) and the promulgation of Law No. 11.343 (2006), which signaled, at the time, the new Brazilian legislation on drugs.

Specifically in the health sector, with the formulation of integral, hierarchical, and regionalized care in mind, the Health Care Network (RAS) was implemented, which works linked to the SUS and must follow its basic precepts, such as the right to citizenship, universal and equal access, and integral citizen care, which serve as premises for the development of actions in the field of public health and in the care of users of alcohol and other drugs (Fertonani et al. 2015). Such actions are organized focused on the population, i.e., they are formulated together with the individual, family, and community, according to their needs, requiring professionals to know the populations for which they are responsible. They must also articulate the various services and professionals so that the network functions as such, with the presence of interdisciplinary teams that communicate and cooperate with each other. This dynamic must guarantee the promotion of health, diagnosis, treatment, prevention, and rehabilitation, through an apparatus that moves away from the hegemonic model of high hierarchization and little communication and prevailing medical knowledge, towards a reorganization molded in intersectoriality and in the sum of the knowledge of the various areas of health (Costa et al. 2015; Fertonani et al. 2015).

From the Health Care Network (RAS), the Psychosocial Care Network (RAPS), instituted by the Ministry of Health and whose focus is on care for people with suffering or mental disorders, as well as those who have problems arising from the use of alcohol and other drugs, is ordered, thus attributing the responsibility for care of these patients to mental health (Machado and Boarini 2013; Ordinance No. 3088, 2011). In general, it is through Primary Health Care (PHC) that these individuals have the main access to the country's health system that, through the Family Health Strategy, they are assisted in their demand in a global manner and inserted in the network. It is recommended to offer services or care based on needs and from active and democratic health care methodologies, including prevention of harmful use of alcohol and other drugs, early diagnosis, treatment of simpler cases, and referral of more complex cases to specialized services (Oliveira and Ronzani 2012).

The specialized devices primarily responsible for serving these users are the Center for Psychosocial Care (CAPS) and the Center for Psychosocial Care – Alcohol and Other Drugs (CAPSad). They are intended to treat the specific demands of users with disorders resulting from the use of substances and that, through individual therapeutic projects, in a territorial manner and aiming the social insertion or reinsertion of its users, promote a development of the potential of patients, away from the hospitalocentric vision in intensive, semi-intensive, and non-intensive treatment regimens (Costa et al. 2015: Ordinance No 3088, 2011). In addition, the RAPS also provides a series of devices that must act jointly and in constant dialogue for better maintenance of the network of services, such as Reception Units (UA), Mobile Emergency Care Services (SAMU), Hospital Care, the SRTs (Residential Therapeutic Services), Psychosocial Rehabilitation Strategies, among others (Costa et al. 2015).

The process of implementation of SUS and all the rationality in health that comes from it is a result of a struggle of forces, with advances and setbacks, especially the constant dispute between the private ideals, that conceive health as a commodity and good to be consumed, and the public, that considers health as a basic right of the citizens. In this struggle, difficulties in implementing RAS and RAPS are observed, as well as co-existing health care rationalities in our public health, which directly interfere in the implementation of programs and actions in the area. In this sense, it is important to understand that the change in the Brazilian health system is still in process and in constant struggle with perspectives and contradictions (Costa et al. 2017).

The Insertion of the Professional in Health Policy Experiences

These conflicting interests in the organization of health supply also fall on the development and establishment of drug policies. Furthermore, the assumptions that their use is an event explained by moralizing ideas and treated only on a biological and criminal level are still an existing reality and very influential in the way the State and society see the problem (Ximenes et al. 2018). Such conceptions, articulated with prohibitionist practices, continue to violate and marginalize in a classist and racist way populations inserted in a context of social vulnerability and extreme poverty, mainly blacks and residents of the periphery. In this way, they are used as scapegoats to explain the enormous social inequalities imposed by the capitalist system and normalized by the State (Ronzani 2018; Ximenes et al. 2018). The irrational ideal of a drug-free society operates using the "War on Drugs" as a weapon, consolidating itself in government policies and laws that, over the years, have shown little change in the repressive content of the fight against illicit substances. The so-called Drug Law (Law No. 11,343, 2006) won the media by abrogating Laws 10,409/2002 and 6,638/1976 and by bringing the differentiation of punishment between users and traffickers, while at the same time reinforcing the repression of unauthorized sales and the illicit drug market with greater penalties related to these acts, compared to the 1976 Law. Without objectifying, however, the amount of drug seized that would represent the distinction between consumption itself and commercialization, the law made it possible for exclusionary conduct aimed at specific social groups to increasingly fill prisons. These determinations were largely responsible for a five-fold increase in the rate of inmates from 2006 to 2014, of which about 67% were black or brown (Alves 2009; Karam 2017; Ximenes et al. 2018). On the other hand, the Law presented significant advances by emphasizing the importance of prevention of misuse, health care, and social reinsertion and allowing less repressive and more humanized alternatives regarding the treatment of users (Alves 2009). Contradictions such as these reveal the constant divergence and dispute of interests of political agents in the formulation of legislation, a picture recently highlighted by Law 13,840 (2019), which amends the Law of 11,343 (2006) and fails to mention the reduction of harm and risks to health present in the latter, legalizes involuntary hospitalizations in hospitals and health units and now formally accepts therapeutic communities for voluntary treatment.

Paradoxical elements are also found among the policies developed, such as considering in PNAD, for example, psychiatric hospitals as a possible place for treatment, a determination incompatible with PAIUAD, which establishes that the provision of care must be performed in extra-hospital devices. Likewise, the great expansion of CAPS and CAPSad to the detriment of the other models of care present at PAIUAD is pointed out as a restriction of investments in only one or another device, which does not match the comprehensive assistance project originally proposed. In view of this, doubts are raised as to whether the operation of CAPSad is a mere transposition of the models of care of CAPS mental health (Costa et al. 2017).

Taking into account, therefore, these mismatches of information in force in the arrangement of the attention network, it is also necessary to consider the professional, who in his daily performance, is responsible for enforcing the conducts provided for by Laws and new policies. Based on these conceptions and having the State as a guarantee and financer of their activities, it is important that the professionals are aware of the laws and the historical process that accompany the care in mental health and in the area of alcohol and other drugs. This is necessary so that a critical view of the whole does not allow the guidelines of the protocols to be merely replicas of practices in daily work and that mismatches or scrapping by antagonistic political actors of Psychiatric Reform become stronger. Costa et al. (2013) had access through their study carried out with agents of the welfare network in the area of alcohol and other drugs in a municipality of Minas Gerais some beliefs regarding the attention network. Although they understand the organization of the network and its functionality, there is a naturalization and acceptance of the processes by professionals who do not raise questions about the network's articulation and other ways it could be organized.

In addition to the necessary interaction of professionals with the network and political sectors that structure it, it is also essential to take a look at the contact that exists between the professional and the drug user who reaches the health services in search of help or treatment. The quality of the relationship that is established between these health agents and the user is of paramount importance for better adherence to the service and greater guarantees of success in treatment. However, several studies indicate that professional-user contact does not always happen in a positive way, because many of them show fear and distrust towards drug-using patients, as well as discredit in the treatment process and little knowledge about the subject, facts considered negative in the quality of care (Chu and Galang 2013; Lev-Ran et al. 2013).

The stigma that exists towards the drug user is perceived through the attitudes and beliefs described and interferes in a significant way with health care, directly influencing treatment, and can also be a barrier that affects basic human needs such as housing, interpersonal relationships, and employment (Sickel et al. 2014). Social stigma is defined by a brand that is given to a person or a group and that grants them a strongly negative and inferior characteristic, opening space for marginalization, and exclusion of this individual or group (Oliveira and Ronzani 2012; Ronzani and Furtado 2010).

In the meantime, cultural conceptions may also endorse that public policies, intentionally or unintentionally, limit opportunities for stigmatized people to access health services, reducing prospects for recovery based solely on perceived unpredictability or threat (Rüsch et al. 2005). In this way, stigma is understood to represent a mechanism capable of producing health inequalities (Hatzenbuehler 2016).

Several researches have been carried out around the world in order to investigate how stigma, attitudes, and beliefs have been shown in the drug–professional relationship, indicating a great interest in the subject and its consequences. In addition to the negative attitudes mentioned above, the researches point to the lack of training in the formation courses on the theme of alcohol and other drugs and the care for the patient user as a major factor responsible for negative beliefs and prejudices, as well as the belief that the situation they present is not of real importance as a user who presents, for example, kidney or coronary problems (Ferreira et al. 2019; Rocha et al. 2013).

More positive attitudes are therefore expected and seen as promising in the development of therapeutic projects, because when professionals show more consideration for the user, they tend to feel more prepared and motivated to work with these people (Ronzani and Furtado 2010). Thus, the awareness of the issue of drugs, the history that goes through it and the constant use of substances by society should be made to the extent that the stigma, along with negative attitudes and beliefs, are rethought and reflected in the same critical line as the historical movements of the last century, moving away from moral judgments and facing the reality of drugs from an ethical perspective of prevention and harm reduction.

Final Considerations

Considering that the topic of drugs has been neglected in the formulation of public policies and health care, being relegated to legal/criminal actions and characterized as a topic full of divergences and debated in various instances of the public sphere, it is necessary to discuss this topic based on more detailed analysis and contextualized in a historical line so that misinformation does not interfere with the proposition of ideas or accumulation of misinterpretations (Laport and Junqueira 2015). However, the deep-rooted conceptions about the illegality of some drugs that stimulate a dichotomy of good and evil, of bad and good, are still very present and, added to monetary and political-conservative interests, leave a narrow space for the real implementation of the care project discussed in the 1980s during the Psychiatric Reform.

The understanding of this panorama is essential for anyone who acts, in some way, in the field of drug policies, especially health professionals who deal directly with users of psychoactive substances. These professionals are extremely necessary in the defense of the assistance model provided for in the SUS norms and in the text of the Policy of Integral Attention to Alcohol and Other Drug Users, in addition to providing in practice the improvement of health and living conditions of users, working on social reinsertion. It is also essential that the work be supported in positive attitudes towards the development of the treatment and the situation the user finds himself in, so that the relationship between professional and patient is established in a consistent manner aiming at the best adherence of this patient to the treatment. To this end, discussions and reflections on the subject of drugs and stigma should be encouraged, as well as the formation processes on the subject and the encouragement of the inclusion of the problem in the curricula of health training courses.

References

Alves, V. S. (2009). Modelos de atenção à saúde de usuários de álcool e outras drogas: Discursos políticos, saberes e práticas. *Cadernos de Saúde Pública [online], 25*(11), 2309–2319. https://doi.org/10.1590/S0102-311X2009001100002.

Carlini, E. A. (2006). A história da maconha no Brasil. *Jornal Brasileiro de Psiquiatria, 55*(4), 314–317. https://doi.org/10.1590/S0047-20852006000400008.

Carneiro, H. (2002). As necessidades humanas e o proibicionismo das drogas no século XX. *Outubro, 6*, 115–128. Retrieved from http://www.neip.info/downloads/t_hen2.pdf.

Chu, C., & Galang, A. (2013). Hospital nurses' attitudes toward patients with a history of illicit drug use. *Canadian-nurse.com, 109*(6), 29–34.

Costa, P. H. A., Colugnati, F. A. B., & Ronzani, T. M. (2015). As redes de atenção aos usuários de álcool e outras drogas: Histórico, políticas e pressupostos. In T. M. Ronzani, P. H. A. Costa, D. C. B. Mota, & T. J. Laport (Eds.), *Redes de Atenção aos Usuários de Drogas - Políticas e Práticas* (pp. 41–66). São Paulo, Brazil: Editora Cortez.

Costa, P. H. A., Laport, T. J., Mota, D. B., & Ronzani, T. M. (2013). A rede assistencial sobre drogas segundo seus próprios atores. *Saúde em Debate, 37*, 110–119. https://doi.org/10.1590/1413-81232015202.20682013.

Costa, P. H. A., Ronzani, T. M., & Colugnati, F. A. B. (2017). "No papel é bonito, mas na prática..." análise sobre a rede de atenção aos usuários de drogas nas políticas e instrumentos normativos da área. *Saúde e Sociedade, 26*(3), 738–750. https://doi.org/10.1590/s0104-12902017170188.

Ferreira, V. L., Goroso, M. E. I., & Ronzani, T. M. (2019). Actitudes, creencias y estigma atribuidos por profesionales de la salud a dependientes de sustancias psicoactivas: una revisión sistemática. *Drugs and Addictive Behavior, 4*(2), 225–245. https://doi.org/10.21501/24631779.3368.

Fertonani, H. P., Pires, D. E. P., Biff, D., & Scherer, M. D. A. (2015). Modelo assistencial em saúde: Conceitos e desafios para a atenção básica brasileira. *Ciência & Saúde Coletiva, 20*(6), 1869–1878. https://doi.org/10.1590/1413-81232015206.13272014.

Franco, G. R., & Rodrigues, M. C. (2014). Ensino de habilidades de vida: uma estratégia de prevenção e promoção da saúde na adolescência. In T. M. Ronzani & P. S. Silveira (Eds.), *Prevenção ao uso de álcool e outras drogas no contexto escolar* (pp. 71–90). Juiz de Fora, Brazil: Editora UFJF.

Hatzenbuehler, M. L. (2016). Structural stigma: Research evidence and implications for psychological science. *American Psychologist, 71*(8), 742–751. https://doi.org/10.1037/amp0000068.

Karam, M. L. (2017). Considerações sobre as políticas criminais, drogas e direitos humanos. In M. D. Vecchia, T. M. Ronzani, F. S. Paiva, C. B. Batista, & P. H. A. Costa (Eds.), *Drogas e direitos humanos: reflexões em tempos de guerra às drogas* (pp. 211–232). Porto Alegre, Brazil: Rede Unida Editora.

Laport, T. J., & Junqueira, L. A. P. (2015). A intersetorialidade nas políticas sobre drogas. In T. M. Ronzani, P. H. A. Costa, D. C. B. Mota, & T. J. Laport (Eds.), *Redes de Atenção aos Usuários de Drogas - Políticas e Práticas* (pp. 67–84). São Paulo, Brazil: Editora Cortez.

Lei No 10.409, de 11 de janeiro de 2002. Dispõe sobre a prevenção, o tratamento, a fiscalização, o controle e a repressão à produção, ao uso e ao tráfico ilícitos de produtos, substâncias ou drogas ilícitas que causem dependência física ou psíquica, assim elencados pelo Ministério da Saúde, e dá outras providências. Retrieved from http://www.planalto.gov.br/ccivil_03/LEIS/2002/L10409.htm#:~:text=LEI%20No%2010.409%2C%20DE%2011%20DE%20JANEIRO%20DE%202002.&text=Disp%C3%B5e%20sobre%20a%20preven%C3%A7%C3%A3o%2C%20o,Sa%C3%BAde%2C%20e%20d%C3%A1%20outras%20provid%C3%AAncias

Lei No 11.343, de 23 de agosto de 2006. Institui o Sistema Nacional de Políticas Públicas sobre Drogas - Sisnad; prescreve medidas para prevenção do uso indevido, atenção e reinserção social de usuários e dependentes de drogas; estabelece normas para repressão à produção não autorizada e ao tráfico ilícito de drogas; define crimes e dá outras providências. Retrieved from http://www.planalto.gov.br/ccivil_03/_ato2004-2006/2006/lei/l11343.htm

Lei No 13.840, de 5 de junho de 2019. Dispõe sobre o Sistema Nacional de Políticas Públicas sobre Drogas e as condições de atenção aos usuários ou dependentes de drogas e para tratar do financiamento das políticas sobre drogas. Retrieved from http://www.planalto.gov.br/ccivil_03/_ato2019-2022/2019/lei/L13840.htm

Lei No 6368, de 21 de outubro de 1976. Dispõe sobre medidas de prevenção e repressão ao tráfico ilícito e uso indevido de substâncias entorpecentes ou que determinem dependência física ou psíquica, e dá outras providências. Retrieved from http://www.planalto.gov.br/ccivil_03/leis/L6368.htm

Lev-Ran, S., Adler, L., Nitzan, U., & Fennig, S. (2013). Attitudes towards nicotine, alcohol and drug dependence among physicians in Israel. *Journal of Substance Abuse Treatment, 44*(1), 84–89. https://doi.org/10.1016/j.jsat.2012.04.001.

Machado, L. V., & Boarini, M. L. (2013). Políticas sobre drogas no Brasil: a Estratégia de Redução de danos. *Psicologia: Ciência e Profissão, 33*(3), 580–595. https://doi.org/10.1590/S1414-98932013000300006.

Maciel, S. C. (2012). Reforma psiquiátrica no Brasil: Algumas reflexões/ Psychiatric reform in Brazil: A few reflections. *Cadernos Brasileiros de Saúde Mental/Brazilian Journal of Mental Health, 4*(8), 73–82.

MacRae, E. (2001). Antropologia: Aspectos Sociais, Culturais e Ritualísticos. In S. D. Seibel & A. Toscano Jr. (Eds.), *Dependência de Drogas* (pp. 25–34). São Paulo, Brazil: Editora Atheneu.

Ministério da Saúde. (1997). *Saúde da Família: uma estratégia para a reorientação do modelo assistencial.* Retrieved from https://bvsms.saude.gov.br/bvs/publicacoes/memorias_saude_familia_brasil.pdf

Ministério da Saúde. (2003). *A Política do Ministério da Saúde para atenção integral de usuários de álcool e outras drogas.* Retrieved from http://portalarquivos2.saude.gov.br/images/pdf/2015/marco/10/A-Pol%2D%2Dtica-do-Minist%2D%2Drio-da-Sa%2D%2Dde-para-Aten%2D%2D%2D%2Do-Integral-ao-Usu%2D%2Drio-de%2D%2D-lcool-e-Outras-Drogas%2D%2D2003-.pdf

Oliveira, M. C., & Ronzani, T. M. (2012). Estigmatização e práticas de profissionais da APS referentes ao consumo de álcool. *Psicologia: Ciência e Profissão, 32*(3), 648–661. https://doi.org/10.1590/S1414-98932012000300010.

Portaria No 3088, de 23 de dezembro de 2011. Institui a Rede de Atenção Psicossocial para pessoas com sofrimento ou transtorno mental e com necessidades decorrentes do uso de crack, álcool e outras drogas, no âmbito do Sistema Único de Saúde (SUS). Retrieved from http://bvsms.saude.gov.br/bvs/saudelegis/gm/2011/prt3088_23_12_2011_rep.html

Prates, J. G., Pinho, P. H., de Oliveira, M. A. F., & Claro, H. G. (2014). A concepção dos enfermeiros de serviços de urgência e emergência sobre o processo saúde-doença na assistência aos usuários de substâncias psicoativas. *Saúde em Debate, 38*(101). https://doi.org/10.5935/0103-1104.20140029.

Resolução No 3 GSIPR/CH/CONAD. (2005). Retrieved from https://www.justica.gov.br/central-de-conteudo/politicas-sobre-drogas/cartilhas-politicas-sobre-drogas/2011legislacaopoliticaspublicas.pdf

Rocha, F. M., Vargas, D., de Oliveira, M. A. F., & Bittencourt, M. N. (2013). Caring for people with psychoactive substance dependence: Nursing student perceptions. *Revista da Escola de Enfermagem da USP, 47*(3), 671–677. https://doi.org/10.1590/S0080-623420130000300021.

Ronzani, T. M. (2018). The context of drug use in the consumer society. In T. M. Ronzani (Ed.), *Drugs and social context: Social perspectives on the use of alcohol and other drugs* (pp. 3–13). https://doi.org/10.1007/978-3-319-72446-1_1.

Ronzani, T. M., & Furtado, E. F. (2010). Estigma Social sobre o uso de álcool. *Jornal Brasileiro de Psiquiatria, 59*(4), 326–332. https://doi.org/10.1590/S0047-20852010000400010.

Rüsch, N., Angermeyer, M. C., & Corrigan, P. W. (2005). Mental illness stigma: Concepts, consequences, and initiatives to reduce stigma. *European Psychiatry, 20*(8), 529–539. https://doi.org/10.1016/j.eurpsy.2005.04.004.

Sickel, A. E., Seacat, J. D., & Nabors, N. A. (2014). Mental health stigma update: A review of consequences. *Advances in Mental Health, 12*(3), 202–215. https://doi.org/10.1080/18374905.2014.11081898.

Vargas, E. V. (2006). Uso de drogas: A alter-ação como evento. *Revista de Antropologia, 49*(2), 581–623. https://doi.org/10.1590/S0034-77012006000200003.

Ximenes, V. M., Paiva, F. S., Moura, J. F., Jr., & Costa, P. H. A. (2018). Drugs and poverty: Interfaces of oppression in the capitalist world. In T. M. Ronzani (Ed.), *Drugs and social context: Social perspectives on the use of alcohol and other drugs* (pp. 49–62). https://doi.org/10.1007/978-3-319-72446-1_4.

Chapter 26
Communities That Care (CTC): Community Prevention Interventions

Daniela Ribeiro Schneider, Charlene Fernanda Thurow, Eric C. Brown, and Sheila Giardini Murta

The Community as an Intervention Lobby

Community can be defined as the space where members of a certain group live together and have common interests, based on sharing basic living conditions, experiences of co-participation in diverse cultural practices, and the establishment of a mutually supportive network of relationships (MacIver and Page 1973). The community is thus a space for social organization and for building and maintaining bonds of sociability (MacIver and Page 1973), whose affective dimension is remarkable, also called attachment to the place (Elali and Medeiros 2011). Consequently, the feeling of community presupposes social cohesion and belonging, associated with the satisfaction of personal needs (Nepomuceno et al. 2017).

Communities have become an essential focus of psychosocial interventions since the 1960s in the USA and the 1970s in Brazil. In the USA, the Prevent Psychiatry movement developed the community interventions, focusing on mental health treatment, with the aim of anticipating the development of psychic disorders, acting on their prevention (Caplan 1980). The actions in health are no longer focused only on sick individuals but are expanded to work on the conditions of possibility of the occurrence of diseases and psychic suffering. Thus, the importance of intervention in the community was discussed as an environment where people live their daily lives, *locus* of production of psychosocial problems, and, at the same time, a potentially therapeutic agent (Gonçalves and Portugal 2012; Schneider 2015).

D. R. Schneider (✉) · C. F. Thurow
Universidade Federal de Santa Catarina, Florianópolis, SC, Brazil

E. C. Brown
University of Miami, Miami, FL, USA

S. G. Murta
Universidade de Brasília, Brasília, DF, Brazil

D. De Micheli et al. (eds.), *Drugs and Human Behavior*,
https://doi.org/10.1007/978-3-030-62855-0_26

In Latin America, and specifically in Brazil, psychosocial interventions of a community character had their origin in Social Psychology and their contributions to the attention to socioeconomic problems and their impacts on the production of the processes of subjectivation and socialization of the population. Thus, the emergence of Latin American and Brazilian community interventions has been related to Critical Social Psychology, which, in turn, has been influenced by Basic Ecclesial Communities and Popular Education, linked to Liberation Theology, community experiences of the Catholic Church in the 1970s, directed to the need to improve the living conditions of people in social vulnerability (Gonçalves and Portugal 2012).

Besides Community Social Psychology, there are in Brazil some other models of intervention: (a) the Community Integrative Therapy, by Adalberto Barreto, as an instrument to build social networks of solidarity to promote life and mobilize resources and skills of individuals, families, and communities (Barreto 2013); (b) the Community Treatment, by Efrem Milanese and Raquel Barros, understood as a process of interventions aimed at promoting the improvement of conditions of people who live in situations of severe psychosocial vulnerability and have problems related to the use of drugs, aiming at improving the living conditions of the local community where these people live (Milanese 2012).

It is interesting to note the robust development of community-based psychosocial experiences in Brazil, especially in the field of Care, whose experiences have much to teach the area. On the other hand, in these Brazilian experiences, a more focused approach to risk and harm prevention is still a shortcoming.

This chapter aims to discuss *Communities That Care* (CTC). This community-based system seeks to bridge the gap between advances in prevention science around the world and the lack of dissemination and implementation in public policies and community actions of evidence-based quality prevention programs (Hawkins et al. 1992, 2002, 2014). In this sense, the CTC is guided by assessing risk and protective factors for young people in the target community, aiming at elaborating a diagnosis. This diagnosis also made a survey of the community's goals and values, which add to the analyzed profile definition. Based on this profile, the community coalition can plan to implement evidence-based prevention programs that best meet that community's specific needs (Brown 2015; Pérez-Gómez and Mejía-Trujillo 2015).

Prevention Systems

The prevention system is a broader approach than the preventive programs themselves, which carry out actions aimed at the specific outcomes foreseen in their logical design. A system implies the articulation of multiple preventive components, taking the community as its territorial base. Systems are thus complex entanglements that include different actions (investigations, interventions, and evaluations) in multiple social systems (community, school, family, and individuals) and encompass diverse preventive strategies and expected outcomes. The prevention system, in this way, intervenes in various spheres of the social structure (individuals, peers, family, school, community) and ends up impacting the cultural values of the community (Pérez-Gómez and Mejía-Trujillo 2015).

Community collaboration is a key element in the prevention system, involving networking and resource sharing, and is defined as "the degree to which community members, representing different sectors of the community, engage in information exchange, activity coordination, and resource sharing to strengthen health prevention" (Brown et al. 2011, p. 185).

This collaboration is consolidated through the organization of community coalitions, which have shown themselves to be a viable mechanism for improving public health results, by empowering a collective movement, involving people from their own territory, the focus of the intervention, in the formulation, analysis, and implementation of preventive actions. Therefore, guided by a holistic multi-domain approach to intervention (e.g., peer groups, families, schools, and communities) and by the coordination of activities in various interested groups (e.g., youth, parents, professionals, program developers) and diverse sectors (e.g., government entities, health, schools, religious groups, media, business) (Greenberg et al. 2005), coalitions should: (a) be representative of the diversity of the community they represent; (b) have clearly defined, focused, and manageable goals; (c) use quality data sources and valid measures to monitor progress and provide timely feedback to stakeholders; (d) encourage a culture of community empowerment for evidence-based interventions; (e) implement interventions faithfully; (f) evaluate the effects of the program on results relevant to the community; and (g) gain collective political commitment to change (Gloppen et al. 2012). The challenge for community health coalitions is to apply these elements of effective operation in an integrated and comprehensive framework that can be sustainable to ensure long-term public health actions on youth health problems and behavior.

Systems need a solid theoretical and conceptual basis that enables changes in the cultural structures of the community, as they are designed to deal with a set of social problems that share common elements, such as the risk factors of local youth (Pérez-Gómez and Mejía-Trujillo 2015). Their flexibility allows for a broad set of strategies through intersectorality, by involving various desired outcomes and carrying out permanent reassessment and reorganization, which ensures the sustainability of a prevention system.

To be effective, the transformation sought by the system must be guided by clear objectives and be articulated by a theory of change, which foresees the inputs, the steps to be followed, and the desired results. Therefore, it needs a formalized structure that enables the execution and monitoring of collective planning and seeks to assess its results (Brown et al. 2011).

Communities That Care

Communities That Care was proposed as a prevention system in the late 1980s by researchers J. David Hawkins and Richard F. Catalano of the University of Washington. It is a manualized system that aims to develop community actions to address adolescent health problems and problem behavior through the construction of strong community coalitions based on the training of actors in their own territory on evidence-based strategies that address specific local needs on violence prevention, drug abuse, and antisocial behaviors (Hawkins et al. 2008a, b, 2009; Brown et al. 2011). It is based on Community-Based Participatory Research (CBPR), which assumes community inclusion at all stages of development and implementation by establishing strong links between community empowerment, prevention, and program implementation (Palinkas and Soydan 2012).

CTC is currently one of the most applied prevention systems in the world, already implemented and tested in its effectiveness in more than 500 communities in the USA (Brown et al. 2007, 2011; Brown 2015) and in other countries in different continents, such as Australia, Canada, Sweden, Germany, Netherlands (Brown 2015). The cultural adaptations of the CTC already performed in Latin American countries, such as Colombia, Chile, and Mexico, with social and economic realities closer to Brazil, were highlighted here, suggesting that this prevention system can be viable and effective in the country.

CTC Theory of Change

CTC proposes in its logic model a theory of change that seeks to guide the prevention system to achieve the desired transformations more effectively, as shown in Fig. 26.1.

In this model of change, the implementation of CTC is based on a sequential set of initiatives and actions, one of the main ones being the adoption of evidence-based prevention. This perspective allows, through the evaluation of the effectiveness of implemented activities, the affirmation of ethics in the process and the social control of public spending. The evidence ensures that the desired results in a preventive strategy or program are achieved (Sloboda and Petras 2014).

The theory of change also foresees as a central element the process of *Community collaboration,* already mentioned above. Similarly, it foresees *community support for preventive actions,* which refers to the willingness of community members to support prevention efforts and the adoption of preventive programs focused on the specific needs of the community. This support is considered a key factor in promoting community prevention policy initiatives (Brown et al. 2011).

Community norms, on the other hand, present in the theory of change, a concern shared expectations in the community of how people should behave within specific roles or situations, such as concerning drug use, cases of violence, and patterns of

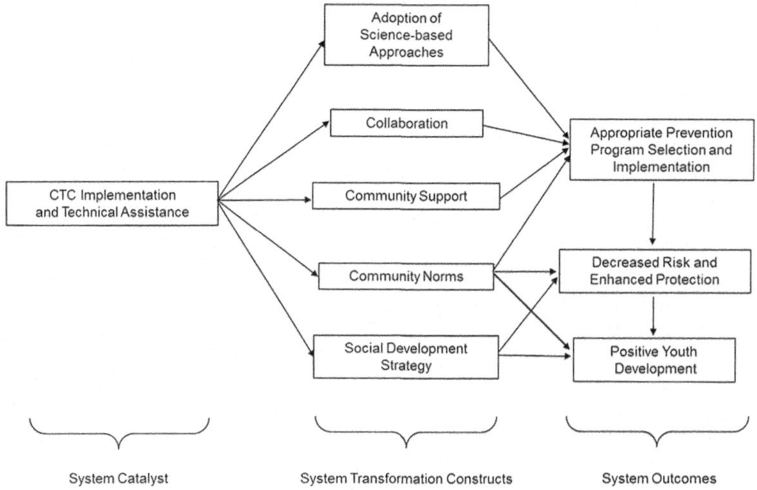

Fig. 26.1 Theoretical model of change in the *Communities That Care* prevention system (adapted from Brown et al. 2011)

interpersonal relationships. The relationship with norms is significant in preventive design, as it involves the permissiveness or lack of permissiveness to young people's behaviors and how to deal with existing differences and conflicts, with influence on the effectiveness of preventive actions (Brown et al. 2011).

The Social Development Model is the base of CTC theory of change (SDM: Catalano and Hawkins 1996; Hawkins et al. 2008a, b), whose strategies describe a chain of causal relationships that, throughout the development process, promote the subject's attachment to the institutions around him, and thus the healthy development of young people in the communities (Brown 2015). According to Arthur et al. (2006) the protective factors developed or reinforced through the social development model involve: (a) expanding social skills in community relations; (b) creating opportunities for the participation of the individual in community actions according to the development phase; (c) recognizing movements and achievements in the pro-social relationship; (d) strengthening affective bonds; (e) elucidating what behaviors are expected in the community relationship. This community mobilization implies the reduction of social disorganization of the community, the promotion of joint work, reciprocity between community members, enabling community involvement to be rewarding by enhancing the experience of belonging, and increasing commitment to prevention initiatives (Brown 2015; Pérez-Gómez and Mejía-Trujillo 2015).

Finally, a catalog of preventive programs with scientific evidence is presented to the community to choose the strategy or program that best suits the reality of local demands, which were raised through the profile of the community and the selection of priority risk factors for intervention. The strategies chosen should aim at minimizing risk and enhancing protective factors, according to the diagnosis made with the youth living in the community, through the application of the *Communities That Care Youth Survey* (CTCYS). The desired outcome is the strengthening of healthy behaviors, increasing the young person's attachment to school, family, and community (Brown et al. 2011; Pérez-Gómez and Mejía-Trujillo 2015).

CTC Implementation Phases

The CTC system is implemented in five cyclical phases, as shown in Fig. 26.2. The initial step involves preparing to receive the intervention. In a behind-the-scenes movement, this phase consists of assessing the community's preparation for change processes and articulating collective actions. Resources and barriers to the implementation of the system are identified, and community leaders are invited as catalysts for the processes that will be initiated. Schools are also activated to enable access to children and young people to carry out a future community diagnosis (Corrêa 2014).

The second phase is the organization of the community council, in which invited members learn about the science of prevention, become involved in working groups, and undergo continuous training; they prepare operationally for the installation of CTC (Hawkins 2006; Hawkins et al. 2002, 2008a, b).

In the third phase, the community profile is built: through the *Communities That Care Youth Survey* (CTCYS), aimed at surveying risk factors and protecting young people in the community, from which the areas of greatest urgency for the intervention are mapped. The community council now establishes priority areas for intervention, choices made from the training offered for interpretation of survey data. Similarly, resources already existing in the community as preventive strategies are

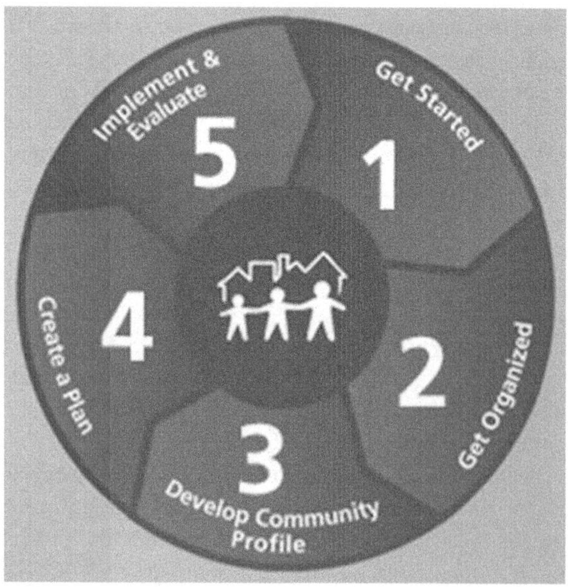

Fig. 26.2 Procedural steps of the CTC. Source: Adapted from the program's official website (https://www.communitiesthatcare.net/)

identified and evaluated (Hawkins 2006; Hawkins et al. 2002, 2008a, b; Sloboda and Petras 2014).

It is in the fourth phase that the strategic action plan is created. The community council defines measurable goals and objectives with a focus on changing the risk factors and behaviors considered problematic; the selection of the program(s) is now carried out. In the USA, this choice often uses the *Blueprints for Healthy Youth Development* website, which offers a catalog of evidence-based US programs with their evaluation and ranking (Hawkins et al. 2002, 2008a, b). For Latin American countries, this is a challenge to be met, as there are few preventive programs already tested for effectiveness, and there is no website that summarizes all the results already produced. In Brazil, we have some programs already culturally adapted, based on the experience of the Ministry of Health, which started in 2013, and whose preventive programs are with effectiveness research in the phase of completion in 2019–2020: Links—Building Collectives, the North American *Good Behavior Game* (for children aged 6 to 10 in Elementary School I); #Tamojunto, the European *Unplugged* (for adolescents aged 13 to 14 in Elementary School II); and Strengthening *Families*, originally the *Strengthening Families Program (*for families in programs to strengthen links in CRAS) (Pedroso et al. 2015). We also have Perae, aimed at reducing alcohol among adolescents, the Australian *School Health and Alcohol Harm Reduction Project (*SHAHRP), adapted by Tatiana de Castro Amato and Ana Regina Noto's team at the Federal University of São Paulo (Amato and Noto 2015). It is possible that there are other programs under development or being adapted in Brazil that have not yet been published or that we have not had access.

The fifth phase is responsible for implementation and evaluation, offering community mobilization all the training for monitoring prevention strategies. These phases are considered cyclical because there is a reassessment of the systematic process. The risk and protection factors of the community are updated every two years, seeking to establish new goals, extending them to other areas to be served in the community territory (Hawkins 2006; Hawkins et al. 2002, 2008a, b; Sloboda and Petras 2014).

Transversely to all these phases, skills are developed that enhance the functioning of the community coalition, aiming at the necessary environmental transformations in interpersonal and intersectoral relations. Such changes are essential to ensure long-term results, as they produce community autonomy (Brown 2015). As Sloboda and Petras (2014, p. 373) point out, "these areas of implementation and dissemination represent leverage points for change at macro (i.e., broad community change), meso (i.e., coalition functioning), and micro (i.e., program delivery to and uptake by youth and families) levels."

CTC Process and Results Research

Based on the premises of evidence-based prevention, the CTC assumes processes of systematic assessment of implementation and results, as well as longitudinal monitoring of some communities, to understand the long-term impact on preventing drug abuse and antisocial behavior among young people (Brown et al. 2009, 2014; Hawkins et al. 2008a, b). Therefore, experimental and quasi-experimental design research conducted in the USA (Hawkins et al. 2008a, b, 2009, 2012; Greenberg et al. 2005) and the UK (Crow et al. 2006; France and Crow 2001, 2005) presented positive results for CTC. For example, some of the results have shown that young people in participating communities are 32% less likely to abuse alcohol than those who did not (Hawkins et al. 2009). Studies on the system implemented in the Netherlands (Jonkman et al. 2005, 2008; Oesterle et al. 2012) have obtained mixed results.

In Colombia, CTC has already had some years of implementation, with process evaluations developed (Pérez-Gómez and Mejía-Trujillo 2015). Likewise, in Chile, where the system was implemented and its process evaluated (Rioseco 2017). In Brazil, the CTCYS instrument is in the process of validation, initially by a master thesis at the University of Brasilia (Corrêa 2014) and now, in a new stage, by Universidade Federal de Santa Catarina. In Spain, this instrument is considered one of the primary surveys for risk and protection factors, in addition to measuring the prevalence of drug use. India and Central American countries such as Guatemala, Honduras, and El Salvador have shown interest in the system. They have initiated the use of some CTC prerogatives in their preventive actions (Pérez-Gómez and Mejía-Trujillo 2015).

The experience of Colombia, reported by Pérez-Gómez and Mejía-Trujillo (2015, p. 728), draws attention to the first four phases, which make the CTC as a preventive strategy that produces "solidarity, awareness of the responsibility for the future of young people, the need to identify the protective and risk factors and to modify them whenever possible and necessary." For this reason, the authors qualify CTC as a promising preventive system for Latin American countries, mainly because of its power to empower communities. Future studies may examine to what extent this premise is realized in the national context.

References

Amato, T., & Noto, A. R. (2015). *Estudo de adaptação e viabilidade de um programa de redução de riscos do consumo de álcool para o contexto de escolas particulares no Brasil* (Doctoral dissertation, Universidade Federal de São Paulo, Brazil). Retrieved from http://hdl.handle.net/11600/41674

Arthur, M. W., Ayers, C. D., Graham, K. A., & Hawkins, J. D. (2006). Mobilizing communities to reduce risk for drug abuse: A comparison of two strategies. In Z. Sloboda & W. J. Bukoski (Eds.), *Handbook of drug abuse prevention* (pp. 129–144). http://sci-hub.tw/10.1007/0-387-35408-5_6 .

Barreto, A. (2013). *Adalberto Barreto: Terapia Comunitária Integrativa*. Retrieved from http://consciencia.net/adalberto-barreto-terapia-comunitaria-integrativa/

Brown, E., Graham, J. W., Hawkins, J. D., Arthur, M. W., Baldwin, M. M., Oesterle, S., & Abbott, R. D. (2009). Design and analysis of the Community Youth Development Study longitudinal cohort sample. *Evaluation Review, 33*(4), 311–334. https://doi.org/10.1177/0193841X09337356.

Brown, E., Hawkins, J. D., Arthur, M. W., Briney, J. S., & Abbott, R. D. (2007). Effects of Communities That Care on prevention services systems: Findings from the community youth

development study at 1.5 years. *Prevention Science, 8*, 180–191. https://doi.org/10.1007/s11121-007-0068-3.
Brown, E., Hawkins, J. D., Rhew, I. C., Shapiro, V. B., Abbott, R. D., Oesterle, S., et al. (2014). Prevention system mediation of Communities That Care effects on youth outcomes. *Prevention Science, 15*(5), 623–632. https://doi.org/10.1007/s11121-013-0413-7.
Brown, E. C. (2015). Mobilizando comunidades para a prevenção da saúde e de problemas de comportamento de jovens. In S. G. Murta, C. Leandro-França, K. B. Santos, & L. Polejack (Eds.), *Prevenção e promoção em saúde mental: fundamentos, planejamento e estratégias de intervenção* (pp. 558–581). Novo Hamburgo, Brazil: Sinopsys.
Brown, E. C., Hawkins, J. D., Arthur, M. W., Briney, J. S., & Fagan, A. A. (2011). Prevention service system transformation using Communities That Care. *Journal of Community Psychology, 39*(2), 183–201. https://doi.org/10.1002/jcop.20426.
Caplan, G. (1980). *Princípios de Psiquiatria Preventiva*. Rio de Janeiro, Brazil: Zahar.
Catalano, R. F., & Hawkins, J. D. (1996). The social development model: A theory of antisocial behavior. In J. D. Hawkins (Ed.), *Cambridge criminology series. Delinquency and crime: Current theories* (pp. 149–197). Cambridge University Press.
Corrêa, A. O. (2014). *Adaptação e validação do Communities That Care Youth Survey (CTCYS) para uma comunidade brasileira: um estudo piloto* (Master's thesis, Universidade de Brasília, Brazil). Retrieved from http://repositorio.unb.br/bitstream/10482/17238/1/2014_ArthurDeOliveiraCorrêa.pdf
Crow, I., France, A., & Hacking, S. (2006). Evaluation of three Communities That Care projects in the UK. *Security Journal, 19*(1), 45–57. https://doi.org/10.1057/palgrave.sj.8350001.
Elali, G. A., & Medeiros, S. T. F. D. (2011). Apego ao lugar. In S. Cavalcante & G. A. Elali (Eds.), *Temas Básicos Em Psicologia Ambiental* (pp. 53–62). Petrópolis, Brazil: Vozes.
France, A., & Crow, I. (2001). *CTC - The story so far: An interim evaluation of Communities That Care*. York: Services for Joseph Rowntree Foundation. Retrieved from http://www.jrf.org.uk/bookshop/eBooks/1859352901.pdf.
France, A., & Crow, I. (2005). Using the "risk factor paradigm" in prevention: Lessons from the evaluation of Communities that Care. *Children & Society, 19*(2), 172–184. https://doi.org/10.1002/chi.866.
Gloppen, K. M., Arthur, M. W., Hawkins, J. D., & Shapiro, V. B. (2012). Sustainability of the Communities That Care prevention system by coalitions participating in the Community Youth Development Study. *Journal of Adolescent Health, 51*(3), 259–264. https://doi.org/10.1016/J.JADOHEALTH.2011.12.018.
Gonçalves, M., & Portugal, F. T. (2012). Alguns apontamentos sobre a trajetória da psicologia social comunitária no Brasil. *Psicologia Ciência e Profissão, 32*, 138–153. https://doi.org/10.1590/S1414-98932012000500010.
Greenberg, M. T., Domitrovich, C. E., Graczyk, P. A., & Zins, J. E. (2005). The study of implementation in school-based preventive interventions: Theory, research, and practice. In M. T. Greenberg & C. Domitrovich (Eds.), *Promotion of mental health and prevention of mental and behavioral disorders*. Retrieved from https://www.researchgate.net/publication/253475340.
Hawkins, J. D. (2006). *Corporate social responsibility: Balancing tomorrow's sustainability and today's profitability*. https://doi.org/10.1057/9780230625815
Hawkins, J. D., Brown, E., Oesterle, S., Arthur, M. W., Abbott, R. D., & Catalano, R. F. (2008a). Early effects of Communities That Care on targeted risks and initiation of delinquent behavior and substance use. *Journal of Adolescent Health, 43*(1), 15–22. https://doi.org/10.1016/J.JADOHEALTH.2008.01.022.
Hawkins, J. D., Catalano, R. F., & Arthur, M. W. (2002). Promoting science-based prevention in communities. *Addictive Behaviors, 27*(6), 951–976. https://doi.org/10.1016/S0306-4603(02)00298-8.
Hawkins, J. D., Catalano, R. F., Arthur, M. W., Egan, E., Brown, E., Abbott, R. D., & Murray, D. M. (2008b). Testing Communities That Care: The rationale, design and behavioral baseline equivalence of the community youth development study. *Prevention Science, 9*(3), 178–190. https://doi.org/10.1007/s11121-008-0092-y.

Hawkins, J. D., Catalano, R. F., & Miller, J. Y. (1992). Risk and protective factors for alcohol and other drug problems in adolescence and early adulthood: Implications for substance abuse prevention. *Psychological Bulletin, 112*(1), 64–105. https://doi.org/10.1037/0033-2909.112.1.64.

Hawkins, J. D., Oesterle, S., Brown, E., Abbott, R. D., & Catalano, R. F. (2014). Youth problem behaviors 8 years after implementing the Communities That Care prevention system. *JAMA Pediatrics, 168*(2), 122. https://doi.org/10.1001/jamapediatrics.2013.4009.

Hawkins, J. D., Oesterle, S., Brown, E., Arthur, M. W., Abbott, R. D., Fagan, A. A., & Catalano, R. F. (2009). Results of a type 2 translational research trial to prevent adolescent drug use and delinquency. *Archives of Pediatrics & Adolescent Medicine, 163*(9), 789. https://doi.org/10.1001/archpediatrics.2009.141.

Hawkins, J. D., Oesterle, S., Brown, E., Monahan, K. C., Abbott, R. D., Arthur, M. W., & Catalano, R. F. (2012). Sustained decreases in risk exposure and youth problem behaviors after installation of the communities that care prevention system in a randomized trial. *Archives of Pediatrics & Adolescent Medicine, 166*(2), 141. https://doi.org/10.1001/archpediatrics.2011.183.

Jonkman, H., Haggerty, K., Steketee, M., Fagan, A. A., Hanson, K., & Hawkins, J. D. (2008). Communities That Care®, core elements and context: Research of implementation in two countries. *Social Development Issues, 30*(3), 42–57.

Jonkman, H., Junger-Tas, J., & Van Dijk, B. (2005). From behind dikes and dunes: communities that care in the Netherlands. *Children & Society, 19*(2), 105–116. https://doi.org/10.1002/chi.865.

MacIver, R. M., & Page, C. H. (1973). Comunidade e sociedade como níveis de organização da vida social. In F. Fernandes (Ed.), *Comunidade e Sociedade*. São Paulo, Brazil: Editora da USP.

Milanese, E. (2012). *Tratamento comunitário. Manual de trabalho I: Conceitos e práticas* (2nd ed.). São Paulo, Brazil: Instituto Empodera.

Nepomuceno, B. B., Barbosa, M. S., Ximenes, V. M., & Cardoso, A. A. V. (2017). Bem-Estar Pessoal e Sentimento de Comunidade: um estudo psicossocial da pobreza. *Psicologia em Pesquisa, 11*(1), 74–83. https://doi.org/10.24879/2017001100100214.

Oesterle, S., Hawkins, J. D., Steketee, M., Jonkman, H., Brown, E., Moll, M., & Haggerty, K. P. (2012). A cross-national comparison of risk and protective factors for adolescent drug use and delinquency in the United States and the Netherlands. *Journal of Drug Issues, 42*(4), 337–357. https://doi.org/10.1177/0022042612461769.

Palinkas, L. A., & Soydan, H. (2012). New horizons of translational research and research translation in social work. *Research on Social Work Practice, 22*(1), 85–92. https://doi.org/10.1177/1049731511408738.

Pedroso, R. T., Abreu, S., & Kinoshita, R. T. (2015). Aprendizagens da intersetorialidade entre saúde e educação na prevenção do uso de álcool e outras drogas. *Textura, 17*(33), 9–24.

Pérez-Gómez, A., & Mejía-Trujillo, J. (2015). Implementação de um sistema preventivo baseado em evidências: perspectivas para a América Latina. In S. G. Murta, C. Leandro-França, K. B. Santos, & L. Polejack (Eds.), *Prevenção e promoção em saúde mental: fundamentos, planejamento e estratégias de intervenção* (pp. 713–732). Novo Hamburgo, Brazil: Sinopsys.

Rioseco, L. C. (2017). *Revisión sistemática de la implementación del sistema Communities That Care en Chile* (Unpublished work). Santiago do Chile: Fundação San Carlos del Maipo.

Schneider, D. R. (2015). Da Saúde Mental à Atenção Psicossocial: Trajetórias da Prevenção e da Promoção de Saúde. In S. Murta et al. (Eds.), *Prevenção e Promoção em Saúde Mental: Fundamentos, Planejamento e Estratégias de Intervenção* (Vol. 1, pp. 34–53). Nova Hamburgo, Brazil: Sinopsys.

Sloboda, Z., & Petras, H. (2014). *Defining Prevention Science*. https://doi.org/10.1007/978-1-4899-7424-2

Chapter 27
Circles of Culture as a Possible Tool for Community Approach to the Phenomenon of Alcohol and Other Drugs Use

Maria Lorena Lefebvre and Telmo Mota Ronzani

Introduction

About 275 million people worldwide used drugs at least once in 2016, which is about 5.6% of the world's population aged 15–64, according to the United Nations Office on Drugs and Crime (UNODC 2018). About 8.4 l of alcohol per capita are consumed per year in the Americas, putting the region second in the world after Europe, where 10.9 l are consumed per year according to the Pan American Health Organization (PAHO 2014).

These data show that the use of alcohol and other drugs is a phenomenon that affects a large sector of the population worldwide, having as causes a multiplicity of factors, among which we find: biological, psychological and environmental, according to Stoltenberg (PAHO 2014), being able to measure the profound impact it has on the quality of life of people and their communities.

Therefore, it is necessary to emphasize the importance of knowing in which environment it takes place, since this makes possible to understand the use and how it relates to socio-historical realities. In relation to this, Paiva and Costa (2017) emphasize the importance of the issue of drug use as a social and cultural expression, closely linked to the social structure and the context in which they take place, and stress that, although it is a unique practice, it is not a single individual choice, it is developed in relation to the context, the substance and the subject.

In this way we can highlight the need to work together with the actors involved and in their territories, in order to understand and address this phenomenon in each

M. L. Lefebvre (✉)
Universidad Nacional de Tucumán, San Miguel de Tucumán, Tucumán, Argentina

T. M. Ronzani
Universidade Federal de Juiz de Fora, Juiz de Fora, MG, Brazil

D. De Micheli et al. (eds.), *Drugs and Human Behavior*,
https://doi.org/10.1007/978-3-030-62855-0_27

particular context, understanding the particular reality of each group and developing relevant strategies with them.

That is why Latin American Community Psychology can make contributions to address this phenomenon in general and from its methodologies in particular as it implies an approach to these practices and their context, from “their interior”. It is a possible work framework, as Montero (1993) states, as it recognizes the importance of the active and participatory character of people in the community to understand the problems of reality within an economic and social structure, as well as the possibility of transforming their reality.

It is in this sense that the Circles of Culture, proposed by Freire (2004), are tools that we consider extremely valuable, since it makes possible an action-reflection, in the words of Toniolo and Henz (2017), in which knowledge and experiences are interwoven (academic and popular) from a problematic dialogue, to reveal a critical conscience, where new knowledge and possibilities of transformation of their realities emerge. A possibility to “say their word”, words that generate culture, knowledge and life, that say a lot about the reality that is lived by the people of the communities, that made possible new “knowledge” and “doings” for the understanding and the approach to the consumption of alcohol and other drugs, while generating a “look and action” from the inside.

In this way, we seek, following Lellis (2015), to be able to approach through the singularity of each situation and work from there the experiences and the understanding of this phenomenon, from its knowledge, its experiences, its links of exchange, so we could build collective and contextualized answers that are viable for each territory.

In summary, the following work will aim to propose, from the Latin American Community Psychology, the Circles of Culture, developed by Freire (2004) as a possible strategy to approach the phenomenon of alcohol and other drugs, in the community approaches. To do so, we will first talk about the relationship between inequality, poverty and Community Psychology in Latin America, which will build the basis of understanding, from where we propose in this opportunity the use of alcohol and other drugs. Next, we will describe the tool: Circles of Culture, its foundation and possible use, so that the proposal of use of alcohol and other drugs in Community Psychology is understood.

Inequality, Poverty and Community Psychology

Use of alcohol and other drugs, as mentioned above, must be thought in context. In our case, we are focusing on Latin America, where our proposal seeks to highlight the importance of building interventions that are close to reality, taking into account, as Ximenes et al. (2015) state, that it is crossed by social, economic and educational inequalities, etc.

In the case of Latin America, according to the Economic Commission for Latin America and the Caribbean ([ECLAC] 2019), inequality between 2002 and 2017 decreased in most Latin American countries because income became more egalitarian overall. However, they clarify that the latest measurements of Gini Coefficient show a halt in this process: in 2002–2008 the average annual decline in the index was 1.3%, in 2008–2014 0.8% and in 2014–2017 0.3%.

Inequalities in the different Latin American countries have historical structural characteristics in common, but present different social formations in each place, in each territory, and differ according to historical, economic, political, cultural, geographical reality, etc. This is due to the fact that the mode of production of material life, as Marx (1844/1960) proposes, conditions the process of social and political life.

Within this dynamic, each territory produced a "social surplus", a surplus that is characterized by new situations of precariousness that lead to "poverty, which is the consequence of an economic policy that combines the production of wealth by the workers and the concentration of income by the owners of the means of production" (Ximenes et al. 2016).

Poverty, as Ximenes et al. (2016) state, is the concrete evidence of social inequalities, since we understand it as the extreme difference in the possibility of access to and distribution of both public and State goods and services, employment, income, among others.

In the case of Latin America, although there was a slight growth in economic development within the capitalist model, this is fragile, since poverty has not yet been eradicated, but rather it is an essential part of sustaining this system (Taaffe 2007), proof of which is that in 2017, according to ECLAC (2019) the number of people living in poverty reached 184 million (30.2% of the population), of which 62 million were in extreme poverty (10.2% of the population), the highest percentage since 2008.

And… Psychology?

For Paredes-Chi and Castillo-Burguete (2018), psychology presented difficulties, for a long time, in dealing with the daily life and development of people in poverty contexts, with the study and deepening of psychosocial processes being unavoidable in order to deal with social inequalities.

It is in this context that Community Psychology emerges in Latin America, with simultaneous processes in several countries: Colombia, Puerto Rico, Brazil, Venezuela, Mexico, Peru, Chile, Dominican Republic, Argentina, approximately in the mid-1970s (other psychological practices had already been carried out in the communities). According to Ortiz (2000), it was born as a response to the crisis affecting that branch of psychology, generating "a praxis in function of social reality, aimed at redefining object, method and theory, as well as the very identity of psychologists with the objective of change and social transformation" (Montero 1993, p. 2).

This simultaneity and complementarity can be observed in the theoretical and practical productions in this field, since the developments made by Marx's writings, Borda's militant sociology, Freire's approach to popular education, Berger and Luckman's social constructionism and participatory action research, among others, were shared (Montero 1993), thus giving it a certain shared identity.

The contributions of Martín-Baró (2011) are also highlighted, as he states that the main task of this psychology branch should be to lead individuals and groups in processes of awareness of reality, of de-ideologization, to understand who they are within society, thus showing the active and protagonist character of the people in the community, seeking to recognize and enhance the capabilities, strengths and possibilities, so that they acquire awareness and control over their lives (Ortiz 2000).

We see here the influence of Marx in his double commitment: with the theoretical knowledge and with the political action, in as much as he understands the theory not as pure speculation, but as comprehension of the social practice and its transforming possibility, understanding it as a product of the groups and their communities, derived from the dynamic and dialectic conception of the human being and his social relations (Ortiz 2000).

Therefore, the role of psychologist in this branch will be to accompany the generation of this social change, being a catalyst, a facilitator (Bennett et al. 1966; Montero 1993, 2004, 2006; Murell 1973; Rappaport 1977) that recognizes the knowledge both of his discipline and of the community, thus giving account of the contributions of Paulo Freire's popular education in this field.

For all these reasons, we consider that Latin American Community Psychology is a fertile and necessary field where strategies can be developed to contribute to the understanding of this phenomenon in particular, while following Guareschi (2009) (in Ximenes et al. 2016) the ethical conception that supports it is highlighted, as it understands the essential of a clear position faced to popular issues and recognizes the importance of the participation of all people involved in the construction of transforming practices for change, essential requirements for the reading and approach that we propose.

The "Place" of Drugs

According to Paiva and Costa (2017) historically drug consumption is commonly observed in our social reality, giving them different functionalities, depending on the socio-cultural context in which this practice is carried out, so it is not strange that it has awakened the economic interest of capitalist societies, becoming one more product to be commercialized, occupying a place within the market (Souza and Medeiros 2015).

This logic, according to them, also argues that use is an individual choice. This choice is supported by a liberal matrix, where the individual is responsible and master of his choices, successes and failures, trying to make invisible the dialectic relationship he has with his social reality, with his group, with his community, seeking in turn to obscure the discussion in relation to social inequalities that generate conditions of possibility and determined contexts for the practices of alcohol and other drug use.

It is for that reason that in order to be able to make approaches from this framework it is necessary to remember, as Parajón (2006) raises, that all human being necessarily exists in a time and space, which constitute his inevitable and necessary social-historical, which is essential part of the complex framework of determinations that operate over him, and that at the same time he constructs and reconstructs. Each group, each community, will have its own characteristics of creation and recreation of these practices, and Latin American Community Psychology is a fertile ground to understand them and design ways to approach them, as it understands, according to Montero (1993) that the community is a dynamic social group, which has a common history from which identification processes are developed because they share needs, problems and interests, generating an interactive network in a given space and time, which differs from the larger society without ceasing to belong to it.

We can see then, how this Psychology branch offers us a possibility of work, being able to make possible an understanding of how the plot of that particular group is carried out in relation to the practices of use of alcohol and other drugs. It is about, as Fernández (1989) proposes, to investigate the multiple meanings and no meanings that circulate in that particular group event, looking for with them to produce new collective productions of sense, understanding themselves as groups-subjects according to Fernández and Del Cueto (1985), as long as they can enunciate something, of the context in which they are inserted, to achieve a creative intervention. As Parajón expressed (2006), it is sought to carry out an approach not only from the visible conducts, but also to ask "from the place in which they are carried out".

In this way, the aim is to take up again the socio-historical reality of each community, of each group that composes it, managing to produce knowledge about what the use of alcohol and other drugs means for them, which can reflect on and question what these practices represent for them, while at the same time generating the possibility of thinking about joint strategies on possible ways of approach, according to their possibilities and limitations, in accordance with what is viable for their territory.

It is for all these reasons that we would like to highlight one aspect, which is to question the extent to which we can only think of it as a merely singular practice. We raise the importance of at least questioning the point of "choice" as the only reason for the use of alcohol and other drugs, thus being able to contemplate other possibilities, to think of other ways of understanding the relationship with it. It is there where we consider pertinent, from this branch of Psychology, to take into account how the conditions of possibility generated by social inequalities and poverty impact on the way these group practices are understood, built and reproduced, according to each particular community.

This is how to build a way of understanding the "place" occupied by the use of alcohol and other drugs in the lives of individuals and communities, taking into account the social structure in which they are inserted. If we understand that the scenario of social inequalities is a central element in which these practices are gestated and reproduced, Community Psychology has the necessary tools to do so, since it understands that it is in those contexts where we have to be, to insert ourselves in them, to work with them, so that knowledge and understanding is a joint construction and shared with those others, the protagonists of those practices, in order to make reflections and actions that enable adequate strategies for this phenomenon.

A Possible Tool: Circles of Culture

It is because of all the above that we have thought of a proposal that contemplates the active participation of all those involved (people from the community and professionals) and the context in which they are inserted with their social, economic and cultural frameworks as unavoidable elements, following how Ximenes et al. (2016) propose the process of work in the communities from this branch of Psychology.

We would like to clarify that there are several methods in Community Psychology, and in view of this Montero (2006) explains that

> Method is not an idol to which offerings must be sacrificed (…) method is the instrument to achieve a goal and that goal is the production of knowledge, which is governed by relations of an epistemological (of knowledge production, of knowledge) and ontological order (that is, according to the nature of the object of knowledge). As said before, method then follows the problem and its object. It is constructed to be able to solve a problem, serving an object (pp. 39–40)

Following these words, we decided to choose this methodology of a participatory nature, as we understand that forms of participation are product of social learning that takes place in specific times and spaces, which must be considered in their determining impact according to Parajón (2006). This makes possible to satisfy our objective as it addresses the socio-historical dimension of users and their communities.

Specifically, we chose the Circles of Culture, created by Freire in 1964, as they contemplate the interweaving of academic and popular knowledge, the problematization and denaturalization of the phenomena that occur in the community while building possible strategies for a particular territory. They were conceived as tools for working in groups, seeking to clarify situations, as well as the search for action itself.

This tool arises in the framework of the "Adult Education Project", in the Popular Culture Movement of Recife. Freire (2004) proposed the term culture, understood as the result of the work of all men, of their creative and recreational efforts, and thus they rediscover themselves as makers of that cultural world and, therefore, capable of transforming it.

The author in his book "Education as practice for freedom" (Freire 2004) describes the Circles of Culture as an active method that proposes an exercise of critical positioning to people, through group discussion of challenging situations, and on which not only reflection but also action is sought. It clarifies that the themes of debates are thought out on the basis of conversations or interviews with people in the community, which are of their interest, while also using drawings or graphics, which are presented in the form of a dialogue. The aim is to help people overcome their naïve understanding of the world and to develop a critical attitude, and to take an active role *in and with* their reality.

It is necessary to know which is the original method, since from it the necessary modifications will be made for each situation. That is why, following what Freire (2004) proposed in the mentioned book, the phases of elaboration and practice that were developed for this method are described below, in a synthetic way:

- Obtaining the vocabulary universe of the groups with which you will work: this is done through informal meetings with people in the community. The material to be worked on is obtained, as well as the richness of people language. This reveals the way in which they perceive their desires, frustrations, beliefs and hopes.
- Selection of the vocabulary universe studied: the most appropriate generating words will be those that present the greatest phonetic richness of the place, those that present the greatest intensity between what they name and what they represent, and the greatest plurality in the commitment of the word to that social, cultural and political reality.
- Creation of typical existential situations of the group to be worked with: these are coded problem-situations, which challenge the groups, and which include elements that must be decoded by them, with coordinator's help. They are local themes that open up perspectives for analysing national and regional problems, which make possible to raise awareness.
- Elaboration of cards that help coordinators in their work: they are guides to orientate the people who coordinate.
- Preparation of cards with the decomposition of the phonetic families that correspond to the generating words: what is emphasized here is the importance of agreeing on criteria, in order to carry out the work in the most similar way possible. And for this, the attitude of the coordinators in relation to the dialogue is essential, in order to ensure that a space for learning and not for "domestication" can be built.

In order to exemplify how community approaches are carried out, and the impact they produce, here we have Freire's words (1989) from his book "The importance of the act of reading":

> Among the many memories I have of the practice of the Culture Circles of St Thomas' debates, I would now like to refer to one that particularly concerns me. We were visiting a Circle in a small fishing community called Monte Mário. […] The group of alphabetizers watched the coding in silence. At a certain moment, four of them stood up, as if they had agreed, and went to the wall where the codification was fixed (the village drawing). They

> watched the coding closely. Then they went to the window of the room where we were. They looked at the world outside. They looked at each other, eyes alive, almost surprised, and, looking again at the coding, they said: "It is Mount Mario. Mount Mario is like that and we didn't know it". Through the coding, those four participants in the Circle "took a distance" from their world and recognized it. In a sense, it was as if they were "emerging" from their world, "coming out" of it, to know it better. (p. 24).

In this way, it is possible to work with the community, based on their own experiences and knowledge, and from there generate processes of action-reflection, which allow decoding the world and being able to "say their word" and then be able to do (Freire 2008). To "say the word", as the author proposes, should not be the privilege of some, but a basic and fundamental right of all, as we are part of society, we constitute it, we form it and we can modify it (or at least it should be).

But… Why and How Could We Do It?

As the title states, the phenomenon of alcohol and other drug consumption was thought possible to be approached from Latin American Community Psychology in general, and from the Circles of Culture in particular, due to two reasons:

The first is based on the possibility of reading, understanding and approaching the phenomenon from the historical-social point of view, and the second is related to the importance of building a unique approach project according to each particular situation.

With regard to the first reason, as we saw above, the phenomenon of consumption can be thought from a Social Model, as developed by Palm (2006), and necessarily analysed from the macro-social aspects, as proposed by Ronzani (2018), since it is necessary to be able to know the context in which the use is carried out in order to be able to develop effective approaches, taking into account the economic, political, social and cultural characteristics, which are expressed and impacted in a different way in each region or country.

As we mentioned, the conditions that generate social inequalities and poverty are "modelling" forms of socio-cultural expression of this segregation, which can be expressed in the consumption of alcohol and other drugs, so it is not enough to investigate only the drugs themselves, as Paiva and Costa (2017) propose, but also the use and meaning that they represent for them.

That is why from Latin American Community Psychology, contributions can be made while working with people involved, with their ways of reading and understanding the world, with their way of linking, while we are inserted in the territories where these practices are produced and reproduced. We start with the knowledge that they have about their reality, which is a useful tool when it comes to understanding the use of drugs in a given context, as well as being able to think of strategies that are relevant to them.

That is why we propose the workshops of the *Círculo de Cultura*, because from there, instances can be generated, as proposed by Freire (2004), so that the people of the community can carry out processes in which meaning emerges, processes of reflection-action are carried out, in which they are problematized in order to decode the reality in which they are inserted, so that they are capable of questioning those socio-historical conditions in which the use of alcohol and other drugs is configured. And, from there, to elaborate a new text, that contains in itself the other previous texts, producing a new process of awareness that makes possible the transforming action; it is about re-constructing other possibilities of being and doing according to their reality.

The second reason was thought of because of the importance of a unique approach to each particular situation.

In fact, mental health laws of Brazil No. 10,216/2001 (Portaria No. 3,088, 2011) and Argentina No. 25,657/2010 (Ministry of Health of Argentina 2010) (both currently with modifications that do not respect this point) detailed the need for accompaniment and construction of an individual therapeutic project for each person who consumes alcohol and other drugs, in order to generate appropriate conditions for possible improvements, because it respected the uniqueness of each person.

Similarly, making an analogy, we believe that it should be done in the community approaches, because each community has a different plot, so it leads to create appropriate tools for each of them.

That is why we proposed as a possible tool, the Circles of Culture, as it seeks to start from the contextual reality of people, to use dialogue and to adapt to each particular situation. As Toniolo and Henz (2017) state, this has always been Freire's premise, since the method does not impose itself on reality, but rather we must start from each new situation, reinventing it,

> the only way anyone can apply, in their context, any of the propositions I made is exactly to remake myself, that is, not to follow me. To follow me, the fundamental thing is not to follow me (Freire and Faundez 2014, p. 41).

In each Culture Circle a new proposal is built for that group, where the premises are analysed and rethought by all the participants being co-authors of the new production, from their contexts, looking for a critical reading of the social, historical, cultural reality, always respecting the logics of each group, in order to be able to better energize the transformation processes.

Thinking about the phenomenon of the use of alcohol and other drugs in particular, we can try, as an example, how they could be put into practice. The people of the community would define the words or initial points (codification), then they would be asked to share their thoughts, meanings, experiences in relation to it (decoding), thus making it possible to listen and analyse together, expanding individual knowledge from a problematic, cooperative dialogue, revealing reality with critical awareness, seeking the collective construction of new knowledge and possible actions (codification) appropriate to their reality.

Final Words

In this chapter we try to explain why the Circles of Culture are a possible strategy for a community approach to the phenomenon of alcohol and other drug consumption, since they aim to generate processes of awareness, understanding this, in the words of Sanders, an American professor who studied Freire in depth, as

> the awakening of consciousness', a change of mentality that involves a realistic and correct understanding of one's place in nature and society; the ability to critically analyse its causes and consequences, and to make comparisons with other situations and possibilities; and an effective and transformative action (Sanders 1968, p. 16).

We consider these processes necessary, since UNODC and PAHO data show that the consumption of alcohol and other drugs is a phenomenon that affects a large sector of the world's population, and it is necessary to understand and address it in the socio-historical contexts in which it takes place.

That is why this tool is proposed from Latin American Community Psychology, from practices in the field of health, fully committed to social and political action, which highlights active participation of people in the community throughout the process, aiming to induce the changes considered necessary, to generate possible alternatives and contextualized to this phenomenon.

References

Bennett, C. C., Anderson, L. S., Cooper, S., Hassol, L., Klein, D. C., & Rosenblum, G. (1966). *Community Psychology: A report of the Boston Conference on the Education of Psychologist for Community Mental Health*. Boston, United States of America: Boston University Press.

Comisión Económica para América Latina y el Caribe. (2019). *La pobreza en América latina*. Retrieved from https://www.cepal.org/es/comunicados/la-pobreza-america-latina-se-mantuvo-estable-2017-pero-aumento-la-pobreza-extrema

Fernández, A. M. (1989). *El campo grupal. Notas para una genealogía*. Buenos Aires, Argentina: Editora Nueva Visión.

Fernández, A. M., & Del Cueto, A. M. (1985). *Lo Grupal 2*. Buenos Aires, Argentina: Editora Búsqueda.

Freire, P. (1989). *A importância do ato de ler*: em três artigos que se complementan/PauloFreire. São Paulo: Autores Asociados: Cortes. Coleção questões da nossa época.

Freire, P. (2004). *La educación como práctica de la libertad*. Buenos Aires: Siglo XXI.

Freire, P. (2008). *Pedagogía de la Autonomía: Saberes necesarios para la práctica educativa*. Buenos Aires, Argentina: Siglo XXI.

Freire, P., & Faundez, A. (2014). *Por una pedagogía de la pregunta: Crítica a una educación basada en respuestas a preguntas inexistentes*. Buenos Aires, Argentina: Siglo XXI.

Lellis, M. (2015). Perspectivas em Psicologia Comunitária e Saúde: A propósito da lei Nacional de Saúde Mental en Sarriera, Saforcada y Alfaro. *Perspectivas Psicossocial na Saúde Comunitária: A comunidade como protagonista* (pp. 89–113). Porto Alegre, Brasil: Sulina.

Martín-Baró, I. (2011). Para uma Psicologia da Libertação. In F. Lacerda Jr. & R. S. L. Guzzo (Eds.), *Psicologia Social para a América Latina* (2nd ed.). Campinas, Brasil: Alínea Editora.

Marx, K. (1844/1960). *Manuscritos económicos y filosóficos de 1844*. Santiago de Chile: Austral.

Ministerio de Salud de la Nación Argentina. (2010). *Ley Nacional de Salud Mental No 26.657/2010*. Retrieved from http://fepra.org.ar/docs/Ley-nacional-salud-mental.pdf

Montero, M. (1993). Entre el asistencialismo y la autogestión: la psicología comunitaria en la encrucijada. *Psychosocial Intervention, 3*(7), 7–20. Rosario, Argentina: Conferencia dictada en el "Encuentro Universitario de Psicología".

Montero, M. (2004). *Introducción a la Psicología Comunitaria*. Buenos Aires, Argentina: Paidós.

Montero, M. (2006). *Hacer para transformar. El método en la psicología comunitaria*. Buenos Aires, Argentina: Paidós.

Murell, S. A. (1973). *Community psychology and social systems*. New York, United State of America: Behavioral Publications.

Organización Panamericana de la Salud. (2014). *Informe mundial de la OMS destaca los impactos negativos del alcohol en la salud.* Retrieved from https://www.paho.org/per/index.php?option=com_content&view=article&id=2684:informe-mundial-de-la-oms-destaca-los-impactos-negativos-del-alcohol-en-la-salud&Itemid=900

Ortiz, A. M. (2000). Notas sobre algunos cuestionamientos teóricos y epistemológicos en relación a un nuevo paradigma para la psicología social comunitaria. In A. G. F. Parajón (Ed.), *Recorridos en Psicología Social Comunitaria: Perspectivas teóricas e intervenciones* (pp. 51–64). Tucumán, Argentina: Universidad Nacional de Tucumán.

Paiva, F., & Costa, E. (2017). Desigualdade Social, Políticas sobre drogas e Direitos Humanos: Uma reflexão sobre a realidades Brasilera. In M. D. Vecchia, T. M. Ronzani, F. S. Paiva, C. B. Batista, & P. H. A. Costa (Eds.), *Drogas e Direitos Humanos: Reflexões em tempos de Guerra às Drogas* (pp. 53–72). Porto Alegre, Brazil: Rede UNIDA.

Palm, J. (2006). *Moral concerns: Treatment staff and users' perspectives on alcohol and other problems* (Doctoral dissertation). Stockholm, Sweden: University of Stockholm.

Parajón, A. G. F. (2006). *El triángulo de las tres "P": Psicología, participación y poder*. Buenos Aires, Argentina: Paidós.

Paredes-Chi, A., & Castillo-Burguete, M. T. (2018). "Caminante no hay (un solo) camino, se hace camino al andar": Investigación acción participativa y sus repercusiones en la práctica. *Revista Colombiana de Sociología, 41*(1), 35–50. https://doi.org/10.15446/rcs.v41n1.66616.

Portaria No 3.088, de 23 de dezembro de 2011. Institui a Rede de Atenção Psicossocial para pessoas com sofrimento ou transtorno mental e com necessidades decorrentes do uso de crack, álcool e outras drogas, no âmbito do Sistema Único de Saúde (SUS). Retrieved from http://bvsms.saude.gov.br/bvs/saudelegis/gm/2011/prt3088_23_12_2011_rep.html

Rappaport, J. (1977). *Community psychology*. New York, United States of America: Holt, Rinehart & Winston.

Ronzani, T. M. (2018). The context of drug use in the consumer society. In T. M. Ronzani (Ed.), *Drugs and social context: Social perspectives on the use of alcohol and other drugs* (pp. 3–13). https://doi.org/10.1007/978-3-319-72446-1_1.

Sanders, T. G. (1968). The Paulo Freire Method. *American Universities Field Staff Report, 15*(1), 4–21.

Souza, P. H. G. F., & Medeiros, M. (2015). Top income shares and inequality in Brazil 1929–2012. *Sociologies in Dialogue, 1*(1), 119–132. https://doi.org/10.20336/sid.v1i1.2.

Taaffe, P. (2007). *Marxismo no mundo de hoje: Respostas sobre a guerra, o capitalismo e o meio ambiente* (Diego Siqueira, Trans). São Paulo, Brazil: Socialismo Revolucionário.

Toniolo, J. M. S. A., & Henz, C. I. (2017). Paulo Freire no âmbito da pesquisa: os círculos dialógicos investigativo formativos como possibilidade de reinvenção dos círculos de cultura e auto(trans)formação permanente com professores. *Inter-Ação, 42*(2), 520–537. https://doi.org/10.5216/ia.v42i2.44026.

United Nations Office on Drugs and Crime. (2018). *Informe mundial sobre las drogas 2018*: resúmen, conclusiones y consecuencias en materia de políticas. Retrieved from https://www.unodc.org/wdr2018/prelaunch/WDR18_ExSum_Spanish.pdf

Ximenes, V. M., Nepomuceno, B. B., Cidade, E. C., & Moura, J. F., Jr. (2016). *Implicações psicossociais da pobreza: Diversidades e resistências*. Fortaleza, Brazil: Expressao Gráfica e Editora.

Ximenes, V. M., Ribeiro, K. G., Pires, R. G., Cardoso, A. V., & Nobre, B. L. (2015). Determinantes sociais da saúde (DSS) na análise da saúde comunitária e suas implicações no estudo da pobreza. In J. C. Sarriera, E. T. Saforcada, & J. Alfaro (Eds.), *Perspectivas Psicosocial na Saúde Comunitaria: A comunidade como protagonista* (pp. 89–113). Porto Alegre, Brazil: Editora Sulina.

Chapter 28
Harm Reduction in the Prevention of Risk Use and Drug Dependence at School

Marcelo Sodelli

Introduction

Since the emergence of AIDS in the early 1980s, the area of prevention of risk use and drug addiction has been under severe criticism. If in the 1970s drug prevention was limited to the prohibitionist stance, synthesized in the simplistic slogan "say no to drugs," from the new problem of HIV prevention (especially in relation to intravenous drug users), it became increasingly evident how much the prohibitionist stance could not achieve its objective of promoting abstinence from drug use (Canoletti & Soares, 2005).

Recent research (Sodelli, 2016) shows that one of the main elements that explains the failure of the prohibitionist approach is precisely what underlies its preventive assumptions: the recommendation of abstinence. Both the prevention and treatment areas, based on the Prohibitionist model, have as their main objective in their interventions to keep (at any price) people in abstinence. From this objective it is easy to understand why in prevention work is restricted to "pedagogy of terror" (prevention through the establishment of fear), while in treatment the binomial abstinence/internal care is maintained.

This chapter aims to present another preventive path: vulnerability reduction actions. To do so, we must first seek an understanding more in tune with the human being's experience with drugs, then we must review the objective of prevention, bringing this action to the field of the possible, to finally present a new preventive posture in the perspective of harm reduction.

M. Sodelli (✉)
Pontifícia Universidade Católica de São Paulo, São Paulo, SP, Brazil
e-mail: msodelli@pucsp.br

D. De Micheli et al. (eds.), *Drugs and Human Behavior*,
https://doi.org/10.1007/978-3-030-62855-0_28

The Human Being and Drug Use

By examining the human condition, from the phenomenological-existential perspective, it is possible to quickly understand why drug use has been present, at least as far as we know, from the oldest civilizations, such as the Phoenicians (4000 B.C.), for example (Seibel and Toscano Jr. 2001). Ancient Egyptian documents describe the production of beer through the fermentation of bread, which continues to this day.

For the existential phenomenology, the human being presents two fundamental ontological conditions: to be mortal (finitude) and to be free (freedom). In everyday life, these two existential conditions are experienced ontologically through the affective dispositions of anguish and guilt. Thus, the human being for being finite and free, a task is placed in his existence; to care for his own existence. Every human being has as his fundamental task to take care of himself, to give meaning to the things of the world. To live life is to experience the abandonment of the natural (we are strangers to nature), no matter how much the human being seeks an instinctive connection with the world, first of all we are crossed by historical narratives. Knowing that it is impossible to transfer the task of taking care of oneself to another, the world can become an inhospitable place, life can be felt as a burden, as a burden one has to carry (Heidegger, 1993).

It is important for us to understand that awareness of our existence is not built up overnight, let alone something that is naturally established. If we look at the existential trajectory of the human being, we can realize that in the beginning, when we are still babies, our degree of consciousness about life is practically nonexistent. We were born completely dependent on other human beings, because surely, if we were not cared for we would suffer. As the years go by, the baby is expected to gain independence in many ways, that with the help of other human beings it becomes a child, adolescent, and adult. In fact, what is expected is nothing more than for that baby to become autonomous and independent after many years, that is, for it to take on the task of taking care of itself. The greatest burden of taking care of oneself is that this task is never finished, when we solve a problem soon another appears, to exist as a human is to be fated to have to deal with oneself forever, with practically no guarantee of what will happen. In fact, the greatest certainty we have in life is paradoxically that life ends, that we are finite. Thus, to take care of existence is to take care of a life traversed by finite time, life is not unlimited, but limited by our death.

Aware of this, the human being can experience intense feelings, such as anguish and despair, pain and boredom. This awareness of having to take care of one's own existence reveals the essential existential vulnerability of the human being. It is from this existential vulnerability that the opening to the possible use of drugs originates. It is in the face of the anguish of the foreign future that the possibility of drug use is opened up as a promise of a more tranquil life. Thus, the use of drugs will reveal itself as one of the possibilities of relief from caring, in the precariousness of life (Sipahi and Vianna 2002). Of course, it is not only through drug use that man seeks relief from having to take care of his own being. Other activities can also provide this feeling, for example, watching a good movie, practicing sports, participating in a religious cult, having a sexual relationship. All these activities can provide us with pleasurable moments, in which we experience an automatic disconnection from our arduous task of caring for our own being, that is, they can cause a change in the state of consciousness.

Historically, it is undeniable that the human being has been dedicated to creating various methods to alter consciousness, such as dancing, fasting, meditation, and even creating activities that put his own life at risk, such as motoring, climbing, and so many other experiences (Sheerer, 1997). This particularity of man's existential condition should not be understood as a failure of the human being, but rather as something that enables the expansion of creativity. It is this human condition that enables us to overcome our own limits and in which resides all our contradiction of being human, because, while we have the potential to create the most beautiful poetry, we are capable of thoughts of acts with extreme barbarities.

Thus, we understand through phenomenological-existential thinking that it is impossible to end the possibility of drug use among human beings, because for this to happen, it would be necessary to modify their own ontological condition. In this way, any effort, whether of a preventive nature to the harmful use of drugs, that universally intends to deny this human possibility, will be doomed to failure.

It becomes possible, then, to consider the issue of drug use as one among so many other possibilities of altering our consciousness, of diminishing suffering and existential anguish. Human history teaches us that the use of drugs is only a way of life. People have always used them, for many different reasons, and no doubt will continue to use them (Toscano Jr. 2001).

Primary Prevention Damage Reduction

Damage Reduction originated in England in 1926 with the recommendations of a report that became known as the "Rolleston Report," which established the right of English doctors to prescribe regular supplies of opiates to drug addicts.

However, it was not until the early 1980s in the Netherlands that the principles of the Damage Reduction (DR) proposal began to be systematized into forms of programs. On the initiative of an association of drug users, a bold proposal was made to combat a hepatitis B epidemic among intravenous drug users (IDUs). Soon after, the Dutch health system adopted this program and began distributing syringes to prevent them from being shared and thus reducing the transmission of the disease among IUDs (Sodelli, 2011).

The RD program has a simple principle: it is a social policy whose priority objective is to mitigate the negative effects of drug use. For example, in relation to injecting drug use, when the difficulty or unwillingness of users to give up the use of the substance is verified, the idea is to create alternatives to reduce the harm caused.

The first point to clarify is the understanding of the harm reduction approach as primary prevention. It is known that prevention can be divided into three modes of intervention:

- Primary prevention refers to work that is done with people (students) who have not yet experienced, or who are at the age at which the use of a licit or illicit drug may possibly begin;
- Secondary prevention aims to reach people who have already experienced or are using drugs occasionally, in order to prevent this pattern of use from becoming problematic or abusive (habitual use);
- Tertiary prevention corresponds to users who already present problems (problematic use, habitual use) and preventive intervention is made so that they do not reach dependency.

In describing these three modes of prevention, we could reflect that the assumptions of the harm reduction approach would be meaningless in primary prevention, since this intervention is suitable for individuals who have not yet had any experience with drug use. We could ask how harm reduction would be possible for people who have not yet used drugs. Or, to find out what preventive work in school would be like, considering a preventive project developed in early childhood education or elementary school. And more: what kind of training would we be proposing to the children?

Considering that the prohibitionist concept is rooted in our educational culture, a widely used tool in the school environment, summarized in the concept "cannot because it cannot," one of the main difficulties would be not knowing which assumption to put in the place of mere prohibition. Possibly, many would argue that if we do not work the concepts of prohibition and abstinence, in primary prevention, among and with those who have not yet experienced any drug, drug consumption would increase considerably in adolescence, running the risk of losing the little control that we still have over young people.

The idea of linking harm reduction as primary prevention is to reaffirm the position that the goal of prevention should not be to end drug use because, as we have already demonstrated, this is an impossible task. Therefore, preventive work that advocates only prohibition of the "can't because it can't" type has proven ineffective in dealing with the problem of drug use. Thus, prevention should, fundamentally, take on the task of intervening in the reduction of the levels of vulnerability to the harmful use of psychoactive substances (Sodelli, 2016).

To work on drug prevention from the perspective of the harm reduction approach in primary prevention is to understand that the best way to deal with the phenomenon of drug use is not to decide and define by others which behaviors are most appropriate and correct. Very different from that is to build, together with the other, possibilities of more authentic choices, more free, reducing vulnerabilities.

From this approach, the behavior of "trying a drug" should not be understood as a failure in primary preventive work, but as a possibility, among others, of human existence. In this way, we could only say that there was a failure in primary preventive intervention if this experimentation evolved into the harmful use of drugs.

All objections to this way of working on prevention are underpinned by the misconception that working on prohibition and abstinence, in primary prevention, contributes to the development of safer behaviors in relation to drug use. We can easily see a contradiction there: how can we expect safer behavior in drug use if we do not even discuss this possibility in primary prevention?

Following our line of argument, the sense of prevention would be to reduce the risks associated with drug use, among which we highlight: pattern of habitual use or dependence, driving under the effect of some psychoactive substance, overdose, sharing syringes or pipes, drug use associated with risky behavior (unprotected sex, extreme sports), violence, etc.

From this perspective, the issue of drug use is understood in a different way: drugs should not be classified a priori as evil substances, but rather as neutral substances. We could only value drugs, in the relationship with man, in this context in which the meaning of use is established, be it recreational, medicinal, harmful, compulsive use, among others.

By linking the harm reduction model to primary prevention, we are proposing much more than a new preventive model: we are offering a model of preventive education. In other words, what man do we want to form and what society do we want to build?

Final Considerations

Not disregarding the strength of the prohibitionist model, we sought, in the phenomenological-existential understanding, arguments to deconstruct this deterministic and fatalistic view of man's relationship with drugs.

Although our phenomenological-existential study cannot be understood as a profound investigation of the human condition, it was enough to reveal to us other possibilities of man's relationship with drugs and to open new alternatives for the development of preventive projects to the harmful use of drugs.

Without a doubt, one of the greatest contributions of this study was the understanding that the idea of ending the use of drugs among human beings is unreal, because for this to happen, it would be necessary to modify the very ontological condition of the Man (the non-transferable task of caring for his own existence). In this way, any effort, whether of a preventive nature or of treatment for the use of drugs, that pretends universally to deny this human possibility, will be doomed to failure.

By arriving through existential phenomenology at the understanding of the impossibility of changing man's existential condition and, consequently, his willingness to use drugs, we identify, in the harm reduction approach, a fertile ground to establish a new preventive objective: to reduce vulnerabilities to harmful drug use. We have thus established a counterpoint to the prohibitionist approach, that is, instead of working only on abstinence and repression, the sense of prevention should be to promote actions that reduce vulnerabilities to harmful drug use. It is in this sense that we understand the intertwining of primary prevention to drug use with the harm reduction approach and, more specifically, in the school setting, the possibility of the permanent construction of a caring network between teacher and student.

In dialogue with interests other than control, prohibition, the sense of preventive practice changes, as does the way in which it is discussed. Therefore, it is not the technician (teacher, psychologist, doctor, etc.) who will determine how the target subject (student, teacher) should prevent himself/herself, but it is the subject himself/herself, after intense reflection, who will question himself/herself, seeking ways and support to reduce his/her vulnerabilities (Sodelli, 2016).

Considering the harm reduction approach in primary prevention, we can ask whether it would not be one of the senses of prevention to make a concrete attempt to contribute to the care of oneself and also the other. Now, to consider this approach is to recognize the importance of enabling the student to build his or her life project, or in other words, to encourage in the student the power of transformation, which we are naming today as the possibility of building his or her full citizenship.

The insistence on advocating the prohibitionist model, the pedagogy of control, the distancing of the sense of educating from the sense of preventing could cost all of us the perpetuation of the inexistence of a genuine work of prevention of the harmful use of drugs in the school environment. That is, the forgetfulness of one of the most proper senses of education: to reduce vulnerabilities.

References

Canoletti, B., & Soares, C. B. (2005). Programas de prevenção ao consume de drogas no Brasil: uma análise da produção científica de 1991 a 2001. *Interface - Comunicação, Saúde e Educação, 9*(16), 115–129. https://doi.org/10.1590/S1414-32832005000100010.

Heidegger, M. (1993). *Ser e o tempo* (4th ed.). Petrópolis: Vozes.

Seibel, S. D., & Toscano, A., Jr. (2001). Conceitos básicos e classificação geral das substâncias psicoativas. In S. D. Seibel & A. Toscano Jr. (Eds.), *Dependência de drogas*. São Paulo: Atheneu.

Sipahi, F. M., & Vianna, F. D. C. (2002). A dependência de drogas e a fenomenologia existencial. *Revista da Associação Brasileira de Daseinsanalyse, 11*, 85–92.

Sodelli, M. (2011). Drogas e ser humano a prevenção do possível. In Conselho Regional de Psicologia da 6ª região (Ed.), *Álcool e outras drogas*. São Paulo: CRPSP.

Sodelli, M. (2016). *Drogas e Prevenção: da desconstrução da postura proibicionista as ações redutoras de vulnerabilidade*. São Paulo: Via Veritas.

Sheerer, S. Dominação Ideológica versus Lazer Psicotrópico (1997). *In: Ribeiro, M.M.; Seibel, D.S. Hegemonia do cinismo* (pp. 287–301). São Paulo: Ed. Memorial.

Toscano, A., Jr. (2001). Um breve histórico sobre o uso de drogas. In S. D. Seibel & A. Toscano Jr. (Eds.), *Dependência de drogas*. Atheneu: São Paulo.

Chapter 29
Prevention and School: Possible Paths in Drug Education

Julia Bernardo, Gelsimar Machado, and Liana Romera

Introduction

The theme of drug use, when related to the prevention of abusive, excessive, or risky use, has undergone intense transformations in recent decades, both in its philosophical bases and concepts, including its multidisciplinarity. Consequently, these changes have impacted how prevention exists as a public policy, as well as the structure of preventive actions and interventions. In terms of discussions on drug prevention, we are currently experiencing a period of transition and change of paradigms, in which old models with outdated characteristics are gradually replaced by new ways of understanding uses and practicing prevention.

Old actions were based on the ratification of untruths consolidated between the lines of moralizing speeches and the dissemination of simplistic actions of informative nature. Such actions included the distribution of pamphlets or frightening messages that proved, over time, to be ineffective. This lack of effectiveness in how to promote prevention opens, to a certain extent, spaces for the construction of new possibilities. We are entering a new era, and, although some stains left by old models still remain, we can already glimpse the construction of new ways of proposing preventive policies and actions.

In general, the understanding of the forms of drug use has changed in recent years. The category of recreational use, for example, adopted by the World Health Organization (WHO) as a form of use in leisure time and space, has been recognized and evidenced as one of the different possibilities of contact with licit and illicit substances, especially among the young population. The change in use

J. Bernardo (✉)
Universidade Federal de São Paulo, Guarulhos, SP, Brazil

G. Machado · L. Romera
Universidade Federal do Espírito Santo, Vitória, ES, Brazil

D. De Micheli et al. (eds.), *Drugs and Human Behavior*,
https://doi.org/10.1007/978-3-030-62855-0_29

categorization also has a direct impact on the ways of promoting preventive actions, revealing the need for updating the planning and implementation of such actions, especially those developed in the educational sphere at its different levels (elementary school, high school, and higher education).

In this sense, this work is developed grounded in a critical reflection on the transformations that have occurred in drug prevention actions, with the objective of bringing to the discussion elements that can contribute to the deconstruction of old paradigms, as well as the construction of new paths that can support drug education actions and policies based on current dialogue and possibilities for more effective interventions.

Thus, we briefly highlight the two main models on which prevention has been based in recent decades, and the process of transition, albeit slow, from the first to the second model. The first model, known as "War on Drugs," was built on the belief in a drug-free society, had a prohibitionist character, and focused on repressing consumption, using fear as an educational strategy for prevention. The second model adopts the "Harm Reduction Prevention," with more emancipatory approaches that take into account the complexities of drug-related factors according to biopsychosocial, rights, and citizenship dimensions (Moreira, Vóvio, & De Micheli, 2015).

Faced with the duality of the War on Drugs and Harm Reduction models, Becoña (2012) argues that the main objective of prevention programs should not be for people not to use drugs, as this would be an idealistic and utopian goal. However, the author understands that it is possible to mitigate risk factors and increase protective factors. Such objectives aim at reducing risky consumption and modifying the contexts of use based on the relationship established between the individual and their social environment. The new perspective indicates that these changes require the construction of personal skills and abilities that allow and legitimize the perception of environments and contexts.

This revision in the concept of drug prevention results from evaluations of prevention programs, which have demonstrated the need for the development of other practices. Contemplating the development of a broader skill set and not only those restricted to non-drug use reveals the necessity of considering actions based on scientific evidence, in addition to including the contextual characteristics of each site, emphasizing the growing influence of this knowledge on the elaboration of prevention programs. In the wake of such changes in how to practice prevention, drug ceases to be the focus of these actions while the individual assumes a central role. Especially in actions elaborated in the educational field, themes related to health promotion and the development of social skills gain greater protagonism.

School, Health Promotion, and Drug Education

The introduction of health topics at school is not so recent. At the late nineteenth century and early twentieth century, in Brazil, preventive practices in schools were based on "hygiene" principles, aimed at improving the sanitary conditions of the population and prescribing behaviors anchored to normative recommendations and training for habit changes, as well as the control and eradication of diseases (Monteiro & Bizzo, 2015).

Parallel to the hygienist movement, during the 1990s, health was introduced into the school curriculum and started to be worked on by teachers and taught to students, with activities designed for transmitting information and teaching attitudes, values, and practices that should be developed within the classroom (Monteiro & Bizzo, 2015). This process is linked to global debates on health promotion, the concept of health from the perspective of quality of life, and the interdisciplinarity of the theme. The First International Conference on Health Promotion in 1986, which culminated in the Ottawa Charter, defines health promotion as a process that seeks to empower the community so that people can actively participate in improving quality of life and health (Buss, 2000; Czeresnia, 2003). Health is seen as a shared responsibility between individuals, the community, and the state, counting on popular participation to identify their needs and aspirations in order for possible actions and changes to make sense in the face of the local reality.

The interface between health and education, recommended in official documents such as the National Drug Policy (Resolução No 3 GSIPR/CH/CONAD, 2005), National Health Promotion Policy (Ministério da Saúde, Secretaria de Vigilância em Saúde, Secretaria de Atenção à Saúde, 2010), and National Curricular Parameters: cross-cutting themes (Ministério da Educação, Secretaria de Educação Fundamental, 1998), has required from professionals of these areas an exercise in communication that could culminate in effective actions within the school (Canoletti & Soares, 2005; Rua & Abramovay, 2001).

The concept that school is an important reference for personal and social development, where young people spend much of their time, is reinforced by several researchers (Albertani & Sodelli, 2014; Moreira et al., 2015; Sodelli, 2010). Furthermore, its role in sharing and problematizing social norms and values favors health promotion (Pedroso & Hamann, 2019). Also, school is one of the most strategic environments for preventive actions, since it aggregates individuals of different ages and characteristics (Ronzani, 2013).

The matter of drugs is intertwined with policies aimed at including health issues in educational contexts, due to its social and health nature. Reducing drug use is essential, considering the increasingly early consumption of these substances among adolescents (Centro Brasileiro de Informações sobre Drogas Psicotrópicas, 2012; Foxcroft & Tsertsvadze, 2011). The health-promoting school emerges grounded in intersectoral cooperation and in the integral nature of health, seeking the participatory involvement of the entire school community and taking into consideration aspects such as cultural adaptation and measures that improve life and social skills (Noto & Moreira, 2006).

In this perspective, the teacher is recognized as a mediator of this process, understanding education as a possible way for teacher and student to build their individual and collective stories (Albertani, 2011; Lopes et al. 2020). Cruz (2011) notes that school is not only a space for learning different subjects but also for creating citizens and social individuals for healthy human relationships, reflection on reality, and construction of life projects. Therefore, school is a privileged territory for developing drug prevention programs (Souza et al., 2015).

Despite the relevance of the topic of drugs and how to handle it in a social context, discussions and preventive actions in the educational environment have been clearly insufficient. Traditionally, interventions involve superficial lectures and sporadic projects, with informative methodology and a unilateral, moralistic, punitive view, minimizing the effectiveness of medium- and long-term preventive actions and contributing to discrediting and trivializing the theme among the youth. The first prevention programs focused on rationality and information, believing that these two tools would be capable of reducing or eliminating drug use among adolescents and young people. This approach was very simplistic and did not consider the numerous factors related to drug use and the behavior of adolescents and young people that go beyond known reasons. In this mediation process, teaching tends to provide students with misleading and uncritical information, with low scientific grounds. Moreover, teachers are often poorly prepared to deal with the topic of drugs (Dallo, 2014; Paiva & Costa, 2014). Time has shown that this rational model has not produced the expected results, causing science to seek new proposals.

Elements for Preventive Actions at School

The distinction between these prevention models is based on changes in the understanding of the very concept of prevention and its objectives, including the practical activities related to possible actions for a given population and context. The interaction between the political and ideological discourses present in the War on Drugs and Harm Reduction models permeates the reflections on drugs and also influences the forms of prevention.

A brief survey on possible actions from a perspective closer to harm reduction, which Carlini-Cotrim (1998) calls "Prevention living with differences," identified five strategies: *scientific knowledge*: providing impartial and scientific information; *affective education*: techniques for developing skills and competencies aimed at improving self-esteem, group interaction, and decision making; *offering alternatives*: structuring social spaces to expand the repertoire of activities connected to work, education, and leisure; *health education:* based on quality of life and education for a healthy life, with activities that raise awareness not only for individual but also for collective health; *changing conditions and teaching:* focused on the school experience and the possibilities/potential of teaching as a process to prepare children and adolescents in an integral way, involving all education actors in ongoing and lasting actions.

In this last model, targeted specifically at educational contexts, actions can be grounded in changing institutional practices, improving the school environment, encouraging social development, providing health services, and involving parents in curricular activities (Carlini-Cotrim, 1998). According to the author, the possibilities linked to Harm Reduction proposals, albeit different, can offer a foundation for student development by providing experiences and contexts in which they can become more responsible, inquisitive, and critical.

Although the understanding of substance use prevention has shown some progress, much remains to be done in terms of practical actions and public policies. Some of the difficulties observed include conceptualizing prevention, understanding the role of the school in this scenario, and sensitizing the educator about the importance of carrying out preventive actions in the school.

There are different ways of referring to the topic, such as use prevention or risky/abusive/inappropriate use, and to the strategies adopted, such as health promotion, health education, drug education, harm reduction, or "say no to drugs." The way of referring to prevention, and what is at stake (preventing use itself or abusive, harmful, or risky use), elucidates some of the assumptions in preventive actions and the bases that guide these actions.

In this chapter, we have adopted the term "drug prevention" broadly, understanding that it represents an interdisciplinary way of interaction. We agree with authors who advocate that prevention programs should follow principles that value life, rather than impose moralistic and repressive views (Bucher, 1992). Actions based on the appreciation of life aim to strengthen individuals and social groups in order to understand drug contexts and uses. They involve health promotion and drug education, as well as part of the group that criticizes the War on Drugs policy, uniting specialists from various areas around the tendency of adopting risk/harm reduction strategies (Canoletti & Soares, 2005; Sodelli, 2010). We also point out the need to bring the concept of education closer to that of prevention, introducing preventive work into the school environment as part of a wider world in which the school context can transform reality. The Harm Reduction approach is closer to this perspective of education in the sense of promoting critical development, decision making skills, and autonomy (Albertani & Sodelli, 2014; Moreira et al., 2015). In the Harm Reduction model, drugs are no longer the main focus, while human beings and their complexity, biopsychosocial dimension, and citizenship become the targets of actions and reflections, along with health promotion and quality of life.

Considering this complexity when referring to the possibilities of prevention in schools, it is important to provide some reflections that corroborate the ideas presented so far. Among the numerous changes that have taken place in the field of drug prevention, which can currently also be called health promotion or drug education, we highlight health assets (Morgan & Ziglio, 2007), which correspond to factors (or resources) that can improve the skills of people, groups, communities, populations, social systems, and/or institutions, aiming at well-being and health, as well as the reduction of inequalities. Health assets can be associated with three levels: personal, community, and organizational or institutional, and the strengthening of each of these levels may happen in a distinct and complementary way, mobilizing and stimulating individual and community empowerment around health promotion policies and strategies.

The approaches adopted in the school environment were proposed by Sodelli (2010) in guidelines that address prevention through actions aimed at reducing vulnerabilities, integrating the notions of vulnerability and harm reduction. These actions are based on three levels: individual (teacher and student), social (context), and programmatic (public and institutional policies). The three plans can be interconnected in possible interventions directed at an education that provides people with a better understanding of themselves, life, and world problems, reducing vulnerabilities.

Regarding the preventive work in schools, Albertani (2011) underlines three axes: the school structure, implicit actions, and explicit actions. Such systematization directs the prevention intrinsic to the educational process toward the development of attitudes and behaviors that permeate different areas of life. In this sense, the school structure must fulfill its role by offering quality education with student participation and teaching that develops personal and social skills, promoting decision making for an autonomous, healthy, and responsible life. Implicit actions correspond to components immersed in the school and curriculum routine that encourage the intellectual, emotional, and social development of its students. Explicit actions are those directly linked to drug prevention and inserted into the other axes according to the sensitivity and knowledge of educators about the context of their students, with openness to reflect on the subject.

We emphasize that drug prevention actions in school contexts will depend both on educational concepts and on the perspective adopted regarding drugs and the direct objectives of the preventive action. Namely, in case the school decides to work within the perspective of harm reduction (even if not so clearly, but rather in more open and emancipatory proposals), other elements still must be considered when thinking about the effectiveness of the actions. Table 29.1 lists a set of important elements for preventive actions, their methods of integration, and possible results, taking into account the direct objectives of these actions:

In Table 29.1, the left column presents action elements, the following two columns show possible actions that may not lead to effective prevention, and the last two indicate preventive school actions that might produce more effective results.

A proposal from a school that seeks the integral development of its students may be in line with harm reduction, but if the preventive action is only informative, it will not be effective in changing student behavior. Prevention promoted through sporadic actions, an annual campaign, for example, may not guarantee continuity or the adoption of new practices and reflections on the subject. A project carried out by individuals outside the school may shift the preventive role to other professionals, in addition to compromising its maintenance, since the school will depend on other people, agencies, and institutions. Despite the complexity of the preventive task, it cannot be seen as an extra school and teaching activity. According to Albertani and Sodelli (2014), the formative role, in terms of developing autonomous and responsible persons who can participate in society, is intrinsic to the teaching practice, and not an accumulation of tasks.

Similarly, actions that usually yield positive results, such as brief interventions (Cruz, 2011), may not be effective if the school does not have the support necessary to train its teachers or space in the school routine to include another project. Implementing a prevention project requires considering the variables and routines of each school context. We also emphasize that prevention for prevention's sake, or

Table 29.1 Elements, methods, and results of preventive actions

Elements	Less effective methods	Possible results	More effective methods	Possible results
Use of information	Consider only the transmission of information	May not promote an effective change in student behavior	Consider scientific information in an activity that promotes life skills	May have better results because they add social personal development
Duration	Sporadic action	Medium- and long-term results are unlikely to be effective	Actions planned to involve the curriculum at all levels of education	Enable integral learning in activities suitable to each stage of the student
Planning and execution	Actions performed by people outside the educational environment	May compromise the continuity and results of the project	Actions carried out by the school community, integrating teachers, students, parents, and local community	Allow the integration of several important actors for the educational and preventive process
Integration and assimilation	Projects and actions adopted as something extra, in addition to other tasks that teachers must fulfill	Projects that are not part of the educational policy plan can be considered an accumulation of tasks	Projects and actions included in the educational policy plan, investing in continuing education	Allow education agents to take on preventive tasks as part of the teaching practice and the school role

just adopting any prevention program in the school context, is not enough to obtain effective results. Poorly conducted prevention might trigger iatrogenic effects, arousing curiosity for drug use, generating stigma and prejudice, and strengthening a simplistic, moralistic, and prohibitionist view.

School activities aimed at reaching more effective prevention outcomes should consider a number of important elements when thinking about prevention, its objectives, and ways of including these actions in the school context. In this regard, we highlight the development of individual and social skills, which are currently referred to and systematized into life skills; the inclusion of activities at all levels of education, adapting the language for each age group; and the assistance of the school community in building actions, in order for them to make sense, be adopted by all, and be incorporated into the educational policy plan and school curriculum, with emphasis on continuing teacher education. The teacher is an important agent for health promotion proposals at school, ensuring they are consistent and part of a larger project, integrated into the school curriculum and going through the various dimensions of the teaching-learning process.

Adapting a project that is coherent with health promotion proposals and health education on drugs requires work directed toward improving skills development so that people can make decisions and choices about their lives that contribute to reducing risks and vulnerabilities and favor individual and collective health

(Albertani, 2011; Czeresnia, 2003; Moreira et al., 2015). In this scenario, reflecting on potential prevention projects entails considering the school, its context, the educational community, the objectives, the method (or ways of including activities), and the evaluation of actions.

Given the various particularities of prevention in school contexts, actions should be assessed based on empirical data, seeking to identify ineffective ones and enhance satisfactory results supported by science. Prevention based on scientific evidence is advocated as the core of communication and dialogue between policy implementers and facilitators of preventive actions in different social spaces, with special emphasis on educational environments at their different levels. We highlight that we call scientific evidence that which is evaluated, followed up, and monitored, and can also be adapted depending on the progress of actions. For a project, action, or program to be evaluated, the real objectives and the method developed must be clear. That being said, we underline that all prevention aimed at non-consumption tends to be ineffective and utopian.

The United Nations Office on Drugs and Crime (2015) has been acting worldwide to support governments and institutions in the process of qualifying their preventive actions, based on the assessment and dissemination of effective practices. Evidence-based practices and scientific studies represent, nowadays, a new way of understanding prevention, and the importance of updating preventive actions must be recognized.

In the last decade, scientific production has pointed out a new positioning in articles addressing the theme of drug prevention and health promotion (Moreira et al., 2015). Although shy, this new perspective already signals transformations and the overcoming of old prevention models in schools, indicating the construction of new ways of working on prevention and health education in the school environment.

In this sense, life skills development programs represent a modality of intervention in the field of prevention, understood more broadly, based on scientific evidence, and resulting from adaptations and updates of old programs, in order to increase the efficacy of drug prevention among adolescents and young people.

Interfaces Between Education and Health: The Contribution of Life Skills

Life skills interventions have gained strength in various fields over the years, including drug prevention programs for the school population. Linking drug prevention to the improvement of personal and interpersonal skills can produce significant results as such skills involve common themes for adolescents that do not explicitly involve the discussion of drugs.

Life skills were adopted by the WHO. Programs for teaching these skills consist of developing emotional, social, and cognitive abilities that can help individuals better deal with everyday conflict situations (Gorayeb, 2002; World Health

Organization, 1997). They comprise 10 basic skills: self-awareness, empathy, effective communication, interpersonal relationships, decision making, problem solving, creative thinking, critical thinking, coping with emotions, coping with stress.

Murta, Prette, and Prette (2010) highlight life skills and social skills as protective factors that minimize the vulnerability to several mental health problems. Studies in Brazil are recent and have been increasing, especially those developed with adolescents aimed at prevention and health promotion (Ministério da Justiça, Secretaria Nacional de Políticas sobre Drogas, 2015; Peres, Grigolo, & Schneider, 2016). International production is more significant. Botvin and Griffin (2014) present an overview of programs based on life skills over 30 years, showing several studies with expressive results directed at different populations. One of the strengths of this approach is to develop skills so individuals can have autonomy in their decisions, especially about whether or not to consume psychoactive substances and under which conditions, in line with the Harm Reduction perspective. Fostering freedom of decision is the role of a progressive educational system that benefits and respects human beings.

As noted, drug prevention actions focused on substances and traditional models produce negligible results. The work with life skills becomes relevant in the educational environment by enabling actions to be formulated according to the specific characteristics of the students, favoring the development of everyday skills in activities that promote social interaction, based on information from scientific studies. In addition, this approach is now encouraged both in the area of health and education, promoting dialogue and interdisciplinarity between them, and representing a possibility to glimpse a common language for building policies and preventive actions.

Final Considerations

When we examine and reflect on the inconsistencies between drug prevention programs in the school environment and on the methods shown to be most promising, we can find several answers as well as questions about the barriers that prevent actions that prove to be effective, in different studies, from being replicated in other experiences and contexts. This discussion can involve political, economic, social, cultural, ideological, and religious issues.

While reaching a common denominator capable of intertwining the many understandings surrounding drug prevention is not possible, many experiences have shown that traditional preventive proposals tend to be ineffective, given how fast society has changed in recent decades in various scenarios. Particularly in the educational sphere, actions must be reconfigured and coherent with the context of the adolescent population, their school routine, the objectives of the preventive action, the concept of teaching, and the perspective of prevention.

References

Albertani, H. M. B. (2011). Prevenção na escola: um novo olhar, uma nova prática. In E. A. Silva & D. De Micheli (Eds.), *Adolescência, uso e abuso de drogas: uma visão integrativa* (pp. 637–656). São Paulo, Brazil: FAP-Unifesp.

Albertani, H. M. B., & Sodelli, M. (2014). Drogas e educação: A escola (real) e a prevenção (possível). In T. M. Ronzani & P. S. Silveira (Eds.), *Prevenção ao uso de álcool e outras drogas no contexto escolar* (pp. 133–155). Juiz de Fora, Brazil: UFJF.

Becoña, E. I. (2012). Ements que debe tener un programa preventivo eficaz. In J. A. G. Castillo & C. L. Sanches (Eds.), *Estrategias de intervención en la prevención de drogodependencias* (pp. 51–74). Madrid, Spain: Editorial Sintesis.

Botvin, G. J., & Griffin, K. W. (2014). Life skills training: Preventing substance misuse by enhancing individual and social competence. *New Directions for Youth Development, 141*, 57–65. https://doi.org/10.1002/yd.20086.

Bucher, R. (1992). *Drogas e drogadição no Brasil*. Porto Alegre, Brazil: Artes Médias.

Buss, P. (2000). Promoção da saúde e qualidade de vida. *Revista Ciência & Saúde Coletiva, 5*(1), 163–177. https://doi.org/10.1590/S1413-81232000000100014.

Canoletti, B., & Soares, C. B. (2005). Programas de prevenção ao consume de drogas no Brasil: uma análise da produção científica de 1991 a 2001. Interface - Comunicação. *Saúde e Educação, 9*(16), 115–129. https://doi.org/10.1590/S1414-32832005000100010.

Carlini-Cotrim, B. (1998). Drogas na escola: prevenção, tolerância e pluralidade. In J. G. Aquino (Ed.), *Drogas na escola: Alternativas teóricas e práticas* (pp. 19–30). São Paulo, Brazil: Summus.

Centro Brasileiro de Informações sobre Drogas Psicotrópicas. (2012). *VI levantamento nacional sobre o consumo de drogas psicotrópicas entre estudantes do ensino fundamental e médio das redes pública e privada de ensino nas 27 capitais brasileiras*. Retrieved from https://www.cebrid.com.br/wp-content/uploads/2012/10/VI-Levantamento-Nacional-sobre-o-Consumo-de-Drogas-Psicotrópicas-entre-Estudantes-do-Ensino-Fundamental-e-Médio-das-Redes-Pública-e-Privada-de-Ensino-nas-27-Capitais-Brasileiras.pdf

Cruz, L. A. N. (2011). As implicações do curso de formação continuada sobre consumo de álcool: Uma proposta de intervenção breve aplicada por professores (Doctoral dissertation, Universidade Estadual Paulista, Marília, São Paulo, Brasil). Retrieved from http://hdl.handle.net/11449/102199

Czeresnia, D. (2003). O conceito de saúde e a diferença entre prevenção e promoção. In D. Czeresnia & C. M. Freitas (Eds.), *Promoção da saúde: Conceitos, reflexões, tendências* (pp. 39–53). Rio de Janeiro, Brazil: Fiocruz.

Dallo, L. (2014). Sensibilização de professores e alunos para a prevenção de uso abusivo de drogas e sexo desprotegido (Doctoral dissertation, Universidade Estadual Paulista, Marília, São Paulo, Brasil). Retrieved from http://hdl.handle.net/11449/110464

Foxcroft, D. R., & Tsertsvadze, A. (2011). Universal school-based prevention programs for alcohol misuse in young people. *Cochrane Systematic Review, 5*, CD009113. https://doi.org/10.1002/14651858.CD009113.

Gorayeb, R. O. (2002). Ensino de habilidades de vida em escolas no brasil. *Psicologia, Saúde & Doenças, 3*(2), 213–217.

Lopes, F. M., Dias, N. M., Mendonça, B. T., Coelho, D. M. V., Andrade, A. L. M., & Micheli, D. D. (2020). What do we know about neurosciences?: Concepts and misunderstandings between the general public and between educators. *Revista Psicopedagogia, 37*(113), 129–143. http://dx.doi.org/10.5935/0103-8486.20200011.

Ministério da Educação, Secretaria de Educação Fundamental. (1998). *Parâmetros curriculares nacionais: Terceiro e quarto ciclos do ensino fundamental: introdução aos parâmetros curriculares nacionais*. Retrieved from http://portal.mec.gov.br/seb/arquivos/pdf/introducao.pdf

Ministério da Justiça, Secretaria Nacional de Políticas sobre Drogas. (2015). *Programa #tamojunto: prevenção na escola: Guia do professor*. Retrieved from http://www.cosemssp.org.br/downloads/TJ-GUIA-PROFESSOR.pdf

Ministério da Saúde, Secretaria de Vigilância em Saúde, Secretaria de Atenção à Saúde. (2010). *Política Nacional de Promoção da Saúde* (3rd ed.). Retrieved from http://www.pmf.sc.gov.br/arquivos/arquivos/pdf/28_01_2016_11.08.42.d8b758b0ec9278e68635ac40fcb82034.pdf

Monteiro, P. H. N., & Bizzo, N. (2015). A saúde na escola: Análise dos documentos de referência nos quarenta anos de obrigatoriedade dos programas de saúde, 1971-2011. História, Ciências. *Saúde – Manguinhos, 22*(2), 411–427. https://doi.org/10.1590/10.1590/S0104-59702014005000028.

Moreira, A., Vóvio, C. L., & De Micheli, D. (2015). Drug abuse prevention in school: Challenges and possibilities for the role of the educator. *Revista de Educação e Pesquisa, 41*(1), 119–134. https://doi.org/10.1590/S1517-97022015011670.

Morgan, A., & Ziglio, E. (2007). Revitalising the evidence base for public health: an assets model. *Promotion & Education, 14*(2), 17–22. https://doi.org/10.1177/10253823070140020701x.

Murta, S. G., Prette, A., & Prette, Z. A. (2010). Prevenção ao sexismo e ao heterossexismo entre adolescentes. *Revista de Psicologia da Criança e do Adolescente, 2*, 73–86.

Noto, A. R., & Moreira, F. G. (2006). Prevenção ao uso indevido de drogas: Conceitos básicos e sua aplicação na realidade brasileira. In D. X. Silveira & F. G. Moreira (Eds.), *Panorama atual de drogas e dependências* (pp. 313–318). São Paulo, Brazil: Editora Atheneu.

Paiva, F. S., & Costa, P. H. A. (2014). Participação juvenil: uma alternativa para se abordar o uso de drogas no espaço escolar. In T. M. Ronzani & P. S. Silveira (Eds.), *Prevenção ao uso de álcool e outras drogas no contexto escolar* (pp. 113–132). Juiz de Fora, Brazil: Editora UFJF.

Pedroso, R. T., & Hamann, E. M. (2019). Adequações do piloto do programa Unplugged#Tamojunto para promoção à saúde e prevenção de drogas em escolas brasileiras. *Ciência & Saúde Coletiva, 24*(2), 371–381. https://doi.org/10.1590/1413-81232018242.32932016.

Peres, G. M., Grigolo, T. M., & Schneider, D. R. (2016). Percepções sobre um programa de prevenção ao uso de drogas nas escolas para o desenvolvimento de habilidades de vida. *Saúde & Transformação Social, 6*(1), 111–123.

Resolução No 3 GSIPR/CH/CONAD. (2005). Retrieved from https://www.justica.gov.br/central-de-conteudo/politicas-sobre-drogas/cartilhas-politicas-sobre-drogas/2011legislacaopoliticaspublicas.pdf

Ronzani, T. M. (2013). Perspectivas de prevenção ao uso de álcool e outras drogas. In T. M. Ronzani (Ed.), *Ações integradas sobre drogas: Prevenção, abordagens e políticas públicas* (pp. 21–35). Juiz de Fora, Brazil: Editora UFJF.

Rua, M. G., & Abramovay, M. (2001). *Avaliação das ações de prevenção às DST/AIDS e uso indevido de drogas nas escolas de ensino fundamental e médio em capitais brasileiras.* Brasília, Brazil: UNESCO.

Sodelli, M. (2010). *Uso de drogas e prevenção: Da desconstrução da postura proibicionista às ações redutoras de vulnerabilidade.* São Paulo, Brazil: Iglu.

Souza, F. B, Andrade, A. L. M., Rodrigues, T. P., Nascimento, M. O. & De Micheli, D. (2015). Evaluation of teachers' conceptions about substance misuse in public and private schools: an exploratory. Estudos e Pesquisas em Psicologia, *15*(3), 1081–1095. http://dx.doi.org/10.12957/epp.2015.19429

United Nations Office on Drugs and Crime. (2015). *International drug prevention standards.* Retrieved from https://www.unodc.org/documents/prevention/UNODC_2013_2015_international_standards_on_drug_use_prevention_E.pdf

World Health Organization. (1997). *Life skills education for children and adolescents in schools: Introduction and guidelines to facilitate the development and implementation of life skills programmes.* Retrieved from https://apps.who.int/iris/bitstream/handle/10665/63552/WHO_MNH_PSF_93.7A_Rev.2.pdf?sequence=1&isAllowed=y

Chapter 30
From Biopolitics to Bioethics: From Vulnerability to Autonomy of Drug Users

João Mendes de Lima Júnior , Antonio Nery Filho, and Camila Vasconcelos

Introduction

The debate that follows in this text is not about the pharmacological characteristics of psychoactive drugs. It aims to reflect on the discourses on drugs and human beings. Strictly speaking, it is a critical reflection about human beings, the power over them, the choices, the vulnerabilities, and the protection. In fact, before that, there is an analytical incursion into how clinical and political discourses, hegemonically, offer their answers aimed at people who use drugs. This is a provocation in terms of paradigmatic challenge or epistemological turn[1]: to produce a substantial shift from *drug-centered* rationality (nature, patterns of use, jurisprudence, effects, etc.), to a rationality where the analysis is centered on the subject (desire, responsibility, self-care, vulnerabilities, autonomy, etc.). The commitment here is to color the debate today made monochromatic.

The relationship between humans and chemicals that alter consciousness for festive, therapeutic or religious purposes is a millennial event. This finding is satisfactorily recorded in vast literature produced by important historians specializing in the subject, such as Escohotado (1998), who even consider that there is a "history within history," a kind of chapter in which drugs are as important as forgotten within the narrative of religions and medicine. It should be considered that each historical moment has built its own senses and answers to the management of the question.

[1] Pinheiro and Martins (2009, p. 19) evoke this principle to produce a review of the concepts and methodologies of studies related to the right to health. The authors suggest that a new approach should focus on the user.

J. M. de Lima Júnior (✉)
Universidade Federal do Recôncavo da Bahia, Santo Antônio de Jesus, BA, Brazil

A. N. Filho · C. Vasconcelos
Universidade Federal da Bahia, Salvador, BA, Brazil

D. De Micheli et al. (eds.), *Drugs and Human Behavior*,
https://doi.org/10.1007/978-3-030-62855-0_30

According to this author, until very recently no one cared about the questions of planting and cultivation, eminently botanical aspects, of plants with psychoactive properties. Recently, the issue has gained a dimension of "planetary catastrophe" to the point of being converted into a "threat" capable of mobilizing against itself broad and even antagonistic segments of specters: capitalists and communists, Christians and Mohammedans, poor and rich, etc. What has aligned the opposites in the same attempt today is what Lima Jr., Silva, Moura, Reinaldo, and Costa (2017, p. 145) called the "moral crusade," aggravated by the fact that the issue was thrown into the dangerous ditch of the "taboos."

Different cultures, as a consequence of the time-space combination, have built up different ways of addressing the issue. It is worth asking: which directions were adopted? What representations were built? What rationalities prevailed? This is a *sine-qua-non* analytical perspective for the purpose of denaturalizing this debate, radically marked by a symbolic dimension. It cannot be denied that throughout history there have been different treatments for the different psychoactive substances. In any case, there has always been a socio-cultural function coated with values, meanings, semiotic variations that compete the debate for a plan of analysis beyond the natural, whether in relation to human behavior or in relation to the chemical characteristics of the substances. Any debate that neglects this finding incurs a simplistic and sterile argument. Therefore, a serene and audacious debate will seek the epistemological complexity that configures the vast field of psychoactive substances and their uses as objects of multidisciplinary knowledge. In fact, there are some aspects in this debate that only orbit exactly in the unnatural dimension, which are: ideology, the senses, the discourses.

Faced with the hegemonic way in which the theme has been currently guided, in which it is captured by a simplistic trap that reduces it to the binomial very bad, the first step to produce the "epistemological turn" in this debate, stems from the effort to intend the displacement of biological rhetoric to the analysis of the discourses that mark the senses present there. In this way, the analytical force is placed in the constitutive rationalities of praxis, and this is far beyond the physiological effects or the chemical dimension of psychoactive substances.

Questioning taboos is an act of the order of civilizing compromise. The path to this can be initiated by dissecting the discourse that constitutes it. For decades of the twentieth century the word "drug" was marked by negative meanings. It became a kind of forbidden word, a danger to be avoided, therefore, excluded from the daily conversations, struck by tricks in the production of narratives. According to Foucault (2012, p. 8), the production of discourse takes place in situations of control, selection, ordering and distribution of meanings that aim to "conjure their powers and dangers." It is a strategy of domination that deprives the risk of "heavy and fearful materiality." It is in discourse and through discourse that some of the main "procedures of exclusion" are manifested, especially in disciplinary societies. Of the exclusion procedures by discourse what stands out most is exactly the "interdiction," the taboo of the word. Since this initial procedure, a combination between desire and power from segments (institutional or not) that seek to materialize mechanisms of domination through the consolidation and maintenance of a certain hegemony has already been manifested. Therefore, it is in speech, and not outside it, that the first battles are fought.

For Foucault (2012, p. 10), "discourse is not simply what translates the struggles or systems of domination, but what, because of what we struggle for, the power we want to seize. Discourse is in itself the element of dispute. It comprises a ring where struggles, injuries, successes and failures, techniques of servitude, etc. occur, which give rise to a "will of truth" translated into the form of rationalities that are wanted to be hegemonic with sufficient force to impose restrictions, sanctions, coercion, which formalize the systems of domination. In turn, the "will of truth" that runs through true discourse imposes itself in such a paradoxically imposing and subtle way that it can mask the truth itself; the will of truth is desire and power, desire for power. Truth itself is beyond the will of truth which, determined by the search for affirmation and domination, alienates the truth itself. The will of truth (desire, power) eclipses truth. As a result of these findings, it is urgent to analyze the discourses that guide the current drug policy by dissecting its components, its rationalities. A paradigmatic turn in this debate would not occur before a dissection of the threads and intersection points of the rationalities that compose the hegemonic discourse.

The Moral Crusades

Escohotado (1998), Lima Jr. et al. (2017) speak of a "moral crusade" against drugs. It is necessary to recover a little of this history and identify the bases of this discourse. According to Escohotado (1998), in spite of the millenary use of alcohol in Christian rituals, the use of substances that alter consciousness for non-ritualistic purposes is now configured as a crime against order or "*against the redención agracy*," a type of event that culminated in the expulsion of symbolic order. The chemical modulation of "animo" becomes a hateful conduct, incurring a crime against the doctrine. The body, a sacred object, could not be altered without the divine consent, beyond what the physiologically induced pleasure, coming from the introduction of chemical substances, becomes abominable, a depravity. A practice that orthodox Christians called "apostasy," that is to say, "…is to despise the prophetic salvation." The crimes against order or doctrine corresponded to the only mode of unforgivable acts. Such a practice is consolidated and pervades the entire Middle Ages. Thus, the first great "crusade" against drugs derives from a dogma of orthodox Christianity which typifies as "sin" all pleasures resulting from chemically induced alterations. Christian discourse founds one of the greatest taboos related to the subject. The dogmatic order manages a disciplinary effect of broad social scope. For Foucault (2012, p. 34), discipline is a principle of control of the production of discourse. According to him, the restrictions and coercion inscribed in the course of the development of a discourse determine the conditions of its functioning. The rules pronounced determine procedures of control by the discourse. In the face of the imperative of a dogma, servile obedience remains undisputed.

A second order of events also significant in this debate is the emergence of a new typology of disorders introduced by Benjamin Rush around 1791 in the USA. Institutional psychiatry in the gestational phase follows the perspective of the natural sciences from the nosographic classification of mental alterations. Rush, a well-known American intellectual, politician, and psychiatrist elevates the dysfunctional use of alcohol to the category of illness. This author frames such behavior in the set of "will disorders." From then on, drunkenness is catalogued as a pathology. The use of drugs that since the Middle Ages was categorized as a sin received a new classification at the end of the eighteenth century, which is now configured as a disease.

The eighteenth century was particularly decisive for the production of a new rationality in relation to health and clinic. For Foucault (2018), this period saw important pillars that built the speeches and medical practices. Among the significant events of that century we can highlight: the birth of social medicine, especially urban medicine in France. At this time, from the needs arising from the heaping up of the burgs, there is a fusion between economic reason, political reason, and health reason. The city planning was exercised through sanitary practices such as, for example, "quarantine" strategies at times of epidemic outbreaks. This exercise of power translates "a political-medical dream of good organization of cities in the 18th century" (p. 156). Moreover, it is also to this century that the author attributes the emergence of the "hospital as a therapeutic tool" (p. 171). Allied to the desire for public hygiene, the hospital fulfilled a mix of different attributes such as social exclusion, vigilance, an ideal place for the exercise of discipline. As far as madness is concerned, until that century there was no systematic practice of hospitalization. Of course, the hospital existed before that, but the novelty in this context is the emergence of "disciplinary mechanisms in the confused space of the hospital that will enable its medicalization"(p. 182). There are some consequences in this context: (a) expansion of the cataloguing of general and mental pathologies; (b) ordering and strengthening of the hospital as a therapeutic institution that reproduces disciplinary mechanisms; (c) strengthening of medical discourse; (d) medicalization of[2] society. While medicine is being strengthened, not without objection, psychiatry is gradually also receiving an exclusive social mandate on madness and deviant behavior classified as pathological. The key to this is precisely the classification system. The initial moment of the era of nosography expansion and improvement, it was then necessary to expand the repertoire. Thus the use of psychoactive substances for non-medical purposes receives the meaning of "addiction" which, according to Carneiro (2002, p. 3), is a fabrication, a construction that is located in the passage between the eighteenth and nineteenth centuries. Besides having inserted a new pathology in the scientific literature of the time, it was Benjamin

[2] The medicalization in Foucault's text should not be understood as the large-scale administration of medicine for an increasing number of diseases. It is the introduction of medical discourse into the general functioning of social practices as in hygiene practices, health surveillance practices, vaccination, and urban space scanning. In other words, it is the effect of medical knowledge determining political actions and social behavior.

Rush himself who led a "doctor-psychiatric" crusade against the then named "disorder of the will" or "impulse control."

Finally, the third great moral crusade sprouts in the legal field, with seeds planted in the nineteenth century but germinated on a global scale from the twentieth century onwards. If the orthodox Christian discourse considered numbness/inebriation a crime against the sacred—therefore, a sin—from the nineteenth century on, its use became part of the catalogue of crimes, illegal conduct liable to penalties, including imprisonment and death penalty in some countries. The restrictions and prohibitions on drugs—as we have seen—were not new in human history. The novelty is that the issue is gaining ground in state policies in all states of the world. An international alignment emerges for prohibition and other forms of legal-penal treatment for the trade and use of psychoactive substances. The prohibitionist discourse is consolidating from emblematic historical markers. In Shanghai, in 1909, the first international conference on the opium trade was held. In The Hague, in 1912, the first "Opium Convention"was held. In the city of Geneva, in 1924, a conference took place whose consequence was the expansion of the concept of narcotic substance[3] as well as the establishment of international control mechanisms for the trade of narcotics, creating new definitions, including for drug trafficking. Finally, in New York in 1961, the UN organized a *Single Convention on Narcotic Drugs*. Gradually, the twentieth century consolidates the prohibitionist discourse, now with a legal framework and severe penal effects. This system of rationality chooses to typify, prohibit, and criminalize some psychoactive substances, but paradoxically protecting some other substances, giving them a configuration of legality. This is not the case here to exhaust these contradictions.

It is thus the triune system of moral crusades against drugs. A moral doctrine is consolidated with three registers: sin, disease, crime. From the taboo of the word to the forbidden object, power mechanisms, disciplinary practices, rules of exclusion, fights, wounds, systems of domination were manifested. Prohibitionism becomes a kind of legendary figure with three heads, three languages, and one signifier that has the same meaning in all three registers. The common element that interconnects these codes and discursive systems is one: the forbidden. While the forbidden becomes manifest, its counterface reveals what is in it of desire and power. Now, from the genealogical point of view, according to Foucault (2012, p. 65), this power embedded in discourse seeks to affirm itself and does so through coercion, restriction, exclusion, and discipline. In turn, the discipline, as a principle of control of discourse, updates the rules establishing the limits of inclusion and exclusion. Both power and discipline exercise dominance, capture, appropriation of the object. Thus, to the extent that the "drug" object has been captured by each of the above

---

[3] It is interesting to note the use of the words "narcotic" (lat. narcociens), "narcotic" and "narcotic" (gr. narkotikós), to designate, indistinctly, all psychoactive substances when, strictly speaking, they should be used to indicate only the Central Nervous System depressants, that is, those capable of producing a reduction in psychic activity, inducing sleep, numbness, numbness, insensitivity. Currently, in order to include all substances, regardless of their pharmacological effect (depressant, stimulant or disorganizer), the use of the expression "psychoactive substances" is suggested.

discourses, for a long time there seemed to be no space and senses outside these frameworks. The discourse being the place of battles it reaches its apex when it neutralizes the noises and dissidences. To all, without exception, the discourse reaches. Thus, it becomes hegemonic. Discourse is the means and end of systems of domination. Discourse is manifested by disciplinary power. Discipline is dialectically a "principle of control of the production of discourse," but also the means by which discourse itself is manifested. Therefore, according to Foucault (2006, p. 28), the discipline is a kind of "multiple anonymous power, pale, without color … a discrete, distributed power; it is a power that functions in a network and whose visibility is found only in the docility and submission of those on whom, in silence, it is exercised." It is precisely there in the discreet gesture of the diagnosis, of the sentence pronounced, in the referral to hospital or to prison that the desire and the power of the prohibitionist discourses, whose will of truth is intended to be unquestionable and irrevocable, is manifested.

The Biopower Over the Body

Since the first signs of changes in medical practices between the senventeenth and nineteenth centuries, a new *modus operandi has been* seen to be sedimented. Since modern medicine is a social practice, it develops a set of "body social technologies" (Foucault, 2018, p. 144). The link between medicine and politics is consolidated with pretensions of squaring the urban space and life in society. Whether in the German version of state medicine, French urban social medicine or the medicine of the English workforce, there are aspects that are repeated as something constitutive. In the first place, medical discourse becomes a reference point for the social order; medicine receives a social mandate that grants it the power to define the architecture of cities (from debates on air circulation and street spacing, water control, standardization of places and ways to treat waste, definition of suitable sites for cemeteries, etc.), but, fundamentally, the social mandate culminated in the appropriation of power over life and death, once attributed to the sacred. Thus, medicine is delegated almost exclusively to the dominion over bodies. As an effect of the consolidation of the new system of wealth production, "society's control over individuals is not operated simply by consciousness or ideology, but begins in the body, with the body… the body is a biopolitical reality. Medicine is a biopolitical strategy" (p. 144), thus inaugurating the era of a "biopower" (p. 152).

What lies at the heart of this new social place of medicine is the exercise of unprecedented power. The biopower, exercised in the record of biopolitics, is the "… power to return life or to cause death." No longer "sovereign" power as a power of death, but the management of life, administered and calculated to ensure the usability and docility of bodies as a strategy for the amplification of the workforce, skills, and life in general. In this sense, it is characterized as "a power whose highest function is no longer to kill, but to invest in life from above" (Foucault, 2018, p. 152). The guarantee of life is the bargaining chip of the body-species transformed into the body-machine, useful to the production system, docile by imposition. It is about postponing death to the extent that a utility value is distributed to living bodies. Capitalism has developed by regulating the bodies inserted in the productive system, adjusting population density, and economic arrangements. Therefore, every effort to maintain life from an investment in bodies does not come from a benevolent gesture, the question is with the utility of bodies.

Medicine has played an important role in the normalization of society. Initially, the normalization of medical practices and knowledge, following the normalization of spaces, then the normalization of life and health. The health and insalubrity criteria parameterized by the medical discourse, i.e., the medicalization of life. Standardization is the effect of a set of power technologies: regulation, control, dominance, discipline. The power over the sick body is transferred to the domain of medicine. It is up to the physician to determine the procedures that reestablish the aptitudes and conditions of health. For Foucault (2010, p. 43), the function of the norm is not to exclude, to reject; being linked to a perspective of transformation, normative power corresponds to a positive technology of power. It is a power that manufactures, that models, that multiplies by its own effects. The norm carries within itself an expectation of power.

There is a discipline arising from medicine, medicalization, which manifests itself on the body of subjects shaping them, determining the forms of use. The discipline, a silent and faceless force, seeks to arbitrate on everything that affects the body. Any intervention on the body must be supported by medical discourse. The food ingested, the substances consumed, the aesthetic modelling, absolutely everything should be with the orientation of the medical discipline. The opposite generates non-conformity, a reason to intensify the mechanisms of domination.

It is possible to establish a direct relationship between biopower and current drug policies. For centuries drug use was an eminently social phenomenon. The regulatory factors were anthropologically constituted. In the middle of the seventeenth century to the eighteenth century the use of psychoactive substances became a medical issue. From then on, from diagnosis to management, all actions started to be determined by medical knowledge. The common man, in this sense, is now never authorized to make use of his own body if this use is not legitimized by the ideals of medicine.

Part of the medical practices directed at the insane is also reproduced in relation to people who use drugs. First of all, psychiatry is given the social mandate to be the guardian of the order regarding everything related to mind and behavior. Madness was not exactly a medical event before the eighteenth century. With the consolidation of psychiatry there is also a definition of competencies and procedures. Psychiatry starts to appropriate the wanderers, the disturbed, the abnormal, the crazy, the drunk, and other users of (other) drugs. With exclusivity, without dissent. Secondly, like the method adopted in relation to madness, there is a set of procedures that consecrate the discourse and power of the doctor in relation to the mad. They are rituals of destitution of the power of the mad subject; obviously they translate the systems of domination. As a result, "… the subject who suffers from it was disqualified as crazy, that is, deprived of all power and all knowledge as to his illness" (Foucault, 2018, p. 211). The first of these ceremonies of removal of power is the rejection of the word, the silencing of the power of speech. The mad subject "… is one whose speech cannot circulate like that of others" (Foucault, 2012, p. 10). In that case, it is not the "forbidden word" as a taboo, the point is that the word becomes null and void. The second ceremony of removal of the power of the madman is the internment. As with imprisonment, the subject's body is now at the controls of a power technology. In the asylar system the whole institutional apparatus converges to domination techniques. The hospital, "… closed space for a confrontation, place of a dispute, institutional field where it is a question of victory and submission" (Foucault, 2018, p. 203). Captured by psychiatric know-how, the subject can no longer be heard or hold power over his body. The combination of these two ceremonies culminates in a "primordial overpower" (p. 203). These technologies of power become the *modus operandi* of psychiatric practices in a general way, manageable in all other modalities of performance. In relation to the users of psychoactive substances the procedures are identical: speech silencing and body domination. This body can be confiscated by guarantees and justifications that a supposed knowledge gives to doctors and operators of the law.

In the case of people who use drugs the systems of domination gain more dense characteristics, since in addition to the volume of power of the medical-psychiatric discourse there is also the summoning of legal knowledge, because, as said before, some psychoactive substances are legally catalogued as illicit. The strategies of "correction" arise from a juridical-psychiatric parallelism. Drug use is in a zone of blurring between illness and crime, for psychiatry and for justice, respectively. In any case, Foucault warns of the need to establish a demarcation "…between sickness and responsibility, between pathological causality and freedom of the legal subject, between therapy and punishment, between medicine and penalty, between hospital and prison". Even if there were a full separation between the discourses, only the administrative problem of framing would be solved, but not the ethics of care.

The Ethics of Life: Bioethics

In a radically different way, as seen in the analyses above, some elements of Bioethics are brought as a synonym of an "epistemological turn" in this debate. In practice, it would be equivalent to changing the focus of analysis from the body-machine to the body-subject. A paradigmatic shift: from domination to autonomy; from focus on substances to focus on human histories and vulnerabilities; from the government of men to the care of themselves; from politics as repression to the politics of responsibility.

A question of principle: to whom does the body of the subject-legal/personal physicist belong? What legitimacy of the State, medicine and justice in determining maneuvers, interventions and uses of the individual body?

The United Nations Educational, Scientific and Cultural Organization's Universal Declaration on Bioethics and Human Rights (UNESCO, 2005) builds a baseline to guide discussions on health interventions. The preamble to the document contains a number of considerations and acknowledgements of which four issues are highlighted here: (a) it considers the capacity of humans to reflect on their existence, avoid danger, and take responsibility; (b) it considers that the progress of science and its applications must be in accordance with respect for human dignity, effective respect for human rights, and fundamental freedoms; (c) it recognizes that health depends not only on scientific and technological advances, but also on psychosocial and cultural aspects; (d) it recognizes that decisions on ethical issues raised by medicine and other life sciences have repercussions on individuals, families, and humanity in general.

Article 5 of the Declaration deals exactly with the theme of *autonomy* and *individual responsibility*. It is considered that: the autonomy of persons with regard to decision-making, as long as they assume their responsibility and respect the autonomy of others, must be respected. In the case of persons incapable of exercising their autonomy, special measures should be taken to protect their rights and interests (UNESCO, 2005, p. 7).

Here is an important point of tension with the hegemonic discourse that materializes the biopower. This part of a tacit premise, a paralogism, a reasoning that has been gestured since Bejamin Rush's first thesis, which merged drug use and impulse disorder into a single conclusion. The thesis was amalgamated and it was not long before the act of using drugs legitimized the loss or suppression of autonomy. In the diapason between drug use and the possible alterations of psychic functions there is still a set of vast confusions such as the common ambiguities between controlled use/recreational use, acute intoxication/harmful use and dependence. Such misconceptions are born from mistakes in premises and also from false premises. Now, starting from the premise that psychoactive drugs generate an impulse disorder that, in turn, compromises superior psychic functions, the conclusion seemed evident: if there is damage in the consciousness of oneself and of the act, then restrictions in autonomy must occur. This is a paralogy, the construction of mistaken conclusions due to inconsistent or false premises.

When the narrative that drug use(s) is the ignition of a pathological picture prevails, the fusion of two of the strongest forms of biopower occurs simultaneously: the psychiatric discourse and the legal discourse. In discussing "*the abnormals*," Foucault (2010, p. 27) already warned of the repercussion of this fusion, which produces punitive power mechanisms with important repercussions on autonomy and individual freedom. These repercussions denature the very essence of the concept of autonomy, that is, the subject's capacity to self-determine, to self-govern. Thus, this approximation of knowledges with undefined boundaries, which frame psychiatric phenomena and legal events, creates an imprecise demarcation between "pathological causality and the freedom of the legal subject, between therapeutics and punishment, between medicine and penalty, between hospital and prison". This is what has been happening hegemonically in Brazilian drug policy, the policies offered are based on the removal of power over oneself, the referral to prison, to hospitals or therapeutic communities. This management re-edits "the great internment," as criticized by Foucault in "*History of Madness*." In any case, what is in dispute is freedom of choice and autonomy. In the case of the drug user, the loss of social autonomy—of autonomy to live—intensifies to the point of being extended to the loss of autonomy over his own body.

More recent studies in the biomedical field already point to inconsistencies in the dopamine hypothesis, which assumed that drug use would produce a generalized disorganization in the reward system and that, therefore, psychically oriented decision-making capacity would be impaired. This was the basis of the justification for the suppression of the subject's autonomy. According to Hart (2014, p. 22), "the fact that someone uses drugs, even if regularly, does not mean that he is addicted." It does not even mean that this person has a problem with drugs. More than that, Bruce Alexander's scientific findings since the 1970s (with the rat park) and the new experiments of Hart, Haney, Foltin, and Fischman (2000) misrepresent the consensus that drug use—such as cocaine/crack—induces the urge to use them pathologically. The drugs, psychoactive or not, produce effect for a certain time. If there is consensus about the curves of pharmacological action of a transitory nature, it is not logical to consider that the alteration of the decision-making capacity is impaired ad infinitum.

The Universal Declaration of Bioethics and Human Rights brings in Article 7 the need to consider "persons incapable of expressing their consent." At no time is there talk of the infinite character of this "incapacity," as much as there is no suggestion of the loss of autonomy, even of people incapable of expressing themselves. On the contrary, it is suggested to consider the "best interests" of that person. This same article also considers the possibility of the right to refuse to participate in medical procedures or experiments. Thus, it is said that:

In accordance with national law, special protection should be granted to persons who are unable to express their consent: (a) authorization for an investigation or medical practice shall be obtained in accordance with the best interests of the person concerned and with national law (UNESCO, 2005, p. 7).

Neves (2006) understands autonomy as the ability of a person to self-determine, refuting any paternalistic protectionism, but health care must be maintained. This theme is central to thinking about the direction of a health policy disconnected from the prerogatives of biopower as an aprioristic condition. The question of autonomy is at the root of the relationship between the supply of care and acceptance or not. Between the clinical protocol for diabetes and the performance of prescribed procedures there is the subject who decides whether or not to follow the recommendations; this is no different in the case of other clinical pictures whose situation is not infectious and which is related to a civilly capable person. Even in more complex situations, such as the acceptance of vaccines, there is no plausible legal argument that compulsorily forces the subject to be vaccinated. What is at stake is, apart from autonomy, the right to refuse. It is not a question of strengthening an anti-vaccination movement, but of pointing out that, as Succi (2018) considers, ethical management in this case involves negotiation, clarification, empowerment, and strengthening of the link between health professionals and the subject to whom the offer is directed.

According to Onocko-Campos and Campos (2006), autonomy corresponds to "a process of co-constitution of a greater capacity of subjects to understand and act on themselves and on the context according to democratically established objectives." Autonomy is a principle and a value, it is built in human relations, it is the fruit of a cumulative process that goes through the individual and collective history of each one. It is not a question of denying relationships and dependencies—as a social isolation—but it corresponds and a new way of agencying the networks of dependency, the context, and the vulnerabilities. Neves (2006) considers that autonomy implies a relationship of alterity in that it requires the "other" to establish conditions for its effective exercise. Autonomy is something that is built in relationships with the "other," a process circumscribed in a given context; it is precisely in this equation that the capacity to act on oneself is forged. The free subject is not the paradoxical subject; the autonomous subject is not the isolated subject. The capacity to decide to act on oneself is one of the most sophisticated effects of evolution, whether with respect to cognitive conditions or with respect to civilizing achievements. Autonomy, as the capacity to act on oneself and on the world, "depends on the subjects' access to information, and more than this depends on their capacity to use this knowledge in a critical exercise of interpretation" (Onocko-Campos & Campos, 2006, p. 671). Here it should be considered that strengthening autonomy is equivalent to *empowering* groups and people.

Let us consider, albeit briefly, these aspects relating to vulnerabilities. The same author considers that human vulnerability (*vulnos* = wound) has a "substantive" face (Onocko-Campos & Campos, 2006, p. 158), ontological, constitutive of the human, inalienable. All, without distinction, have some susceptibility to being wounded. What establishes the substantive dimension in this perspective of analysis is exactly the fact that there is a universal condition of the living. But, on the other hand, there is also an "adjective" perspective, which applied to groups, communities and people qualifies the particular condition of each reality, even if it is contingent, provisional, and also demands particular attention and management.

Strengthening the autonomy of the person, therefore, it is possible to produce, as an effect, the reduction of adjective vulnerability, that is, the characteristic that the person carries—momentarily or not—that makes him/her more susceptible to being hurt, or, in the case of the study in question, with significant difficulty to protect him/herself from physical or moral aggressions, promoted along the vulneration processes, primordial objective of a practice based on bioethical foundations.

About Vulnerability and Protective Bioethics

All human beings are exposed to risk factors and suffering. Freud (1930/1996, p. 93), when analyzing "civilization," considers that suffering is a constant; it stems from various sources, such as the realization of the superiority of the forces of nature in the face of reduced human capacities, but also derives from the certainty of the fragility of the human body itself. Moreover, unease is the product of civilizing events such as pressure and/or inadequacy to the rules that adjust social relations in the difficult balance between family, states and society. Thus, states Freud (p. 83),

> Life, as we find it, is too hard for us; it gives us many sufferings, disappointments and impossible tasks. In order to bear it, we cannot dispense with palliative measures. There are perhaps three such measures: powerful derivatives, which make us shed light on our misfortune; substitute satisfactions, which diminish it; and *toxic substances*, which make us insensitive to them.

Freud considers that malaise is a universal and inevitable condition; no one suffers its consequences on a greater or lesser scale. It is a condition of living beings. The curious thing about this observation is the note about the measures to mitigate suffering that include the use of toxic substances to reduce sensitivity to pain. In this Freudian finding there are two issues that interest us and that are related to the theme analyzed here. First, the universal character of malaise in civilization, which can also be considered "noun" to the extent of its universality and inevitability. Secondly, the realization that the use of palliative resources is part of the human repertoire of attempts to alleviate suffering, that is, the use of "oxic substances" or psychoactive substances is an alternative historically built by human beings, to alleviate their "wounds" and the sufferings that result from them. Contrary to hygienist rationality, the use of psychoactive drugs is something too human, regardless of the legal character of the specific substances. The denial of this evidence only reveals contempt for the senses and subjective functions of drug use with respect to its ontological and anthropological dimensions; effectively it does not favor anything in the quest to build a protective *ethos*.

From this perspective, the epistemological shift here towards caring for people who use drugs, which moves from biopower to bioethics, implies focusing on vulnerabilities as the focus of special attention, and not on psychoactive substances as the center of politics and care. It is neither the legal norm nor the decontextualized clinical protocol that offer protection to the subject, but what is announced as a promising horizon is the possibility of reestablishing the subject's capacity to act on himself and on the context. For this, it is necessary to recognize, value, and strengthen their autonomy. A new ethical perspective emerges from this: it is only man, who has the power to destroy everything, who is responsible and zealous for vulnerability; in the face of threats of deterioration and death, it is up to him to take care of vulnerability in his society. And in the face of deterioration, it is up to him to take care of the vulnerable, the wounded. According to Schramm (2017), there are individuals and populations susceptible to being wounded and vulnerable. According to the author, they are subjects "who are not able to protect themselves or who do not have any support that comes from their family, the group to which they belong, the State or society itself." In this sense, Bioethics of Protection can be considered as a reflection prone to dialogue with the State, requiring the latter to take care of the vulnerable subjects, but only intervening when necessary:

From this perspective, the State would therefore have the role of intervening, offering the necessary protection to the vulnerable subjects; but, on the other hand, it would not have the role of "intervenor" and "protector" in all cases where its action is not required by the needs of helpless citizens, that is, in cases where the citizen is able to "take care of himself." Otherwise, the Democratic State can become a State of Exception, morally questionable for intervening where it should not (Schramm, 2007).

The perception of vulnerability, however, be it in degree of susceptibility or actual occurrence, does not allow the State or humans themselves to appropriate the autonomies of others, even under the argument of care. It allows for monitoring, guidance, dialogue and the enhancement of the autonomy of those to whom attention is directed. Contrary to this is the usurpation of autonomy, the weakening of decision-making and the silencing of the voice of the wounded person.

In these terms, a public policy directed at people who use drugs, which focuses on the biochemical aspect of the use, added to the pretension of cancelling their speeches and decisions, focuses on an epistemological misunderstanding, and obscures the other determinants. The biopower-inspired standard intervention subtracts from the subject the possibility of dealing with his vulnerabilities from his own resources, powers, and self-directed solutions; instead, it empties the subject's power while holding him hostage to another who captures and dominates him as he considers his weakness and inability to make decisions. This perspective builds a discursive game in which the promise of protection stems from the confiscation of autonomy; that is, practices designed to "protect the subject" are confused with the emptying of self-determination and culminate in the surrender of the subject.

In this sense, the offer of protection focuses on an injury; autonomy is harmed and, thus, the subject's vulnerability is intensified by the removal of his power. Of course, an approach inspired by bioethical assumptions should initially avoid producing additional injuries, which is what the principle of "non-maleficence" assumes. Care for the vulnerable or vulnerable subject is ethically committed to be a non-violent act; autonomy is not a bargaining chip in the pursuit of protection and care. Vulnerability as a principle requires an ethical position to be taken that is capable of producing initial positive action to recognize this condition in itself, but also to create strategies to reduce the subjective vulnerabilities, that is to say, the processes of vulnerability. What exposes the individual to potential risk of injury is his or her vulnerability, not his or her autonomy; therefore, actions aimed at protecting the individual should be aimed at controlling vulnerability, without damaging their autonomy.

While substantive vulnerability—which makes up the human condition—reaches everyone in equal proportions, adjective vulnerability characterizes special situations where people and groups are in significantly more unprotected conditions, and are therefore even more susceptible to injury. Kottow (2003, p. 72) considers that besides the vulnerability that is inherent to human existence, there are people and groups affected by special conditions of unprotection, helplessness, harm, that is, unfavorable conditions that make them even more vulnerable. If universal vulnerability—noun—has a primary ontological dimension, adjective vulnerability has a secondary origin. In this author's understanding, acquired or secondary vulnerability is marked by the destitution of capacities. Thus, "this secondary type has specific causes, and therefore cannot be neutralized by the mere extension of the protective mantle. Displaced people need corrective solutions… an effort to reduce or eliminate this disablement, and, therefore, to reduce their secondary vulnerability…" In a way, several authors converge on the idea that this protection should derive from strengthening the autonomy or empowerment of the vulnerable, which should be synchronized with actions that seek to remove the causes of vulnerability.

The contributions of bioethical reflections bring a new horizon for the analysis of the relationship between humans and drugs. In the first place, the focus is not on drugs as a substance, but on the subject as a being of desires and powers. Second, at the center of concern is the recognition and pursuit of mitigating adjective vulnerabilities, very different from the failed fight against drug use. Thus, one must seek to combat the vulnerable contexts. Thirdly, in this paradigm the action of protection does not coincide with the emptying of autonomy and subjectivation, inseparable consequences of biopower practices. In short, the forceful idea of what has been called here the "epistemological turn" is in close harmony with what was said by Nery and Flach (2017): Biopower engenders efforts from the perspective of maintaining the hegemony of the biomedical model that strengthens the discipline, normalization, and medicalization of "deviants," dehydrating resistances and producing silencing of human suffering; bioethics inspires dislocation in the way of producing daily care; this requires questioning reality from the perspective of social transformation, and not just the mere social reproduction of hegemonic practices. Thus, still following the reasoning of these authors, the exit from the field of bioethics invokes a State with a commitment to intervene to protect the vulnerable, but without producing the "*iatrogeny of good,*" *that* is, without imploding freedom, autonomy and justice.

Final Considerations

Paraphrasing Caetano Veloso,[4] where they want the simple. The relationship between humans and drugs has a decassilaba dimension, complex, irreducible to simplistic or reductionist rhetoric. In this study, far from depriving psychoactive drugs of value, we seek new points of view capable of resignifying them in the history of humans, recognizing them as appeasers of suffering in the face of finitude, presenting perspectives that unveil vulnerabilities and strengthen humanistic discourses to the detriment of those merely reductive of autonomy. If for a long time the consumption of psychoactive drugs was situated in the sphere of silence, at another time it became a mediator between the earth and the divine in the religious dimension. This is how the word religion, "religare," taught us its origin, in order to later submit to the tyranny of rules and laws, of knowledge and domination over bodies, culminating in the demonizing and favoring logic of unbearable controls, depriving men and women of their autonomy.

[4] In the song "Quereres" (1984), the author writes: where you want the free, decassílabo.

More recently, in the face of the promises pronounced by the sciences, without the consequent responsibilities with the protection of life in the future, Bioethics emerged as a field, involving the various dimensions of human knowledge, announced through the necessary and indispensable approach between science and the humanities. In this sense, the purpose of this reflection was to signal the possibility of restoring to humans the hegemony of choices, far from the discourses that insist on the usurpation of their autonomies, under the argument of eventual submission of humans to drugs, in an impossible equation. Bioethics and its theoretical instruments are understood as fundamental to the indispensable epistemological turn. Far from the reducing certainties in the field of the "Ethics of Life," one can doubt, formulate the informable, propose that, as Silveira and Moreira (2006) stated, the opposite of dependency is not abstinence; the opposite of dependency is freedom; recognize that the use of a drug, even if it is, today, crack, is not a use for death, but a use to live and endure the unbearable. It is possible, therefore, in the face of this perception, the establishment of care that respects the moral integrity of the subjects, dialoguing with their conditions in search of the supposed health, without annulling their voices. If the use of drugs concerns the context and not the personification of an inanimate entity that subsumes people, abruptly removing them in a politics without bioethical reflections brings a sequence of dehumanizing errors. Under certain circumstances, compulsory abstinence can lead to death. Harm reduction, whether a clinical strategy or a political proposal, is fundamentally a proposal that respects bioethical reflection, because it is essentially sustained by the recognition of the Other as a Subject. Subject of Rights and Duties. There is still a long way to go. This text falls in this direction.

References

Carneiro, H. (2002). *A fabricação do vício*. Retrieved from http://www.neip.info/downloads/t_hen1.pdf

Escohotado, A. (1998). *Historia General de las Drogas*. Madrid, Spain: Alianza Editorial, S.A.

Foucault, M. (2006). *O poder psiquiátrico*. São Paulo, Brazil: Martins Fontes.

Foucault, M. (2010). *Os Anormais*. São Paulo, Brazil: Martins Fontes.

Foucault, M. (2012). *A ordem do Discurso*. São Paulo, Brazil: Loyola.

Foucault, M. (2018). *Microfísica do Poder*. São Paulo, Brazil: Paz e Terra.

Freud, S. (1930/1996). Mal-Estar na Civilização. In *Obras Psicológicas Completas de Sigmund Freud. Edição Standard Brasileira* (Vol. Vol. 21). Rio de Janeiro, Brazil: Imago.

Hart, C. (2014). *Um preço muito alto*. Rio de Janeiro, Brazil: Zahar.

Hart, C., Haney, M., Foltin, R. W., & Fischman, M. W. (2000). Alternative reinforcers differentially modify cocaine self-administration by humans. *Behavioural Pharmacology, 11*(1), 87–91. https://doi.org/10.1097/00008877-200002000-00010.

Kottow, M. H. (2003). Comentários sobre bioética, vulnerabilidade e proteção. In V. Garrafa & L. Pessini (Eds.), *Bioética: Poder e injustiça*. São Paulo, Brazil: Edições Loyola.

Lima, J. M., Jr., Silva, E. A., Moura, Y. G., Reinaldo, A. M. S., & Costa, I. I. (2017). Os desafios do cuidado em saúde para a formação em álcool e outras drogas baseada nos direitos humanos. In M. D. Vecchia, T. M. Ronzani, F. S. Paiva, C. B. Batista, & P. H. A. Costa (Eds.), *Drogas e Direitos Humanos: Reflexões em tempos de Guerra às Drogas* (pp. 141–167). Porto Alegre, Brazil: Rede UNIDA.

Nery, A. F., & Flach, P. (2017). Os sujeitos e a exclusão: das práticas de cuidado à iatrogenia dos movimentos de resistência. In M. D. Vecchia, T. M. Ronzani, F. S. Paiva, C. B. Batista, & P. H. A. Costa (Eds.), *Drogas e Direitos Humanos: Reflexões em tempos de Guerra às Drogas*. Porto Alegre, Brazil: Rede UNIDA.

Neves, M. P. (2006). Sentidos da vulnerabilidade: Característica, condição, princípio. *Revista Brasileira de Bioética, 2*(2), 157–172.

Onocko-Campos, R. T., & Campos, G. W. S. (2006). Co-construção de autonomia: O sujeito em questão. In G. W. S. Campos, M. C. S. Minayo, M. Akerman, M. Drumond Jr., & Y. M. Carvalho (Eds.), *Tratado de Saúde Coletiva*. Editora Hucitec: São Paulo, Brazil.

Pinheiro, R., & Martins, P. H. (2009). *Avaliação em saúde na perspectiva do usuário: Abordagem multicêntrica*. Rio de Janeiro, Brazil: CEPESC/UMS-UERJ; Recife, Brazil: Editora Universitária UFPE; São Paulo, Brazil: ABRASCO.

Schramm, F. R. (2007). Proteger os vulnerados e não intervir aonde não se deve. *Revista Brasileira de Bioética, 3*(3), 377–389.

Schramm, F. R. (2017). A bioética de proteção: Uma ferramenta para a avaliação das práticas sanitárias? *Ciência & Saúde Coletiva, 22*(5), 1531–1538.

Silveira, D. X., & Moreira, F. G. (2006). *Panorama atual de drogas e dependência*. São Paulo, Brazil: Ateneu.

Succi, R. C. M. (2018). Vaccine refusal: What we need to know. *Jornal de Pediatria, 94*(6), 574–581. https://doi.org/10.1016/j.jped.2018.01.008.

United Nations Educational, Scientific and Cultural Organization. (2005). *Universal declaration on bioethics and human rights*. Retrieved from http://portal.unesco.org/en/ev.php-URL_ID=31058&URL_DO=DO_TOPIC&URL_SECTION=201.html

Part V
Special Topics

Chapter 31
Socio-Cultural Aspects of the Use of Psychoactive Substances

Rubens Espejo da Silva

Introduction

While certain individuals "use drugs," others "use psychoactive substances." Here is a substantial difference and mine starting point for this essay. The leak line determining the production of certain "subjects" and therefore of a certain type of society. In other words, as through the regulations on the uses and abuses, whether they are made by the State or by the culture of a people—we find the senses socially produced by the discursive practices[1] on the consumption of drugs and their consequences in our lives.

Anyway, for such an undertaking, we have travelled a few paths: (1) What can be a definition of the term drug; (2) Examples of uses in the history and formation of Brazil, and its social reverberations; (3) What powers and disciplines operate in the subjectivation and objectification of people, as we classify and name the people who chose to use drugs; (4) And, finally, and perhaps most importantly, we will always counter the hegemonic discursive practices— we will serve as diaries of writers, artists, and thinkers—seeking to express the delights of the uses, the rebelliousness, the pains and delights of assuming oneself as a person who uses drugs, as deviant from the established norms.

[1] "We adopt the term *Discursive Practices* in preference to speech. We preserve the term speech to speak of the institutionalized use of language and sign systems of the linguistic type" (Davies & Harré, 2007, apud Spink, 2010). "Discursive practice is understood as the ways in which people, through language, produce meaning and position themselves in everyday social relationships - and the institutionalized use of language - when we speak from ways of speaking appropriate to certain domains of knowledge, psychology for example" (Spink, 2010, p. 27).

R. E. da Silva (✉)
Universidade Paulista, São Paulo, SP, Brazil

D. De Micheli et al. (eds.), *Drugs and Human Behavior*,
https://doi.org/10.1007/978-3-030-62855-0_31

We seek through the works of historian Henrique Carneiro (2018) the sociocultural questions of the use from psychoactive substances, and the philosopher Michel Foucault (2018), more specifically in the book "The Abnormals," our dialogue as a theoretical basis on the need to classify and correct those that can be corrected. A struggle of discursive counter positions, on one side the monsters, on the other, we, only humans—too human—and, what we should keep in mind, said Friedrich Nietzsche: "Whoever fights monstrosities must take care that he does not also become a monster. And if you look long into an abyss, the abyss also looks into you" (Nietzsche, 2005, p. 70). But which monsters do we talk about in our society?

Overview of the Social Construction of the Term "Drugs"

Drugs are more than present in the history of mankind; they have fed, accompanied on journeys, transformed realities, relieved pains, served wars, and still referred to the sacred and the profane. Let us see the importance of a drug in battles: "In the sixth century B.C., Cyrus the Great from Persia ordered his troops to take wine as an antidote to infection and disease. Caesar and Napoleon Bonaparte had this belief too" (Kladstrup, 2002, p. 13). Drugs are constitutive of societies, both in times of peace and war. For the anthropologist Gilberto Velho:

> To study drugs is to study society. The use of drugs is a universal phenomenon, in all societies there is alteration of the state of consciousness, every society deals with it, it can deal more or less deliberately, it can deal through explicit rituals, clear or perhaps not necessarily so explicit; but in any society, through music, through partying, through religion, there are clear situations of systematic alteration of consciousness, with passages from one state to another (Velho & Fiore, 2008, p. 129).

Rules and laws define: "what" and "how much" we can put into our epidermis. In other words, in the last two centuries this millennial story of drug use has become a kind of horror tale—we talk about the War on Drugs; "Nowadays the word drug is loaded with ideology - true moral panic" (Carneiro, 2018, p. 29). Perhaps this is why we choose to use the acronym SPA—Psychoactive Substances—because it is necessary to euphemize the term. For an epistemic disobedience,[2] we adopt here the term drug, assuming all the negativity that this word carries. But in the end, what are drugs for the living species of the planet, in this case us humans:

> Drugs are subjective *objects*, they produce subjectivities, they are techniques of self, humorous, cognitive or sensory modulators, they are plasmators of mental and corporal states, thus serving, in the history of civilizations, as some of the most efficient instruments for creating experiences, whose contents, far from being only objective pharmacological

[2] Without disobedience there is no opposition to coloniality. Without opposition to coloniality, there is no opposition to the multiple unequal and discriminatory relations derived from the central dichotomy of the modern European paradigm—human x non-human: who is the subject of knowledge x who is its object; who deserves to be heard x who should be silenced; who deserves to live x bodies, lives that do not matter [...] (Santos, 2018, p. 7).

> determination, are vehicles for deep senses, symbolic, and imaginary meanings—besides the "pure" effects of the drug, there is a set of culturally significant effects (Carneiro, 2018, pp. 30–31).

Techniques of itself,[3] in our opinion, can be a term that does not moralize the subject, because a technique, whatever it may be, aims at a result, requires procedures. But it still does not explain—or rather—does not say what we seek through drug use:

> The drugs satisfy very different needs: peace or energy, trance or euphoria, concentration or anesthesia. But the common denominator that is sought in all is the diffuse sensation of well-being. Or even something beyond well-being, an excess of well-being, a great well-being (Carneiro, 2018, p. 28).

This may be one of the main aspects of Zarathustra, the prophet without God, said so: "but all pleasure wants eternity - or deep, deep eternity! "(Nietzsche, 2011, p. 218). This is the paradox, eternal pleasure and deep pleasure are forbidden. Having said this: "a drug is not only a certain compound with certain pharmacological properties" (Escohotado, 1997, p. 27). For Vargas (2008), a etymology drug is controversial—it may have come from the Latin *drogia, the* Iranian *daruk, the* Arabic *durâwa*, the Celtic *druko,* but what has the best shelter seems to *derive* from the Dutch *drogbe vate,* which means "barrels of dry things." According to Henrique Carneiro, "the drug comes from the Dutch droog, which means dry products and was used from the 16th to the 18th centuries to designate a set of natural substances used mainly in food and medicine" (Carneiro, 2005, p. 11). It, the drug, overflows any conceptualization.

Among Grapes and Cassava: Small Reports of the Presence of Alcoholic Beverages in Brazil

When the three ships commanded by Pedro Álvares Cabral and the entourage of Portuguese invaded our lands, they brought food and utensils, but also wines. "The wine and water were delivered daily. Each man on board was entitled to a daily Canada (1.4 litre) of wine - stored in about 200 barrels on each ship" (Bueno, 1998, p. 41). Navigating was necessary, living was imprecise, drinking was necessary. It is important to stress and repeat: each man was entitled to almost two bottles of wine a day! Nowadays the vast majority of bottles of wine contain 750 mL

. After almost five centuries, the amount of "adequate" consumption has changed. It has decreased drastically. For the World Health Organization (WHO) the limits

[3] "In the Greco-Latin era, the use of all the "technologies of self" served the purpose of managing, administering, accounting, and judging oneself in order to live better and achieve peace of mind (the "tranquility of the soul" of Seneca) and happiness. The use of pharmaceuticals, as well as food, bathing or walking, served to "balance the moods," subject to the dietary indications of self-care, and each one should therefore be the doctor of himself, especially of his soul" (Carneiro, 2008, p. 66).

for safe, normal, low-risk consumption are: "two doses"[4] a day and no more than 5 days a week (Kalinowski & Humphreys, 2016). Still using wine as an example, we talk about a maximum of 200 mL, two glasses. About the limits and needs, who defines them?

> The effects of drugs are the result of mankind's millennial habit of consuming them since prehistoric times. The empirical knowledge of the effects of plants is one of the great cultural repertoires of practically all peoples, to the point that their consumption has become almost a definition by antonomasia of habit. The limit of consumption, habit, attachment, passion, and addiction is always determined by the particular context of each epoch and society (Carneiro, 2018, p. 52).

It is important to point out that when the Portuguese entered, they did not find the original peoples in abstinence. There were no "abstinent Indians." Here in Brazil, cauim, caxiri, chicha, caiçuma are some of the generic names that Amerindian peoples used to refer to their fermented beverages - "Cauim term of Tupi origin can also be obtained in corn, manioc (cassava), algarobo, fruits or even honey diluted in water (the so-called mead)" (Sztutman, 2008, p. 222).

According to Dias (2008, p. 210), "caxiri and cachaça are equated in indigenous practice and thought, as the groups themselves define the consumption styles and communication possibilities that beverages establish between humans and the supernatural world". Therefore, there are standards and rules for consuming alcoholic beverages among indigenous people, and the abuses or inadequacies of consumption usually come from beverages purchased in cities (cachaça, cognac, wine, beer, whisky) (Dias, 2008). From this "improper" use comes inappropriate drunkenness: "It causes disunity and fights in the family and among friends; it causes accidents; it diminishes the productivity of the families; it makes the Indian lose/forget his culture; when a lot of cachaça is drunk the caxiri is left aside" (Dias, 2008, p. 211).

The abuse of alcoholic beverages by the Indians has a close connection with the drug-food binomial, and this idea is evident in the words of a cacique Palikur: "it is that many Indians do not know how to drink because they want to fill their bellies with cachaça as if it were food" (Dias, 2008, p. 211). It is noted that the use of psychoactive substances is millenary and is confused with the act of eating—food for body and soul—"Every civilization needs food luxuries and a series of stimulants, "dopants" (Braudel, 1989, apud Carneiro, 2018, p. 351).

From the culture of the native peoples to the State, let us see what the Statute of the Indian says—Law No. 6.001 of December 19, 1973, more specifically in Art. 58—they constitute crimes against Indians: paragraph III—to propitiate, by any means, the acquisition, use and dissemination of alcoholic beverages, in tribal groups or among non-integrated Indians. Penalty—detention from 6 months to 2 years. This is the State and its rules—aiming to punish and control the bodies.

---

[4] "The World Health Organization (WHO) adopts as a standard dose measure the equivalent of approximately 10–12 g of ethanol (corresponding to a 330 mL beer can, or a 100 mL wine glass, or a 30 mL distillate dose)" (Health and Alcohol Information Centre, 2019).

Finally, it is impossible to talk about drug use without its historical and geographical location—the "terroir"[5] of our vicissitudes. After all, to talk about culture and drug history is also to talk about its regulations (Carneiro, 2018), but also about its social consumption. From grape to wine, a noble and expensive drink, the delight of the elites' consumption, and, when used in measure—this is the possible abusive use of a certain substance. From sugarcane and the like we have the cachaça—the pinga—a cheap drink, accessible to any social class, one drank a lot, this is the "drunken pinguço."

About the Thirst of the Soul and Those Who Thirst to Eat: Between the Norms and the Production of the Abnormals

Breakfast, chocolate as dessert, wine or beer to forget the long and exhausting day of senseless work, which will be repeated the next day. This is the *absurd*[6] life that cries out for what is inebriated, for the overflowing of the normal and instituted. Between December 29, 1919 and January 4, 1920, it was written at the Hospício Nacional de Alienados in Rio de Janeiro:

> This question of alcohol, which affects me, because I have drunk a lot and, like everyone else, I have to attribute my crises of madness to it, although I know well that it is not the main factor, it helps me to reflect why doctors do not find in love, from the lowest, most carnal, to its highest form, unfolding in a true mysticism, in a divinization of the beloved object; why - I ask - is it not also a factor of madness? (Barreto, 2010, p. 68).

The above excerpt was taken from the "Diário do Hospício" of writer Lima Barreto, hospitalized with the diagnosis of alcoholism. Lima Barreto did not deny the excessive use, but the most relevant, he stated categorically that the drug, in this case alcohol, was not the main cause of his illnesses. There were others.

> The accusations of drugs (unduly generalized in this imprecise plural) of "destroying personality" by creating "inner worlds" that would isolate human beings from their fellow men are refuted by all the anthropological evidence that shows the aggregating role of alcohol and other drugs in countless societies, including the Western one (Carneiro, 2018, p. 61).

The same person who got drunk wildly is no different from the one who wrote the book "O Triste Fim de Policarpo Quaresma" and so many other classics of national literature. The freedom to consume some types of drugs is forbidden, but limits are also set for the consumption of those that are legal, "normal" limits. Limits that the

---

[5] The French term terroir is reminiscent of terrain, but the concept is much broader. It is the set of natural conditions of each vineyard: the terrain, the soil, the drainage, the nutrients there, the microclimate, the altitude, the slope, the exposure to the sun (Alzer & Braga, 2007, p. 148).

[6] "The absurdity is born from this confrontation between the human call and the irrational silence of the world. This is what we must not forget. This is what we must cling to, for every consequence of a life can be born of it. The irrational, the human nostalgia and the absurdity that arises from their encounter, these are the three characters of the drama that must necessarily end all logic that an existence is capable of" (Camus, 2010, p. 39).

"abnormal" insists on exceeding. It is important to stress what is the norm. For Foucault:

> The standard carries a claim to power. The norm is not simply a principle, it is not even a principle of intelligibility; it is an element from which a certain exercise of power is founded and legitimized. Controversial concept," says Canguilhem. Perhaps we could say political. In any case - (…), the norm brings with it both a principle of qualification and a principle of correction. The norm does not have the function of excluding, rejecting. On the contrary, it is always linked to a positive technique of intervention and transformation, to a kind of normative power (Carneiro, 2018, p. 43).

Therefore, we have a knowledge that supports decisions about the abnormals, in short, that besides producing human products, qualifies them. The delinquents, the rabble,[7] the drunkards who do not drink in moderation, all these beings become "*anomalous*," points outside the curve of a fair and straight life, deviant from the normal, susceptible to correction, healing, hospitalization or detention. For Rose (2011), to operate this normative power, to dictate such rules and norms, we need *experts* in human behavior:

> We have seen a proliferation of experts in human conduct over the past hundred years; economists, managers, accountants, lawyers, advisors, therapists, doctors, anthropologists, political scientists, social policy experts, and so on. But I would say that the "unification" of subjectivation regimes in terms of the self has much to do with the emergence of a particular form of positive experts of the human being-those of the psy disciplines, with their "generosity." By "generosity," I mean that contrary to traditional views of the exclusivity of professional knowledge, the psy disciplines have been happy, even eager, to "surrender" to lend their vocabularies, explanations, and forms of judgment to other professional groups and to implant them in their clients (p. 55).

Having presented the reasoning and arguments of the psychology and psychiatry, we feel the need to involve ourselves in this process, and to observe and dialogue with a contradiction that basically constitutes us, namely: a need to heal the other without there being anything in the other to be healed. Obviously this is not an axiom, but a way to denounce the "legitimate" use and abuse of these knowledge producers of docile and useful bodies. It is relevant to say that: the knowledge of these various techniques exercises the power to produce subjectivities and objectivities that are in us or that define who we are in society. Márcio Alves da Fonseca in his studies about Foucault, more specifically about the processes that affect the individual, gives us the subsidies to understand the "subtle" difference between these two concepts. What is called modes of objectification, has the effect of producing a docile and useless object. In the modes of subjectivation, what is produced is a subject attached to a determined identity (Fonseca, 2011). Subjective "drug addict and criminal", subject "sick and chemical dependent."

---

[7]According to the sociologist Jessé Souza "an entire class of individuals, not only without cultural and economic capital to any significant extent, but devoid of it, this is the fundamental aspect of the social, moral, and cultural preconditions that allow this appropriation" (Souza, 2018, p. 27).

It is important to escape the socially imposed stigma, to break unjust laws, in short, to produce an antithesis of the discursive practice of zeal for health and well-being, in order to satisfy the "Hunger of the Soul" (Alencar, 2018). In an attempt to override everything that devours them, some people do not run away from the struggle. Taking this place of contention by storm—they, the people who use drugs, write, and prophesy!

One of these writings took place between 1901 and 1902, in a cabin by the sea called "House of Pleasure," it follows: "I am therefore presented to the public as an animal stripped of all feeling, unable to sell its soul for a daisy. I was not Werther, I will not be Faust. Who knows? Syphilitic and alcoholics may be the men of the future" (Gauguin, 1997, p. 11). The rebel and visionary written is part of the diary entitled "Before and After" by the painter Paul Gauguin. When he could no longer paint, he wrote the diary. He died alone and sick on May 8, 1903. Visionary because a century later, in 1991 the first president of Russia, Boris Yeltsin, was elected - this was the symbol of a head of State affected by excessive alcohol use - "In the Yeltsin period, perhaps there was never a head of state so drunk in official solemnities" (Carneiro, 2018, p. 342).

The scenario so far is known in many homes, present since the beginning of our culture, used by the elite and the rabble, by the head of state, by people on the street, in short—the consumption of alcohol has expressive numbers, especially when talking about its lethality. The 2018 World Health Organization report presents impressive numbers on the seriousness of alcohol consumption, and they are them:

> Alcohol-related diseases cause 3 million deaths per year, are responsible for 5.1% of the global burden of disease expressed in DALYs (Disability-adjusted life year) and continue to be, globally, one of the leading causes / risk factors for health problems. According to recent benchmarking, alcohol was the seventh risk factor for death and disability in 2016 and the leading risk factor among the 15–49-year-old population (World Health Organization, 2018, p. 126).[8]

We present how the fine weave of a net that captures some and not others is composed. We do not deny the discursive production of these overflows of limits, of the "bad" use of technology of itself—but so far we only speak of the unmeasured, the lack of temperance, all within the legality, the regulatory and lenient permission of the State.

[8] The harmful use of alcohol causes three million deaths per year is responsible for 5.1% of the global burden of disease expressed in DALYs (Chap. 4) and continues to be one of the leading risk factors for poor health globally. Currently available data presented in this report indicate some progress in reducing the harmful use of alcohol in some WHO regions, but the reduction is still insufficient to improve the situation dramatically. According to the most recent estimates in comparative risk assessment, alcohol was the seventh leading risk factor for deaths and disability in 2016 and the top risk factor among the world's population aged 15–49 years (GBD 2016 Alcohol Collaborators, 2018).

Criminals, Patients, and Junkies: The Social Event of the Culture of Prohibition!

The use of drugs is part of the human condition, the polysemy of the term drugs would be worthy of another study, but here we propose to talk about its negative affection in society. The association of the term "drug" with illicit drugs is the fruit of an *event* that has been perpetuated since the nineteenth century, and that has taken on worldwide proportions since the twentieth century. As has already been said, to talk about drugs is to talk about their regulations—that is prohibitionism as an event. For Foucault:

> The event is neither substance nor accident, neither quality nor process; the event is not of the order of the bodies. However, it is not immaterial; it is always within the realm of materiality that it is effective; it has its place and consists of the relationship, coexistence, dispersion, cutting, accumulation, selection of material elements; it is neither the act nor the property of a body; it is produced as the effect of a material dispersion (Foucault, 2014, p. 54).

Events produce diverse materialities, produce subjectivities, but in this case, the act of prohibiting the use of certain drugs—they take and imprison lives, rather than protecting them. Our purpose is not to explain or detail prohibitionism and its harmful consequences, but rather to problematize how the context of the illegality of some substances, such as marijuana, cocaine, and heroin, linked to certain socioeconomic conditions produce peculiar types of subjects.

Within this context of classifying criminals, sick and immoral we have the example of resistance from William Burroughs in the book Junky. Burroughs states that his psychoanalysis sessions removed inhibitions and anxieties, helped him to be free, that is, to live as he wanted, accepted his sexual orientation, but his analyst after a while dismissed him classifying him as "degenerate and outlawed" (Burroughs, 1984, p. 14).

William Burroughs was gay, one of the icons of the Beat Generation alongside Jack Keroauc and Allen Ginsberg, in this autobiographical book, narrates his experiences with heavy drugs, especially the injectable use of heroin. He publicly assumes his sexual orientation, as well as the use and abuse of drugs and, not satisfied, makes a counterpoint to medical knowledge through the senses produced by drug use:

> I never regretted my experience with drugs. I think I am in better health now, having taken heavy drugs at various times in my life, than I would be if I had never been addicted. When you stop growing, you die. An addict never stops growing. Most users usually cut off their addiction periodically, which involves shrinking the body and replacing the drug-dependent cells. I learned the junk equation. Heavy drugs are not a way to increase the pleasure of living. Junk is not a cheap drug. It's a way of life. (Burroughs, 1984, pp. 15–16).

Burroughs was American, white and the son of a rich, traditional family. He died at 83 in 1997. This resistance through literature runs counter to traditional forms of governing bodies, after all, we need to create the means to diagnose and separate the sick from the criminal, and here we have a division, jail for some, hospice for others, sometimes both in the figure of the judicial asylums. We found clues about this division in the class of January 8, 1975, contained in the book *The Abnormals*:

> The harsh office of punishment is thus altered by the beautiful office of healing. And that alteration which serves, among other things, the psychiatric examination. We have gone from the legal problem of responsibility to another problem. Is the individual dangerous? Is he sensitive to criminal sanctions? Is it curable and readaptable? In other words, the criminal sanction should henceforth have as its object, not a subject of law held responsible, but a correlative element of a technique that consists in putting aside, dangerous individuals, in caring for those who are sensitive to the criminal sanction, in order to cure them or readapt them. In other words, it is a technique of normalization that from now on will have to deal with the individual delinquent (Foucault, 2018, pp. 21–22).

To use drugs in the biomedical perspective is to take risks in exchange for an ephemeral, dangerous and worst, deadly pleasure—to use drugs would be a crime against oneself—so it is up to the State and its tentacles to protect us from ourselves.

Marijuana: I Smoke, You Smoke, They Do Not Smoke!

Cannabis sativa, better known as marijuana, is one of the oldest plants in humanity. Anthropological and archaeological studies indicate that it may have been the first plant cultivated because nothing was lost of it: "the oil extracted from the seeds, the fiber from the stalks and the psychoactivity found in the flowers have been elements harnessed by numerous societies over the ages" (Bennett, Osburn, 1995, apud Saad, 2019, p. 15). According to Luiza Saad (2019) researcher and activist of the National Network of Antiprohibitionist Feminists (RENFA), "the cultivation and uses of marijuana are millenary; its prohibition is very recent. Less than 100 years ago it was started towards its criminalization" (p. 15). Marijuana is the most consumed illicit drug on the planet today, and its consumption has been increasing in recent years. According to the United Nations Office on Drugs and Crime (UNODC, 2018, p. 42):

> Cannabis remains the most widely used drug in the world. The UNODC estimates that approximately 3.9 per cent (range: 3.4–4.8 per cent) of the global population aged 15–64 used cannabis at least once in 2016: about 192.2 million people (range: 165.8 million–234.1 million). The number of cannabis users estimated for 2016 is 16 percent higher than the number estimated for 2006 (UNODC, 2018).[9]

At this point we need to make a reflection, if to obtain information from recent research on alcohol we use the reports of the World Health Organization (WHO), at the other end, for marijuana, we look at the United Nations Office on Drugs and Crime. Drugs are a health issue, a security issue, but mainly a "Hegemony of

[9] Cannabis continues to be the most widely used drug worldwide. UNODC estimates that roughly 3.9 percent (range: 3.4–4.8 per cent) of the global population aged 15–64 years used cannabis at least once in 2016: some 192.2 million people (range: 165.8 million–234.1 million). The number of cannabis users estimated for 2016 is 16 per cent higher than the number estimated for 2006.

Cynicism" (Ribeiro & Seibel, 1997). Therefore, and according to the figures above, we have a range between 165 and 234 million criminal people, after all they chose to smoke marijuana in societies that forbid it.

The debate on the uses of marijuana has been expanding in Brazilian society, an example of this was the holding on June 1, 2019 of the 11th Marijuana March.[10] The march grows every year. We experienced thousands of people marching in the city of São Paulo for legalization, decriminalization and the end of the War on Drugs, with the motto—for the people alive and free LEGALIZE. If to imagine a Brazilian society that accepts the various uses of marijuana (medicinal, recreational, and economic) the difficulties are Herculean, who will say other drugs that are taboo, such social panic, we speak of cocaine in its aspirated version and crack the smoked version.

Cocaine: The Elegant White Powder on the Nose

Sigmund Freud experienced and caused to experience the sudden exaltation and the sensation of lightness provided by the ingestion of cocaine. In July 1884 he described the experiment in a scientific article about his own coca use:

> I have been experimenting and studying, myself and others, the effect of coca on the healthy human body. My conclusions are fundamentally in line with Mantegazza's description of the effect of coca leaves. The first time I took 0.05g of *cocainum muritaticum* in a 1% solution of water was when I was feeling slightly unwell due to fatigue. This solution is quite viscous, somewhat opalescent, and has a strange aromatic odor. At first it has a bitter taste, which later gives way to a series of very pleasant and aromatic flavors: dry cocaine salt has the same smell and taste, but to a more concentrated degree. A few minutes after ingesting the cocaine, one experiences sudden exaltation and a sensation of lightness. The lips and palate have whitish mucous membranes, followed by a sensation of warmth in the same areas (Associação Psicanalítica de Porto Alegre, 2004, p. 110).

However, the pursuit of eternal pleasure, of deep pleasure, resulted in problems for Freud. The use of cocaine provided him with such well-being that on January 24, 1895 he wrote a letter reporting on the physical ailments to which "the excesses of cocaine in the left nostril had produced a copious amount of thick pus" (Alencar, 2018, p. 70). From the Andes to Europe, from the 19th to the twenty-first century, the flow only increases, according to the UNODC:

> In 2016, it is estimated that the overall number of cocaine users last year increased by almost 7 percent to 18.2 million (range: 13.9–22.9 million), with the number reported increasing in many regions. More than half of all cocaine users reside in the Americas, mostly in North America (34 percent of the global total), and almost a quarter reside in Europe, mostly in Western and Central Europe (about a fifth of the global total) (UNODC, 2018, p. 33).

[10] I have participated in the march since 2017—This year I was in the March's dissemination groups and the estimates of the organizers and partners were over 120,000 people.

We present Freud's writings, as well as highlighting cocaine-consuming regions, to say that culturally: cocaine in its aspirated form is an elite drug and has been called an elegant addiction, however "threatening" it is to healthy humans,

> Among so many drugs that threatened a healthy "race," there were the so-called elegant social vices, so determined by their origin and who used them. Cocaine, for example, had been brought by "rich boys from foreign countries" and introduced into "elegant environments" where it was consumed by "imitation, curiosity and chic". Together with her "elder sister", morphine, "they began to infiltrate powerfully into all the layers of society [...] as a fearful flagello for individuals, for collectivity, for eugenics" (Pernambuco & Botelho, 1924, apud Saad, 2019, p. 77).

This is one side of the coca leaf, or rather, cocaine. There is another, far from being inelegant, that was produced by society, but mainly by the media as repugnant, terrifying, and mortifying, but mainly dehumanizing. Here is cocaine in its inhaled, smoked version, Crack and its social exclusion.

The Media: From the Production of Bodies with Human Absence

If psy knowledge plays an important role in the taxonomy of uses and users, the media have a fundamental role in the socio-cultural process of producing stigma and amplifying prejudices about drug use, especially crack. Igor de Souza Rodrigues researched and analyzed the publications of some of the newspaper's statements to Folha de São Paulo, and they were: "Addicts leave 'favela' of cracolândia"; "Cracolândia has again 'procession'[11]of addicts after action by the city hall"—On September 27, 2013—the same newspaper brings the comment of a "drug expert" who says: "When you come across a 'craqueiro' (person homeless who use crack a lot) holding a pipe and proposes a change of life, you are talking only with a body. The human being who existed there is absent at that moment. It is a conversation in the void" (Rodrigues, 2016, pp. 290–296).

These "bodies of human absence" and "unable to dialogue" have some basic characteristics and are in certain "terroirs" of the city—ready to be "reaped.' 'According to research conducted by the Oswaldo Cruz Foundation and published in the book Crack and social exclusion,

> The profile of crack users in use scenes is composed of 80% of men in their 20s and 30s; eight out of ten are black; eight out of ten have not reached high school; 40% live on the street; 49% are egressors from the prison system (Garcia, 2016, p. 13).

Here is the thick "thin" web of the net that captures black and poor people.

Finally, the media produces events that meet a society that has great difficulties in rethinking itself, especially on the issue of drug use. A society and culture with a

[11] Procession can also be understood as flow, that is, the movement of pilgrimage made by the users as they travel through the territory, the blocks of the city center.

punitive, moralistic, and hygienic stamp. In January 2012, Datafolha conducted a survey on what the population thought of the hospitalizations against the will of the users, and the result was reported by the media: "It is almost unanimous: 9 out of 10 Brazilians think that crack addicts should be hospitalized for treatment even if they don't want to" (Marinheiro, 2012). In 2017, 5 years later, the same newspaper reports: "Four out of five in São Paulo defend forced hospitalization for crack users" (Bergamo, 2017). Finally, the act of repressing and punishing the uses and abuses is encouraged by the media, strengthening the prohibitionist cosmology.[12]

Final Considerations

I, you, he, we, you, they; we are the constituents of this society, producers and the resultant of diverse cultures. We are the objects for application and use of techniques, we are either governable and disciplined or unruly of self and undisciplined—some users of drugs, others more elegant, only make use of psychoactive substances. In this essay we go through some aspects of this social construction in relation to the culture of drug use. Through research, history, diaries, and social theories, all with the intention of demonstrating the complex labyrinth to which there are several threads of Ariadne: the thread of humanities such as sociology, anthropology, and history disputing spaces with traditional knowledge reserved for the area of health, the thread of writers and artists vociferating an existential and poetic place for the unmeasured, the thread of denunciations in the face of the massive production of abject bodies carried out by the media, and passive of all types of human rights violations.

We are and we live in this dichotomous society, which operates rationally in a binary way, normal versus abnormal, healthy versus crazy, drug addicts versus users of psychoactive substances, adherents to the paradigm of abstinence versus harm reducers. Manichaeist and positivist culture that cannot think beyond good and evil and medicine leaflet. To paraphrase Cazuza, we need a society that is less old fashioned and cowardly, and in the days of a Bolsonarist government, which potentialized hatred and recruited prejudice against the different, this would be of the order of utopia. Therefore, we must resist, inside and out. Let us seek to build heterotopic ways[13] within our bodies, as described in the beautiful epigraph From the Book of

[12] "The prohibitionist perspective, in its origin, is based on moral precepts that conceive drug consumption as a criminal practice that should be punished as the imprisonment of "criminals" and "immoral" (Silva, 2017, p. 241).

[13] Heterotopias are, perhaps, Foucault's central and most solid reflection on a science that would bring us clues to think of certain spaces, "other spaces," "counter-spaces," "different spaces that are the contestation of the spaces where we live," locatable, but outside other localities … these "places without places" that Foucault will erect his thought about the spaces that actually exist, but that subvert the order of all the other spaces existing in one and that trimmed to this one, even in the geographical circumstance, embarrass the understanding of the very order of things, discourses and powers (Foucault, 2009, apud Oliveira, 2019, pp. 82–84).

Drugs: Uses and abuses challenges and prejudices (Escohotado, 1997): "From the skin to the inside begins my exclusive jurisdiction. I choose what may or may not cross this border. I am a sovereign state and the limits of my skin are much more sacred than the confines of any country."

No doubt we ended up with absences, missing the electronic music parties and the relationship with psychedelic drugs (LSD), the medicine of the forest with its powerful plants (ayahuasca), but mainly tobacco. To mitigate the lack, we close the chapter with a thought of the Romanian philosopher Emil Cioran: "It is not God, but the Pain that enjoys the advantages of ubiquity. In the crucial moments of life, the help of cigarettes is more effective than that of the Gospels" (Cioran, 2011, p. 73).

References

Alencar, R. (2018). *A fome da alma: Psicanálise, drogas e pulsão na modernidade*. São Paulo, Brazil: Benjamim Editorial.

Alzer, C., & Braga, D. (2007). *Vinhos: A arte de escolher um bom vinho*. Rio de Janeiro, Brazil: Senac.

Associação Psicanalítica de Porto Alegre. (2004). *Über Coca. 100–157*. Retrieved from http://www.appoa.org.br/uploads/arquivos/revista_26_3.pdf

Barreto, L. (2010). *Diário do hospício e o cemitério dos vivos*. São Paulo, Brazil: Cosac Naify.

Bergamo, M. (2017, May 23). Quatro em cada cinco em SP defendem internação à força para usuários de Crack. *Folha de São Paulo*. Retrieved from http://m.folha.uol.com.br/cotidiano/2017/06/1889949-quatro-em-cada-cinco-em-sp-defendem-internacao-a-forca-de-usuarios-de-crack.shtml

Bueno, E. (1998). *A viagem do descobrimento: a verdadeira história da expedição de Cabral*. Rio de Janeiro, Brazil: Objetiva.

Burroughs, W. S. (1984). *Junky Drogado*. São Paulo, Brazil: Brasiliense.

Camus, A. (2010). *O Mito de Sísifo*. Rio de Janeiro, Brazil: Bestbolso.

Carneiro, H. (2005). Transformações do significado da palavra "droga": Das especiarias coloniais ao proibicionismo contemporâneo. In R. P. Venâncio & H. Carneiro (Eds.), *Álcool e drogas na história do Brasil* (pp. 11–28). São Paulo, Brazil: Alameda.

Carneiro, H. (2008). Autonomia ou heteronomia nos estados alterados de consciência. In B. C. Labate, S. L. Goulart, & M. Fiori (Eds.), *Drogas e cultura: Novas perspectivas* (pp. 65–90). Salvador, Brazil: EDUFBA.

Carneiro, H. (2018). *Drogas: A história do proibicionismo*. São Paulo, Brazil: Autonomia Literária.

Centro De Informações Sobre Saúde E Álcool. (2019). *Álcool e saúde dos brasileiros: panorama 2019*. Retrieved from https://cisa.org.br/images/upload/Panorama_Alcool_Saude_CISA2019.pdf

Cioran, E. (2011). *Silogismos da Amargura*. Rio de Janeiro, Brazil: Rocco.

Dias, L. F. (2008). *Usos e abusos de bebidas alcoólicas segundo os povos Indígenas do Uaçá*. Salvador, Brazil: EDUFBA.

Escohotado, A. (1997). *O Livro das Drogas: Usos e abusos, desafios e preconceitos*. São Paulo, Brazil: Dynamis.

Fonseca, M. A. (2011). *Michel Foucault e a constituição do sujeito*. São Paulo, Brazil: EDUC.

Foucault, M. (2014). *A Ordem do Discurso: aula inaugural no Collège de France, pronunciada em 2 de dezembro de 1970*. São Paulo, Brazil: Edições Loyola.

Foucault, M. (2018). *Os Anormais: Curso no Collège de France (1974–1975)*. São Paulo, Brazil: WMF - Martins Fontes.

Garcia, L. (2016). Apresentação Senad/MJ. In *Ministério da Justiça e Cidadania, Secretária Nacional de Políticas sobre Drogas. Crack e Exclusão Social* (pp. 11–16). Retrieved from http://www.aberta.senad.gov.br/medias/original/201702/20170214-115213-001.pdf
Gauguin, P. (1997). *Antes e Depois*. Porto Alegre, Brazil: LP&M.
Kalinowski, A., & Humphreys, K. (2016). Governmental standard drink definitions and low-risk alcohol consumption guidelines in 37 countries. *Addiction, 111*(7), 1293–1298. https://doi.org/10.1111/add.13341.
Kladstrup, D. (2002). *Vinho & guerra: Os franceses, os nazistas e a batalha pelo maior tesouro da França*. Rio de Janeiro, Brazil: Zahar.
Marinheiro, V. (2012, January 25). 90% aprovam internação involuntária. *Folha de São Paulo*. Retrieved from http://www1.folha.uol.com.br/fsp/cotidiano/22009-90-aprovam-internacao-involuntaria.shtml
Nietzsche, F. W. (2005). *Além do Bem e do Mal: Prelúdio a uma filosofia do futuro*. São Paulo, Brazil: Companhia das Letras.
Nietzsche, F. W. (2011). *Assim Falou Zaratustra: Um livro para todos e para ninguém*. São Paulo, Brazil: Companhia das letras.
Oliveira, L. B. F. (2019). *Uma sala-de-estar na Cracolândia de São Paulo ou uma heterotopia De Braços Abertos*. Master's thesis, Pontifícia Universidade Católica de São Paulo, Brazil. Retrieved from https://tede2.pucsp.br/handle/handle/22358
Ribeiro, M. D., & Seibel, S. D. (1997). *Drogas: Hegemonia do cinismo*. São Paulo, Brazil: Memorial.
Rodrigues, I. (2016). Crack, a noia da mídia. In *Ministério da Justiça e Cidadania, Secretária Nacional de Políticas sobre Drogas. Crack e Exclusão Social* (pp. 287–304). Retrieved from http://www.aberta.senad.gov.br/medias/original/201702/20170214-115213-001.pdf
Rose, N. (2011). *Inventando nossos selfs: Psicologia, poder e subjetividade*. São Paulo, Brazil: Vozes.
Saad, L. (2019). *"Fumo de Negro": A criminalização da maconha no pós-abolição*. Salvador, Brazil: EDUFBA.
Santos, V. M. (2018). Notas desobedientes: decolonialidade e a contribuição para crítica feminista à ciência. *Psicologia & Sociedade, 30,* 1–11. https://doi.org/10.1590/1807-0310/2018v30200112.
Silva, E. (2017). Políticas Públicas sobre drogas no Brasil: aspectos históricos e contextuais. In R. Figueiredo, M. Fefferman, & R. Adorno (Eds.), *Drogas & sociedade contemporânea: Perspectivas para além do proibicionismo* (pp. 239–262). São Paulo, Brazil: Instituto de Saúde.
Souza, J. (2018). *A Ralé Brasileira* (3th ed.). São Paulo, Brazil: ContraCorrente.
Spink, M. J. (2010). *Linguagem e produção de sentidos no cotidiano*. Rio de Janeiro, Brazil: Centro Edelstein de Pesquisas Sociais.
Sztutman, R. (2008). Cauim, substância e efeito: sobre o consumo de bebidas fermentadas entre os ameríndios. In B. C. Labate, S. L. Goulart, & M. Fiori (Eds.), *Drogas e cultura: Novas perspectivas* (pp. 219–250). Salvador, Brazil: EDUFBA.
United Nations Office on Drugs and Crime. (2018). *World Drug Report 2018: Analysis of drug markets opiates, cocaine, cannabis, synthetic drugs*. Retrieved from https://www.unodc.org/wdr2018/prelaunch/WDR18_Booklet_3_DRUG_MARKETS.pdf
Vargas, E. V. (2008). Fármacos e outros objetos sócio-tecnicos: Notas para uma genealogia das drogas. In B. C. Labate, S. L. Goulart, & M. Fiori (Eds.), *Drogas e cultura: Novas perspectivas* (pp. 24–40). Salvador, Brazil: EDUFBA.
Velho, G., & Fiore, M. (2008). O Consumo de psicoativos como campo de pesquisa e de intervenção política. In B. C. Labate, S. L. Goulart, & M. Fiori (Eds.), *Drogas e cultura: Novas perspectivas* (pp. 123–140). Salvador, Brazil: EDUFBA.
World Health Organization. (2018). *Global status report on alcohol and health 2018*. Retrieved from https://apps.who.int/iris/bitstream/handle/10665/274603/9789241565639-eng.pdf?ua=1

Chapter 32
Digital Games, Shopping, Sex, and Other Addictions: Neuropsychological and Behavioral Correlates

Richard Alecsander Reichert, Fernanda Calixto, Andressa Melina Becker da Silva, Gabriella Di Girolamo Martins, Beatriz Cortese Barbugli, Adriana Scatena, Renata Thurler Lessa, Denise De Micheli, and André Luiz Monezi Andrade

Introduction

The concept of addiction is complex and dynamic and does not explicitly refer to dependency on substances with the potential to generate changes in the body and alter perceptions and behavior (Andrade & De Micheli, 2017; De Micheli, Andrade, Silva, & Souza-Formigoni, 2016). Over the last decades, new forms of addiction or behavioral excesses have been proposed. This concept encompasses habits that occur with intensity, frequency, and in contexts that can generate or intensify physical and emotional health problems (Davis, Patton, & Jackson, 2017; Grant, Potenza, Weinstein, & Gorelick, 2010; Petri, 2016).

Behaviors such as playing, buying, having sex, exercising, and using technologies are generally considered to be forms of entertainment and obtaining socially approved or tolerated pleasurable sensations (Almeida, Andrade, Cruz, & De Micheli, 2018; Almeida, De Micheli, & Andrade, 2017). These habits, however, can characterize a disorder when they occur in excess, causing social and health damage (Petri, 2016). These behaviors are considered dependencies when they are recurrent and provide pleasure and relief from aversive sensations, with failures in inhibition,

R. A. Reichert
Universidade do Vale do Itajaí, Itajaí, SC, Brazil

F. Calixto
Universidade Federal de São Carlos, São Carlos, SP, Brazil

A. M. B. da Silva
Universidade de Sorocaba, Sorocaba, SP, Brazil

G. D. G. Martins · B. C. Barbugli · R. T. Lessa · A. L. M. Andrade (✉)
Pontifícia Universidadre Católica de Campinas, Campinas, SP, Brazil

A. Scatena · D. De Micheli
Universidade Federal de São Paulo, São Paulo, SP, Brazil

D. De Micheli et al. (eds.), *Drugs and Human Behavior*,
https://doi.org/10.1007/978-3-030-62855-0_32

and that endures even if there are damages in the family, school or university, work, interpersonal relationships, and other areas of life. In short, dependence is defined as a process in which people emit certain behaviors in order to achieve states of pleasure or relief from unpleasant sensations, with failures in inhibition of behaviors that generally persist despite adverse consequences. The recurrence of these behaviors is associated with a picture of clinically significant suffering (Alavi et al., 2012; Bedendo, Andrade, Opaleye, & Noto, 2017; Cho et al., 2019; Messina, Fuentes, Scanavino, & Parsons, 2014).

The literature suggests a relationship between these addiction and disorders associated with substance use (Andrade et al., 2017). This occurs because there is a certain similarity between the neurobiological components, behavioral aspects, and clinical characteristics of these psychopathologies (Andrade, Bedendo, Enumo, & De Micheli, 2018). As an example, we can cite the recurrent emission of certain behaviors despite adverse consequences, reduced self-control and emotional responses that predispose to engagement in certain activities, besides the possible development of tolerance and physiological abstinence (Andrade, Abrahao, Goeldner, & Souza-Formigoni, 2011). In other words, considered non-chemical dependencies, they follow the pattern of substance dependencies, which start with positive reinforcement (e.g., pleasurable sensations, more significant social interaction) and are maintained by negative reinforcement (e.g., attenuating social pressure, relieving stress, alleviating anxiety), escaping the control of individuals (Lopes et al., 2020; Yamauchi, Andrade, Pinheiro, Enumo, & De Micheli, 2019). As the frequency and intensity of behaviors gradually increase, they correlate with a series of personal and social losses and, in many cases, are associated with psychiatric comorbidities. Given this, these issues have been characterized as emerging public health concerns, as they can significantly affect people's lives (Abrahao, Quadros, Andrade, & Souza-Formigoni, 2012; Andrade et al. 2021; De Micheli et al. 2020; Di Nicola et al. 2015; Grant, Brewer, & Potenza, 2006; Grant & Chamberlain, 2016; Messina et al. 2014; Villella et al. 2011). This chapter aims to describe the clinical characteristics and neuropsychological and behavioral aspects of compulsivity in digital games, shopping, sex, and other addictions.

Digital Games

Recently, virtual games have become more frequent, especially among young audiences. The proper use of these tools, besides being a form of entertainment, favors the improvement of some cognitive aspects. On the other hand, the exacerbated involvement in such activities may imply in socio-emotional cognitive damage to individuals. This type of behavior has been considered an addictive behavior and represents an emerging concern in public health since it is associated with psychophysical problems, such as fatigue, sleep disturbances, and symptoms of anxiety and depression (Choi et al., 2017; Festl, Scharkow, & Quandt, 2012; Gentile et al., 2017; Männikkö, Billieux, & Kääriäinen, 2015).

Box 32.1 Diagnostic Criteria for Internet Gambling Disorder (Source: Gentile et al., 2017; Wartberg, Kriston, & Thomasius, 2017)
Diagnostic Criteria

1. Excessive game-related concern.
2. Symptoms of abstinence, such as irritability, anxiety, or sadness when not playing.
3. Development of tolerance, characterized by the need for more time dedicated to games.
4. Unsuccessful attempts to control involvement in games.
5. Reduced interest in alternative activities, caused by engaging in games.
6. Continuity of involvement in games, despite adverse consequences.
7. Omission or distortion of game-related information in the family and other areas.
8. Use of games as a means of escape or avoidance of aversive situations or emotional states.
9. Losses in relationships, professional activities or various opportunities arising from involvement in games.

It is important to emphasize that the constant use of games cannot, in isolation, lead to a diagnosis. Despite the real correlation, there are differences between pathological use and the high frequency of games. To be considered a disorder, this engagement must be associated with clinically significant losses in the lives of the subjects (Gentile et al., 2017).

The study by Wartberg et al. (2017) analyzed the variables associated with disorders related to involvement in digital games and found a higher prevalence among male subjects, minors, with less involvement in social activities and interpersonal relationships and with higher levels of anxiety and depression. Eijnden, Koning, Doornwaard, van Gurp, and ter Bogt (2018) identified symptoms such as reduced psychosocial well-being and low school performance. Also, Männikkö et al. (2015) relate gambling disorders to lower life satisfaction, low self-esteem, and self-efficacy, shyness, anxiety, and impulsiveness. Therefore, it is noted that gambling addiction can develop from other psychological problems such as anxiety, social phobia, and depression (Table 32.1).

Neuroimaging studies indicate that compulsivity in games has neurobiological similarities with other behavioral excesses, such as changes in structures and functions related to reward processing, cognitive control, and behavioral inhibition. Structurally, the gray matter volume and cortical thickness in prefrontal areas such as the dorsolateral prefrontal cortex and striated correlate with the duration of involvement and dependence in games, cognitive deficits, and severity of the frame. Functionally, the involvement of prefrontal areas and reduced serotonin levels are associated with lower behavioral inhibition and control of impulses and severity of

Table 32.1 Functional analysis of digital game dependency

Context/ background	Answers	Consequences	Processes	Effects
Pressure from parents Problems at school Low self-esteem Relationship difficulties	Playing on the internet	Contact with new people Virtual social interaction	Positive reinforcement	Wellness Increased self-esteem
		Distancing from family and peers Avoidance of social contact in real life Mitigation of family and social pressure	Negative reinforcement (escape/ escape)	Relief

the condition. Also, changes in dopaminergic pathways have been associated with the constant search for rewards in activities such as games. Because of this, some theoretical models associate dopamine activity with motivational circuits underlying pathological gambling. These characteristics are common to other types of behavioral dependence, such as substance dependence (Andrade & De Micheli, 2017; Choi et al., 2017; Grant et al., 2006).

Some of the therapeutic interventions conducted in studies investigating the area include psychoeducation about the harmful effects of compulsive gambling; parental guidance, focusing on environmental management, and reducing contact with games when the picture is presented in adolescents (Gentile et al., 2017; Zajac, Ginley, Chang, & Petry, 2017).

The literature signals the need for more comprehensive models for understanding these behaviors, which consider both the aspects of games and the psychological characteristics of players and their motivations, especially in adolescence, which is a period marked by various physical, cognitive, emotional, and social changes. In this phase, accurately, these behaviors can generate significant and lasting consequences, so it is important to know the variables involved to enable the development of effective intervention strategies (Eijnden et al., 2018; Wartberg et al., 2017). To better understanding of compulsive gambling behavior, Gentile et al. (2017) suggest further research with the aim of (a) identify the risk factors that predispose the installation and maintenance of this behavior; (b) analyze its clinical course, including the development period and duration; (c), examine psychiatric comorbidities in order to verify whether compulsivity in gambling is a symptom of other conditions or should be described as an independent disorder; and (d) conduct controlled studies to test the effectiveness of treatments and expand the number of available evidence.

Shopping

The act of buying has developed among ancient civilizations and is still maintained today as a form of acquisition of goods, distraction, and pleasure. However, although ordinary and necessary, this behavior can become problematic. Compulsiveness in purchasing was first described at the beginning of the twentieth century. In the 1990s, there was a growing clinical interest in compulsive purchasing behavior, which became the focus of attention and agenda of discussions and scientific publications in several countries. It is a phenomenon defined by excessive concern, irresistible desires, and immoderate engagement in activities related to purchasing (Mattos et al., 2016; Müller, Reinecker, Jacobi, Reisch, & de Zwaan, 2005; Tavares, Lobo, Fuentes, & Black, 2008; Villella et al., 2011; Zadka & Olajossy, 2016).

Box 32.2 Diagnostic Criteria of Compulsivity in Purchasing (Source: Tavares et al., 2008; Villella et al., 2011)
Diagnostic Criteria

1. Excessive concern or impulse to buy, indicated by at least one of the criteria:
   (a) Frequent worry, intrusive thoughts, and irresistible impulses to buy.
   (b) Purchases for more extended periods than intended, of unnecessary items or beyond what the financial conditions allow.
2. Concerns, impulses, or behaviors concerning shopping cause clinically significant suffering and damage, interfere with daily operation, and generate financial problems.
3. Excessive buying behavior does not only occur during periods of hypomania or mania.

There are several characteristics in common between compulsive buying behavior and substance dependence, such as obsessive need or compulsion to consume, loss of self-control, progressive increase in consumption, among others (Zadka & Olajossy, 2016). As with the use of substances, it is necessary to distinguish "normal purchases" from uncontrolled behavior (pathological) of purchasing, since, similarly, purchases can occur in certain situations, without damage to the subjects. This distinction is made based on levels of personal concern and distress and the development of adverse consequences (Maraz, Griffiths, & Demetrovics, 2016; Tavares et al., 2008).

Studies suggest that this behavior appears as a non-assertive strategy to deal with negative feelings, a factor that contributes to its installation and maintenance. It is an impulsive response to aversive emotional reactions, which interferes with daily functioning, as it can generate or intensify psychological, social, occupational, and

Table 32.2 Functional analysis of compulsivity in purchasing

Context/ background	Answers	Consequences	Processes	Effects
Personal problems Relationship difficulties Aversive emotional responses	Buy	Acquisition of new belongings	Positive reinforcement	Wellness Increased self-esteem
		Distraction Temporary away from everyday problems	Negative reinforcement (escape/escape)	Relief

financial problems. Surveys estimate its prevalence between 6% and 7%, with higher propensity among young people and growing in the adult population (Müller, Mitchell, & de Zwaan, 2015; Nicolai, Darancó, & Moshagen, 2016; Roberts, Yaya, & Manolis, 2014) (Table 32.2).

Nicolai et al. (2016) point out that compulsive purchasing is related to behavioral inhibition deficits, i.e., impulsiveness, which intensifies in the presence of unpleasant emotional responses. In this case, this outcome may come from maladaptive *coping*, using Escape, a process explained by the Motivational *Coping* Theory (Skinner & Zimmer-Gembeck, 2016). According to Nicolai et al. (2016), this may be an explanation for the fact that excessive shopping episodes usually occur after contrary affections. Given this, Müller et al. (2015) report that there is a high prevalence of psychiatric comorbidities (such as anxiety and depression) among people seeking treatment for problems arising from pathological purchases. Maraz, van den Brink, and Demetrovics (2015) identified compulsive shoppers as younger, less educated, mostly female, with higher levels of impulsiveness and obsessive-compulsive symptoms, reduced levels of well-being and self-esteem, and more likely to use substances. According to Mattos et al. (2016), the evaluation of these variables and the verification of concomitant psychiatric disorders favors better interventions and prognosis.

Zadka and Olajossy (2016) list as characteristics associated with compulsory purchase: (1) *hedonistic motivation*, referring to the pleasant emotional components (such as the feeling of pleasure) elicited after the act of buying, as well as the absence of aversive emotional responses (such as guilt); (2) *impulsive motivation*, related to impulse disorders, which, in behavioral terms, refers to the tendency to respond to immediate boosters without considering the delayed aversive stimuli (long-term consequences); (3) *compensatory motivation*, when the items purchased serve as stimuli that, in a certain way, increase self-esteem; and (4) *compulsive motivation, which* considers covert behaviors as intrusive thoughts and anxiety symptoms that lead to shopping as a strategy to reduce tension. Also, the authors cite the constant incentive to consumerism as a factor associated with compulsive shopping, which is influenced by the materialistic culture, the emergence of many new shopping malls, and the excess of advertising and apology for exacerbated consumption in public places and diverse media.

The etiology of pathological purchase is still little known. Most researches point to a similarity of shopping compulsion with other behavioral dependencies, such as desire reactions triggered by certain related stimuli (clues). Among the neurobiological components associated with compulsive purchasing behavior, studies indicate a correlation with neuroanatomic regions such as the ventral striated, the accumbens nucleus, the orbitofrontal cortex, the cingulate cortex, the amygdala, and the hippocampus. Several studies have focused on the reduction in the activity of the prefrontal cortex in compulsive buyers. This area is responsible for crucial functions such as decision making, situation analysis, stimulus interpretation, and behavioral inhibition. People who exhibit pathological purchasing behaviors generally experience a worsening of assertive decision making and deficits in risk assessment skills (Trotzke, Starcke, Pedersen, & Brand, 2014; Zadka & Olajossy, 2016).

Therapeutic recommendations in cases of compulsory purchasing include interventions that seek to identify enforcers related to purchasing patterns. At the same time, self-management strategies are recommended, such as finding other ways to experience pleasure (Koran & Aboujaoude, 2014).

Despite the considerable attention given to compulsive purchasing behavior, empirical research to prove the effectiveness of treatment interventions is still scarce. Better planning of a multidimensional approach that takes into account the variables presented that play a central role in the installation and maintenance of this behavior is still necessary. Studies indicate that cognitive-behavioral models are promising, but more evidence is still needed in order to understand this issue and to formulate more effective strategies for prevention and treatment (Granero et al., 2017; Müller et al., 2015).

Sex

Sex addiction is also known as a hypersexuality disorder and can cause severe problems for people, with consequences similar to other addictive disorders. Data show that its prevalence worldwide is around 3–6%. Subjects who are compulsive about sexual activities report obsessive thoughts and behaviors as well as intense sexual fantasies. This category encompasses problematic behaviors such as excessive masturbation, *cybersex* (*cybersex*, virtual sexual activities), exacerbated use of pornography, among others (Karila et al., 2014; Wéry & Billieux, 2017).

The characteristics of compulsive sexual behavior are related to difficulties in controlling excessive or inappropriate sexual fantasies and intense sexual desires or behaviors that generate damage to daily functioning. In other words, these are public or private responses common to all people, but occurring at high frequency and intensity and/or in inappropriate contexts, causing social harm and physical and emotional health of individuals.

Box 32.3 Diagnostic Criteria for Sex Dependence (Source: Goodman, 1990; Silveira, Vieira, Palomo, & Silveira, 2000)
Diagnostic Criteria

1. Frequent involvement in sexual activities more often or for longer than initially intended.
2. Unsuccessful attempts to reduce or control this sexual behavior.
3. Excessive time spent on activities related to this sexual behavior.
4. Give up social, occupational, or recreational activities as a result of this sexual behavior.
5. Continuity of sexual activity despite often presenting social, financial, psychological, or physical problems caused by such behavior.
6. Increasing the need to increase the frequency or intensity of this sexual activity to achieve the same levels of pleasure.
7. Restlessness or irritation at the impossibility of exercising this sexual activity.

The problematic engagement in online sexual activities, or cybersex, is characterized by the excessive use of virtual technologies in order to obtain sexual pleasure, negatively impacting the lives of individuals. There is no consensual definition of this disorder in the scientific literature, as well as its evaluation and diagnosis. It is a concept that encompasses several other distinct virtual behaviors (Wéry & Billieux, 2017).

There are common aspects of compulsive sexual behavior and substance use disorders, mainly concerning neural components. Although there are still gaps and the need for more research and evidence, studies demonstrate similarities in the functioning of neurotransmitters, such as dopamine and serotonergic systems (involved in behavioral activation and inhibition), which may contribute to the development and maintenance of specific characteristics that cover both disorders. Neuroimaging research indicates that reactivity to stimuli is relevant to addiction and contributes to desires, impulses, and relapses. Studies suggest that regions such as the ventral striated, anterior cingulate cortex, and amygdala are related to this reactivity and constitute a fissure circuit. In addition, among sexually compulsive subjects, a correlation was observed between the degree of habituation (after repeated exposure to certain stimuli, such as sexual images) and the preference for sexual novelties. This information corroborates theories that relate dependence to greater salience or sensitivity to certain stimuli, which are responsible for a higher frequency and/or intensity of behaviors in search of such enhancers (Kraus, Voon, & Potenza, 2016; Kühn & Gallinat, 2016; Wéry & Billieux, 2017).

Hypersexuality is a pattern of multidimensional behavior. Its etiology is multifactorial and may involve the presence of psychiatric comorbidities, substance-induced disorders (by the use of amphetamines, for example), neuropathological disorders (such as frontal lobe syndrome, referring to lesions in the frontal region of the brain, with implications in behavior control), among other factors. Studies on the psychobiology of hypersexuality suggest that among the neurobiological aspects that influence the etiology of this disorder are frontal lesions, related to failures in inhibition of behavior and impulsive hypersexual response; striatic lesions, associated with the intermittent firing of response patterns; and temporal limbic lesions, which may result in sexual appetite disorders, including changes in the direction of sexual desire. In addition, many neurotransmitters are involved in their pathogenesis, such as dopamine and noradrenaline, which play a role in brain reward pathways (Asiff et al., 2018; Stein, Hugo, Oosthuizen, Hawkridge, & van Heerden, 2000).

As with other behavioral dependencies, the indicated treatment for compulsion or sexual dependence should combine pharmacological and psychological approaches, with due attention to possible correlated psychiatric comorbidities. Evidence-based psychotherapies, such as cognitive-behavioral therapy and acceptance and commitment therapy, appear to be useful for the treatment of problems related to compulsive sexual behavior, as well as pharmacological treatments, with serotonergic reuptake inhibitors (e.g., fluoxetine, sertraline, and citalopram) and opioid antagonists (e.g., naltrexone), are effective in reducing associated symptoms. However, more controlled and large-scale studies are still needed to test and formulate more effective intervention strategies (Karila et al., 2014; Wéry & Billieux, 2017).

Smartphones, Internet, and Virtual Social Networks

People devote an increasing amount of time to the use of technologies such as mobile devices, as they enable instantaneous communication, socialization through virtual networks, quick access to information, and various forms of entertainment. Many times, however, this habit is associated with losses in the quality of life of the subjects (Andrade et al. 2021; Andrade, Kim, Scatena, Enes, Enumo, & De Micheli, 2020; Andrade, Kim, Caricati, et al., 2020; Andrade, Scatena, Martins, et al. 2020; Cruz, Scatena, Andrade, & De Micheli, 2018). It is stated that the exacerbated use of cell phones is possibly the most prevalent non-pharmacological behavioral dependence of the twenty-first century. This excessive use is due to the great variety of tools made available by the devices, mainly by Internet access (Andrade, Scatena, Bedendo, et al. 2020; Roberts et al., 2014).

The main characteristics of excessive use of the Internet and virtual social networks concern psychological dependence: desire to access the network, lack of control over use, irritation when use is stopped, and euphoria when access is resumed. There is a fixation on virtual life, low interest in face-to-face life, and neglect of healthy living habits, such as sleep and food, and off-line relationships. Internet and virtual social network dependent individuals experience symptoms such as irritation, bad mood, and tension when they do not have access to the network; and feelings such as guilt, shame, and frustration can arise from social isolation, neglected daily obligations, and unsuccessful attempts to avoid or reduce Internet use. For this reason, the term "nomophobia" arose from the expression "*no-mobile*," which means "without a cell phone," and "phobos," of Greek origin, which means phobia or fear. Thus, nomophobia means anguish or fear of the subject being without access to a mobile phone, computer, and/or Internet. This preference for virtual life and the low engagement in activities in face-to-face life may generate or intensify social problems, such as family, academic, and professional relationships, and health, such as sleep and food-related losses (Fortim & Araujo, 2013; Kardefelt-Winther, 2014; Oliveira, Barreto, El-Aouar, Souza, & Pinheiro, 2017).

Studies associate these behavioral excesses with psychosocial factors and psychiatric comorbidities. There are correlations with a range of psychological disorders, such as stress, anxiety, depression, impulsiveness, attention deficit, and hyperactivity, among others (Abreu, Karam, Góes, & Spritzer, 2008; Cerniglia et al. 2017; Choi et al. 2019; Grant, Lust, & Chamberlain, 2019; Oliveira-Pinheiro et al. 2020; Pluhar, Kavanaugh, Levinson, & Rich, 2019; Tereshchenko & Kasparov, 2019).

Regarding the neuropsychological aspects of Internet addiction and virtual social networks, changes are observed in several brain regions, mainly in the frontal and striated cortex. Studies show structural and functional impairment of regions in the brain related to reward processing, memory, and cognitive control (Park, Han, & Roh, 2016) (Table 32.3).

There is an alternative perspective, *Escape Theory*, which considers the dependency on the use of cell phones and their tools a secondary problem, which emerges as a strategy to deal with more significant problems, such as boredom, low self-esteem, interpersonal relationship problems, among others (as seen in other behavioral dependencies). This view suggests that the excessive use of the cell phone favors the user not to focus on disconcerting issues; as a way to escape or evade their problems. In view of this, identifying the root of the problem is the way to a more effective treatment. This perspective is also known as *compensatory use*, which considers the excessive use of the Internet as a strategy of escape from real-life issues, used by individuals in order to alleviate dysphoric moods. In this sense, due

Table 32.3 Functional analysis of Internet dependency and virtual social networks

Context/background	Answers	Consequences	Processes	Effects
Pressure from the family Low self-esteem Relationship difficulties Personal problems (financial, for example)	Accessing the internet and virtual social networks	Contact with new people Virtual social interaction Facilitation of interpersonal communication	Positive reinforcement	Wellness Increased self-esteem
		Avoidance of social contact in real life Mitigation of family and social pressure Deviating from real-life problems	Negative reinforcement (escape/escape)	Relief

to the lack of interpersonal relationships and other enforcers in real everyday life, the use of the Internet and access to virtual social networks emerge as a form of socialization, thus compensating for psychosocial problems (Kardefelt-Winther, 2014; Roberts et al., 2014).

Therapeutic interventions in cases of Internet addiction are similar to those conducted in cases of online gambling compulsion. Thus, establishing the enforcers related to Internet access, the events that evoke compulsive use, and the strengthening of alternative and incompatible patterns become the focus of analysis and intervention. As mentioned, in many cases, the compulsive use of the Internet occurs with individuals who present losses in interpersonal relationships. In such cases, psychotherapies with a focus on promoting social skills can favor real, healthier social interactions and, as a consequence, can produce a reduction in *online* interactions.

Physical Exercises

Physical exercise is encouraged as one of the World Health Organization's recommendations to maintain health, prevent disease, and improve quality of life (World Health Organization, 2010). However, its excesses can be harmful, bringing consequences not only for the body but also for emotional health, as well as any other dependency (Marques et al., 2019).

Dependence on physical exercise presents itself as excessive behavior, manifested by physiological, tolerance and abstinence symptoms, and psychological, such as anxiety and depression (Hausenblas & Downs, 2002). Its main characteristics are the practice of exercises more than once during the day; increase in the frequency and intensity of the practice, prioritizing it over other activities; development of tolerance about the quantity and frequency of exercises practiced; mood changes, such as irritability, anxiety, depression, when in abstinence; the practice of exercises to get around the symptoms of abstinence; continuity of the practice even if injured; changes in diet and other habits of life for better performance in physical practice (Marques et al., 2019).

Weinstein and Weinstein (2014) research found that exercise dependence has a compulsive dimension, including rewarding aspects. According to these authors, studies with laboratory animals have shown that physical exercises such as running are associated with the release of endorphins and cannabinoids and activation of the dopamine reward system, thus contributing to stress reduction. Genetic studies suggest that genes control the preference for naturally rewarding behaviors such as exercise. There are also psychological reward factors such as habituation, social support, stress relief, abstinence prevention, and anxiety reduction. It is also possible that there are comorbidities, such as psychiatric disorders, eating disorders or substance use (Bedendo, Andrade, & Noto, 2015; Bedendo, Opaleye, Andrade, & Noto, 2013; Oliveira, Andrade, & De Micheli, 2016).

The work of Baekeland (1970), the first one on physical exercise addiction, showed that athletes who trained from 3–4 days a week, when deprived of their practice, presented increased anxiety, sexual tension, and night awakenings, diminishing well-being and social coexistence. However, it is valid to emphasize that dependence on physical exercise does not affect only athletes, but it is likely to happen to any individual (Marques et al., 2019).

Final Considerations

In the same way that use and dependence on substances, behaviors such as compulsive engagement in games, shopping, sex, and other activities are correlated to some personal and contextual variables. Given this, an addendum to the fact that correlation does not imply a causal relationship is necessary. The correlation of specific behaviors with environmental or neurobiological variables does not mean that factor A is the cause of the B phenomenon. The literature presents, for example, the correlation between behavioral excesses and losses in interpersonal relationships. What is the basis? Is the engagement (considered compulsive) in certain activities the cause of socio-emotional cognitive problems? Or do cognitive-socio-emotional problems lead to behavioral dependencies as strategies to deal with life adversities? All behavior is multidetermined, so all factors must be identified and considered for a more comprehensive understanding and for the formulation of more effective intervention strategies that, above all, take into account the singularities of the subjects.

It is also important to emphasize that these habits (substance use, games, shopping, sex, physical exercise, among others) are typical behaviors and can only be considered problematic when they cause clinically significant damage. Therefore, education, prevention, and treatment programs should rethink concepts such as "addiction" and "dependency" and consider their multifactorial and the different forms of manifestation. The problem is not restricted to taboo and morally sanctioned issues (such as drug use), but also to behaviors tolerated, approved, and even encouraged by society. However, many of these behaviors that have become public health concerns, given their potential aggravating factors, still go unnoticed by families and health and education professionals.

Besides pointing out the relevance of studying and building evidence on interventions in cases of non-chemical compulsions, this text sought to establish that, regardless of the topography presented, all forms of compulsion have characteristics in common that cause similar social, personal, and financial losses. It is worth noting that compulsive gambling, compulsive use of the Internet, excessive purchases through *online* channels, and even access to sex through pornography are impulsive patterns made possible through facilitated access to technologies and the Internet. In this way, the very healthy generalized use of technologies (that is, without excesses and so as not to cause losses) becomes a challenge in a society increasingly technological and connected.

References

Abrahao, K. P., Quadros, I. M. H., Andrade, A. L. M., & Souza-Formigoni, M. L. O. (2012). Accumbal dopamine D2 receptor function is associated with individual variability in ethanol behavioral sensitization. *Neuropharmacology, 62*(2), 882–889. https://doi.org/10.1016/j.neuropharm.2011.09.017.

Abreu, C., Karam, R., Góes, D., & Spritzer, D. (2008). Dependência de internet e de jogos eletrônicos: uma revisão. *Revista Brasileira de Psiquiatria, 30*(2), 156–167. https://doi.org/10.1590/S1516-44462008000200014.

Alavi, S., Ferdosi, M., Jannatifard, F., Eslami, M., Alaghemandan, H., & Setare, M. (2012). Behavioral addiction versus substance addiction: Correspondence of psychiatric and psychological views. *International Journal of Preventive Medicine, 3*(4), 290–294.

Almeida, D. E. R. G., Andrade, A. L. M., Cruz, F. D., & De Micheli, D. (2018). Perception of freedom in leisure among substance users and nonusers. *Psico-USF, 23*(1), 13–24. https://doi.org/10.1590/1413-82712018230102.

Almeida, D. E. R. G., De Micheli, D., & Andrade, A. L. M. (2017). O lazer e o uso de substâncias entre adolescentes: uma revisão integrativa. *Estudos e Pesquisas em Psicologia, 17*(3), 970–988. https://doi.org/10.1590/1413-82712018230102.

Andrade, A. L. M., Abrahao, K. P., Goeldner, F. O., & Souza-Formigoni, M. L. O. (2011). Administration of the 5-HT2C receptor antagonist SB-242084 into the nucleus accumbens blocks the expression of ethanol-induced behavioral sensitization in Albino Swiss mice. *Neuroscience, 189*, 178–186. https://doi.org/10.1016/j.neuroscience.2011.05.028.

Andrade, A. L. M., Bedendo, A., Enumo, S. R. F., & De Micheli, D. (2018). Brain development in adolescence: General aspects and update. *Adolescência e Saúde, 15*(Supl. 1), 62–67. Retrieved from: https://www.adolescenciaesaude.com/detalhe_artigo.asp?id=759#.

Andrade, A. L. M., & De Micheli, D. (2017). *Inovações no Tratamento de Dependência de Drogas* (1st ed.). Rio de Janeiro, Brazil: Atheneu.

Andrade, A. L. M., Enumo, S. R. F., Passos, M. A. Z., Vellozo, E. P., Shoen, T. H., Kulik, M. A., Niskier, S. R., et al. (2021). Problematic Internet Use, Emotional Problems and Quality of Life Among Adolescents. *Psico-USF, 26*(1), 41–51. http://dx.doi.org/10.1590/1413-82712021260104.

Andrade, A. L. M., Kim, D. J., Caricati, V. V., Martins, G. D. G., Kirihara, I. K., Barbugli, B. C., et al. (2020). Validity and reliability of the Brazilian version of the smartphone addiction scale-short version for university students and adult population. *Estudos de Psicologia (Campinas), 37*, e190117. https://doi.org/10.1590/1982-0275202037e190117.

Andrade, A. L. M., Kim, D. J., Scatena, A., Enes, C. C., Enumo, S. R. F., & De Micheli, D. (2020). Validity and Reliability of the Brazilian Version of the Smartphone Addiction Scale-Long Version (SAS-LV). Trends in Psychology, in press. https://doi.org/10.1007/s43076-020-00046-y.

Andrade, A. L. M., Scatena, A., Bedendo, A., Enumo, S. R. F., Dellazzana-Zanon, L. L., Prebianchi, H. B., et al. (2020). Findings on the relationship between internet addiction and psychological symptoms in Brazilian adults. *International Journal of Psychology*. https://doi.org/10.1002/ijop.12670.

Andrade, A. L. M., Scatena, A., Martins, G. D. G., de Oliveira Pinheiro, B., da Silva, A. B., Enes, C. C., et al. (2020). Validation of smartphone addiction scale-short version (SAS-SV) in Brazilian adolescents. *Addictive Behaviors, 110*, 106540.

Andrade, A. L. M., Teixeira, L. R. D. S., Zoner, C. C., Niro, N. N., Scatena, A., & Amaral, R. A. D. (2017). Fatores associados à Depressão Pós-Parto em mulheres em situação de vulnerabilidade social. *SMAD, Revista Eletrônica Saúde Mental Álcool e Drogas, 13*(4), 196–204. https://doi.org/10.11606/issn.1806-6976.v13i4p196-204.

Asiff, M., Sidi, H., Masiran, R., Kumar, J., Das, S., Hatta, N., & Alfonso, C. (2018). Hypersexuality as a neuropsychiatric disorder: The neurobiology and treatment options. *Current Drug Targets, 19*(12), 1391–1401. https://doi.org/10.1017/s1092852900012657.

Baekeland, F. (1970). Exercise deprivation: Sleep and psychological reactions. *Archives of Genetic Psychiatry, 22*(4), 365–369. https://doi.org/10.1001/archpsyc.1970.01740280077014.

Bedendo, A., Andrade, A. L. M., & Noto, A. R. (2015). Sports and substance use in high school students different perspectives of this relationship. *SMAD Revista Eletrônica Saúde Mental Álcool e Drogas, 11*(2), 85–96. https://doi.org/10.11606/issn.1806-6976.v11i2p85-96.

Bedendo, A., Andrade, A. L. M., Opaleye, E. S., & Noto, A. R. (2017). Binge drinking: A pattern associated with a risk of problems of alcohol use among university students. *Revista Latino-Americana de Enfermagem, 25*, e2925–e2933. https://doi.org/10.1590/1518-8345.1891.2925.

Bedendo, A., Opaleye, E. S., Andrade, A. L. M., & Noto, A. R. (2013). Heavy episodic drinking and soccer practice among high school students in Brazil: The contextual aspects of this relationship. *BMC Public Health, 13*(1), 247. https://doi.org/10.1186/1471-2458-13-247.

Cerniglia, L., Zoratto, F., Cimino, S., Laviola, G., Ammaniti, M., & Adriani, W. (2017). Internet addiction in adolescence: Neurobiological, psychosocial and clinical issues. *Neuroscience & Biobehavioral Reviews, 76*, 174–184. https://doi.org/10.1016/j.neubiorev.2016.12.024.

Cho, S. B., Su, J., Kuo, S. I., Bucholz, K. K., Chan, G., Edenberg, H. J., et al. (2019). Positive and negative reinforcement are differentially associated with alcohol consumption as a function of alcohol dependence. *Psychology of Addictive Behaviors, 33*(1), 58. https://doi.org/10.1037/adb0000436.

Choi, B., Huh, S., Kim, D., Suh, S., Lee, S., & Potenza, M. (2019). Transitions in problematic internet use: A one-year longitudinal study of boys. *Psychiatry Investigation, 16*(6), 433–442. https://doi.org/10.30773/pi.2019.04.02.1.

Choi, J., Cho, H., Kim, J., Jung, D., Ahn, K., Kang, H., et al. (2017). Structural alterations in the prefrontal cortex mediate the relationship between internet gaming disorder and depressed mood. *Scientific Reports, 7*(1), 1–10. https://doi.org/10.1038/s41598-017-01275-5.

Cruz, F. A. D., Scatena, A., Andrade, A. L. M., & De Micheli, D. (2018). Evaluation of internet addiction and the quality of life of Brazilian adolescents from public and private schools. *Estudos de Psicologia (Campinas), 35*(2), 193–204. https://doi.org/10.1590/1982-02752018000200008.

Davis, P., Patton, R., & Jackson, S. (Eds.). (2017). *Addiction: Psychology and treatment*. Hoboken, NJ: Wiley.

De Micheli, D., Andrade, A. L. M., Silva, E. A., & Souza-Formigoni, M. L. O. (2016). *Drug abuse in adolescence* (1st ed.). New York: Springer. https://doi.org/10.1007/978-3-319-17795-3.

De Micheli, D., Andrade, A., & Galduróz, J. C. (2020). Limitations of DSM-5 diagnostic criteria for substance use disorder in adolescents: what have we learned after using these criteria for several years? *Brazilian Journal of Psychiatry*, in press. https://doi.org/10.1590/1516-4446-2020-1151.

Di Nicola, M., Tedeschi, D., De Risio, L., Pettorruso, M., Martinotti, G., Ruggeri, F., et al. (2015). Co-occurrence of alcohol use disorder and behavioral addictions: Relevance of impulsivity and craving. *Drug and Alcohol Dependence, 148*, 118–125. https://doi.org/10.1016/j.drugalcdep.2014.12.028.

Eijnden, R., Koning, I., Doornwaard, S., van Gurp, F., & ter Bogt, T. (2018). The impact of heavy and disordered use of games and social media on adolescents' psychological, social, and school functioning. *Journal of Behavioral Addictions, 7*(3), 697–706. https://doi.org/10.1556/2006.7.2018.65.

Festl, R., Scharkow, M., & Quandt, T. (2012). Problematic computer game use among adolescents, younger and older adults. *Addiction, 108*(3), 592–599. https://doi.org/10.1111/add.12016.

Fortim, I., & Araujo, C. (2013). Aspectos psicológicos do uso patológico de internet. *Boletim - Academia Paulista de Psicologia, 33*(85), 292–311.

Gentile, D. A., Bailey, K., Bavelier, D., Brockmyer, J. F., Cash, H., Coyne, S. M., et al. (2017). Internet Gaming Disorder in children and adolescents. *Pediatrics, 140*(Supplement 2), S81–S85. https://doi.org/10.1542/peds.2016-1758H.

Goodman, A. (1990). Addiction: Definition and implications. *Addiction, 85*(11), 1403–1408. https://doi.org/10.1111/j.1360-0443.1990.tb01620.x.

Granero, R., Fernández-Aranda, F., Mestre-Bach, G., Steward, T., Baño, M., Agüera, Z., et al. (2017). Cognitive behavioral therapy for compulsive buying behavior: Predictors of treatment outcome. *European Psychiatry, 39*, 57–65. https://doi.org/10.1016/j.eurpsy.2016.06.004.

Grant, J., Brewer, J., & Potenza, M. (2006). The neurobiology of substance and behavioral addictions. *CNS Spectrums, 11*(12), 924–930. https://doi.org/10.1017/S109285290001511X.

Grant, J., & Chamberlain, S. (2016). Expanding the definition of addiction: DSM-5 vs. ICD-11. *CNS Spectrums, 21*(4), 300–303. https://doi.org/10.1017/S1092852916000183.

Grant, J., Lust, K., & Chamberlain, S. (2019). Problematic smartphone use associated with greater alcohol consumption, mental health issues, poorer academic performance, and impulsivity. *Journal of Behavioral Addictions, 8*(2), 335–342. https://doi.org/10.1556/2006.8.2019.32.

Grant, J., Potenza, M., Weinstein, A., & Gorelick, D. (2010). Introduction to behavioral addictions. *The American Journal of Drug and Alcohol Abuse, 36*(5), 233–241. https://doi.org/10.3109/00952990.2010.491884.

Hausenblas, H. A., & Downs, D. S. (2002). Relationship among sex, imagery, and exercise dependence symptoms. *Psychology of Addiction Behavior, 16*(2), 169–172.

Kardefelt-Winther, D. (2014). A conceptual and methodological critique of internet addiction research: Towards a model of compensatory internet use. *Computers in Human Behavior, 31*, 351–354. https://doi.org/10.1016/j.chb.2013.10.059.

Karila, L., Wery, A., Weinstein, A., Cottencin, O., Petit, A., Reynaud, M., & Billieux, J. (2014). Sexual addiction or hypersexual disorder: Different terms for the same problem? A review of the literature. *Current Pharmaceutical Design, 20*(25), 4012–4020. https://doi.org/10.2174/13816128113199990619.

Koran, L., & Aboujaoude, E. (2014). Treating compulsive buying disorder. *Current Treatment Options in Psychiatry, 1*(4), 315–324. https://doi.org/10.1007/s40501-014-0024-3.

Kraus, S., Voon, V., & Potenza, M. (2016). Should compulsive sexual behavior be considered an addiction? *Addiction, 111*(12), 2097–2106. https://doi.org/10.1111/add.13297.

Kühn, S., & Gallinat, J. (2016). Neurobiological basis of hypersexuality. *International Review of Neurobiology, 129*, 67–83. https://doi.org/10.1016/bs.irn.2016.04.002.

Lopes, F. M., Dias, N. M., Mendonça, B. T., Coelho, D. M. V., Andrade, A. L. M., & Micheli, D. D. (2020). What do we know about neurosciences?: Concepts and misunderstandings between the general public and between educators. Revista Psicopedagogia, *37*(113), 129–143. http://dx.doi.org/10.5935/0103-8486.20200011

Männikkö, N., Billieux, J., & Kääriäinen, M. (2015). Problematic digital gaming behavior and its relation to the psychological, social and physical health of Finnish adolescents and young adults. *Journal of Behavioral Addictions, 4*(4), 281–288. https://doi.org/10.1556/2006.4.2015.040.

Maraz, A., Griffiths, M. D., & Demetrovics, Z. (2016). The prevalence of compulsive buying: A meta-analysis. *Addiction, 111*(3), 408–419. https://doi.org/10.1111/add.13223.

Maraz, A., van den Brink, W., & Demetrovics, Z. (2015). Prevalence and construct validity of compulsive buying disorder in shopping mall visitors. *Psychiatry Research, 228*(3), 918–924. https://doi.org/10.1016/j.psychres.2015.04.012.

Marques, A., Peralta, M., Sarmento, H., Loureiro, V., Gouveia, É. R., & de Matos, M. G. (2019). Prevalence of risk for exercise dependence: A systematic review. *Sports Medicine, 49*(2), 319–330. https://doi.org/10.1007/s40279-018-1011-4.

Mattos, C., Kim, H., Requião, M., Marasaldi, R., Filomensky, T., Hodgins, D., & Tavares, H. (2016). Gender differences in compulsive buying disorder: Assessment of demographic and psychiatric comorbidities. *PLoS One, 11*(12), e0167365. https://doi.org/10.1371/journal.pone.0167365.

Messina, B., Fuentes, D., Scanavino, M. T., & Parsons, J. T. (2014). Neuropsicologia da dependência de sexo e outras dependências não químicas. In D. Fuentes, L. Malloy-Diniz, C. Camargo, & R. Cosenza (Eds.), *Neuropsicologia: teoria e prática* (2nd ed., pp. 249–255). Porto Alegre, Brazil: Artmed.

Müller, A., Mitchell, J., & de Zwaan, M. (2015). Compulsive buying. *The American Journal on Addictions, 24*(2), 132–137. https://doi.org/10.1111/ajad.12111.

Müller, A., Reinecker, H., Jacobi, C., Reisch, L., & de Zwaan, M. (2005). Pathologisches kaufen: Eine literaturübersicht. *Psychiatrische Praxis, 32*(1), 3–12. https://doi.org/10.1055/s-2003-814965.

Nicolai, J., Darancó, S., & Moshagen, M. (2016). Effects of mood state on impulsivity in pathological buying. *Psychiatry Research, 244*, 351–356. https://doi.org/10.1016/j.psychres.2016.08.009.

Oliveira, B. P., Andrade, A. L. M., & De Micheli, D. (2016). Relação entre os níveis de atividade física e qualidade de vida no uso de drogas em adolescentes. *SMAD. Revista Eletrônica Saúde Mental Álcool e Drogas, 12*(3), 178–187. https://doi.org/10.11606/issn.1806-6976.v12i3p178-187.

Oliveira, T., Barreto, L., El-Aouar, W., Souza, L., & Pinheiro, L. (2017). Cadê meu celular? Uma análise da nomofobia no ambiente organizacional. *Revista De Administração De Empresas, 57*(6), 634–635. https://doi.org/10.1590/s0034-759020170611.

Oliveira Pinheiro, B., Monezi Andrade, A. L., Lopes, F. M., Reichert, R. A., de Oliveira, W. A., da Silva, A. M. B., & De Micheli, D. (2020). Association between quality of life and risk behaviors in Brazilian adolescents: An exploratory study. *Journal of Health Psychology*, in press. https://doi.org/10.1177%2F1359105320953472.

Park, B., Han, D., & Roh, S. (2016). Neurobiological findings related to internet use disorders. *Psychiatry and Clinical Neurosciences, 71*(7), 467–478. https://doi.org/10.1111/pcn.12422.

Petri, N. M. (2016). *Behavioral addictions: DSM-5 and beyond.* Oxford, UK: Oxford University Press. https://doi.org/10.1093/med/9780199391547.001.0001.

Pluhar, E., Kavanaugh, J., Levinson, J., & Rich, M. (2019). Problematic interactive media use in teens: Comorbidities, assessment, and treatment. *Psychology Research and Behavior Management, 12*, 447–455. https://doi.org/10.2147/PRBM.S208968.

Roberts, J., Yaya, L., & Manolis, C. (2014). The invisible addiction: Cell-phone activities and addiction among male and female college students. *Journal of Behavioral Addictions, 3*(4), 254–265. https://doi.org/10.1556/JBA.3.2014.015.

Silveira, D., Vieira, A., Palomo, V., & Silveira, E. (2000). Validade de critério e confiabilidade da versão brasileira de uma escala de rastreamento para dependência de sexo. *Revista Brasileira de Psiquiatria, 22*(1), 04–10. https://doi.org/10.1590/S1516-44462000000100003.

Skinner, E. A., & Zimmer-Gembeck, M. J. (2016). *The development of coping: Stress, neurophysiology, social relationships, and resilience during childhood and adolescence*. Cham, Switzerland: Springer. https://doi.org/10.1007/978-3-319-41740-0.

Stein, D., Hugo, F., Oosthuizen, P., Hawkridge, S., & van Heerden, B. (2000). Neuropsychiatry of hypersexuality. *CNS Spectrums, 5*(1), 36–46. https://doi.org/10.1017/s1092852900012657.

Tavares, H., Lobo, D., Fuentes, D., & Black, D. (2008). Compras compulsivas: uma revisão e um relato de caso. *Revista Brasileira de Psiquiatria, 30*(suppl 1), S16–S23. https://doi.org/10.1590/S1516-44462008005000002.

Tereshchenko, S., & Kasparov, E. (2019). Neurobiological risk factors for the development of internet addiction in adolescents. *Behavioral Sciences, 9*(6), 62. https://doi.org/10.3390/bs9060062.

Trotzke, P., Starcke, K., Pedersen, A., & Brand, M. (2014). Cue-induced craving in pathological buying. *Psychosomatic Medicine, 76*(9), 694–700. https://doi.org/10.1097/psy.0000000000000126.

Villella, C., Martinotti, G., Di Nicola, M., Cassano, M., La Torre, G., Gliubizzi, M. D., Messeri, I., Petruccelli, F., Bria, P., Janiri, L., & Conte, G. (2011). Behavioural addictions in adolescents and young adults: Results from a prevalence study. *Journal of Gambling Studies, 27*(2), 203–214. https://doi.org/10.1007/s10899-010-9206-0.

Wartberg, L., Kriston, L., & Thomasius, R. (2017). The prevalence and psychosocial correlates of internet gaming disorder. *Deutsches Aerzteblatt Online., 114*(25), 419–424. https://doi.org/10.3238/arztebl.2017.0419.

Weinstein, A., & Weinstein, Y. (2014). Exercise addiction-diagnosis, bio-psychological mechanisms and treatment issues. *Current Pharmaceutical Design, 20*(25), 4062–4069. https://doi.org/10.2174/13816128113199990614.

Wéry, A., & Billieux, J. (2017). Problematic cybersex: Conceptualization, assessment, and treatment. *Addictive Behaviors, 64*, 238–246. https://doi.org/10.1016/j.addbeh.2015.11.007.

World Health Organization. (2010). *Global recommendations on physical activity for health.* Retrieved from https://apps.who.int/iris/bitstream/handle/10665/44399/9789241599979_eng.pdf;jsessionid=3DCE1A5AD3B61137A30F017185494668?sequence=1

Yamauchi, L. M., Andrade, A. L. M., Pinheiro, B. O., Enumo, S. R. F., & De Micheli, D. (2019). Evaluation of the social representation of the use of alcoholic beverages by adolescents. *Estudos de Psicologia (Campinas), e180098*, 36. https://doi.org/10.1590/1982-0275201936e180098.

Zadka, Ł., & Olajossy, M. (2016). Compulsive buying in outline. *Psychiatria Polska, 50*(1), 153–164. https://doi.org/10.12740/PP/44010.

Zajac, K., Ginley, M., Chang, R., & Petry, N. (2017). Treatments for internet gaming disorder and internet addiction: A systematic review. *Psychology of Addictive Behaviors, 31*(8), 979–994. https://doi.org/10.1037/adb0000315.

Chapter 33
The Biopsychosocial Impact of Abusive Use of Digital Media

Gabriella Di Girolamo Martins, Veronica Vidotto Caricati, Beatriz Cortese Barbugli, Caroline Matilde da Silva Ribeiro, Fernanda Beatriz Hodar Lobato, Adriana Scatena, Renata Thurler Lessa, Denise De Micheli, and André Luiz Monezi Andrade

Introduction

Sociologist Zygmunt Bauman refers to society as a liquid, which is related in many social fields, which used to happen only in small groups. Nowadays, with technological advances such as the Internet and other digital media, these small groups have become part of a large network that does not have physical and visual contact, but rather requests for friendship or break-ups (block/exclude), thus giving rise to relationships that are rare in solid integration, considered a protective factor for healthy development (Bauman 2007; Kuss et al. 2018).

Currently, there are about 4.4 billion Internet users in the world, with China in first place with 721.4 million users, followed by India with 462.1; the USA 286.9; and Brazil in fourth place with 139.1 million users. However, among these countries, Brazil is second concerning the insertion of the Internet, reaching 66.4% of the population; the USA at 88.5%; China reaches 52.2%; and India 34.8%. Therefore, it is noted that, although Brazil is in fourth place in the ranking of Internet users, there is a greater perpetuation in the population about China and India (Internet World Stats 2020).

In Brazil, a survey conducted in households by the Regional Center for Studies for the Development of the Information Society (2018; Young and Abreu 2019) on digital cognition revealed that about 126.9 million Brazilian individuals currently use the Internet, mainly through the *smartphone*. Furthermore, the data show that, for the first time in 7 years, half of the rural area and the populations of layers D and E are connected, thus reaffirming its dissemination. Besides, another study reported

G. D. G. Martins · V. V. Caricati · B. C. Barbugli · C. M. da Silva Ribeiro · F. B. H. Lobato · R. T. Lessa · A. L. M. Andrade (✉)
Pontifícia Universidadre Católica de Campinas, Campinas, SP, Brazil

A. Scatena · D. De Micheli
Universidade Federal de São Paulo, São Paulo, SP, Brazil

D. De Micheli et al. (eds.), *Drugs and Human Behavior*,
https://doi.org/10.1007/978-3-030-62855-0_33

that socioeconomic classes C, D, and E had the highest growth rate in *smartphone* use since 2004 (Forsman and Nordmyr 2015), thus being a form of connection that had an infiltration rate of over 100%. With its multiple applications, this device has innovated the new digital era, proving to be effective nanotechnology at the very heart of the fourth industrial revolution (Andrade et al. 2020a, b, c).

A study developed by Spanish researchers indicated that among the 874 adolescents evaluated, 90.7% prefer the *smartphone* to connect to the Internet because of its ease, accessibility, and portability (Ruiz-Palmero et al. 2016; Sánchez-Carbonell et al. 2008). These data indicate how the new interactions are grounded in interactivity, developed through the interests of mass communication. The significant beneficiary ends up being, therefore, who develops such virtual strategies taking the public to a limited regime that can trigger a dependence on it, making people also hostages of the commercialization of *smartphones*.

The implications of digital development in the twenty-first century reveal that all individuals are or will soon be in constant interaction with the Internet. Thus, one can understand *smartphone* as the phenomenon that has accelerated and modified the way individuals relate socially, once interactions have become mobile and portable. It is also worth mentioning that even with a minimum distance (room and bedroom, for example), this resource is already used as a means of communication.

In this scenario, it has been widely discussed about the advantages and disadvantages that the Internet offers to the population in general, reaching all social environments (Andrade et al. 2020d, 2021). The communication network until the 1950s, created and used exclusively for military purposes, over the years has spread rapidly, becoming a digital medium (Internet) for public use (Goethals et al. 2000). It has spread in such a way that today it is understood in a global dimension on which scholars share positive and negative points of view about its use. However, research has already confirmed that the excessive use of it can cause physical and psychic comorbidities to the individual who uses it and is therefore already considered a serious public health problem in several countries (Cerniglia et al. 2017; Kuss et al. 2018).

At this juncture, some scholars discuss the care needed to navigate digital media, as revealed by Vadher et al. (2019). In their study, 16.3% of the sample presented problematic use of the Internet and 3% of IA. Participants with problematic use were more likely to have worse quality of sleep and worse quality of life, thus the Internet, despite being somewhat beneficial on the one hand, its excessive use can lead to physical and psychic pathologies both for the individual who uses it and for those who live with it.

Based on this, the EU KIDS online project conducted a study with more than 25 European countries, and in turn, identified that adolescents between 11 and 16 years old are prone to addiction, a phase in which young people achieve greater independence about their online behaviors, which can be understood as a risk factor for Internet addiction, given that this age group is more vulnerable (Kuss et al. 2018). Among the adolescents who participated in the study, 12% reported that they do not succeed in trying to reduce Internet use time; 13% agreed that they spend less time than should with family/friends; 16% said "surf" when they are not interested in something; and finally, 5% reported not eating or sleeping due to Internet use (United Nations Children's Fund, Office of Research - Innocenti, London School of Economics and Political Science 2016).

These data demonstrate that the Internet is impacting the daily lives of adolescents both socially and psychologically, making it necessary to understand better the excessive and alienated use of the multiple languages of the Internet (Dimitrakopoulou 2013). Remembering that this has already happened in another *zeitgeist* (*spirit of the time*), in the revolution of 1930, as evidenced in the film "Modern Times." Charles Chaplin acts, in all cinematic screens, evidencing the abuse of human repetitive movements, where Taylorism and Fordism reinforce the idea of alienation. This context raises the question of the importance of identifying problems related to the excessive use of digital media, of formulating effective strategies for prevention and treatment, and of the participation of parents in this process of intelligent and healthy use of technology.

Features and Criteria of Internet Dependency Diagnostics

The Diagnostic and Statistical Manual of Mental Disorders ([DSM-V], American Psychiatric Association 2013) has not yet included in its specifications the Internet dependency disorder due to some limitations, such as cultural differences, age groups, and methodological designs of the research. However, it has already included in its appendix—determined to designate future studies for diseases—gambling addiction. The International Statistical Classification of Diseases and Health-Related Problems ([ICD-11], World Health Organization 2019) already includes *gaming disorder* in its manual and has included Internet Gaming Disorder in its appendices as a condition for further study. Although there are no standardized protocols so far, some authors have already entered a consensus on features to assist in this process:

- Excessive concern about the Internet.
- We need to increase the time connected (online) to have the same satisfaction.
- Display repeated efforts to decrease Internet usage time.
- Display irritability and depression.
- When the use of the Internet is restricted, it presents emotional ability (the Internet as a form of emotional regulation).
- Stay more connected (online) than scheduled.
- They are lying to others about the number of hours connected.

In order to be considered a dependency, the individual must meet at least five of these seven criteria. These criteria can be found on the website *Internet Addiction and New Technologies* and were developed from professionals (psychologists, psychiatrists) who have obtained a high demand from individuals with such dependency. Furthermore, these criteria were developed based on outpatient and office experience (Young and Abreu 2019).

Some researchers discuss its etiology based on the "*Reward Deficiency Syndrome," that* is, understanding that there is a shortage of serotonergic and dopaminergic receptors that leads to a higher rate of synaptic catabolism by dopamine. Thus, these individuals with less satisfaction seek for greater stimulation of the brain "reward center" (Blum et al. 2008; Winkler et al. 2013). These findings corroborate Brand et al. (2014) research, which demonstrates, through neuroimaging techniques in individuals with Internet dependence, neurofunctional changes in regions such as the prefrontal cortex, suggesting the influence of neurobiological factors.

Regarding the epidemiology of IA there are studies in the literature showing that its prevalence ranges from 5% to almost 38% (Wartberg et al. 2016; Cruz et al. 2018; Yang et al. 2018). The data also reveal a significant variation within the same country, for example, in China, ranging from 13.7% to 37.2% (Guo et al. 2018; Yang et al. 2018). Such variations demonstrate the difficulty of measuring such a construct and refer to the importance of new studies in the area, with a robust methodological structure.

Other studies also support the association between IA and substance abuse due to common symptoms such as compulsivity, abstinence, tolerance, and some functional limitations (Petry et al. 2014). This theory is in line with research by Wartberg et al. (2016) and Morioka et al. (2017) that revealed in their studies an association between alcohol and excessive use of the Internet due to brain activation stimulated by both IA and substance use. This activation occurs in the so-called reward system or local brake, responsible for the regulation of emotions and compulsive behavior (Andrade and De Micheli 2016; De Micheli et al. 2016; Giedd 2016; Greenberg and Paivio 2003).

Association Between Internet Addiction and Comorbidities

Some exploratory studies already bring essential data on the excessive use of Internet associated with depression, anxiety, and sleep disorder, with prevalence in the age group of young adults, age group of greater vulnerability due to the maturation process (Vadher et al. 2019; Andrade et al. 2018; Malak and Khalifeh 2018; Machado et al. 2018; Yang et al. 2018; Wu et al. 2016).

A study developed in China by Li et al. (2017) identified the prevalence of 8.1% of IA in a sample of 1015 participants. Also, the data indicated an association between Internet usage time and symptoms of anxiety and depression. Insomnia was associated with 60.6% of Internet use and 44.8% of depressed people, corroborating the study by Karacic and Oreskovic (2017) conducted in Germany ($N = 667$). In this study, the authors identified a negative correlation between Internet use time and quality of life and mental health aspects, besides the fact that 39% of their sample had Internet dependence.

Intervention and Treatment for Internet Addiction

In a meta-analysis developed by Winkler et al. (2013) on treatment for IA, it was concluded that the primary forms of intervention are: counseling programs, cognitive-behavioral therapy (CBT) and drug intervention, with a *follow-up* range of 1.5–6 months, and among the 16 articles included, six were done in groups. In this work, no concomitant intervention between psychopharmacology and psychotherapy was inserted, but more recent studies report that the integration between treatments can be cumulative and provide a greater reduction of symptoms for psychiatric conditions (Zhu et al. 2009).

From the perspective of these researchers, it is concluded that among those participants who received some type of intervention, there was no significant difference between psychopharmaceuticals and psychotherapy. Both were positive in reducing IA symptoms, time spent online, anxiety, and depression. It must be taken into account that this study was developed throughout the process with few articles, none of which was concomitant in the treatments, with only five randomized clinical trials and 11 that did not have a control group.

Table 33.1 shows some interventions used in the number of sessions and the main results obtained by them. The *follow-up/follow-up* time of the interventions was quite diversified, ranging from 30 days to 6 months. Regarding the type of instrument to evaluate the interventions, the *Internet Addiction Test* (IAT), translated and validated in Brazil in 2012, was more used to assess the standard of Internet use. Nevertheless, all studies pointed out as inclusion criteria that had some degree of IA (Conti et al. 2012).

In general, the results indicated that the main treatments for IA were: psychoeducational program, cognitive-behavioral therapy, psychological intervention, family intervention, and electroacupuncture. The preference for cognitive-behavioral therapy is noted, although there are other interventions (Kim et al. 2018; Young 2013). Also, these treatments to treat individuals with DI are still in progress, since this disorder is still being studied and discussed within the scientific literature and therefore is not included in the current version of DSM-5.

Some studies use electroacupuncture and psychological intervention as a treatment for IA from scientific bases. Research demonstrates the existence of a neuropsychological basis in which the abusive use of substances inhibits the cascade of brain reward, which are complex reactions involving various neurotransmitters and structures in the limbic system. In this sense, activation of the mesolimbic dopaminergic pathway occurs, which begins in the ventral tegmental area and ends in the dopamine D2 receptors in the cell membranes of neurons located in the *accumbens* nucleus and the hippocampus, producing a sensation of pleasure and well-being.

The main neurochemical pathways involved in this process are: serotonergic (5-HT), encephalinergic (Enk), GABAergic (GABA), and dopaminergic (DA). When there is a deficit or blockage in this system, the individual often uses substances (alcohol, cigarettes) and develops compulsive behaviors that lead to the practice of activities that put his life at risk. In this sense, electroacupuncture is used to alter the inhibition function and relieve the comorbidities associated with addiction (Andrade and De Micheli 2017). Neuropsychological literature shows that,

Table 33.1 Main interventions for users with Internet dependence

Author	Symptoms	N	Follow-up	Method	Results
Ke and Wong (2018)	Internet addiction	Students (13–18 years)	1 month	Eight sessions (psychological intervention program—Internet use for youths—PIP-IU-Y)	Reduced-intensity of symptoms after the sessions. The effect was maintained during the follow-up
Kim (2018)	Internet addiction	17 teenagers (12–17 years old)	1 month	8 CBT sessions	Cognitive-behavioral therapy (CBT) was useful for adolescents with problematic Internet use, depression, and anxiety. Effect maintained in follow-up
Tas and Ayas (2018)	Internet addiction	24 adolescents	45 days	RCT with two arms consisting of 10 sessions. Group: psychoeducational program and control	The psychoeducational program has been effective in reducing psychological symptoms and Internet addiction. The effect remained during the follow-up
Yang (2017)	Internet addiction	48 participants (18–30 years)	45 days	RCT with three arms. Group: electroacupuncture, psychological intervention, the control group	Both interventions, psychological and electroacupuncture, had a positive effect in particular on psychological experiences and behavioral expressions, impulsivity control, and protection of brain neurons
Young (2013)	Internet addiction	128 participants (no age)	1–3–6 months	12 CBT sessions	Reduced-intensity of the symptoms after the sessions, with 95% of the sample being able to control the crack after the intervention. After 6 months, 78% still maintained their anxiety and stress levels lower than baseline levels

RCT randomized clinical trial; *CBT* cognitive-behavioral therapy besides demonstrating positive results, the integration of both interventions can substantially improve the outcomes of IA (Andrade et al. 2014; Winkler et al. 2013; Blum et al. 2008; Malhotra et al. 2007).

The preference for CBT comes from positive results related to other dependencies. This approach works on understanding feelings and thoughts concerning problem behavior as well as helping the patient to chart strategies for possible relapses (Rangé and Marlatt 2008). Thus, the therapy will work from the identification of problem behavior through maladaptive cognitions, negative beliefs, and distortions that contribute to the pathological use of digital media (Young 2007). It is important to emphasize that the effectiveness of the treatment is closely related to the patient's engagement with the psychotherapeutic process (Lindenberg et al. 2017).

Final Considerations

The use of the Internet and its technologies in the daily life of individuals are becoming more and more indispensable and do not necessarily have a pathological component since they are often used as a coping strategy against stressful events (Gonçalves et al. 2021). However, some authors have concluded that using the Internet for communication and moving away from real life entails a poor adaptation (Kraut et al. 1998; Kardefelt-Winther 2014). Therefore, it is necessary to evaluate the context in which the individual is inserted, the damage and the intensity that comes from its intense use (De Micheli 2020). Despite the increasing amount of scientific work, there is still a lack of consensus among researchers and a deficit in instruments for assessing the dependence on digital media. As a result, treatments are restricted to those familiar and associated with addictions, where there is a positive outcome in treatment, such as CBT for substance use disorders.

In contemporary times, studies reveal that the predominant use of the Internet is through the smartphone. Therefore, research is suggested regarding the relationship of the individual with this electronic device. It is up to the researchers to elaborate on an implementation protocol specialized in this area, allied to the public sphere, mainly in the health areas. The application of worldwide campaigns that have Internet users as their audience can also contribute to a greater awareness of the subject among the population. In short, it is necessary to have a clinical look so that something is done to find common aspects among the symptoms of these individuals who suffer from such disorder in order to develop strategies and protocols of treatment and prevention based on scientific evidence.

References

American Psychiatric Association. (2013). *Diagnostic and statistical manual of mental disorders, fifth edition*. Arlington, TX: Author.

Andrade, A. L. M., Bedendo, A., Enumo, S. R. F., & Micheli, D. (2018). Brain development in adolescence: General aspects and update. *Adolescência e Saude, 15*(Supl. 1), 62–67.

Andrade, A. L. M., & De Micheli, D. (2017). *Inovações no Tratamento de Dependência de Drogas* (1st ed.). Rio de Janeiro: Atheneu.

Andrade, A. L. M., & De Micheli, D. (2016). *Innovations in the treatment of substance addiction* (1st ed.). New York: Springer. https://doi.org/10.1007/978-3-319-43172-7.

Andrade, A. L. M., De Micheli, D., & Fisberg, M. (2014). Cognitive aspects of fetal alcohol syndrome in Young adults: Two case studies. *Interação em Psicologia, 17*(2), 217–223.

Andrade, A. L. M., Enumo, S. R. F., Passos, M. A. Z., Vellozo, E. P., Shoen, T. H., Kulik, M. A., Niskier, S. R., et al. (2021). Problematic Internet Use, Emotional Problems and Quality of Life Among Adolescents. *Psico-USF, 26*(1), 41-51. http://dx.doi.org/10.1590/1413-82712021260104.

Andrade, A. L. M., Kim, D. J., Caricati, V. V., Martins, G. D. G., Kirihara, I. K., Barbugli, B. C., et al. (2020a). Validity and reliability of the Brazilian version of the smartphone addiction scale-short version for university students and adult population. *Estudos de Psicologia, 37*, e190117. https://doi.org/10.1590/1982-0275202037e190117.

Andrade, A. L. M., Kim, D. J., Scatena, A., Enes, C. C., Enumo, S. R. F., & De Micheli, D. (2020d). Validity and Reliability of the Brazilian Version of the Smartphone Addiction Scale-Long Version (SAS-LV). *Trends in Psychology*, in press. https://doi.org/10.1007/s43076-020-00046-y.

Andrade, A. L. M., Scatena, A., Bedendo, A., Enumo, S. R. F., Dellazzana-Zanon, L. L., Prebianchi, H. B., et al. (2020b). Findings on the relationship between internet addiction and psychological symptoms in Brazilian adults. *International Journal of Psychology, 55*(6), 941–950. https://doi.org/10.1002/ijop.12670.

Andrade, A. L. M., Scatena, A., Martins, G. D. G., De Oliveira Pinheiro, B., Da Silva, A. B., Enes, C. C., et al. (2020c). Validation of smartphone addiction scale-short version (SAS-SV) in Brazilian adolescents. *Addictive Behaviors, 110*, 106540. https://doi.org/10.1016/j.addbeh.2020.106540.

Bauman, Z. (2007). *Vida líquida*. Rio de Janeiro, Brazil: Jorge Zahar.

Blum, K., Chen, A. L., Chen, T. J., Braverman, E. R., Reinking, J., Blum, S. H., et al. (2008). Activation instead of blocking mesolimbic dopaminergic reward circuitry is a preferred modality in the long-term treatment of reward deficiency syndrome (RDS): A commentary. *Theoretical Biology and Medical Modelling, 5*, 24. https://doi.org/10.1186/1742-4682-5-24.

Brand, M., Young, K. S., & Laier, C. (2014). Prefrontal control and internet addiction: A theoretical model and review of neuropsychological and neuroimaging findings. *Frontiers in Human Neuroscience, 8*, 375. https://doi.org/10.3389/fnhum.2014.00375.

Cerniglia, L., Zoratto, F., Cimino, S., Laviola, G., Ammaniti, M., & Adriani, W. (2017). Internet addiction in adolescence: Neurobiological, psychosocial and clinical issues. *Neuroscience & Biobehavioral Reviews, 76*, 174–184. https://doi.org/10.1016/j.neubiorev.2016.12.024.

Conti, M. A., Jardim, A. P., Hearst, N., Cordás, T. A., Tavares, H., & Abreu, C. N. (2012). Avaliação da equivalência semântica e consistência interna de uma versão em português do Internet Addiction Test (IAT). *Archives of Clinical Psychiatry, 39*(3), 106–110. https://doi.org/10.1590/S0101-60832012000300007.

Cruz, F. A. D., Scatena, A., Andrade, A. L. M., & De Micheli, D. (2018). Evaluation of internet addiction and the quality of life of Brazilian adolescents from public and private schools. *Estudos de Psicologia, 35*(2), 193–204. https://doi.org/10.1590/1982-02752018000200008.

De Micheli, D., Andrade, A. L. M., Silva, E. A., & Souza-Formigoni, M. L. O. (2016). *Drug abuse in adolescence* (1st ed.). New York: Springer. https://doi.org/10.1007/978-3-319-17795-3.

De Micheli, D., Andrade, A., & Galduróz, J. C. (2020). Limitations of DSM-5 diagnostic criteria for substance use disorder in adolescents: what have we learned after using these criteria for several years? Brazilian Journal of Psychiatry, in press. https://doi.org/10.1590/1516-4446-2020-1151.

Dimitrakopoulou, V. (2013). European public health policies and interventions for detecting and deterring internet addictive behaviors in adolescents. *International Journal of Child and Adolescent Health, 6*(4), 455. https://doi.org/10.1556/2006.5.2016.085.

Forsman, A. K., & Nordmyr, J. (2015). Psychosocial links between internet use and mental health in later life: A systematic review of quantitative and qualitative evidence. *Journal of Applied Gerontology, 36*(12), 1471–1518. https://doi.org/10.1177/0733464815595509.

Giedd, J. N. (2016). The amazing teen brain. *Scientific American, 312*(6), 32–37.
Goethals, K., Aguiar, A., & Almeida, E. (2000). *História da Internet* (Master's thesis, Universidade do Porto, Porto, Portugal). Retrieved from https://paginas.fe.up.pt/~mgi97018/historia.html
Gonçalves, M. F., Bedendo, A., Andrade, A. L. M., & Noto, A. R. (2021). Factors associated with adherence to a web-based alcohol intervention among college students. *Estudos de Psicologia (Campinas), 38*, e190134. https://doi.org/10.1590/1982-0275202138e190134.
Greenberg, L. S., & Paivio, S. C. (2003). *Working with emotions in psychotherapy (vol. 3, The Practicing Professional)*. New York: The Guilford Press.
Guo, L., Luo, M., Wang, W. X., Huang, G. L., Xu, Y., Gao, X., et al. (2018). Association between problematic internet use, sleep disturbance, and suicidal behavior in Chinese adolescents. *Journal of Behavioral Addictions, 7*(4), 965–975. https://doi.org/10.1556/2006.7.2018.115.
Internet World Stats. (2020). *Internet users in the world by regions*. Retrieved from https://www.internetworldstats.com/stats.htm
Karacic, S., & Oreskovic, S. (2017). Internet addiction and mental health status of adolescents in Croatia and Germany. *Psychiatria Danubina, 29*(3), 313–321.
Kardefelt-Winther, D. (2014). A conceptual and methodological critique of internet addiction research: Towards a model of compensatory internet use. *Computers in Human Behavior, 31*, 351–354. https://doi.org/10.1016/j.chb.2013.10.059.
Ke, G. N., & Wong, S. F. (2018). Outcome of the psychological intervention program: Internet use for youth. *Journal of Rational-Emotive and Cognitive-Behavior Therapy, 36*(2), 187–200. https://doi.org/10.1007/s10942-017-0281-3.
Kim, S. H., Yim, H. W., Jo, S. J., Jung, K. I., Lee, K., & Park, M. H. (2018). The effects of group cognitive behavioral therapy on the improvement of depression and anxiety in adolescents with problematic internet use. *Journal of the Korean Academy of Child and Adolescent Psychiatry, 29*(2), 73–79. https://doi.org/10.5765/jkacap.2018.29.2.73.
Kraut, R., Patterson, M., Lundmark, V., Kiesler, S., Mukophadhyay, T., & Scherlis, W. (1998). Internet paradox: A social technology that reduces social involvement and psychological Well-being? *American Psychologist, 53*(9), 1017–1031. https://doi.org/10.1037/0003-066X.53.9.1017.
Kuss, D. J., Kanjo, E., Crook-Rumsey, M., Kibowski, F., Wang, G. Y., & Sumich, A. (2018). Problematic mobile phone use and smartphone addiction across generations: The roles of psychopathological symptoms and smartphone use. *Journal of Technology in Behavioral Science, 3*, 141–149. https://doi.org/10.1007/s41347-017-0041-3.
Li, J. B., Lau, J. T., Mo, P. K., Su, X. F., Tang, J., Qin, Z. G., & Gross, D. L. (2017). Insomnia partially mediated the association between problematic internet use and depression among secondary school students in China. *Journal of Behavioral Addictions, 6*(4), 554–563. https://doi.org/10.1556/2006.6.2017.085.
Lindenberg, K., Szasz-Janocha, C., Schoenmaekers, S., Wehrmann, U., & Vonderlin, E. (2017). An analysis of integrated health care for internet use disorders in adolescents and adults. *Journal of Behavioral Addictions, 6*(4), 579–592. https://doi.org/10.1556/2006.6.2017.065.
Machado, M. D. R., Bruck, I., Antoniuk, S. A., Cat, M. N. L., Soares, M. C., & Silva, A. F. D. (2018). Internet addiction and its correlation with behavioral problems and functional impairments: A cross-sectional study. *Jornal Brasileiro de Psiquiatria, 67*(1), 34–38. https://doi.org/10.1590/0047-2085000000181.
Malak, M. Z., & Khalifeh, A. H. (2018). Anxiety and depression among school students in Jordan: Prevalence, risk factors, and predictors. *Perspectives in Psychiatric Care, 54*(2), 242–250. https://doi.org/10.1111/ppc.12229.
Malhotra, A. K., Lencz, T., Correll, C. U., & Kane, J. M. (2007). Genomics and the future of pharmacotherapy in psychiatry. *International Review of Psychiatry, 19*(5), 523–530. https://doi.org/10.1080/09540260701563460.
Morioka, H., Itani, O., Osaki, Y., Higuchi, S., Jike, M., Kaneita, Y., et al. (2017). The association between alcohol use and problematic internet use: A large-scale nationwide cross-sectional study of adolescents in Japan. *Journal of Epidemiology, 27*(3), 107–111. https://doi.org/10.1016/j.je.2016.10.004.

Petry, N. M., Rehbein, F., Gentile, D. A., Lemmens, J. S., Rumpf, H. J., Mößle, T., et al. (2014). An international consensus for assessing internet gaming disorder using the new DSM-5 approach. *Addiction, 109*(9), 1399–1406.

Rangé, B. P., & Marlatt, G. A. (2008). Terapia cognitivo-comportamental de transtornos de abuso de álcool e drogas. *Brazilian Journal of Psychiatry, 30*(Suppl. 2), s88–s95. https://doi.org/10.1590/S1516-44462008000600006.

Ruiz-Palmero, J., Sánchez-Rodríguez, J., & Trujillo-Torres, J. M. (2016). Utilización de Internet y dependencia a teléfonos móviles en adolescentes. *Revista Latinoamericana de Ciencias Sociales, Niñez y Juventud, 14*(2), 1357–1369. https://doi.org/10.11600/1692715x.14232080715.

Sánchez-Carbonell, X., Beranuy, M., Castellana, M., Chamarro, A., & Oberst, U. (2008). La adicción a Internet y al móvil: ¿moda o trastorno? *Adicciones, 20*(2), 149–159.

Tas, I., & Ayas, T. (2018). Effects of psychoeducational program for reducing psychological symptoms on internet addiction among adolescents. *Education and Science, 43*(196), 257–279. https://doi.org/10.15390/EB.2018.7652.

United Nations Children's Fund, Office of Research–Innocenti, London School of Economics and Political Science. (2016). *Global kids online: Research synthesis, 2015–2016*. Retrieved from www.globalkidsonline.net/synthesis

Vadher, S. B., Panchal, B. N., Vala, A. U., Ratnani, I. J., Vasava, K. J., Desai, R. S., & Shah, A. H. (2019). Predictors of problematic internet use in school going adolescents of Bhavnagar, India. *International Journal of Social Psychiatry, 65*(2), 151–157. https://doi.org/10.1177/0020764019827985.

Wartberg, L., Brunner, R., Kriston, L., Durkee, T., Parzer, P., Fischer-Waldschmidt, G., et al. (2016). Psychopathological factors associated with problematic alcohol and problematic internet use in a sample of adolescents in Germany. *Psychiatry Research, 240*, 272–277. https://doi.org/10.1016/j.psychres.2016.04.057.

Winkler, A., Dörsing, B., Rief, W., Shen, Y., & Glombiewski, J. A. (2013). Treatment of internet addiction: A meta-analysis. *Clinical Psychology Review, 33*(2), 317–329. https://doi.org/10.1016/j.cpr.2012.12.005.

World Health Organization. (2019). *International statistical classification of diseases and related health problems, eleventh revision*. Retrieved from https://icd.who.int/browse11/l-m/en

Wu, A. M., Li, J., Lau, J. T., Mo, P. K., & Lau, M. M. (2016). Potential impact of internet addiction and protective psychosocial factors onto depression among Hong Kong Chinese adolescents–direct, mediation and moderation effects. *Comprehensive Psychiatry, 70*, 41–52. https://doi.org/10.1016/j.comppsych.2016.06.011.

Yang, J., Guo, Y., Du, X., Jiang, Y., Wang, W., Xiao, D., et al. (2018). Association between problematic internet use and sleep disturbance among adolescents: The role of the child's sex. *International Journal of Environmental Research and Public Health, 15*(12), 2682. https://doi.org/10.3390/ijerph15122682.

Yang, Y., Li, H., Chen, X. X., Zhang, L. M., Huang, B. J., & Zhu, T. M. (2017). Electroacupuncture treatment for internet addiction: Evidence of normalization of impulse control disorder in adolescents. *Chinese Journal of Integrative Medicine, 23*(11), 837–844. https://doi.org/10.1007/s11655-017-2765-5.

Young, K. S. (2007). Cognitive behavior therapy with internet addicts: Treatment outcomes and implications. *Cyberpsychology & Behavior, 10*(5), 671–679. https://doi.org/10.1089/cpb.2007.9971.

Young, K. S. (2013). Treatment outcomes using CBT-IA with internet-addicted patients. *Journal of Behavioral Addictions, 2*(4), 209–215. https://doi.org/10.1556/jba.2.2013.4.3.

Young, K. S., & Abreu, C. N. (2019). *Internet addiction in children and adolescents: Risk factors, assessment and treatment*. New York: Springer.

Zhu, T. M., Jin, R. J., & Zhong, X. M. (2009). Clinical effect of electroacupuncture combined with psychologic interference on patient with internet addiction disorder. *Chinese Journal of Integrated Traditional and Western Medicine, 29*(3), 212–214.

Chapter 34
History of Violence and Emotional Regulation as Risk Factors for Substance Use Disorders among Women

Jaluza Aimèe Schneider and Luisa Fernanda Habigzang

Introduction

Although the highest prevalence of drug use, in general, is among the male population, a significant increase in women with substance use disorders in recent decades has been identified worldwide (International Narcotics Control Board [INCB] 2017). It is noteworthy that the abuse of tranquilizers and opioids, without medical orientation, is already evidenced more frequently in the female population (United Nations Office on Drugs and Crime [UNODC] 2018). In Brazil, it was found that the consumption of alcohol by women increased significantly between 2006 and 2018, while the consumption of the same substance by men remained stable in this period (Vigitel Brazil 2018). Regarding the use of crack at the national level, which is a public health problem, it was estimated that around 21% of users were women (Bastos and Bertoni 2014). Given the current context of drug use by the female population, the need to discuss biopsychosocial characteristics, including their different vulnerabilities, with a view to specialized prevention and treatment care, based on scientific evidence, is highlighted (Butler et al. 2017; Moraes et al. 2018; UNODC 2016).

Among the main specificities of the female population, it is observed the consumption of drugs a lot with greater frequency and the tendency for them to have a greater negative clinical, physical, and psychic consequences, resulting from the use of the substance earlier (Guimarães et al. 2017; INCB 2017; Lejuez et al. 2007). In comparison with male users, the female population tends to have higher rates of sexual risk behaviors, higher probability of carrying Human Immunodeficiency Virus (HIV) and other Sexually Transmitted Infections (STIs) (Guimarães et al. 2017; Vernaglia et al. 2017; UNODC 2018). Women also have higher levels of

J. A. Schneider (✉) · L. F. Habigzang
Pontifícia Universidade Católica do Rio Grande do Sul,
Porto Alegre, Rio Grande do Sul, Brazil

D. De Micheli et al. (eds.), *Drugs and Human Behavior*,
https://doi.org/10.1007/978-3-030-62855-0_34

impulsivity and *craving* symptoms and trend to have lower adherence to treatment for substance use disorders (Balbinot et al. 2016; Lejuez et al. 2007; Maciel et al. 2017). Moreover, the stigma and social exclusion experienced by women are significantly greater than in the male population (Medeiros et al. 2018; Moraes et al. 2018; UNODC 2016; Vernaglia et al. 2017). This issue is related to the social judgments about the roles attributed to the female gender that are linked to greater prejudice and perception of drug use by women as an immoral behavior, generating in the users themselves, beliefs of self-accountability, and self-blame about their condition (Medeiros et al. 2017; Souza et al. 2014).

Among the main risk factors for the initiation and maintenance of drug use by women, traumatic experiences throughout life, such as having been the victim of different types of violence, are highlighted (Guimarães et al. 2017; Madruga et al. 2017; UNODC 2018). The history of violence and the trauma resulting from such experiences are associated with higher rates of emotional deregulation and impulsiveness, which further increases the vulnerability of this population to substance abuse (Weiss et al. 2013). In this perspective, substance use becomes a poorly adaptive strategy for the alleviation of negative emotions, using consumption as a coping to deal with emotional suffering (Westphal et al. 2017). In light of these aspects, this chapter aims to discuss the evidence on the history of violence and emotional deregulation as risk factors for the development and maintenance of substance use disorder in women.

Current Surveys

Traumatic experiences, resulting from violence situations, are widely discussed in the literature on substance use, with evidence of high rates of posttraumatic stress disorder (PTSD) as a consequence (Mandavia et al. 2016; Westphal et al. 2017). High rates of trauma are observed in drug users regardless of gender. However, research aimed at understanding the incidence and consequences of different types of violence among substance users has intensified, enabling the identification of specific characteristics of male and female drug users about their traumatic experiences.

Studies that aim to identify and understand the violence experienced by women who use substances highlight the high rate of child abuse and gender-based violence. Child maltreatment is described as actions that occur in a relationship of responsibility or power that can result in harm to the health, development, and dignity of the child and adolescent, including neglect and psychological, physical, and/or sexual abuse (World Health Organization [WHO] 2016). Violence against women, on the other hand, consists of any violent action based on gender inequality that may result in psychological, physical, sexual, or property damage to women (WHO 2013). In this perspective, a study conducted with 2120 Brazilian women demonstrated that witnessing violence in childhood, which is a form of psychological mistreatment, significantly increased the probability of cocaine use in adulthood

(Madruga et al. 2017). In the USA, a study of 20,089 women indicated that being a victim of gender-based violence increased the probability of developing a substance use disorder 2.5 to 3.6 times later (Walsh et al. 2015). Also in relation to gender-based violence, women who were victims after the age of 45 were 5 times more likely to have substance-related problems (Walsh et al. 2015).

On gender specificities related to the history of violence among drug users, it is observed, for example, the higher prevalence and the greater impact of sexual violence on substance use in the female population (Halpern et al. 2018; Sanvicente-Vieira et al. 2019; Vernaglia et al. 2017). According to the study by Sanvicente-Vieira et al. (2019), men who used crack had higher levels of child abuse related to physical abuse, while women had higher levels of emotional neglect and sexual abuse. A survey of crack users in six cities, in different regions of Brazil, identified the highest number of significant reports of history of sexual violence among women compared to men in the same study (Vernaglia et al. 2017). It should be noted that the results of a meta-analysis in the randomized effects model showed that, among men and women, histories of physical and sexual abuse increased the risk of having problems related to drug use by 74% and 73%, respectively (Halpern et al. 2018). However, the same study indicated that gender only had a moderating effect on sexual abuse, underscoring the greater vulnerability of the female population compared to the male victim of child sexual abuse in developing substance use disorder (Halpern et al. 2018).

The history of violence is also a risk factor for relapses after treatment for substance use disorder. More severe rates of emotional neglect have been related to increased risk of relapse in cocaine use after treatment among men and women (Hyman et al. 2008). It is noteworthy that only in the female population was the greater severity of the history of emotional abuse and sexual abuse in childhood related to cocaine use in greater quantity after treatment (Hyman et al. 2008). The increased risk may be related to the fact that users of substances with a history of trauma are more likely to engage in impulsive behaviors, indicating greater deficits in the regulation of emotions (Weiss et al. 2013; Wolff et al. 2016).

Emotional regulation skills are strategies, behavioral and cognitive, which assist in coping with intrusive, intense, and suffering emotions, (Gross 2002; Linehan 2018). The difficulty or inability to deal with intense and unpleasant emotional experiences can cause significant harm in different areas of an individual's life, and having skillful ways to regulate emotions becomes fundamental to their social functioning and well-being (Izard 2010; Mennin and Farach 2007). It is important to emphasize that the abilities to regulate emotions do not aim at emotional suppression, but at obtaining functional and adaptive behavioral strategies to deal with them according to the individual's life context (Izard 2010; Gross 2002). Among the main emotional regulation skills are clarity and emotional awareness, impulse control, and acceptance of emotions (Gross 2002).

Few strategies to regulate emotions can lead to an increase in impulsive behaviors that generate negative consequences, such as the use of substances themselves (Aldao et al. 2010; Axelrod et al. 2011). Corroborating this idea, research identified that college students with high levels of negative emotional experiences were more likely to use alcohol to manage their suffering (Veilleux et al. 2014). Cocaine use was also observed as a management of stress related to interpersonal conflicts (Waldrop et al. 2007). It is understood that the expectation that the substance will alleviate unpleasant emotions becomes an important predictor for the continued use of the drug, despite the negative consequences of its use. Similarly, the belief in relief from suffering favors not learning new functional coping strategies that are not harmful (Shadur and Lejuez 2015; Vujanovic et al. 2016; Westphal et al. 2017). In this sense, it has already been observed that users of different substances were not concerned with learning to deal with the memories and feelings related to trauma when compared to non-users of drugs (Clark et al. 2014). This issue was also addressed in an American study in which, among women, cocaine use was one of the main coping strategies used to deal with daily stressors, suggesting the absence of motivation to learn alternative and adaptive ways (Waldrop et al. 2007). Therefore, not having skills ways to deal with emotional suffering is considered an important risk factor for substance use (Dingle et al. 2018; Price et al. 2012).

Emotional regulation strategies have gender-related specificities that highlight the differences in vulnerabilities to substance use in the female population. A literature review indicated that women are more likely to believe that they will not be able to cope with their intense emotions, and more often seek impulsive and unadaptive handling to regulate their emotions, such as drug use and other harmful behaviors, such as excessive eating and self-mutilation (Nolen-Hoeksema 2012). The frequency of cocaine use among women has already been associated with a decrease in alternative behavioral and resolution responses to daily stressors among women (Waldrop et al. 2007). According to Giusti and Zilberman (2017), girls are more likely to start using the substance to alleviate unpleasant emotions or ease symptoms of psychiatric comorbidities, which is not so strongly observed among boys. In the same perspective, a study showed that women who used alcohol were more likely to drink as a response to their negative emotions than men, and also that the presence of comorbidity, such as depression or anxiety disorder, increased the probability of using alcohol to deal with the suffering symptoms of their psychopathologies (Karpyak et al. 2016).

Among individuals with trauma resulting from violence situations, evidence indicates that emotional deregulation is considered an indirect or mediating influence on substance consumption (Mandavia et al. 2016; Weiss et al. 2013). A study conducted with crack users observed that the presence of traumatic events during life significantly increased the difficulties in regulation their emotions and, consequently, increased the search for substance consumption (McDermott et al. 2009). Among women victims of violence, substance use was associated with PTSD symptoms only among those with emotional deregulation (Tull et al. 2015). The differences in emotional regulation skills between men and women who were victims of child abuse, with and without substance use problems, were assessed in a study conducted in Germany (Wolff et al. 2016). The results indicated greater emotional deregulation among those who used some substance, in addition to the positive correlation between the increased deficit of regulation of emotions and the severity of physical and emotional neglect and abuse (Wolff et al. 2016).

One of the main hypotheses in the specialized literature suggests that among individuals with a history of trauma the substance is used as a form of self-medication, thus considered a non-adaptive management to deal with their emotions (Clark et al. 2014; Dass-Brailsford and Safilian 2017; Westphal et al. 2017). According to this hypothesis, for individuals who do not have behavioral and cognitive skills abilities to deal with unpleasant emotions, the effect of the drug becomes an immediate resolution to diminish or avoid suffering and, consequently, a strong booster for maintaining consumption (Cafure 2016; Shadur and Lejuez 2015). There is evidence that individuals with substance use disorders and PTSD had higher levels of emotional deregulation in the specific dimensions of clarity and emotional acceptance, as well as difficulties in engaging in long-term goal-oriented behaviors and controlling impulsive behaviors (Weiss et al. 2013).

In order to decrease impulsive and harmful behavior, the teaching of emotional regulation skills is established as an intervention to learn new behavioral repertoires to deal with emotions considered unpleasant. For Axelrod et al. (2011), the development of emotional regulation skills allows the individual to choose more effective behaviors to deal with his emotions, instead of using the substance as his only alternative. Thus, increasing the frequency of emission of adaptive behaviors and also decreasing the actions that cause harm to the individual, including functional management of emotions, can strongly contribute to the prevention and treatment of women drug users who have been victims of violence (Cloitre et al. 2010; Linehan 2018; Mennin and Farach 2007).

Currently, promising results are evident in studies on interventions to teach and train emotional regulation skills for women who are victims of substance abuse disorders. A randomized study identified that women with chronic trauma due to child abuse benefited strongly from training in emotional regulation skills, along with a focus on stress tolerance and interpersonal effectiveness (Cloitre et al. 2010). Weiss et al. (2013) emphasize the importance of *mindfulness* strategies for the female drug user population with a history of mistreatment, aim that from the awareness of emotions the victims increase the power of choice of their behaviors. In view of these aspects, the relevance of evidence-based interventions aimed at teaching emotion regulation skills to women users of substances who have been victims of violence is highlighted.

Final Considerations

According to the United Nations (UNODC 2018), one-third of the world's substance users are women, which is also assumed to be underestimated. This underscores the need for evidence-based discussions that enable critical and scientific understanding of the numerous gender specificities of substance use disorders. To this end, this chapter sought to briefly discuss two important risk factors that are prominent in the female substance-using population: the history of violence and emotional deregulation.

From existing data on the subject, it is suggested that having emotional regulation skills increases the likelihood that women with a history of violence will be able to cope with trauma-related suffering with functional and healthy behavior. In this way, interventions with a focus on increasing emotional regulation can be configured as a form of substance abuse prevention and treatment for women who are victims of different types of violence.

References

Aldao, A., Nolen-Hoeksema, S., & Schweizer, S. (2010). Emotion-regulation strategies across psychopathology: A meta-analytic review. *Clinical Psychology Review, 30*(2), 217–237. https://doi.org/10.1016/j.cpr.2009.11.004.

Axelrod, S. R., Perepletchikova, F., Holtzman, K., & Sinha, R. (2011). Emotion regulation and substance use frequency in women with substance dependence and borderline personality disorder receiving dialectical behavior therapy. *The American Journal of Drug and Alcohol Abuse, 37*(1), 37–42. https://doi.org/10.3109/00952990.2010.535582.

Balbinot, A. D., Horta, R. L., Soares, J. D. C., Brasil, R. A., Poletto, S., & Teixeira, M. B. (2016). Hospitalizações por uso de drogas não se alteram com uma década de Reforma Psiquiátrica. *Revista de Saúde Pública, 50*, 1–9. https://doi.org/10.1590/S1518-8787.2016050006085.

Bastos, F. I. P. M., & Bertoni, N. (Eds.). (2014). *Pesquisa nacional sobre o uso de crack: quem são os usuários de crack e/ou similares do Brasil? Quantos são nas capitais brasileiras?* Retrieved from https://www.arca.fiocruz.br/handle/icict/10019

Butler, A. J., Rehm, J., & Fischer, B. (2017). Health outcomes associated with crack-cocaine use: Systematic review and meta-analyses. *Drug & Alcohol Dependence, 180*, 401–416. https://doi.org/10.1016/j.drugalcdep.2017.08.036.

Cafure, B. (2016). Uma visão analítico-comportamental do uso de cocaína. *Universitas Humanas, 12*(1). https://doi.org/10.5102/univhum.v12i1.3336.

Clark, C. B., Reiland, S., Thorne, C., & Cropsey, K. L. (2014). Relationship of trauma exposure and substance abuse to self-reported violence among men and women in substance abuse treatment. *Journal of Interpersonal Violence, 29*(8), 1514–1530. https://doi.org/10.1177/0886260513507138.

Cloitre, M., Stovall-McClough, K. C., Nooner, K., Zorbas, P., Cherry, S., Jackson, C. L., Gan, W., & Petkova, E. (2010). Treatment for PTSD related to childhood abuse: A randomized controlled trial. *The American Journal of Psychiatry, 167*(8), 915–924. https://doi.org/10.1176/appi.ajp.2010.09081247.

Dass-Brailsford, P., & Safilian, C. M. (2017). Integrated approaches to treating psychological trauma and substance abuse in women: An update. *Trauma & Acute Care, 2*(2), 1–4. https://doi.org/10.21767/2476-2105.100041.

Dingle, G. A., Neves, D. D. C., Alhadad, S. S., & Hides, L. (2018). Individual and interpersonal emotion regulation among adults with substance use disorders and matched controls. *British Journal of Clinical Psychology, 57*(2), 186–202. https://doi.org/10.1111/bjc.12168.

Giusti, J. S., & Zilberman, M. N. (2017). A mulher e os transtornos relacionados a substâncias: uma perspectiva feminina. In A. Gigliotti & A. Guimarães (Eds.), *Adição, dependência, compulsão e impulsividade* (pp. 241–254). Rio de Janeiro, Brasil: Rubio.

Gross, J. J. (2002). Emotion regulation: Affective, cognitive, and social consequences. *Psychophysiology, 39*(3), 281–291. https://doi.org/10.1017/S0048577201393198.

Guimarães, R. A., de Castro, V. D. O. L., Stabile, A. C., Motta-Castro, A. R. C., Santos Carneiro, M. A., Araujo, L. A., et al. (2017). Gender differences in patterns of drug use and sexual risky behaviour among crack cocaine users in Central Brazil. *BMC Psychiatry, 17*(1), 412. https://doi.org/10.1186/s12888-017-1569-7.

Halpern, S. C., Schuch, F. B., Scherer, J. N., Sordi, A. O., Pachado, M., Dalbosco, C., et al. (2018). Child maltreatment and illicit substance abuse: A systematic review and meta-analysis of longitudinal studies. *Child Abuse Review, 27*(5), 344–360. https://doi.org/10.1002/car.2534.

Hyman, S. M., Paliwal, P., Chaplin, T. M., Mazure, C. M., Rounsaville, B. J., & Sinha, R. (2008). Severity of childhood trauma is predictive of cocaine relapse outcomes in women but not men. *Drug and Alcohol Dependence, 92*(1–3), 208–216. https://doi.org/10.1016/j.drugalcdep.2007.08.006.

International Narcotics Control Board (2017). *Annual report*. Retrieved from https://www.incb.org/documents/Publications/AnnualReports/AR2017/Annual_Report/E_2017_AR_ebook.pdf

Izard, C. E. (2010). The many meanings/aspects of emotion: Definitions, functions, activation, and regulation. *Emotion Review, 2*(4), 363–370. https://doi.org/10.1177/1754073910374661.

Karpyak, V. M., Biernacka, J. M., Geske, J. R., Abulseoud, O. A., Brunner, M. D., Chauhan, M., et al. (2016). Gender-specific effects of comorbid depression and anxiety on the propensity to drink in negative emotional states. *Addiction, 111*(8), 1366–1375. https://doi.org/10.1111/add.13386.

Lejuez, C. W., Bornovalova, M. A., Reynolds, E. K., Daughters, S. B., & Curtin, J. J. (2007). Risk factors in the relationship between gender and crack/cocaine. *Experimental and Clinical Psychopharmacology, 15*(2), 165–175. https://doi.org/10.1037/1064-1297.15.2.165.

Linehan, M. (2018). *Treinamento de habilidades em DBT: Manual de terapia comportamental dialética para o terapeuta*. Porto Alegre, Brasil: Artmed.

Maciel, L. Z., Tractenberg, S. G., Viola, T. W., Araújo, R. B., & de Oliveira, R. G. (2017). Craving e dependência de crack: diferenças entre os gêneros. *Psicologia Argumento, 33*(81), 258–265. https://doi.org/10.7213/psicol.argum.33.081.AO03.

Madruga, C. S., Viana, M. C., Abdalla, R. R., Caetano, R., & Laranjeira, R. (2017). Pathways from witnessing parental violence during childhood to involvement in intimate partner violence in adult life: The roles of depression and substance use. *Drug and Alcohol Review, 36*(1), 107–114. https://doi.org/10.1111/dar.12514.

Mandavia, A., Robinson, G. G., Bradley, B., Ressler, K. J., & Powers, A. (2016). Exposure to childhood abuse and later substance use: Indirect effects of emotion dysregulation and exposure to trauma. *Journal of Traumatic Stress, 29*(5), 422–429. https://doi.org/10.1002/jts.22131.

McDermott, M. J., Tull, M. T., Gratz, K. L., Daughters, S. B., & Lejuez, C. W. (2009). The role of anxiety sensitivity and difficulties in emotion regulation in posttraumatic stress disorder among crack/cocaine dependent patients in residential substance abuse treatment. *Journal of Anxiety Disorders, 23*(5), 591–599. https://doi.org/10.1016/j.janxdis.2009.01.006.

Medeiros, K. T., Maciel, S. C., Santos, L. F., & Sousa, P. F. (2018). Traçando o perfil de uma amostra de usuárias de crack em tratamento. *Revista de Psicologia da IMED, 10*(1), 160–174. https://doi.org/10.18256/2175-5027.2018.v10i1.2730.

Medeiros, K. T., Maciel, S. C., & Sousa, P. F. D. (2017). A mulher no contexto das drogas: Representações sociais de usuárias em tratamento. *Paidéia, 27*, 439–447. https://doi.org/10.1590/1982-432727s1201709.

Mennin, D., & Farach, F. (2007). Emotion and evolving treatments for adult psychopathology. *Clinical Psychology: Science and Practice, 14*(4), 329–352. https://doi.org/10.1111/j.1468-2850.2007.00094.x.

Moraes, M. E. F., Roso, A., & Lara, M. P. D. (2018). Gênero como uma categoria de análise nos estudos brasileiros sobre mulheres e consumo de crack. *Gerais: Revista Interinstitucional de Psicologia, 11*(1), 11–25. https://doi.org/10.36298/gerais2019110103.

Nolen-Hoeksema, S. (2012). Emotion regulation and psychopathology: The role of gender. *Annual Review of Clinical Psychology, 8*, 161–187. https://doi.org/10.1146/annurev-clinpsy-032511-143109.

Price, C. J., Wells, E. A., Donovan, D. M., & Rue, T. (2012). Mindful awareness in body-oriented therapy as an adjunct to women's substance use disorder treatment: A pilot feasibility study. *Journal of Substance Abuse Treatment, 43*(1), 94–107. https://doi.org/10.1016/j.jsat.2011.09.016.

Sanvicente-Vieira, B., Rovaris, D. L., Ornell, F., Sordi, A., Rothmann, L. M., Niederauer, J. P. O., et al. (2019). Sex-based differences in multidimensional clinical assessments of early-abstinence crack cocaine users. *PLoS One, 14*(6), e0218334. https://doi.org/10.1371/journal.pone.0218334.

Shadur, J. M., & Lejuez, C. W. (2015). Adolescent substance use and comorbid psychopathology: Emotion regulation deficits as a transdiagnostic risk factor. *Current Addiction Reports, 2*(4), 354–363. https://doi.org/10.1007/s40429-015-0070-y.

Souza, M. R. R., Oliveira, J. F., & Nascimento, E. R. (2014). A saúde de mulheres e o fenômeno das drogas em revistas brasileiras. *Texto & Contexto Enfermagem, 23*(1), 92–100. https://doi.org/10.1590/S0104-07072014000100011.

Tull, M. T., Bardeen, J. R., DiLillo, D., Messman-Moore, T., & Gratz, K. L. (2015). A prospective investigation of emotion dysregulation as a moderator of the relation between posttraumatic stress symptoms and substance use severity. *Journal of Anxiety Disorders, 29*, 52–60. https://doi.org/10.1016/j.janxdis.2014.11.003.

United Nations Office on Drugs and Crime. (2016). *Guidelines on drug prevention and treatment for girls and women*. Retrieved from https://www.unodc.org/documents/drug-prevention-and-treatment/unodc_2016_drug_prevention_and_treatment_for_girls_and_women_E.pdf

United Nations Office on Drugs and Crime. (2018). *World report 2018*. Retrieved from https://reliefweb.int/sites/reliefweb.int/files/resources/WDR18_Booklet_1_EXSUM.pdf

Veilleux, J. C., Skinner, K. D., Reese, E. D., & Shaver, J. A. (2014). Negative affect intensity influences drinking to cope through facets of emotion dysregulation. *Personality and Individual Differences, 59*, 96–101. https://doi.org/10.1016/j.paid.2013.11.012.

Vernaglia, T. V. C., Leite, T. H., Faller, S., Pechansky, F., Kessler, F. H. P., Cruz, M. S., & Brazilian Crack Group. (2017). The female crack users: Higher rates of social vulnerability in Brazil. *Health Care for Women International, 38*(11), 1170–1187. https://doi.org/10.1080/07399332.2017.136700.

Vigitel Brazil. (2018). *Surveillance of risk and protective factors for chronic diseases by telephone survey: estimates of frequency and sociodemographic distribution of risk and protective factors for chronic diseases in the capitals of the 26 Brazilian states and the Federal District in 2018*. Retrieved from http://portalarquivos2.saude.gov.br/images/pdf/2019/julho/25/vigitel-brasil-2018.pdf

Vujanovic, A. A., Bonn-Miller, M. O., & Petry, N. M. (2016). Co-occurring posttraumatic stress and substance use: Emerging research on correlates, mechanisms, and treatments—introduction to the special issue. *Psychology of Addictive Behaviors, 30*(7), 713. https://doi.org/10.1037/adb0000222.

Waldrop, A. E., Back, S. E., Brady, K. T., Upadhyaya, H. P., McRae, A. L., & Saladin, M. E. (2007). Daily stressor sensitivity, abuse effects, and cocaine use in cocaine dependence. *Addictive Behaviors, 32*(12), 3015–3025. https://doi.org/10.1016/j.addbeh.2007.07.006.

Walsh, K., Keyes, K. M., Koenen, K. C., & Hasin, D. (2015). Lifetime prevalence of gender- based violence in US women: Associations with mood/anxiety and substance use disorders. *Journal of Psychiatric Research, 62*, 7. https://doi.org/10.1016/j.jpsychires.2015.01.002.

Weiss, N. H., Tull, M. T., Anestis, M. D., & Gratz, K. L. (2013). The relative and unique contributions of emotion dysregulation and impulsivity to posttraumatic stress disorder among substance dependent inpatients. *Drug & Alcohol Dependence, 128*(1), 45–51. https://doi.org/10.1016/j.drugalcdep.2012.07.017.

Westphal, M., Aldao, A., & Jackson, C. (2017). Emotion dysregulation in comorbid posttraumatic stress disorder and substance use disorders: A narrative review. *Military Psychology, 29*(3), 216–233. https://doi.org/10.1037/mil0000157.

Wolff, S., Holl, J., Stopsack, M., Arens, E. A., Höcker, A., Staben, K. A., et al. (2016). Does emotion dysregulation mediate the relationship between early maltreatment and later substance dependence? findings of the CANSAS study. *European Addiction Research, 22*(6), 292–300. https://doi.org/10.1159/000447397.

World Health Organization. (2013). *Global and regional estimates of violence against women: Prevalence and health effects of intimate partner violence and non-partner sexual violence.* Retrieved from http://apps.who.int/iris/bitstream/10665/85239/1/9789241564625_eng.pdf

World Health Organization. (2016). *Inspire: Seven strategies for ending violence against children.* Retrieved from https://apps.who.int/iris/bitstream/handle/10665/207717/9789241565356-eng.pdf?sequence=1

Chapter 35
Therapeutic Use of Hallucinogens

Victor Distefano Wiltenburg , Dianne da Rocha Prado, and Fúlvio Rieli Mendes

Introduction

Hallucinogenic substances of natural origin have been used by humans for millennia for various purposes, including mystical, spiritual, religious, therapeutic, and recreational uses. Since the nineteenth century, scientists has also started to isolate such compounds and synthesize analogues of the hallucinogens known until then, as well as new molecules with hallucinogenic potential, being the diethylamide of the lysergic acid (LSD) the best known example. Researches carried out in the 1950s and 1960s showed the therapeutic potential of several hallucinogens such as LSD, dimethyltryptamine (DMT), psilocybin, mescaline, among others for several clinical conditions (Kyzar et al. 2017; Rucker et al. 2018). At the same time, the use of these hallucinogenic substances for recreational purposes by hippies and counterculture groups grew enormously, causing authorities around the world to turn their attention to their regulation. Despite the medical potential demonstrated and evidence that these substances produced low risk of addiction and little damage to health, compared to legal drugs such as alcohol and tobacco, hallucinogens were classified as potentially dangerous drugs and began to have their use prohibited. An important milestone in these government policies was the inclusion of LSD, DMT, psilocybin, along with marijuana and other hallucinogenic substances in the Schedule 1 of the Controlled Substances Act adopted in the USA in 1970 and the United Nations Convention on Psychotropic Substances in 1971 (Nutt et al. 2013).

As a result, studies of hallucinogenic drugs have declined tremendously since 1970, even because of the difficulty in obtaining permits to study these substances. However, in the last 10–15 years there has been a growing resurgence of interest in

V. D. Wiltenburg · D. da Rocha Prado · F. R. Mendes (✉)
Universidade Federal do ABC, São Bernardo do Campo, SP, Brazil
e-mail: fulvio.mendes@ufabc.edu.br

D. De Micheli et al. (eds.), *Drugs and Human Behavior*,
https://doi.org/10.1007/978-3-030-62855-0_35

hallucinogens. According to Doblin et al. (2019), there are more studies with psychedelics occurring today than at any other time in history. Perhaps this is not true in terms of the absolute number of publications, but certainly contemporary studies rely on more solid data and use more rigorous methodologies to evaluate the therapeutic potential of hallucinogens. It is noteworthy that current clinical studies evaluate the effectiveness of hallucinogens in diseases difficult to treat, including chronic pain, mood disorders (depression and anxiety, including treatment-resistant depression), post-traumatic stress disorder, among others (De Gregorio et al. 2018; Santos et al. 2018; Muttoni et al. 2019; Rucker et al. 2016) In addition, the benefits of hallucinogens have been evaluated to improve the mood and psychological condition of patients suffering from terminal illness and anxiety associated with life-threatening diseases, and to reduce the risk of suicide in vulnerable individuals (Garcia-Romeu et al. 2016; Muttoni et al. 2019). Furthermore, as paradoxical as it may seem, studies have suggested that hallucinogens are promising agents to help in the treatment of drug dependence, such as alcohol, tobacco, cocaine, heroin, etc. (Mendes and Prado 2017; Morgan et al. 2017; Winkelman 2014). It is interesting to note that in many current studies the so-called microdoses are used, i.e., doses much lower than those generally used for recreational purposes. In addition, a large number of clinical studies have been based on assisted therapy, where the experimental drug is associated with some type of psychosocial therapy and patients receive constant support from medical and research teams.

Hallucinogenic substances belong to different classes with quite distinct chemical structures and mechanisms of action (Garcia-Romeu et al. 2016). The classical hallucinogens, also known as psychedelics, are serotonin receptor agonists, and they induce hallucinogenic effect due mainly to the stimulation of receptors of subtype 5-HT_{2A}. LSD, DMT, and psilocybin belong to this group. A second group represented by ecstasy (MDMA) acts by inhibiting the reuptake of serotonin and dopamine; while a third group is formed by dissociative anesthetics, agents such as ketamine that are antagonists to NMDA-type glutamate receptors. Hallucinogenic drugs that act by other mechanisms are treated as atypical hallucinogens, such as ibogaine, which acts on multiple targets, and salvinorin A, a kappa opioid receptor agonist. Table 35.1 provides a summary of the substances addressed in this chapter, containing their chemical structures, mechanisms of action, and main therapeutic indications with scientific support.

In this chapter, we will describe the main hallucinogenic substances with therapeutic potential in neurological and psychiatric diseases, with emphasis on the most recent studies. The historical aspects of the use of each substance will also be addressed, discussing its mechanisms of action and the general effects produced. In addition, although this is not the focus of the chapter, we will comment on the mystical and religious use of some of the hallucinogens and cite their use as agents of creativity or other peculiar uses, when appropriate.

Table 35.1 Chemical structure, class and form of acquisition, mechanisms of action, and main therapeutic indications of the hallucinogens treated in the chapter

Drugs	Chemical structure	Source and chemical class	Mechanisms of action	Main therapeutic indications with scientific support
Lysergic acid diethylamide	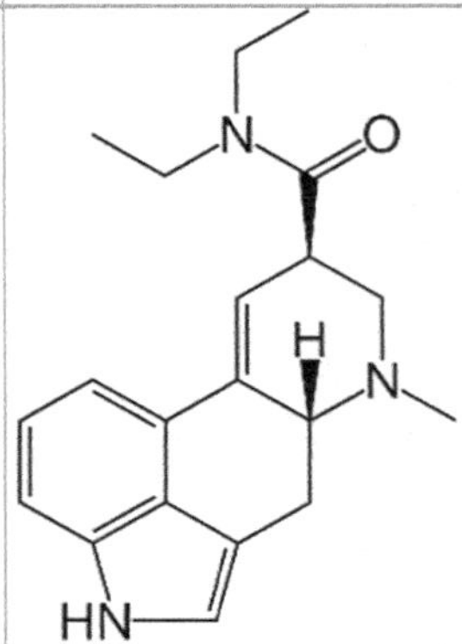	Indolic alkaloid synthetically produced from lysergic acid, obtained from ergotamine hydrolysis, present in rye ergot fungus	Serotonergic agonist with affinity for 5-HT1A, 5-HT2A, and 5-HT2C; acts to a lesser extent on dopaminergic receptors	Treatment of anxiety and mood disorders, depression, addictions, in particular alcohol dependency
Dimethyltryptamine	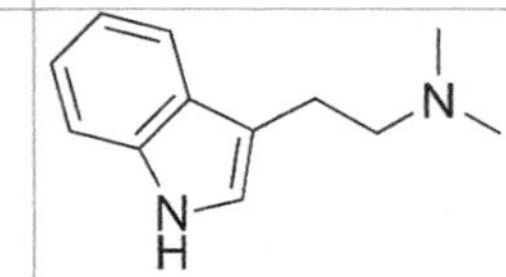	Indolic alkaloid present in several plants, such as *Psychotria viridis*, used in the preparation of ayahuasca	Serotonergic agonist (5-HT1A, 1B, 1D and 5-HT2A and 2C receptors), acts to a lesser extent on other targets	Depression and drug addiction, especially of alcohol
Psilocybin	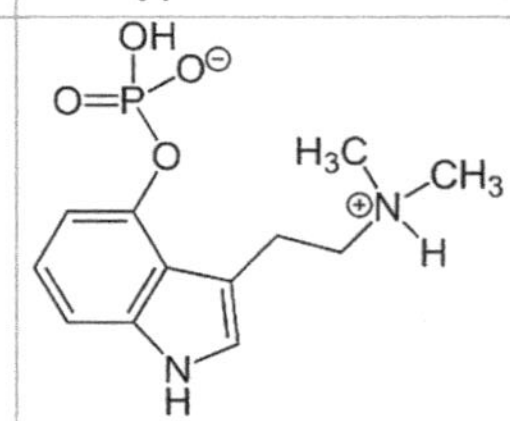	Indolic alkaloid found in several mushroom species of the genus *Psilocybe*	Serotonergic agonist with high affinity for 5-HT2A receptors and moderate affinity for 5-HT1A and 5-HT2C	Anxiety and antidepressant agent, treatment of obsessive compulsive disorder and tobacco and alcohol dependence

(continued)

Table 35.1 (continued)

Drugs	Chemical structure	Source and chemical class	Mechanisms of action	Main therapeutic indications with scientific support
Mescaline	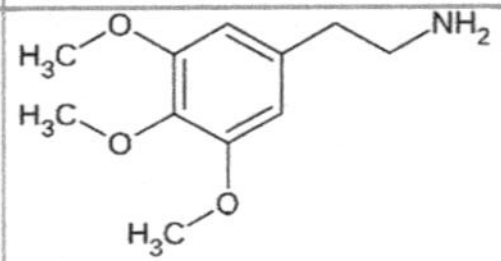	Alkaloid present in some species of cacti such as peyote (*Lophophora williamsii*) and San Pedro (*Echinopsis pachanoi*)	Serotonergic agonist with high affinity for 5-HT2C receptors, moderate for 5-HT2A and 5-HT2B and dopaminergic modulator	Proposed for the treatment of depression, anxiety, obsessive compulsive disorder and substance dependence
Methylenedioxy-methamphetamine	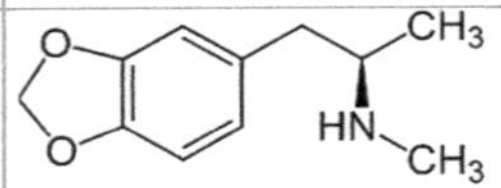	Synthetic methamphetamine derivative	Inhibits the reuptake of catecholamines, facilitating its release. Also acts as a 5-HT1 and 5-HT2 serotonergic agonist	Depression, anxiety and post-traumatic stress disorder
Ketamine	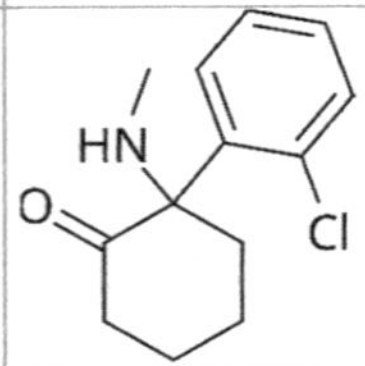	Synthetic substance	Powerful NMDA receptor antagonist, acts with less affinity on opioid receptors, monoamine transporters, among others	Anesthetic, pain relief and depression, especially treatment-resistant depression
Ibogaine	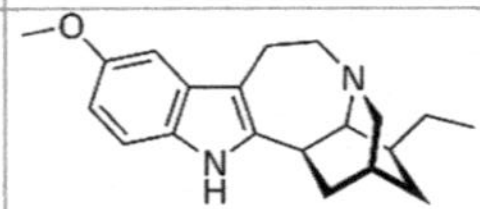	Alkaloid present in the root of iboga (*Tabernanthe iboga*)	Has affinity for NMDA receptors, kappa opioid receptors, sigma-type receptors, and nicotinic receptors, besides being a 5-HT2A receptor agonist	Treatment of addiction, especially for opioids
Salvinorin A	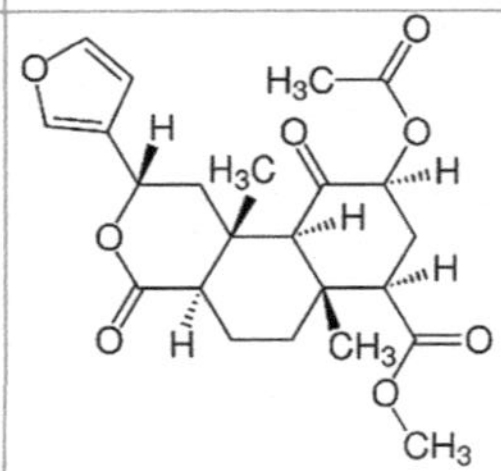	Neoclerodan diterpene derived from *Salvia divinorum*	Selective agonist of kappa opioid receptors and allosteric modulator of CB1	Analgesic, presents pre-clinical evidence for the treatment of addiction, in particular of stimulant drugs

Source: elaborated by the authors

Lysergic Acid Diethylamide (LSD)

LSD or LSD25, despite being the most famous and most studied hallucinogen in the world, is still considered a new drug, since it is a synthetic substance, while natural psychedelics have been inserted into human culture for thousands of years. First synthesized in 1938 by the Swiss chemist Albert Hoffmann, LSD remained relatively unknown to the general public for years. It was only from the 1950s that its use became popular, crossing scientific, political, and artistic spheres. At that time the substance became widely used by spiritual and religious leaders, researchers, and artists around the world and was also part of U.S. government programs such as the project MK-Ultra, among others (Ketchum 2006; Smith et al. 2014).

Research from the 1950s and 1960s played a relevant role in the better understanding of LSD. Its chemical, pharmacological, and pharmacokinetic properties, among other characteristics studied in this period are addressed in a review by Passie et al. (2008). LSD acts primarily as a serotonergic agonist, and its hallucinogenic effects are attributed, especially to 5-HT_{2A} receptor stimulation. However, other studies suggest a potent action of LSD in dopaminergic and adrenergic receptors (Halberstadt 2015; Nichols 2004). It is interesting to mention that, according to Schmid et al. (2015), LSD can generate increased levels of prolactin, oxytocin, and epinephrine in patients under the effect of the drug, suggesting that its effects are broader than originally believed. Regarding its toxicity, no neurotoxic effects were found, nor were deaths related to its use (Passie et al. 2008), but side effects are common, such as disorientation, anxiety, bad trips, among others. It is important to mention that in the mainstream media it is common to find news about deaths related to LSD, however, these are usually due to indirect effects, such as consequences of perceptual changes in reality by the user and other substances ingested together, with recreational purposes.

Although LSD studies have remained in "hibernation" due to the prohibition of the use and production of the substance in several regions of the world, recently, research has again emerged in the scientific community with information about this substance and its therapeutic potential. Several clinical indications for LSD are described, including from relief for headaches to treatment for anxiety and mood disorders, depression, addictions, among others (Tupper et al. 2015). Peter Gasse was one of the pioneers in the recent wave investigating the properties of LSD. His group conducted a double-blind randomized study with 12 patients who suffered from anxiety associated with life-threatening diseases, such as terminal cancer, AIDS, among others. In this study, the patients underwent psychotherapy sessions associated with a dose of 200 μg of LSD, besides to a group that received a subperceptual dose of 20 μg. The results were promising, with patients treated with the highest dose reporting a reduction in anxiety in 77.8% of cases and an improvement in quality of life in 66.7% in relation to themselves (Gasser et al. 2015).

The use of LSD as a treatment for alcohol addiction is among the main therapeutic uses studied. A meta-analysis conducted in 2012 with a total of 536 participants showed that individuals treated with a dose of LSD combined with conventional addiction treatments, such as hospitalization and psychotherapy, had a significant decrease in the use of alcohol compared to the control group not treated with psychedelic (Krebs and Johansen 2012). A recent systematic review indicated, despite the great heterogeneity among the studies included, that LSD presents therapeutic potential to reduce psychiatric symptoms, especially in alcoholism (Fuentes et al. 2020). Another study assessing the self-report of 444 participants suggests a correlation between the use of classic hallucinogens, especially LSD, in reducing abuse of cannabis, stimulant, and opioid (Garcia-Romeu et al. 2020).

In a systematic review, it was concluded that hallucinogens with serotonergic mechanisms, such as LSD, have the ability to reduce the recognition of negative emotions, possibly via modulation of amygdala activity, a neuroanatomical region traditionally related to the perception and recognition of emotions. In addition, a promising benefit is proposed in patients with impaired recognition of emotions in facial expressions, an aspect considered fundamental in social cognition and which mood and anxiety disorders are associated with their deficit (Rocha et al. 2019).

Since the beginning of research with hallucinogens, there has been accumulated evidence that they have the capacity to decrease the oscillatory power of the central nervous system, predominantly in the low frequency bands and an increase in the frequency of alpha rhythms (Fink 2004). However, it was only in the last years that LSD started to be studied using more modern neuroimaging techniques, such as magnetoencephalography, functional magnetic resonance, among others. It is interesting that these techniques have shown some compatibility with the physiological reports of LSD users, such as increased blood flow in the visual cortex and decreased alpha waves in these regions, in addition to a large increase in the network communication related to the primary visual cortex, which suggests the relationship with perceptual changes in vision and hallucinations experienced by users (Carhart-Harris et al. 2016a). Other studies have also shown that hallucinogens alter patterns in brain waves and the default mode networking, opening new avenues for studies of the possible potential of these drugs (Liechti 2017).

Finally, it is relevant to comment on an issue that is progressing rapidly in the media and online forums: the use of microdoses. Microdose is the intake of sub-threshold LSD doses, i.e. the user should not present and experience any apparent physiological change. Microdoses vary among users, however, the optimal dose is generally considered to be between 6 and 25 μg. The main benefits cited by users are increased focus, improved mood, improved ability to cope with life's difficulties, and improved creativity, which could be why they are increasingly been used in environments where creativity is a special point, such as the artistic environment. Despite the growing increase in the use of microdoses to these purposes, few studies have been conducted on this subject, with recent work indicating safety (Family et al. 2020). Some works suggest that LSD can improve suggestibility and creative imagination in healthy women (Carhart-Harris et al. 2015) and may evoke a greater emotional response to music (Kaelen et al. 2015), however, other studies have not found significant differences due to micro-dosage (Family et al. 2020). In 2019, a study involving 278 microdosers of LSD, psilocybin, or both was published. Although some findings are controversial and discussed by the authors as limitations of the study, statistical analysis of the data indicated an improvement in mood (26.6%) and focus (14.8%) of participants, although an increase in physical discomfort (18%) and anxiety (6.7%) was also observed, which suggests the need for new research with scientific rigor on this subject (Anderson et al. 2019).

N, N-dimethyltryptamine (DMT) and Ayahuasca

DMT is an indolic alkaloid widely found in nature, present in several plants, but also described as an endogenous molecule in animals (Carlini 2003). The main genera of plants containing DMT include: *Phalaris, Delosperma, Acacia, Desmodium, Mimosa, Virola,* and *Psychotria,* although DMT has also been found in apparently innocuous sources, such as leaves of citrus plants (Servillo et al. 2012). DMT has an affinity for 5-$HT_{1A,\ 1B,\ 1D}$ and 5-HT_{2A} and $_{2C}$ receptors, and it is a potent hallucinogen when used by parenteral route at a dosage of 25 mg (Callaway et al. 1996). There is great speculation about the role of DMT in naturally occurring altered states of consciousness such as psychosis, dreams, creativity, imagination, spiritual phenomena, and near-death experiences (Callaway 1988; Strassman 2001).

There is no consensus on where the synthesis of endogenous DMT occurs and its action on the human organism remains unknown. Strassman (2001) proposed that DMT is synthesized by the pineal gland, produced at specific moments of human existence, such as birth and death, however, other studies propose that DMT may be synthesized by the adrenal glands and lung, where have been reported high levels of indolethylamine N-methyltransferase, the enzyme responsible for its synthesis (Thompson et al. 1999; Thompson and Weinshilboum 1998).

Many plant species are used to alter states of consciousness, whether for recreational or syncretic purposes. Among these, the genera *Psychotria* and *Mimosa* are present in the preparation of beverages considered sacred for religious and therapeutic purposes, such as ayahuasca and jurema wine. Ayahuasca is originally used by indigenous people in shamanic rituals and is generally prepared by decoction of two plants native to the Amazon region, the bark and stem of *Banisteriopsis caapi* and the leaves of *Psychotria viridis. P. viridis* presents DMT in its composition, while *B. caapi* has alkaloids with β-carboline structure (harmine, harmaline, and tetrahydroharmine) that present inhibitory action on monoamine oxidase (MAO) (McKenna 2004). Jurema or *ajucá* wine is consumed in northeastern Brazil by indigenous tribes. It is generally prepared from the fermentation process of plants of the Mimosaceae family, mainly jurema-preta (*Mimosa tenuiflora*), with the addition of seeds of *Peganum harmala* (Camargo 2014; Gaujac et al. 2013). Similar to the plants used in the preparation of ayahuasca, *M. tenuiflora* presents DMT in its composition, while the seed of *P. harmala* has alkaloids with β-carboline structure (Hemmateenejad et al. 2006). The hallucinogenic effect of both beverages occurs due to the synergism of the substances in the plants used, i.e., the inhibition of intestinal MAO facilitates the absorption of DMT, which is responsible for the hallucinogenic effects (Callaway et al. 1999; Carlini 2003; McKenna 2004).

Although research on pure DMT is mainly on its physiological and psychotomimetic effects, which are essential for understanding its endogenous role, the rapid growth of ayahuasca as a cultural phenomenon in relation to its healing reports has provoked curiosity about its possible toxic and therapeutic effects. Among the possible toxic effects resulting from the consumption of ayahuasca, dehydration due to recurrent episodes of nausea, vomiting, and diarrhea stands out, with hypertension, tachycardia, mydriasis, palpitation, euphoria, and even aggressive excitation being common, with serotonergic syndrome possibly the most serious effect (Callaway et al. 1999; Meres Costa et al. 2005). Several studies have been conducted to investigate the neurophysiological, neuroendocrine, cardiovascular, biochemical, and immunological impact of acute ayahuasca administration on healthy volunteers (Santos 2013; Santos et al. 2011, 2012). These studies suggest that acute administration of ayahuasca in the clinical setting to healthy volunteers is safe and tolerable (Santos 2013). In addition, the impact of repeated ayahuasca use was evaluated in a longitudinal study with 127 users and 115 controls, and no evidence of psychological maladjustment, mental health deterioration, or cognitive dysfunction was found in the group of ayahuasca users (Bouso et al. 2012).

Since DMT is a substance for illicit use and controlled sale, much of the current research has used ayahuasca, whose ceremonial use is legalized in Brazil and other countries. Recent studies suggest that psychedelics, such as ayahuasca, have promising antidepressant, anxiolytic, and anti-addictive effects. Barbosa et al. (2005) reported reductions in anxiety and depression symptoms in nine participants after their first ayahuasca intake, assessing the initial and short-term mood, 1–4 days before their first ayahuasca experience, and 1–2 weeks after that experience. Semi-structured interviews and a structured psychiatric scale were used and both individuals reported behavioral changes in the sense of assertiveness, serenity, and vivacity/joy. In 2016, a clinical trial evaluated the antidepressant effect in 17 patients with Major Depression Disorder (MDD) after administration of a single dose of ayahuasca (Sanches et al. 2016). Changes in severity of depression were assessed before, during, and after the session through the Montgomery–Asberg and Hamilton Depression Scales. An antidepressant effect was observed in the 1 h after administration, lasting significantly for 21 days. Palhano-Fontes et al. (2019) conducted the first double-blind, placebo-controlled clinical trial in the treatment of MDD with ayahuasca in 29 patients at the Onofre Lopes University Hospital of the Federal University of Rio Grande do Norte. Changes in the severity of depression were evaluated using the Montgomery–Asberg and Hamilton Depression Scales on days 1, 2, and 7, after administration of a single dose of placebo or ayahuasca adjusted to contain 0.36 mg/kg DMT. The antidepressant effect in the group that received ayahuasca was significant when compared to the placebo on all the days observed.

Observational studies have reported remission of alcohol use, changes in behavior, mood, and improved outlook on life after ayahuasca use (Barbosa et al. 2016; Callaway et al. 1996; Fábregas et al. 2010; Halpern et al. 2008). Fábregas et al. (2010) reported that the effects were preserved in 1 year of monitoring, this result being observed in individuals who use the beverage in a community inserted in a preserved area of the Amazon rain forest, but not in individuals who use it in an urban group located in the city of Rio Branco, capital of the state of Acre, in the northern region of Brazil. A preliminary observational study in Canada concluded that ayahuasca may also have contributed to statistically significant reductions in the use of alcohol, tobacco, and cocaine, but not of marijuana and opiates among participants (Thomas et al. 2013). Jiménez-Garrido et al. (2020) conducted a longitudinal study with two subgroups of ayahuasca users: new users (*näive*) and long-term users. The study showed that new users showed clinical improvement in psychiatric conditions after 6 months, evaluated by questionnaires, while long-term users showed lower rates of depression and higher scores for quality of life, compared to the *näive* group.

Oliveira-Lima et al. (2015) conducted a pre-clinical study where the development of ethanol-induced behavioral sensitization was evaluated in mice. The work showed that ayahuasca was able to block ethanol sensitization in the animals. Another study evaluated the effect of ayahuasca, as well as the isolated effects of the species *P. viridis* and *B. caapi* on the ethanol-induced conditioned place preference in mice (Cata-Preta et al. 2018). Ayahuasca or the extract of each species was administered before ethanol during the conditioning sessions, and it was observed that ayahuasca was able to block the development of conditioned preference, while separately the extracts had no significant effect. In addition, the effects of a post-conditioning treatment were evaluated in the ethanol paired environment and all extracts blocked the ethanol-induced conditioned place preference.

Liester and Prickett (2012) present four hypotheses to explain the possible biochemical, physiological, psychological, and transcendental mechanisms by which ayahuasca can exert its positive effects on drug dependence. The *biochemical hypothesis* suggests that ayahuasca has anti-addictive properties through the reduction of dopamine in the mesolimbic pathway, as a result of its effects on serotonergic receptors, since DMT is a potent 5-HT_{2A} receptor agonist, its action results in a decrease in the release of dopamine in the mesolimbic, mesocortical, and nigrostriatal pathways. In addition, ayahuasca users have high levels of prolactin, which is a possible indication of a reduction in dopamine that negatively modulates the release of this hormone. The *physiological hypothesis* suggests that the reduction in dopamine levels in the mesolimbic pathway interferes with the synaptic plasticity associated with the development and maintenance of dependence. The *psychological hypothesis* suggests that ayahuasca treats addiction through the resolution of traumas, encouraging understanding of potential outcomes of choices and improving decision-making. Finally, the *transcendental hypothesis* suggests that ayahuasca treats dependence through facilitated transcendental experience; these aspects of the experience may include visions of a spiritual reality, altering the notion of time and space, ineffability, intuitive insights, and feelings of oneness with the universe. A recently published review discusses the potentiality of ayahuasca and other serotonergic hallucinogens in the treatment of psychiatric disorders and comments on the neurochemical effects possibly related to their therapeutic actions (Santos and Hallak 2020).

Although endogenous DMT does not have a well-defined role, ayahuasca as a therapeutic option has proven to be a promising aid in the treatment of depression, anxiety, and drug addiction, however, other controlled clinical studies are needed to prove the efficacy and safety of this beverage for the treatment of these diseases. In addition, it is essential to evaluate the importance of religion and the context of use in the treatment of addiction, anxiety, and depression, as well as the adverse effects resulting from long-term chronic use of DMT.

Psilocybin

Psilocybin is an indolic alkaloid found in several mushroom species of the *Psilocybe* genus, the best known species being *Psilocybe mexicana*, known as magic mushroom or sacred mushroom due to its entheogenic effect. Another very common species is *Psilocybe cubensis*, which occurs in several American countries. These magic mushrooms were already used for many centuries by the primitive American people, especially by the Mayans and Aztecs for healing purposes and also in religious and social ceremonies, but have only recently been studied by modern science (Schultes et al. 2001).

In addition to their uses in spiritual and ritualistic rituals, *Psilocybe* mushrooms are used for recreational purposes, and are widely cultivated for that. Psilocybin is a tryptamine with LSD-like properties, and in the body it is converted to psilocin (4-hydroxy-dimethylamine) which acts mainly as a strong 5-HT_{2A} agonist, with moderate effect on subtypes 5-HT_{1A} and 5-HT_{2C} (Daniel and Haberman 2017; Garcia-Romeu et al. 2016).

Numerous studies with psilocybin date back to the 1950s and 1960s, but in recent years several clinical studies have been conducted on the drug (Daniel and Haberman 2017; Garcia-Romeu et al. 2016). Evidence indicates that psilocybin use is relatively safe, especially when it occurs with moderate doses and in controlled environments. Adverse reactions from psilocybin use are mild in low doses and tend to go away rapidly. They include increased heart rate and blood pressure, headache, disorientation, transient anxiety, and a feelings of fear (Garcia-Romeu et al. 2016; Studerus et al. 2011). Hallucinogenic effects are usually transient, but the change in perception of consciousness is maintained for weeks or months and according to some authors may explain the prolonged effect obtained with the use of acute doses of psilocybin for the treatment of certain psychiatric conditions. A recent online survey of psilocybin users found that the effects perceived as negative most reported by participants were bad trip and thinking distortions, usually associated with consumption of high doses or combinations with other substances (Bienemann et al. 2020).

Among the several therapeutic indications for which psilocybin has been proposed, it is worth to mention its use for patients with anxiety and depression associated with terminal or life-threatening diseases. A pilot study was conducted with patients at an advanced stage of cancer and diagnosis of generalized anxiety related to the disease (Grob et al. 2011). In this study, participants were divided into two randomized groups, one treated with psilocybin at 0.2 mg/kg and the other with niacin (vitamin B6, 250 mg) as a placebo and after a few weeks the treatment was reversed with subjects acting as their own control. Although the results are not very clearly presented the authors suggest that the degree of anxiety and depression was reduced after treatment with psilocybin when compared with niacin (Grob et al. 2011). In turn, Ross et al. (2016) conducted a similar study with a larger sample of 29 patients with cancer-related anxiety and depression. In this study, participants were divided into two groups receiving niacin (250 mg) or psilocybin (0.3 mg/kg) concomitantly with psychotherapy and in a cross-sectional scheme, i.e., treatment was reversed after 7 weeks. The results indicate that administration of a single dose of psilocybin was sufficient to produce a rapid and sustained anxiolytic and antidepressant effect in patients with cancer-related psychological distress (Ross et al. 2016).

In another study, patients with unipolar depression resistant to conventional treatments were selected, and the treatment was performed with two doses of psilocybin (10 and 25 mg) separated for a period of 7 days, concomitant to psychological support before, during and after each treatment session with psilocybin (Carhart-Harris et al. 2016b; Carhart-Harris et al. 2018). The authors report that the depressive symptoms were reduced, compared to the baseline evaluation, 1 week, 3 and 6 months after the treatment with the highest dose, without serious adverse events; however, there was no control group in this study and the authors point out that new studies with a more rigorous design are needed to better examine the therapeutic potential of psilocybin in depression. On the other hand, a study that evaluated the effect of various doses and treatment regimens with psilocybin and psilocin in laboratory animals found no evidence of antidepressant action, but the authors consider that other animal models may be needed for translational studies with the drug (Jefsen et al. 2019). It is also worth mentioning a literature-based theoretical study that suggests that the combination of psilocybin and mindfulness meditation could be a promising new treatment for depression, acting through complementary mechanisms (Heuschkel and Kuypers 2020).

The effectiveness of psilocybin was also evaluated in patients with obsessive compulsive disorder. In this study, nine patients received up to four doses of psilocybin (from 25 to 300 μg/kg) spaced at least 1 week and were evaluated by the obsessive compulsive Yale-Brown scale, showing significant reduction in the score 24 h after treatment (Moreno et al. 2006).

A few studies have also evaluated the use of psilocybin for the dependence of legal drugs such as alcohol and tobacco. Johnson et al. (2014) selected 15 tobacco addicts for an intervention that initially consisted of a 4-week period of cognitive-behavioral therapy followed by psilocybin administration in weeks 5, 7, and 13. According to the authors, 80% of participants remained abstinent after 6 months of treatment, suggesting that this treatment is quite promising compared to other approaches whose typical success rate is below 35% (Johnson et al. 2014). In a similar study, ten participants diagnosed as alcohol-dependent were selected and subjected to psychosocial treatment for 4 weeks and then received one or two doses of psilocybin separated by a 4-week interval, in addition to the psychosocial intervention. Not all participants completed the study and the results were moderate, but they suggested a reduction in alcohol consumption by all participants after psilocybin compared to baseline and to post-psychosocial treatment condition, i.e., before the psilocybin administration (Bogenschutz et al. 2015).

In summary, the scientific literature indicates that psilocybin is a very safe drug when used in moderate doses and suggests that the assisted therapy with a single dose or interval doses of psilocybin is very promising for the treatment of conditions such as anxiety and depression related to the advanced-stage cancer, as well as in the treatment of alcohol and tobacco dependence, especially when combined with some type of psychosocial therapy.

Mescaline

Mescaline (3,4,5-trimethoxyphenylethylamine) is a psychoactive substance present in the Peyote cactus (*Lophophora williamsii*) found in Central and South America and the San Pedro cactus (*Echinopsis pachanoi*, syn. *Trichocereus pachanoi*), also known as *Wachuma,* occurring in Andean countries of South America, and also found in smaller quantities in other American cacti. Peyote has been used by native peoples of Mexico for more than 5700 years due to its psychedelic properties, and it has been recorded in archeological sites dating from 5800 to 6000 years (Cassels and Sáez-Briones 2018; De Gregorio et al. 2018). Peyote is also called the divine cactus or sacred cactus by native Americans and members of groups who make its use in religious ceremonies. They believe that the ingestion of peyote facilitates communication with God or divine entities thanks to its power to make the individual transcend the boundaries of earth, space, and time (Olive 2009). Its medicinal use by Native American people includes the relief of toothache, fever, rheumatism, treatment of alcoholism, and other addictions, among other uses (Shultes 1938, as cited in Dinis-Oliveira et al. 2019). Its preparation consists of cutting small discs from the cactus, which after dried can be chewed or used in the preparation of peyote tea. However, peyote has an intense bitter taste and produces nausea in most people, which explains why it is common to use gelatine capsules containing the cactus powder to avoid the bitter taste, especially among those who use it recreationally.

Mescaline was first identified and isolated in 1896 by Arthur Heffter and then synthesized by Ernst Späth in 1919. Mescaline acts similarly to other serotonergic hallucinogens, acting as an agonist for 5-HT_2 receptors, especially the 5-HT_{2C} subtype, and to a lesser extent for 5-HT_{2A} and 5-HT_{2B} subtypes (Cassels and Sáez-Briones 2018; Dinis-Oliveira et al. 2019). It has also been reported that mescaline increases the release and/or reuptake of serotonin and presents mild dopaminergic activity. Mescaline has low lipophilicity compared to other hallucinogens of the same class, and as a consequence crosses the blood–brain barrier with greater difficulty, and higher doses are needed to produce similar effects to other hallucinogens (Páleníček et al. 2008). On the other hand, its effects last longer than those of other similar hallucinogens, such as psilocybin and LSD. It is also relevant to mention that peyote has several mescaline-like alkaloids and it is postulated that some of them also contribute to its hallucinogenic effects, as well as some of its metabolites also appear to be biologically active. For a review on pharmacokinetics and pharmacodynamics aspects of mescaline, it is suggested to read Dinis-Oliveira et al. (2019).

According to this review published by Dinis-Oliveira et al. (2019), the use of mescaline has been proposed for the treatment of depression, anxiety, obsessive compulsive disorder, and drug addiction. In addition, members of the *Native American Church* report that mescaline is used to relieve symptoms of alcohol withdrawal and to reduce relapse (recurrence) rates of use (Dinis-Oliveira et al. 2019; Winkelman 2014). A study conducted by Halpern et al. (2005) with members of the

Native American Church concluded that there is no evidence of cognitive or psychological impairment among regular peyote users within the religious context. However, controlled clinical studies supporting the use of mescaline for the treatment of drug addiction and other psychiatric conditions are still lacking.

In summary, the available literature indicates that mescaline, at higher concentrations than other serotonergic hallucinogens, produces hallucinogenic effects with a slower onset and longer duration, acting mainly as a 5-HT_{2C} agonist. Furthermore, mescaline apparently does not produce cognitive and psychological damage when used by practitioners within religious contexts, but its therapeutic potential still needs to be better examined.

3,4- *Methylenedioxy-Methamphetamine* (MDMA)

MDMA or ecstasy, as it is best known, is a methamphetamine derivative first synthesized in 1912 by the German chemist Anton Kollsch and patented by the pharmaceutical industry Merck. Although this potent psychotropic remained forgotten for many years, its use became popular in the scientific world in the 1970s through the US psychiatrist Leo Zeff, which introduced it into his psychotherapy practices as did other therapists later. In the following years, MDMA became popular for recreational use, this time under the popular name of "ecstasy," "molly," or "candy," becoming one of the main drugs used in the scenario of clubs and electronic parties. It is worth mentioning that in this chapter, the therapeutic use of this substance will be approached based on research and practices in which only its pure form was used, because, with the growing increase in the use of MDMA, countless substances (contaminants and adulterants) began to be added in its composition in order to cheapen the drug or enhance its effects. Among the contaminants commonly mixed with MDMA are caffeine, ephedrines, cocaine, other amphetamine derivatives, hallucinogens in general, among others (Cole et al. 2002; Sherlock et al. 2008; Togni et al. 2015).

Pharmacologically, MDMA has general common properties of both hallucinogens and amphetamine stimulants, acting primarily as a potent catecholamine reuptake inhibitor, but also facilitating the release of catecholamines and serotonin in the synaptic cleft. With the recent resurgence of research involving hallucinogens, the concern regarding the toxicity of MDMA has also returned. However, this issue is still approached in a contradictory and non-homogeneous way, mainly due to the divergence between the academic-scientific environment and the mainstream media. Studies conducted both in animals and humans show that although there is evidence of serotonergic depletion generated by MDMA and loss of cognitive performance as memory and attention, the use of controlled doses and in assisted environments with the necessary support presents evidence of certain safety (Doblin et al. 2014; Parrott et al. 2013; Parrott 2014).

Great part of data and research related to clinical use of MDMA precedes the classification of MDMA as a Schedule 1 drug in the classification of narcotic drugs, which includes drugs with high potential for addiction and undetermined toxicity. The group of Peter Gasser has contributed valuable information to the scientific community, with a total of 171 participants being treated for different mental disorders between 1988 and 1993 and assessed on the long term under the joint treatment of MDMA and psycholytic and/or psychedelic therapy. Of these, 121 participants answered the final follow-up questionnaire, of which 84.3% reported an improvement in quality of life, and more than 90% claimed an improvement in the disorder they were being treated for (Gasser 1994).

In recent years, the great interest by general public and the growing number of studies on hallucinogens have brought MDMA to the spotlight again. This substance is one of the most researched as potential treatment for Post-traumatic Stress Disorder (PTSD) and possibly in the most advanced phase of study and clinical use among hallucinogens with this capacity, in addition to therapeutic potential for depression and anxiety (Holland 2001). The most recent clinical studies with MDMA have focused on the treatment of PTSD, especially among those resistant to conventional treatments. In a study of patients diagnosed with PTSD the participants were divided into two groups: the control group received placebo ($n = 8$) and the experimental group ($n = 12$) administration of 125 mg of MDMA as the main dose, added of 62.5 mg 2 h later (Mithoefer et al. 2011). Each session with the hallucinogen lasted approximately 8 h and was interrupted in 4 weeks under double-blind conditions. Additionally, 11 psychotherapy sessions were performed in the weeks without the drug, totaling 2 months of intervention. The results were promising, succeeding in a significant reduction in the CAPS scale (instrument that assists the professional in the correct diagnostic evaluation of PTSD) in the group that received MDMA compared to the placebo group, 4 days after each session and 2 months after the second session. It is interesting to note that 4 days after the second session, 10 of the 12 participants who received MDMA had a significant decrease in the CAPS scale, against 2 in 8 of the placebo group (Mithoefer et al. 2011).

Following a similar protocol and with the same doses, another double-blind randomized study divided the participants into two groups, one received the total dose of the hallucinogen ($n = 8$), while the other group ($n = 4$) received a sub-perceptual dose of the hallucinogen. The group that received the full dose reported an improvement in PTSD although it showed no statistically significant difference when analyzed the CAPS pre- and post-treatment scale. Finally, the researchers conclude that the results obtained with three sessions guided and assisted by the hallucinogen were more effective than two sessions (Oehen et al. 2013).

It is important to highlight the important role played by the Multidisciplinary Association for Psychedelic Studies (MAPS, http://www.maps.org), a non-profit organization that since 1986 has been actively promoting research and developing new practices using hallucinogens and cannabinoids. MAPS has been promoting research with serious and responsible groups, following great scientific criteria. MAPS is currently investigating the potential of MDMA-associated therapies for a possible cure for PTSD, as well as chronic and social anxiety and cases of depression (Johnson 2018). Its results are promising, and in a pilot study nearly 80% of participants no longer presented the criterion for PTSD after the end of treatment, which consisted of two sessions with MDMA and a follow-up period of 1 month (Ot'alora et al. 2018). It is also interesting to note that MDMA treatment is in phase 3 clinical stage and the study is carried out in partnership with the US Armed Forces for the treatment of war veterans, in addition to being accompanied by the Food and Drug Administration (Johnson 2018; Mithoefer et al. 2019).

Finally, a recent study showed that MDMA can influence the critical period of some emotional aspects (Nardou et al. 2019). The critical period is a stage of development in which the nervous system is extremely sensitive to specific environmental stimuli, becoming important for the learning and maturation of brain circuits. Thus, numerous research groups around the world seek to encourage the reopening of these critical periods for therapeutic purposes. Romain Nardou's group showed evidence that the regulation of oxytocin-mediated synaptic plasticity in the nucleus accumbens establishes a critical period for social reward learning, and a single dose of MDMA is able to modulate this reopening by interacting with oxytocin (Nardou et al. 2019). These findings corroborate research in the field and give additional incentive to researchers and enthusiasts of the potential of this substance and to understand the pathogenesis of certain neurodevelopmental diseases and psychopathologies, especially PTSD.

Ketamine

The history of ketamine begins with the synthesis of phencyclidine in March 1956 by Dr. Harold Maddox, a chemist at the American laboratory Parke & Davis (Maddox et al. 1965). Initial studies revealed that this substance produced varied effects depending on the animal species and the dosage used. In rodents, hyperactivity was frequently observed, while in dogs and monkeys a more sedative effect was observed (Chen et al. 1959). In all animal species tested, large doses resulted in a cataleptic or general anesthetic response, while even higher dosages resulted in the development of convulsions. Potential therapeutic uses in humans considered at the time included pre- and post-operative analgesia, surgical anesthesia, and treatment of mental disorders (Domino 1964, 2010).

Subsequently, the Parke & Davis laboratory continued to develop phencyclidine analogues that would have similar pharmacological activities without the adverse effects observed in humans with the drug, such as manic episodes, hallucinations, and delirium. As part of this effort, ketamine was discovered in 1965, and despite its similar chemical structure to phencyclidine, initial studies suggested that it had fewer adverse effects in humans, providing safe and effective sedation, analgesia and amnesia (Harari and Netzer 1994; Jansen 2004). Its action is mainly explained by acting as a potent antagonist to N-methyl-D-aspartate (NMDA) glutamate receptors (Haas and Harper 1992), reducing the excitability of the central nervous system. Ketamine is currently used as a dissociative anesthetic mainly in veterinary medicine although it can also be used in clinics and is approved by regulatory agencies in several countries around the world. Among the main limitations of ketamine are its psychotomimetic and dissociative effects, including hallucinations, changes in mood and affection, confusion, and the potential to generate abuse and dependence (Tyler et al. 2017), which makes its use in humans limited and quite controlled.

The potential of ketamine to treat psychiatric disorders was first reported by Khorramzadeh and Lotfy (1973). In 1974, in Argentina its use was combined with psychoanalytic therapy (Fontana and Loschi 1974). During this period, doctors in Mexico began to use it in group psychotherapy, combining psychoanalytical techniques with indigenous Mexican healing ceremonies (Roquet 1974). In recent years, ketamine has become a promising candidate as an antidepressant drug in the treatment of Major Depression Disorder (MDD), including treatment-resistant depression (TRD) with a lower clinical onset than conventional antidepressants (Abdallah et al. 2015; Zanos et al. 2016).

To date, more than 100 clinical trials related to ketamine and depression have been recorded in the U.S. National Library of Medicine (ClinicalTrials.gov) database. In 2000, the first double-blind, placebo-controlled clinical trial in the treatment of MDD was conducted at Yale University (Berman et al. 2000). In this study, seven patients underwent 2 days of treatment at intervals of at least 1 week and were treated with ketamine hydrochloride (0.5 mg/kg—intravenous route) or saline solution for 40 min. After administration, the patients completed the Hamilton and Beck Depression Assessment Scales, the Visual Analogue Scale, and the Psychiatric Brief Assessment Scale at different time intervals, and the results indicated a significant improvement in depressive symptoms within 72 h after administration of ketamine hydrochloride compared to patients who received the placebo, suggesting the antidepressant potential of ketamine and reinforcing the need for further studies. Other studies were conducted with a similar approach, for example, Zarate et al. (2012) conducted a study with 15 individuals with bipolar depression types I and II. Treatment with a simple intravenous dose of ketamine (0.5 mg/kg) produced a rapid and robust response in patients, confirming previous data obtained by the same group in another sample of patients (Diazgranados et al. 2010). The same group had also demonstrated the efficacy of ketamine in patients with TRD (Zarate et al. 2006). Several other studies also support the rapid and persistent effect of ketamine for the treatment of depression, including depression in anxious patients and TRD (Voineskos et al. 2020).

In 2018, a randomized clinical trial evaluated the effect of ketamine in 80 patients diagnosed with MDD and suicidal ideation using the Montgomery–Åsberg Depression Rating Scale, Beck Depression Inventory, and Profile of Mood States (Grunebaum et al. 2018). The treatment produced a significant anti-suicide response rate of 55% in 24 h after intravenous administration of 0.5 mg/kg ketamine hydrochloride when compared to the administration of midazolam (0.02 mg/kg in 100 mL of saline solution). Recently, a secondary analysis was performed by Phillips et al. (2020) with data from 31 patients from a double-blind, placebo-controlled randomized clinical trial in the treatment of TRD with ketamine. The results suggest that ketamine is capable of reducing suicidal ideation in individuals with TRD, with the effects being more prolonged after repeated administration.

Ketamine is available in the form of two enantiomers: the S(+) and R(−) configurations. S(+) ketamine has approximately five times more affinity for the NMDA receptor than the R(−) form (Vollenweider et al. 1997) and it is postulated that in equimolar doses, S(+) ketamine promotes greater analgesic and anesthetic activity with fewer psychotomimetic effects than the racemic mixture and the R(−) form, providing similar clinical benefits with fewer adverse effects (Muller et al. 2016). It is worth noting that the hypothesis that S(+) ketamine provides better antidepressant efficacy than racemic ketamine under controlled conditions has not yet been confirmed in a clinical trial. Moreover, the possibility that different mechanisms of action may be involved in obtaining anesthetic, analgesic, sedative, and antidepressant activity with ketamine remains debatable.

In addition to its antidepressant effects, a single sub-anesthetic dose of racemic ketamine hydrochloride (0.5 mg—intravenous route), administered for 40 min in 26 patients with TRD, and in a second study three times a week for 12 days in nine patients also with TRD, produced a significant reduction in the probability of suicide, lasting for 12 days (Price et al. 2009). Patients were evaluated 2 h before and 24 h after administration of the substance through the Montgomery–Åsberg Depression Rating Scale and the Implicit Association Test, a performance-based measure of association between concepts useful in assessing suicide.

The potential of ketamine on the treatment of drug dependence was evaluated by a double-blind randomized clinical trial in which 90 heroin-dependent were distributed in two groups that received existential psychotherapy combined with a high dose (2.0 mg/kg) or a low dose (0.2 mg/kg) of intramuscular ketamine (Krupitsky et al. 2002). After the first 2 years of follow-up, a higher rate of abstinence, larger and lasting reductions in craving, and a positive change in the unconscious nonverbal emotional attitude were observed in individuals who were treated with a high dose of ketamine, compared to the group that received a low dose of this substance.

The efficacy, safety, and tolerability of ketamine use for the treatment of mood disorders are discussed in a review by Abdallah et al. (2015) and a meta-analysis of the studies conducted is presented by Coyle and Laws (2015). The enthusiasm in the psychiatric research community is notorious for the possible discovery of a new class of antidepressants with a distinct mechanism from conventional antidepressants that act on monoamine neurotransmission systems. Recently, several clinical studies have been conducted with a ketamine analogue, esketamine, administered in the form of nasal spray for the treatment of depression and schizophrenia (Popova et al. 2019; Canuso et al. 2018). However, there are doubts about the adverse effects resulting from the chronic use of ketamine and concerns because it is a substance with potential for abuse. Thus, the challenge remains to establish an effective protocol that maintains the clinical antidepressant effect of ketamine observed in acute administration, while there is long-term safety, specifically regarding the potential for neurological and urological toxicity, as well as induction of substance use disorders.

Ibogaine

Ibogaine is one of the alkaloids present in the root of the iboga (*Tabernanthe iboga*), an African bush native to the central-west coast of Africa. Historically, the iboga root was used as a physical and mental invigorant, along with aphrodisiac properties. Although its use in ritualistic and spiritual contexts in Africa, especially in the Bwiti religion, is made from the ingestion of the plant root, in this chapter we will discuss the use of isolated ibogaine alkaloid. The ibogaine was isolated in 1900 by Édouard Landrin who carried out several experiments on animals to evaluate its effects on the circulatory, respiratory, muscular, and nervous systems (Landrin 1905). Since that time, Landrin already observed the therapeutic potential of this alkaloid as a cardiac regulator, appetite stimulator and for its neurasthenic effects (Landrin 1905). Recently, the world scientific and cultural scene has focused its attention on the detoxifying properties of ibogaine (Brown 2013).

Ibogaine is a tryptamine (monoamine alkaloid found in plants, fungi, and animals and chemically related to the amino acid tryptophan) and acts on different neurotransmission systems in the central nervous system. It presents affinity for NMDA receptors, kappa opioid receptors, sigma-type receptors, and nicotinic receptors, besides being a 5-HT_{2A} receptor agonist. Its metabolite noribogaine acts as a potent inhibitor of serotonin reuptake (Maillet et al. 2015), decreases dopamine levels, interacting in its absorption, besides increasing the metabolization of this neurotransmitter (Glick et al. 2001; Wells et al. 1999).

The toxicity of iboga and its active compounds is the subject of studies and concern for the Western scientific community since the discovery of the plant. In high doses, the consumption of iboga or its alkaloid ibogaine, as well as its metabolite noribogaine, may induce toxicity in the cardiovascular system and neurotoxic effects, and there are reports of deaths related to its use (Kubiliene et al. 2008; Popik and Glick 1996).

The consumption of iboga root is linked to several therapies; however, what has most attracted the attention of the academic-scientific environment is its use as a detoxifier and to treat drug addiction. Ibogaine has shown promising effects in animal models of dependence, such as self-administration, conditioned preference, among others. Its anti-addictive potential so far has been evaluated mainly in the case of opioids (Cappendijk et al. 1994; Leal et al. 2003), but other studies also suggest that ibogaine is useful to treat dependence on other substances of abuse. In this sense, studies using the model of self-administration in rodents showed a decrease in the self-administration behavior of morphine (Glick et al. 1991, 1994), cocaine (Glick et al. 1994), amphetamine (Maisonneuve et al. 1992), methamphetamine (Pace et al. 2004), and alcohol (Rezvani et al. 1995).

Recently, a considerable increase in the number of studies in humans has been observed. In a clinical study of 33 opioid-dependent patients, 29 (88%) showed a drastic reduction in the signs of abstinence from the drug after sessions of assisted psychotherapy with an acute dose of approximately 20 mg/kg of ibogaine (Alper et al. 1999). Another study also focused on opioid detoxification found that the 32 participants showed a reduction in opioid withdrawal symptoms, in addition to an improvement in depressive symptoms, months after treatment, which consisted of acute use of 800 mg fixed-dose ibogaine within a treatment that lasted between 12 and 14 days, including counseling sessions, therapies, and a period of detoxification (Mash et al. 2001). In other research using internationally consolidated metrics such as COWS (Clinical Opioid Withdrawal Scale), SOWS (Subjective Opioid Withdrawal Scale), and BSCS (Brief Substance Craving Scale), a significant reduction in the effects of the abstinence syndrome was found, in addition to the increased abstinence time experienced by participants who were treated with a dose between 18 and 20 mg/kg of alkaloid (Malcolm et al. 2018).

In another study, 75 users of alcohol, cannabis, cocaine, and crack were followed for treatment in rehabilitation clinics for addicts in Brazil, using cognitive-behavioral therapy in combination with ibogaine treatment. In total, the 75 users participated in 134 sessions with alkaloid use, most of which received between 1 and 3 doses of approximately 17 mg/kg, and 61% of the participants were able to remain abstinent from drug use during the follow-up questionnaires, and no fatalities or serious clinical adversities were observed. Those treated with only one dose of ibogaine reported a mean abstinence time of 5.5 months, while those treated with multiple sessions had a mean abstinence of 8.4 months. Thus, this study suggests that treatment with ibogaine is effective in prolonging periods of abstinence in users, but stresses that for safety reasons the use of ibogaine should be conducted in appropriate clinics with experienced and qualified professionals (Schenberg et al. 2014).

Finally, it is interesting to mention 18-methoxycoronaridine (18-MC), a synthetic derivative of ibogaine, first synthesized in 1996. 18-MC presents promising results in diminishing the reinforcing capacity of a variety of drugs of abuse, including cocaine, nicotine, methamphetamine, and alcohol, in addition to reducing the levels of extracellular dopamine in the nucleus accumbens (Glick et al. 1998, 2006), a region known as reward pathway and closely related to biological mechanisms of dependence. Furthermore, 18-MC does not produce the side effects such as tremors, bradycardia, and neurotoxicity reported for ibogaine (Glick et al. 2000; Molinari et al. 1996), making it an interesting target for future research on the therapeutic potential of drug dependence.

Salvinorin A: *Salvia divinorum*

Salvia divinorum, commonly called "pastora," "sage," or just "salvia," is a plant of the mint family (Lamiaceae) and of the same genus as *Salvia officinalis*, an aromatic and medicinal species. It comes from a small region of Mexico, Oaxaca, region of the Mazatec Indians. *Salvia divinorum* has been used by the Mazatec culture for centuries for ritualistic and therapeutic purposes, as a medicine to treat diarrhea, headaches, rheumatism, anemia, among others (Zawilska and Wojcieszak 2013). However, it was only in 1939 that it became known in the academic-scientific community (Johnson 1939). Its main psychoactive component is salvinorin A, a neoclerodan diterpene that was isolated only in 1982 (Ortega et al. 1982) and whose properties were confirmed in 1994 (Siebert 1994).

Pharmacologically, salvinorin A acts differently from most of the substances mentioned in this chapter, since it does not have affinity for 5-HT_{2A} serotonin receptor (Roth et al. 2002). More recent research, both in animals and in vitro, shows that salvinorin A acts as a selective agonist for kappa opioid receptors (Butelman et al. 2010; Maqueda et al. 2016; Roth et al. 2002), in addition to acting as an allosteric modulator for endocannabinoid type 1 receptor (Braida et al. 2008; Coffeen and Pellicer 2019). Activation of kappa opioid receptor is related to reduction of synaptic dopamine in the nucleus accumbens and caudate/putamen (Ebner et al. 2010), this effect being the opposite of those of drugs such as cocaine and amphetamine, which increase dopamine release in these regions and in the mesolimbic pathway, or reward pathway (Volkow et al. 2002).

Currently, an increasing use of salvia as a substance for recreational use is observed, due to the easy access and similar effect to other better known hallucinogens, which has also contributed to the increased interest in the scientific community, as has been observed for other hallucinogenic drugs. In this scenario, research focusing on the therapeutic potential of salvia has emerged. The analgesic and anti-inflammatory potential of salvia has been explored (Coffeen and Pellicer 2019), as well as its potential in the treatment of addiction to stimulants, in view of its action on kappa opioid receptors. It has been reported that kappa opioid receptor agonists have anti-addictive potential in drug use (Prisinzano et al. 2008). A study of an experimental kappa agonist drug showed its ability to prevent brain changes observed after chronic cocaine use in rodents (Tomasiewicz et al. 2008). Another study showed that salvinorin A blocked motor sensitivity generated by cocaine intake by rats (Chartoff et al. 2008).

A series of studies sought to better elucidate the behavioral and physiological effects of salvinorin A, these addressed in a review by Garcia-Romeu et al. (2016). It is relevant to mention that although traditional use by Mexican shamans is in the form of drinking or chewing the leaves, in recreational use *Salvia divinorum* is commonly used by inhalation or smoking (Cunningham et al. 2011). Some research has shown that inhaled use leads to intense psychomimetic effects and increases levels of cortisol and prolactin (Ranganathan et al. 2012). Dissociative effects are reported, in which the user has the perception of detachment from reality (Maqueda et al. 2015) with intense perceptual changes (Addy et al. 2015). On the other hand, inhalation has not produced effects commonly observed with other recreational substances, such as LSD and other hallucinogens for which anxiogenic effects are reported (MacLean et al. 2013) or changes in blood pressure and heart rate (Addy 2012; Johnson et al. 2011; Ranganathan et al. 2012).

Due to the effects of salvinorin A resulting in decreased activation of the mesolimbic dopaminergic pathway, recreational use of salvia is not expected to be associated with addiction. In an online survey, 155 users of the plant were evaluated with a scale that measures the severity of addiction to a drug (SDS, Severity of Dependence Scale). No respondents completed the requirements for addiction related to salvia use (Sumnall et al. 2011). In another online survey, this time with

500 participants, using the DSM-IV criteria for drug abuse and dependence, nobody was qualified as suffering substance abuse disorders (Baggott et al. 2010).

In the case of *Salvia divinorum*, ritualistic use or the search for mystical effects is an important factor in users' experiences, both for recreational and therapeutic purposes. Consistent with indigenous uses, laboratory references indicate that the use of salvinorin A can generate experiences with mystical or spiritual aspects (MacLean et al. 2013). Spiritual experiences such as shamanic experiences, out-of-body experience, contact with entities, and change in perception of reality are reported by users of salvia (Nygård 2007). It is interesting that the diversity of experiences under the effects of hallucinogens, especially salvia, which presents an atypical mechanism of action, gives us open questions about the importance of biological aspects of drugs in the experiences, as reported by Addy et al. (2015). In this way, opportunities are opened for future research regarding the role and functions of the kappa opioid system and other mechanisms in the human organism and the study of consciousness.

Marijuana

Marijuana or Cannabis (*Cannabis sativa*) is possibly the most studied psychoactive plant by humans. Its use as a medicinal plant is millenary and marijuana is probably the most used drug in the world for recreational purposes. The main active compounds of marijuana are cannabidiol and delta-9-tetrahydrocannabinol (Δ^9-THC), the latter being mainly responsible for its psychoactive effects. The recreational use of marijuana is illicit in Brazil, but its use has been decriminalized in several countries and the approval of its medical use has grown worldwide. Despite being part of the list of prohibited substances with restricted therapeutic use (schedule 1) there are numerous studies that indicate that marijuana, or its active constituents, is effective for the treatment of various diseases and clinical conditions, such as neuropathic pain, epilepsy, multiple sclerosis, post-traumatic stress disorder, against nausea in patients undergoing chemotherapy, to improve appetite in patients with cancer and HIV, among other uses (Garcia-Romeu et al. 2016). Recently, several drugs containing marijuana extract, its isolated constituents (mainly cannabidiol), or synthetic analogues have been developed, but there is also the prescription of marijuana as a cigarette or preparations of marijuana oil with enriched cannabidiol content. Despite several scientific evidences, there is still a lot of resistance from some governments and part of society, which makes it difficult to register marijuana medicines. The therapeutic use of marijuana medicines has recently been approved in Brazil, but its cultivation remains prohibited in the country Ministério da Saúde 2019.

Because we have a wide literature available with easily accessible publications and because it is not a classic hallucinogen, we have chosen not to address marijuana in this chapter. For an overview of the therapeutic use of marijuana or its active ingredients, the following recent reviews are recommended: Amin and Ali (2019), Bonaccorso et al. (2019), Hoch et al. (2019), White (2019).

Final Considerations

This chapter showed that despite the growing interest in the therapeutic use of hallucinogens and the existence of clinical studies, most studies on psychedelic substances still date back to the 1950s and 1960s, and much of the information on the effects and mechanisms of action of these substances are still dependent on pioneering studies. However, some of these studies are not easily accessible and sometimes they used methodologies that would not be accepted today, and it is important to better understand the risks and potentials of such substances based on current evidence. On the other hand, numerous studies have been published on the last few years about the pharmacological properties of hallucinogens, including controlled clinical studies, with growing evidence of the efficacy and safety of some of these substances, especially ketamine, LSD, DMT, and psilocybin. These substances have proven promising for the treatment of various psychiatric conditions, such as mood disorders and drug addiction, when used under controlled conditions and under medical supervision. Even so, new clinical studies with larger samples of patients are needed, within well planned protocols that allow the evaluation of fundamental issues such as dose, treatment time, possible adverse effects, and limitations of use. Finally, it is important to keep in mind that the therapeutic use of hallucinogenic substances is still an incipient promise and that it will probably take some years before these options become available.

References

Abdallah, C. G., Sanacora, G., Duman, S. R., & Krystal, J. H. (2015). Ketamine and rapid-acting antidepressants: A window into a new neurobiology for mood disorder therapeutics. *Annual Review of Medicine, 344*(6188), 1173–1178. https://doi.org/10.1126/science.1249098.

Addy, P. H. (2012). Acute and post-acute behavioral and psychological effects of salvinorin A in humans. *Psychopharmacology, 220*(1), 195–204. https://doi.org/10.1007/s00213-011-2470-6.

Addy, P. H., Garcia-Romeu, A., Metzger, M., & Wade, J. (2015). The subjective experience of acute, experimentally-induced Salvia divinorum inebriation. *Journal of Psychopharmacology, 29*(4), 426–435. https://doi.org/10.1177/0269881115570081.

Alper, K. R., Lotsof, H. S., Frenken, G. M. N., Luciano, D. J., & Bastiaans, J. (1999). Treatment of acute opioid withdrawal with ibogaine. *American Journal on Addictions, 8*(3), 234–242. https://doi.org/10.1080/105504999305848.

Amin, M. R., & Ali, D. W. (2019). Pharmacology of medical Cannabis[eBook]. In A. Bukiya (Ed.), *Recent advances in cannabinoid physiology, advances in experimental medicine and biology* (Vol. 1162). Cham: Springer. https://doi.org/10.1007/978-3-030-21737-2_8.

Anderson, T., Petranker, R., Christopher, A., Rosenbaum, D., Weissman, C., Dinh-Williams, L.-A., et al. (2019). Psychedelic microdosing benefits and challenges: An empirical codebook. *Harm Reduction Journal, 16*(1), 43. https://doi.org/10.1186/s12954-019-0308-4.

Baggott, M. J., Erowid, E., Erowid, F., Galloway, G. P., & Mendelson, J. (2010). Use patterns and self-reported effects of Salvia divinorum: An internet-based survey. *Drug and Alcohol Dependence, 111*(3), 250–256. https://doi.org/10.1016/j.drugalcdep.2010.05.003.

Barbosa, P. C. R., Giglio, J. S., & Dalgalarrondo, P. (2005). Altered states of consciousness and short-term psychological after-effects induced by the first time ritual use of ayahuasca in an

urban context in Brazil. *Journal of Psychoactive Drugs, 37*(2), 193–201. https://doi.org/10.1080/02791072.2005.10399801.
Barbosa, P. C. R., Strassman, R. J., Da Silveira, D. X., Areco, K., Hoy, R., Pommy, J., et al. (2016). Psychological and neuropsychological assessment of regular hoasca users. *Comprehensive Psychiatry, 71*, 95–105. https://doi.org/10.1016/j.comppsych.2016.09.003.
Berman, R. M., Cappiello, A., Anand, A., Oren, D. A., Heninger, G. R., Charney, D. S., & Krystal, J. H. (2000). Antidepressant effects of ketamine in depressed patients. *Biological Psychiatry, 47*(4), 351–354. https://doi.org/10.1016/S0006-3223(99)00230-9.
Bienemann, B., Ruschel, N. S., Campos, M. L., Negreiros, M. A., & Mograbi, D. C. (2020). Self-reported negative outcomes of psilocybin users: A quantitative textual analysis. *PLoS One, 15*(2), e0229067. https://doi.org/10.1371/journal.pone.0229067.
Bogenschutz, M. P., Forcehimes, A. A., Pommy, J. A., Wilcox, C. E., Barbosa, P., & Strassman, R. J. (2015). Psilocybin-assisted treatment for alcohol dependence: A proof-of-concept study. *Journal of Psychopharmacology, 29*(3), 289–299. https://doi.org/10.1177/0269881114565144.
Bonaccorso, S., Ricciardi, A., Zangani, C., Chiappini, S., & Schifano, F. (2019). Cannabidiol (CBD) use in psychiatric disorders: A systematic. *Neurotoxicology, 74*, 282–298. https://doi.org/10.1016/j.neuro.2019.08.002.
Bouso, J. C., González, D., Fondevila, S., Cutchet, M., Fernández, X., Ribeiro Barbosa, P. C., et al. (2012). Personality, psychopathology, life attitudes and neuropsychological performance among ritual users of ayahuasca: A longitudinal study. *PLoS One, 7*(8), e42421. https://doi.org/10.1371/journal.pone.0042421.
Braida, D., Limonta, V., Capurro, V., Fadda, P., Rubino, T., Mascia, P., et al. (2008). Involvement of κ-opioid and Endocannabinoid system on Salvinorin A-induced reward. *Biological Psychiatry, 63*(3), 286–292. https://doi.org/10.1016/j.biopsych.2007.07.020.
Brown, T. (2013). Ibogaine in the treatment of substance dependence. *Current Drug Abuse Reviews, 6*(1), 3–16. https://doi.org/10.2174/15672050113109990001.
Butelman, E. R., Rus, S., Prisinzano, T. E., & Kreek, M. J. (2010). The discriminative effects of the κ-opioid hallucinogen salvinorin a in nonhuman primates: Dissociation from classic hallucinogen effects. *Psychopharmacology, 209*(2), 253–262. https://doi.org/10.1007/s00213-009-1771-5.
Callaway, J. C. (1988). A proposed mechanism for the visions of dream sleep. *Medical Hypotheses, 26*(2), 119–124. https://doi.org/10.1016/0306-9877(88)90064-3.
Callaway, J. C., McKenna, D. J., Grob, C. S., Brito, G. S., Raymon, L. P., Poland, R. E., et al. (1999). Pharmacokinetics of Hoasca alkaloids in healthy humans. *Journal of Ethnopharmacology, 65*(3), 243–256. https://doi.org/10.1016/S0378-8741(98)00168-8.
Callaway, J. C., Raymon, L. P., Hearn, W. L., McKenna, D. J., Grob, C. S., Brito, G. S., & Mash, D. C. (1996). Quantitation of N,N-dimethyltryptamine and harmala alkaloids in human plasma after oral dosing with ayahuasca. *Journal of Analytical Toxicology, 20*(6), 492–497. https://doi.org/10.1093/jat/20.6.492.
Camargo, M. T. L. A. (2014). Contribuição ao estudo Etnofarmacobotânico da bebida ritual de religiões afrobrasileiras denominada “vinho da Jurema” e seus aditivos psicoativos. *Revista Do Núcleo de Estudos de Religião e Sociedade, 26*, 1–20.
Canuso, C. M., Singh, J. B., Fedgchin, M., Alphs, L., Lane, R., Lim, P., et al. (2018). Efficacy and safety of intranasal esketamine for the rapid reduction of symptoms of depression and suicidality in patients at imminent risk for suicide: Results of a double-blind, randomized, placebo-controlled study. *American Journal of Psychiatry, 175*(7), 620–630. https://doi.org/10.1176/appi.ajp.2018.17060720.
Cappendijk, S. L. T., Fekkes, D., & Dzoljic, M. R. (1994). The inhibitory effect of norharman on morphine withdrawal syndrome in rats: Comparison with ibogaine. *Behavioural Brain Research, 65*(1), 117–119. https://doi.org/10.1016/0166-4328(94)90080-9.
Carhart-Harris, R. L., Kaelen, M., Whalley, M. G., Bolstridge, M., Feilding, A., & Nutt, D. J. (2015). LSD enhances suggestibility in healthy volunteers. *Psychopharmacology, 232*(4), 785–794. https://doi.org/10.1007/s00213-014-3714-z.

Carhart-Harris, R. L., Bolstridge, M., Rucker, J., Day, C. M. J., Erritzoe, D., Kaelen, M., & Nutt, D. J. (2016b). Psilocybin with psychological support for treatment-resistant depression: An open-label feasibility study. *The Lancet Psychiatry, 3*(7), 619–627. https://doi.org/10.1016/S2215-0366(16)30065-7.

Carhart-Harris, R. L., Bolstridge, M., Rucker, J., Watts, R., Erritzoe, D. E., Kaelen, M., & Nutt, D. J. (2018). Psilocybin with psychological support for treatment-resistant depression: Six-month follow-up. *Psychopharmacology, 235*, 399–408. https://doi.org/10.1007/s00213-017-4771-x.

Carhart-Harris, R. L., Muthukumaraswamy, S., Roseman, L., Kaelen, M., Droog, W., Murphy, K., et al. (2016a). Neural correlates of the LSD experience revealed by multimodal neuro-imaging. *Proceedings of the National Academy of Sciences, 113*(17), 4853–4858. https://doi.org/10.1073/pnas.1518377113.

Carlini, E. A. (2003). Plants and the central nervous system. *Pharmacology Biochemistry and Behavior, 75*, 501–512. https://doi.org/10.1016/S0091-3057(03)00112-6.

Cassels, B. K., & Sáez-Briones, P. (2018). DARK classics in chemical neuroscience: Mescaline. *ACS Chemical Neuroscience, 9*(10), 2448–2458. https://doi.org/10.1021/acschemneuro.8b00174.

Cata-Preta, E. G., Serra, Y. A., Moreira-Junior, E. d. C., Reis, H. S., Kisaki, N. D., Libarino-Santos, M., et al. (2018). Ayahuasca and its DMT- and β-carbolines - containing ingredients block the expression of ethanol-induced conditioned place preference in mice: Role of the treatment environment. *Frontiers in Pharmacology, 9*, 561. https://doi.org/10.3389/fphar.2018.00561.

Chartoff, E. H., Potter, D., Damez-Werno, D., Cohen, B. M., & Carlezon, W. A. (2008). Exposure to the selective κ-opioid receptor agonist salvinorin A modulates the behavioral and molecular effects of cocaine in rats. *Neuropsychopharmacology, 33*(11), 2676–2687. https://doi.org/10.1038/sj.npp.1301659.

Chen, G., Ensor, C. R., Russell, D., & Bohner, B. (1959). The pharmacology of 1-(1-phenylcyclohexyl) piperidine-HCl. *Journal of Pharmacology and Experimental Therapeutics, 127*(3), 241–250.

Coffeen, U., & Pellicer, F. (2019). Salvia divinorum: From recreational hallucinogenic use to analgesic and anti-inflammatory action. *Journal of Pain Research, 12*, 1069–1076. https://doi.org/10.2147/jpr.s188619.

Cole, J. C., Bailey, M., Sumnall, H. R., Wagstaff, G. F., & King, L. A. (2002). The content of ecstasy tablets: Implications for the study of their long-term effects. *Addiction, 97*(12), 1531–1536. https://doi.org/10.1046/j.1360-0443.2002.00222.x.

Coyle, C. M., & Laws, K. R. (2015). The use of ketamine as an antidepressant: A systematic review and meta-analysis. *Human Psychopharmacology, 30*(3), 152–163. https://doi.org/10.1002/hup.2475.

Cunningham, C. W., Rothman, R. B., & Prisinzano, T. E. (2011). Neuropharmacology of the naturally occurring κ-opioid hallucinogen salvinorin a. *Pharmacological Reviews, 63*(2), 316–347. https://doi.org/10.1124/pr.110.003244.

Daniel, J., & Haberman, M. (2017). Clinical potential of psilocybin as a treatment for mental health conditions. *Mental Health Clinician, 7*(1), 24–28. https://doi.org/10.9740/mhc.2017.01.024.

De Gregorio, D., Enns, J. P., Nuñez, N. A., Posa, L., & Gobbi, G. (2018). D-lysergic acid diethylamide, psilocybin, and other classic hallucinogens: Mechanism of action and potential therapeutic applications in mood disorders. *Progress in Brain Research, 242*, 69–96. https://doi.org/10.1016/bs.pbr.2018.07.008.

Diazgranados, N., Ibrahim, L., Brutsche, N. E., Newberg, A., Kronstein, P., Khalife, S., et al. (2010). A randomized add-on trial of an N-methyl-D-aspartate antagonist in treatment-resistant bipolar depression. *Archives of General Psychiatry, 67*(8), 793–802. https://doi.org/10.1001/archgenpsychiatry.2010.90.

Dinis-Oliveira, R. J., Pereira, C. L., & da Silva, D. D. (2019). Pharmacokinetic and pharmacodynamic aspects of peyote and mescaline: Clinical and forensic repercussions. *Current Molecular Pharmacology, 12*(3), 184–194. https://doi.org/10.2174/1874467211666181010154139.

Doblin, R., Greer, G., Holland, J., Jerome, L., Mithoefer, M. C., & Sessa, B. (2014). A reconsideration and response to Parrott AC (2013) "human psychobiology of MDMA or 'ecstasy':

An overview of 25 years of empirical research". *Human Psychopharmacology, 29*, 105–108. https://doi.org/10.1002/hup.2389.
Doblin, R. E., Christiansen, M., Jerome, L., & Burge, B. (2019). The past and future of psychedelic science: An introduction to this issue. *Journal of Psychoactive Drugs, 51*(2), 93–97. https://doi.org/10.1080/02791072.2019.1606472.
Domino, E. F. (1964). Neurobiology of phencyclidine (Sernyl), a drug with an unusual spectrum of pharmacological activity. *International Review of Neurobiology, 6*, 303–347. https://doi.org/10.1016/S0074-7742(08)60772-2.
Domino, E. F. (2010). Taming the ketamine tiger. *Anesthesiology, 113*(3), 678–684. https://doi.org/10.1097/ALN.0b013e3181ed09a2.
Ebner, S. R., Roitman, M. F., Potter, D. N., Rachlin, A. B., & Chartoff, E. H. (2010). Depressive-like effects of the kappa opioid receptor agonist salvinorin A are associated with decreased phasic dopamine release in the nucleus accumbens. *Psychopharmacology, 209*(2), 241–252. https://doi.org/10.1007/s00213-010-1836-5.
Fábregas, J. M., González, D., Fondevila, S., Cutchet, M., Fernández, X., Barbosa, P. C. R., et al. (2010). Assessment of addiction severity among ritual users of ayahuasca. *Drug and Alcohol Dependence, 111*(3), 257–261. https://doi.org/10.1016/j.drugalcdep.2010.03.024.
Family, N., Maillet, E. L., Williams, L. T. J., Krediet, E., Carhart-Harris, R. L., Williams, T. M., et al. (2020). Safety, tolerability, pharmacokinetics, and pharmacodynamics of low dose lysergic acid diethylamide (LSD) in healthy older volunteers. *Psychopharmacology, 237*, 841–853. https://doi.org/10.1007/s00213-019-05417-7.
Fink, M. (2004). EEG and human psychopharmacology. *Annual Review of Pharmacology, 9*(1), 241–258. https://doi.org/10.1146/annurev.pa.09.040169.001325.
Fontana, A. E., & Loschi, J. A. (1974). Antidepressive therapy with C1 581. *Acta Psiquiatrica y Psicologica de America Latina, 20*(1), 32–39.
Fuentes, J. J., Fonseca, F., Elices, M., Farré, M., & Torrens, M. (2020). Therapeutic use of LSD in psychiatry: A systematic review of randomized-controlled clinical trials. *Frontiers in Psychiatry, 10*, 943. https://doi.org/10.3389/fpsyt.2019.00943.
Garcia-Romeu, A., Davis, A. K., Erowid, E., Erowid, F., Griffiths, R. R., & Johnson, M. W. (2020). Persisting reductions in cannabis, opioid, and stimulant misuse after naturalistic psychedelic use: An online survey. *Frontiers in Psychiatry, 10*, 955. https://doi.org/10.3389/fpsyt.2019.00955.
Garcia-Romeu, A., Kersgaard, B., & Addy, P. H. (2016). Clinical applications of hallucinogens: A review. *Experimental and Clinical Psychopharmacology, 24*(4), 229–268. https://doi.org/10.1037/pha0000084.
Gasser, P. (1994). Psycholytic therapy with MDMA and LSD in Switzerland. *MAPS Newsletter, 5*(3), 3–7.
Gasser, P., Kirchner, K., & Passie, T. (2015). LSD-assisted psychotherapy for anxiety associated with a life-threatening disease: A qualitative study of acute and sustained subjective effects. *Journal of Psychopharmacology, 29*(1), 57–68. https://doi.org/10.1177/0269881114555249.
Gaujac, A., Martinez, S. T., Gomes, A. A., de Andrade, S. J., Pinto, A. d. C., David, J. M., et al. (2013). Application of analytical methods for the structural characterization and purity assessment of N,N-dimethyltryptamine, a potent psychedelic agent isolated from Mimosa tenuiflora inner barks. *Microchemical Journal, 109*, 78–83. https://doi.org/10.1016/j.microc.2012.03.033.
Glick, S. D., Kuehne, M. E., Raucci, J., Wilson, T. E., Larson, D., Keller, R. W., & Carlson, J. N. (1994). Effects of iboga alkaloids on morphine and cocaine self-administration in rats: Relationship to tremorigenic effects and to effects on dopamine release in nucleus accumbens and striatum. *Brain Research, 657*(1–2), 14–22. https://doi.org/10.1016/0006-8993(94)90948-2.
Glick, S. D., Maisonneuve, I. M., & Szumlinski, K. K. (2000). 18-Methoxycoronaridine (18-MC) and ibogaine: Comparison of antiaddictive efficacy, toxicity, and mechanisms of action. *Annals of the New York Academy of Sciences, 914*, 369–386. https://doi.org/10.1111/j.1749-6632.2000.tb05211.x.

Glick, S. D., Maisonneuve, I. M., Visker, K. E., Fritz, K. A., Bandarage, U. K., & Kuehne, M. E. (1998). 18-Methoxycoronardine attenuates nicotine-induced dopamine release and nicotine preferences in rats. *Psychopharmacology, 139*(3), 274–280. https://doi.org/10.1007/s002130050716.

Glick, S. D., Rossman, K., Steindorf, S., Maisonneuve, I. M., & Carlson, J. N. (1991). Effects and aftereffects of ibogaine on morphine self-administration in rats. *European Journal of Pharmacology, 195*(3), 341–345. https://doi.org/10.1016/0014-2999(91)90474-5.

Glick, S. D., Maisonneuve, I. M., Hough, L. B., Kuehne, M. E., & Bandarage, U. K. (2006). (±)-18-Methoxycoronaridine: A novel Iboga alkaloid congener having potential anti-addictive efficacy. *CNS Drug Reviews, 5*(1), 27–42. https://doi.org/10.1111/j.1527-3458.1999.tb00084.x.

Glick, S. D., Maisonneuve, I. M., & Szumlinski, K. K. (2001). Chapter 2 mechanisms of action of ibogaine: Relevance to putative therapeutic effects and development of a safer iboga alkaloid congener. *Alkaloids: Chemistry and Biology, 56*, 39–53. https://doi.org/10.1016/S0099-9598(01)56006-X.

Grob, C. S., Danforth, A. L., Chopra, G. S., Hagerty, M., McKay, C. R., Halberstad, A. L., & Greer, G. R. (2011). Pilot study of psilocybin treatment for anxiety in patients with advanced-stage cancer. *Archives of General Psychiatry, 68*(1), 71–78. https://doi.org/10.1001/archgenpsychiatry.2010.116.

Grunebaum, M. F., Galfalvy, H. C., Choo, T. H., Keilp, J. G., Moitra, V. K., Parris, M. S., et al. (2018). Ketamine for rapid reduction of suicidal thoughts in major depression: A midazolam-controlled randomized clinical trial. *American Journal of Psychiatry, 175*(4), 327–335. https://doi.org/10.1176/appi.ajp.2017.17060647.

Haas, D. A., & Harper, D. G. (1992). Ketamine: A review of its pharmacologic properties and use in ambulatory anesthesia. *Anesthesia Progress, 39*(3), 61–68.

Halberstadt, A. L. (2015). Recent advances in the neuropsychopharmacology of serotonergic hallucinogens. *Behavioural Brain Research, 277*, 99–120. https://doi.org/10.1016/j.bbr.2014.07.016.

Halpern, J. H., Sherwood, A. R., Hudson, J. I., Yurgelun-Todd, D., & Pope, H. G. (2005). Psychological and cognitive effects of long-term peyote use among native Americans. *Biological Psychiatry, 58*(8), 624–631. https://doi.org/10.1016/j.biopsych.2005.06.038.

Halpern, J. H., Sherwood, A. R., Passie, T., Blackwell, K. C., & Ruttenber, A. J. (2008). Evidence of health and safety in American members of a religion who use a hallucinogenic sacrament. *Medical Science Monitor: International Medical Journal Of Experimental And Clinical Research, 14*(8), 15–22.

Harari, M. D., & Netzer, D. (1994). Genital examination under ketamine sedation in cases of suspected sexual abuse. *Archives of Disease in Childhood, 70*(3), 197–199. https://doi.org/10.1136/adc.70.3.197.

Hemmateenejad, B., Abbaspour, A., Maghami, H., Miri, R., & Panjehshahin, M. R. (2006). Partial least squares-based multivariate spectral calibration method for simultaneous determination of beta-carboline derivatives in Peganum harmala seed extracts. *Analytica Chimica Acta, 575*(2), 290–299. https://doi.org/10.1016/j.aca.2006.05.093.

Heuschkel, K., & Kuypers, K. P. C. (2020). Depression, mindfulness, and psilocybin: Possible complementary effects of mindfulness meditation and psilocybin in the treatment of depression. A review. *Frontiers in Psychiatry, 11*, 224. https://doi.org/10.3389/fpsyt.2020.00224.

Hoch, E., Niemann, D., von Keller, R., Schneider, M., Friemel, C. M., Preuss, U. W., et al. (2019, February 1). How effective and safe is medical cannabis as a treatment of mental disorders? A systematic review. *European Archives of Psychiatry and Clinical Neuroscience, 269*, 87–105. https://doi.org/10.1007/s00406-019-00984-4.

Holland, J. (Ed.). (2001). *Ecstasy: The complete guide: A comprehensive look at the risks and benefits of MDMA*. Rochester, NY: Park Street Press.

Jansen, K. (2004). *Ketamine: Dreams and realities*. Sarasota, FL: Multidisciplinary Association for Psychedelic Studies.

Jefsen, O., Højgaard, K., Christiansen, S., Elfving, B., Nutt, D., Wegener, G., & Müller, H. (2019). Psilocybin lacks antidepressant-like effect in the Flinders sensitive line rat. *Acta Neuropsychiatr, 31*(4), 213–219. https://doi.org/10.1017/neu.2019.15.

Jiménez-Garrido, D. F., Gómez-Sousa, M., Ona, G., Dos Santos, R. G., Hallak, J. E. C., Alcázar-Córcoles, M. A., & Bouso, J. C. (2020). Effects of ayahuasca on mental health and quality of life in naïve users: A longitudinal and cross-sectional study combination. *Scientific Reports, 10*, 4075. https://doi.org/10.1038/s41598-020-61169-x.

Johnson, C. (2018). *Magic medicine : A trip through the intoxicating history and modern-day use of psychedelic plants and substances*. Beverly, MA: Fair Winds Press.

Johnson, J. (1939). The elements of Mazatec witchcraft. *Etnologiska Studier, 9*, 128–150.

Johnson, M. W., Garcia-Romeu, A., Cosimano, M. P., & Griffiths, R. R. (2014). Pilot study of the 5-HT2AR agonist psilocybin in the treatment of tobacco addiction. *Journal of Psychopharmacology, 28*(11), 983–992. https://doi.org/10.1177/0269881114548296.

Johnson, M. W., MacLean, K. A., Reissig, C. J., Prisinzano, T. E., & Griffiths, R. R. (2011). Human psychopharmacology and dose-effects of salvinorin A, a kappa opioid agonist hallucinogen present in the plant Salvia divinorum. *Drug and Alcohol Dependence, 115*(1–2), 150–155. https://doi.org/10.1016/j.drugalcdep.2010.11.005.

Kaelen, M., Barrett, F. S., Roseman, L., Lorenz, R., Family, N., Bolstridge, M., et al. (2015). LSD enhances the emotional response to music. *Psychopharmacology, 232*(19), 3607–3614. https://doi.org/10.1007/s00213-015-4014-y.

Ketchum, J. S. (2006). *Chemical warfare secrets almost forgotten: A personal story of medical testing of army volunteers with incapacitating chemical agents during the cold war (1955-1975)*. Santa Rosa, CA: Chembooks.

Khorramzadeh, E., & Lotfy, A. O. (1973). The use of ketamine in psychiatry. *Psychosomatics, 14*(6), 344–346. https://doi.org/10.1016/S0033-3182(73)71306-2.

Krebs, T. S., & Johansen, P. Ø. (2012, July). Lysergic acid diethylamide (LSD) for alcoholism: Meta-analysis of randomized controlled trials. *Journal of Psychopharmacology, 26*, 994–1002. https://doi.org/10.1177/0269881112439253.

Krupitsky, E., Burakov, A., Romanova, T., Dunaevsky, I., Strassman, R., & Grinenko, A. (2002). Ketamine psychotherapy for heroin addiction: Immediate effects and two-year follow-up. *Journal of Substance Abuse Treatment, 23*(4), 273–283. https://doi.org/10.1016/S0740-5472(02)00275-1.

Kubiliene, A., Marksiene, R., Kazlauskas, S., Sadauskiene, I., Razukas, A., & Ivanov, L. (2008). Acute toxicity of ibogaine and noribogaine. *Medicina, 44*(12), 984–988.

Kyzar, E. J., Nichols, C. D., Gainetdinov, R. R., Nichols, D. E., & Kalueff, A. V. (2017). Psychedelic drugs in biomedicine. *Trends in Pharmacological Sciences, 38*(11), 992–1005. https://doi.org/10.1016/j.tips.2017.08.003.

Landrin, A. (1905). *De L'Iboga Et de L'Ibogaine*. Whitefish, MT: Kessinger Publishing.

Leal, M. B., Michelin, K., Souza, D. O., & Elisabetsky, E. (2003). Ibogaine attenuation of morphine withdrawal in mice: Role of glutamate N-methyl-D-aspartate receptors. *Progress in Neuro-Psychopharmacology and Biological Psychiatry, 27*(5), 781–785. https://doi.org/10.1016/S0278-5846(03)00109-X.

Liechti, M. E. (2017). Modern clinical research on LSD. *Neuropsychophasrmacology, 42*, 2114–2127. https://doi.org/10.1038/npp.2017.86.

Liester, M. B., & Prickett, J. I. (2012). Hypotheses regarding the mechanisms of ayahuasca in the treatment of addictions. *Journal of Psychoactive Drugs, 44*(3), 200–208. https://doi.org/10.1080/02791072.2012.704590.

MacLean, K. A., Johnson, M. W., Reissig, C. J., Prisinzano, T. E., & Griffiths, R. R. (2013). Dose-related effects of salvinorin A in humans: Dissociative, hallucinogenic, and memory effects. *Psychopharmacology, 226*(2), 381–392. https://doi.org/10.1007/s00213-012-2912-9.

Maddox, V. H., Godefboi, E. F., & Parcell, R. F. (1965). The synthesis of phencyclidine and other 1-Arylcyclohexylamines. *Journal of Medicinal Chemistry, 8*(2), 230–235. https://doi.org/10.1021/jm00326a019.

Maillet, E. L., Milon, N., Heghinian, M. D., Fishback, J., Schürer, S. C., Garamszegi, N., & Mash, D. C. (2015). Noribogaine is a G-protein biased κ-opioid receptor agonist. *Neuropharmacology, 99*, 675–688. https://doi.org/10.1016/j.neuropharm.2015.08.032.

Maisonneuve, I. M., Keller, R. W., & Glick, S. D. (1992). Interaction of ibogaine and d-amphetamine: In vivo microdialysis and motor behavior in rats. *Brain Research, 579*(1), 87–92. https://doi.org/10.1016/0006-8993(92)90745-U.

Malcolm, B. J., Polanco, M., & Barsuglia, J. P. (2018). Changes in withdrawal and craving scores in participants undergoing opioid detoxification utilizing Ibogaine. *Journal of Psychoactive Drugs, 50*(3), 256–265. https://doi.org/10.1080/02791072.2018.1447175.

Maqueda, A. E., Valle, M., Addy, P. H., Antonijoan, R. M., Puntes, M., Coimbra, J., et al. (2015). Salvinorin-A induces intense dissociative effects, blocking external sensory perception and modulating interoception and sense of body ownership in humans. *International Journal of Neuropsychopharmacology, 18*, 12), 1–12),14. https://doi.org/10.1093/ijnp/pyv065.

Maqueda, A. E., Valle, M., Addy, P. H., Antonijoan, R. M., Puntes, M., Coimbra, J., et al. (2016). Naltrexone but not Ketanserin antagonizes the subjective, cardiovascular, and neuroendocrine effects of Salvinorin-A in humans. *The International Journal of Neuropsychopharmacology, 19*(7), pyw016. https://doi.org/10.1093/ijnp/pyw016.

Mash, D. C., Kovera, C. A., Pablo, J., Tyndale, R., Ervin, F. R., Kamlet, J. D., & Lee Hearn, W. (2001). Chapter 8 Ibogaine in the treatment of heroin withdrawal. In *Alkaloids: Chemistry and Biology* (Vol. 56, pp. 155–171). Amsterdam: Elsevier. https://doi.org/10.1016/S0099-9598(01)56012-5.

McKenna, D. J. (2004). Clinical investigations of the therapeutic potential of ayahuasca: Rationale and regulatory challenges. *Pharmacology and Therapeutics, 102*(2), 111–129. https://doi.org/10.1016/j.pharmthera.2004.03.002.

Mendes, F. R., & Prado, D. R. (2017). Uso da fitoterapia no tratamento da dependência de drogas. In *Inovações no tratamento de dependência de drogas* (pp. 53–70). Rio de Janeiro, Brazil: Atheneu.

Meres Costa, M. C., Figueiredo, M. C., & De Santos Cazenave, S. O. (2005). Ayahuasca: Uma abordagem toxicológica do uso ritualístico. *Revista de Psiquiatria Clinica, 32*(6), 310–318. https://doi.org/10.1590/S0101-60832005000600001.

Ministério da Saúde, Agência Nacional de Vigilância Sanitária. (2019). *Resolução da Diretoria Colegiada - RDC N° 327*. Retrieved from http://www.in.gov.br/en/web/dou/-/resolucao-da-diretoria-colegiada-rdc-n-327-de-9-de-dezembro-de-2019-232669072

Mithoefer, M. C., Feduccia, A. A., Jerome, L., Mithoefer, A., Wagner, M., Walsh, Z., et al. (2019). MDMA-assisted psychotherapy for treatment of PTSD: Study design and rationale for phase 3 trials based on pooled analysis of six phase 2 randomized controlled trials. *Psychopharmacology, 236*, 2735–2745. https://doi.org/10.1007/s00213-019-05249-5.

Mithoefer, M. C., Wagner, M. T., Mithoefer, A. T., Jerome, L., & Doblin, R. (2011). The safety and efficacy of ±3,4-methylenedioxymethamphetamine- assisted psychotherapy in subjects with chronic, treatment-resistant posttraumatic stress disorder: The first randomized controlled pilot study. *Journal of Psychopharmacology, 25*(4), 439–452. https://doi.org/10.1177/0269881110378371.

Molinari, H. H., Maisonneuve, I. M., & Glick, S. D. (1996). Ibogaine neurotoxicity: A re-evaluation. *Brain Research, 737*(1–2), 255–262. https://doi.org/10.1016/0006-8993(96)00739-1.

Moreno, F., Wiegand, C., Taitano, E., & Delgado, P. (2006). Safety, tolerability, and efficacy of psilocybin in 9 patients with obsessive-compulsive disorder. *The Journal of Clinical Psychiatry, 67*(11), 1735–1740. https://doi.org/10.4088/jcp.v67n1110.

Morgan, C., McAndrew, A., Stevens, T., Nutt, D., & Lawn, W. (2017). Tripping up addiction: The use of psychedelic drugs in the treatment of problematic drug and alcohol use. *Current Opinion in Behavioral Sciences, 13*, 71–76. https://doi.org/10.1016/j.cobeha.2016.10.009.

Muller, J., Pentyala, S., Dilger, J., & Pentyala, S. (2016). Ketamine enantiomers in the rapid and sustained antidepressant effects. *Therapeutic Advances in Psychopharmacology, 6*(3), 185–192. https://doi.org/10.1177/2045125316631267.

Muttoni, S., Ardissino, M., & John, C. (2019). Classical psychedelics for the treatment of depression and anxiety: A systematic review. *Journal of Affective Disorders, 258*, 11–24. https://doi.org/10.1016/j.jad.2019.07.076.

Nardou, R., Lewis, E. M., Rothhaas, R., Xu, R., Yang, A., Boyden, E., & Dölen, G. (2019). Oxytocin-dependent reopening of a social reward learning critical period with MDMA. *Nature, 569*, 116–120. https://doi.org/10.1038/s41586-019-1075-9.

Nichols, D. E. (2004). Hallucinogens. *Pharmacology and Therapeutics, 101*(2), 131–181. https://doi.org/10.1016/j.pharmthera.2003.11.002.

Nutt, D. J., King, L. A., & Nichols, D. E. (2013). Effects of schedule I drug laws on neuroscience research and treatment innovation. *Nature Reviews Neuroscience, 14*(8), 577–585. https://doi.org/10.1038/nrn3530.

Nygård. (2007). *Listening to the sage: The experience of learning from the Salvia divinorum altered state*. (Doctoral Dissertation, Institute of Transpersonal Psychology; Palo Alto, CA).

Oehen, P., Traber, R., Widmer, V., & Schnyder, U. (2013). A randomized, controlled pilot study of MDMA (±3,4- Methylenedioxymethamphetamine)-assisted psychotherapy for treatment of resistant, chronic post-traumatic stress disorder (PTSD). *Journal of Psychopharmacology, 27*(1), 40–52. https://doi.org/10.1177/0269881112464827.

Olive, M. F. (2009). Peyote and mescaline. In *Drugs, the straight facts [book series]* (p. 93). New York: Chelsea House Publishers.

Oliveira-Lima, A. J., Santos, R., Hollais, A. W., Gerardi-Junior, C. A., Baldaia, M. A., Wuo-Silva, R., et al. (2015). Effects of ayahuasca on the development of ethanol-induced behavioral sensitization and on a post-sensitization treatment in mice. *Physiology and Behavior, 142*, 28–36. https://doi.org/10.1016/j.physbeh.2015.01.032.

Ortega, A., Blount, J. F., & Manchand, P. S. (1982). Salvinorin, a new trans-Neoclerodane Diterpene from Sa/via divinorum (Labiatae). *Journal of the Chemical Society, Perkin Transactions, 1*, 2505–2508. https://doi.org/10.1039/P19820002505.

Ot'alora, G. M., Grigsby, J., Poulter, B., Van Derveer, J. W., Giron, S. G., Jerome, L., et al. (2018). 3,4-Methylenedioxymethamphetamine-assisted psychotherapy for treatment of chronic posttraumatic stress disorder: A randomized phase 2 controlled trial. *Journal of Psychopharmacology, 32*(12), 1295–1307. https://doi.org/10.1177/0269881118806297.

Pace, C. J., Glick, S. D., Maisonneuve, I. M., He, L. W., Jokiel, P. A., Kuehne, M. E., & Fleck, M. W. (2004). Novel iboga alkaloid congeners block nicotinic receptors and reduce drug self-administration. *European Journal of Pharmacology, 492*(2–3), 159–167. https://doi.org/10.1016/j.ejphar.2004.03.062.

Páleníček, T., Balíková, M., Bubeníková-Valešová, V., & Horáček, J. (2008). Mescaline effects on rat behavior and its time profile in serum and brain tissue after a single subcutaneous dose. *Psychopharmacology, 196*(1), 51–62. https://doi.org/10.1007/s00213-007-0926-5.

Palhano-Fontes, F., Barreto, D., Onias, H., Andrade, K. C., Novaes, M. M., Pessoa, J. A., & Araújo, D. B. (2019). Rapid antidepressant effects of the psychedelic ayahuasca in treatment-resistant depression: A randomized placebo-controlled trial. *Psychological Medicine, 49*(4), 655–663. https://doi.org/10.1017/S0033291718001356.

Parrott, A. C. (2014, March). MDMA is certainly damaging after 25 years of empirical research: A reply and refutation of Doblin et al. (2014). *Human Psychopharmacology, 29*, 109–119. https://doi.org/10.1002/hup.2390.

Parrott, A. C., Lock, J., Adnum, L., & Thome, J. (2013). MDMA can increase cortisol levels by 800% in dance clubbers. *Journal of Psychopharmacology, 27*, 113–114. https://doi.org/10.1177/0269881112454231.

Passie, T., Halpern, J. H., Stichtenoth, D. O., Emrich, H. M., & Hintzen, A. (2008). The pharmacology of lysergic acid diethylamide: A review. *CNS Neuroscience and Therapeutics, 14*, 295–314. https://doi.org/10.1111/j.1755-5949.2008.00059.x.

Phillips, J. L., Norris, S., Talbot, J., Hatchard, T., Ortiz, A., Birmingham, M., et al. (2020). Single and repeated ketamine infusions for reduction of suicidal ideation in treatment-resistant depression. *Neuropsychopharmacology, 45*, 606–612. https://doi.org/10.1038/s41386-019-0570-x.

Popik, P., & Glick, S. D. (1996). Ibogaine, a putatively anti-addictive alkaloid. *Drugs of the Future, 21*(11), 1109–1115.

Popova, V., Daly, E. J., Trivedi, M., Cooper, K., Lane, R., Lim, P., et al. (2019). Efficacy and safety of flexibly dosed esketamine nasal spray combined with a newly initiated oral antidepressant in treatment-resistant depression: A randomized double-blind active-controlled study. *American Journal of Psychiatry, 176*(6), 428–438. https://doi.org/10.1176/appi.ajp.2019.19020172.

Price, R. B., Nock, M. K., Charney, D. S., & Mathew, S. J. (2009). Effects of intravenous ketamine on explicit and implicit measures of suicidality in treatment-resistant depression. *Biological Psychiatry, 66*(7), 522–526. https://doi.org/10.1016/j.biopsych.2009.04.029.

Prisinzano, T. E., Tidgewell, K., & Harding, W. W. (2008). κ opioids as potential treatments for stimulant dependence. In *Drug Addiction: From Basic Research to Therapy, 7* (pp. 231–245). https://doi.org/10.1007/978-0-387-76678-2_15.

Ranganathan, M., Schnakenberg, A., Skosnik, P. D., Cohen, B. M., Pittman, B., Sewell, R. A., & D'Souza, D. C. (2012). Dose-related behavioral, subjective, endocrine, and psychophysiological effects of the κ opioid agonist Salvinorin A in humans. *Biological Psychiatry, 72*(10), 871–879. https://doi.org/10.1016/j.biopsych.2012.06.012.

Rezvani, A. H., Overstreet, D. H., & Leef, Y. W. (1995). Attenuation of alcohol intake by Ibogaine in three strains of alcohol-preferring rats. *Pharmacology, Biochemistry and Behavior, 52*(3), 615–620. https://doi.org/10.1016/0091-3057(95)00152-M.

Rocha, J. M., Osório, F. L., Crippa, J. A. S., Bouso, J. C., Rossi, G. N., Hallak, J. E. C., & dos Santos, R. G. (2019). Serotonergic hallucinogens and recognition of facial emotion expressions: A systematic review of the literature. *Therapeutic Advances in Psychopharmacology, 9*, 1–11. https://doi.org/10.1177/2045125319845774.

Roquet, S. (1974). Operacion Mazateca: Estudio de hongos y otras plantas allucinoganas—Mexicanastratamiento psicotherapeutico depsicosintesis [Th e Mazateca operation: A study of hallucinogenic plants and mushrooms—Mexican psychotherapeutic psychosynthesis]. In *Cidade do Mexico*. Mexico: Associacion Albert Schweitzer.

Ross, S., Bossis, A., Guss, J., Agin-Liebes, G., Malone, T., Cohen, B., et al. (2016). Rapid and sustained symptom reduction following psilocybin treatment for anxiety and depression in patients with life-threatening cancer: A randomized controlled trial. *Journal of Psychopharmacology, 30*(12), 1165–1180. https://doi.org/10.1177/0269881116675512.

Roth, B. L., Baner, K., Westkaemper, R., Siebert, D., Rice, K. C., Steinberg, S. A., et al. (2002). Salvinorin A: A potent naturally occurring nonnitrogenous κ opioid selective agonist. *Proceedings of the National Academy of Sciences of the United States of America, 99*(18), 11934–11939. https://doi.org/10.1073/pnas.182234399.

Rucker, J. J. H., Iliff, J., & Nutt, D. J. (2018). Psychiatry & the psychedelic drugs. Past, present & future. *Neuropharmacology, 142*, 200–218. https://doi.org/10.1016/j.neuropharm.2017.12.040.

Rucker, J. J. H., Jelen, L. A., Flynn, S., Frowde, K. D., & Young, A. H. (2016). Psychedelics in the treatment of unipolar mood disorders: A systematic review. *Journal of Psychopharmacology, 30*(12), 1220–1229. https://doi.org/10.1177/0269881116679368.

Sanches, R. F., De Lima Osório, F., Santos, R. G. D., Macedo, L. R. H., Maia-De-Oliveira, J. P., Wichert-Ana, L., et al. (2016). Antidepressant effects of a single dose of ayahuasca in patients with recurrent depression a SPECT study. *Journal of Clinical Psychopharmacology, 36*(1), 77–81. https://doi.org/10.1097/JCP.0000000000000436.

Santos, R. G. (2013). Safety and side effects of Ayahuasca in humans-an overview focusing on developmental toxicology. *Journal of Psychoactive Drugs, 45*(1), 68–78. https://doi.org/10.1080/02791072.2013.763564.

Santos, R. G., Bouso, J. C., Alcázar-Córcoles, M. Á., & Hallak, J. E. C. (2018). Efficacy, tolerability, and safety of serotonergic psychedelics for the management of mood, anxiety, and substance-use disorders: A systematic review of systematic reviews. *Expert Review of Clinical Pharmacology, 11*(9), 889–902. https://doi.org/10.1080/17512433.2018.1511424.

Santos, R. G., Grasa, E., Valle, M., Ballester, M. R., Bouso, J. C., Nomdedéu, J. F., et al. (2012). Pharmacology of ayahuasca administered in two repeated doses. *Psychopharmacology, 219*(4), 1039–1053. https://doi.org/10.1007/s00213-011-2434-x.

Santos, R. G., & Hallak, J. E. C. (2020). Therapeutic use of serotoninergic hallucinogens: A review of the evidence and of the biological and psychological mechanisms. *Neuroscience and Biobehavioral Reviews, 108*, 423–434. https://doi.org/10.1016/j.neubiorev.2019.12.001.

Santos, R. G., Valle, M., Bouso, J. C., Nomdedéu, J. F., Rodríguez-Espinosa, J., McIlhenny, E. H., et al. (2011). Autonomic, neuroendocrine, and immunological effects of Ayahuasca. *Journal of Clinical Psychopharmacology, 31*(6), 717–726. https://doi.org/10.1097/jcp.0b013e31823607f6.

Schenberg, E. E., De Castro Comis, M. A., Chaves, B. R., & Da Silveira, D. X. (2014). Treating drug dependence with the aid of ibogaine: A retrospective study. *Journal of Psychopharmacology, 28*(11), 993–1000. https://doi.org/10.1177/0269881114552713.

Schmid, Y., Enzler, F., Gasser, P., Grouzmann, E., Preller, K. H., Vollenweider, F. X., et al. (2015). Acute effects of lysergic acid diethylamide in healthy subjects. *Biological Psychiatry, 78*(8), 544–553. https://doi.org/10.1016/j.biopsych.2014.11.015.

Schultes, R., Hofmann, A., & Ratsch, C. (2001). *Plants of the gods: Their sacred, healing, and hallucinogenic powers*. Rochester, NY: Healing Arts Press.

Servillo, L., Giovane, A., Balestrieri, M. L., Cautela, D., & Castaldo, D. (2012). N-methylated tryptamine derivatives in citrus genus plants: Identification of N, N, N -trimethyltryptamine in bergamot. *Journal of Agricultural and Food Chemistry, 60*(37), 9512–9518. https://doi.org/10.1021/jf302767e.

Sherlock, K., Wolff, K., Hay, A. W., & Conner, M. (2008). Analysis of illicit ecstasy tablets: Implications for clinical management in the accident and emergency department. *Emergency Medicine Journal, 16*(3), 194–197. https://doi.org/10.1136/emj.16.3.194.

Siebert, D. J. (1994). *Salvia divinorum* and salvinorin A: New pharmacologic findings. *Journal of Ethnopharmacology, 43*(1), 53–56. https://doi.org/10.1016/0378-8741(94)90116-3.

Smith, D. E., Raswyck, G. E., & Dickerson Davidson, L. (2014). From Hofmann to the Haight Ashbury, and into the future: The past and potential of lysergic acid Diethlyamide. *Journal of Psychoactive Drugs, 46*(1), 3–10. https://doi.org/10.1080/02791072.2014.873684.

Strassman, R. (2001). *DMT: The spirit molecule*. Rochester, NY: Park Street Press.

Studerus, E., Kometer, M., Hasler, F., & Vollenweider, F. X. (2011). Acute, subacute and long-term subjective effects of psilocybin in healthy humans: A pooled analysis of experimental studies. *Journal of Psychopharmacology, 25*(11), 1434–1452. https://doi.org/10.1177/0269881110382466.

Sumnall, H. R., Measham, F., Brandt, S. D., & Cole, J. C. (2011). *Salvia divinorum* use and phenomenology: Results from an online survey. *Journal of Psychopharmacology, 25*(11), 1496–1507. https://doi.org/10.1177/0269881110385596.

Thomas, G., Lucas, P., Capler, N. R., Tupper, K. W., & Martin, G. (2013). Ayahuasca-assisted therapy for addiction: Results from a preliminary observational study in Canada. *Current Drug Abuse Reviews, 6*(1), 30–42. https://doi.org/10.2174/15733998113099990003.

Thompson, M. A., Moon, E., Kim, U. J., & Weinshilboum, R. M. (1999). Human indolethylamine N-methyl-transferase (INMT) pharmacogenetics: CDNA and gene cloning and chromosomal localization. *Clinical Pharmacology and Therapeutics, 65*(2), 171. https://doi.org/10.1016/S0009-9236(99)80216-1.

Thompson, M. A., & Weinshilboum, R. M. (1998). Rabbit lung indolethylamine N-methyltransferase: cDNA and gene cloning and characterization. *Journal of Biological Chemistry, 273*(51), 34502–34510. https://doi.org/10.1074/jbc.273.51.34502.

Togni, L. R., Lanaro, R., Resende, R. R., & Costa, J. L. (2015). The variability of ecstasy tablets composition in Brazil. *Journal of Forensic Sciences, 60*(1), 147–151. https://doi.org/10.1111/1556-4029.12584.

Tomasiewicz, H. C., Todtenkopf, M. S., Chartoff, E. H., Cohen, B. M., & Carlezon, W. A. (2008). The kappa-opioid agonist U69,593 blocks cocaine-induced enhancement of brain stimulation reward. *Biological Psychiatry, 64*(11), 982–988. https://doi.org/10.1016/j.biopsych.2008.05.029.

Tupper, K. W., Wood, E., Yensen, R., & Johnson, M. W. (2015). Psychedelic medicine: A re-emerging therapeutic paradigm. *CMAJ, 187*(14), 1054–1059. https://doi.org/10.1503/cmaj.141124.

Tyler, M. W., Yourish, H. B., Ionescu, D. F., & Haggarty, S. J. (2017). Classics in chemical neuroscience: Ketamine. *ACS Chemical Neuroscience, 8*, 1122–1134. https://doi.org/10.1021/acschemneuro.7b00074.

Voineskos, D., Daskalakis, Z. J., & Blumberger, D. M. (2020). Management of treatment-resistant depression: Challenges and strategies. *Neuropsychiatric Disorders Treatment, 16*, 221–234. https://doi.org/10.2147/NDT.S198774.

Volkow, N. D., Fowler, J. S., Wang, G.-J., & Goldstein, R. Z. (2002). Role of dopamine, the frontal cortex and memory circuits in drug addiction: Insight from imaging studies. *Neurobiology of Learning and Memory, 78*(3), 610–624.

Vollenweider, F. X., Leenders, K. L., Scharfetter, C., Antonini, A., Maguire, P., Missimer, J., & Angst, J. (1997). Metabolic hyperfrontality and psychopathology in the ketamine model of psychosis using positron emission tomography (PET) and [18F]fluorodeoxyglucose (FDG). *European Neuropsychopharmacology, 7*(1), 9–24. https://doi.org/10.1016/S0924-977X(96)00039-9.

Wells, G. B., Lopez, M. C., & Tanaka, J. C. (1999). The effects of ibogaine on dopamine and serotonin transport in rat brain synaptosomes. *Brain Research Bulletin, 48*(6), 641–647. https://doi.org/10.1016/S0361-9230(99)00053-2.

White, C. M. (2019). A review of human studies assessing Cannabidiol's (CBD) therapeutic actions and potential. *Journal of Clinical Pharmacology, 59*, 923–934. https://doi.org/10.1002/jcph.1387.

Winkelman, M. (2014). Psychedelics as medicines for substance abuse rehabilitation: Evaluating treatments with LSD, peyote, Ibogaine and Ayahuasca. *Current Drug Abuse Reviews, 7*, 101–116. https://doi.org/10.2174/1874473708666150107120011.

Zanos, P., Moaddel, R., Morris, P. J., Georgiou, P., Fischell, J., Elmer, G. I., et al. (2016). NMDAR inhibition-independent antidepressant actions of ketamine metabolites. *Nature, 533*(7604), 481–486. https://doi.org/10.1038/nature17998.

Zarate, C. A., Brutsche, N. E., Ibrahim, L., Franco-Chaves, J., Diazgranados, N., Cravchik, A., et al. (2012). Replication of Ketamine's antidepressant efficacy in bipolar depression: A randomized controlled add-on trial. *Biological Psychiatry, 23*, 1), 1–1), 7. https://doi.org/10.1038/jid.2014.371.

Zarate, C. A., Singh, J. B., Carlson, P. J., Brutsche, N. E., Ameli, R., Luckenbaugh, D. A., et al. (2006). A randomized trial of an N-methyl-D-aspartate antagonist in treatment-resistant major depression. *Archives of General Psychiatry, 63*(8), 856–864. https://doi.org/10.1001/archpsyc.63.8.856.

Zawilska, J. B., & Wojcieszak, J. (2013). Salvia divinorum: From Mazatec medicinal and hallucinogenic plant to emerging recreational drug. *Human Psychopharmacology, 28*(5), 403–412. https://doi.org/10.1002/hup.2304.

Chapter 36
Medicinal Use of Cannabis: Evidence and Therapeutic Implications

Anderson Nazareno Matos

Introduction

It is impossible to deny, there is more and more discussion on marijuana nowadays. Several countries are regulating domestic markets and offering new universes regarding the possible uses of the plant. The West experiences adult, medicinal, and industrial use in different degrees of freedom. Uruguay was a pioneer in 2013 in an experiment in which the state regulates the production process, allowing self-cultivation and cooperative clubs, as well as sale in pharmacies for adult use. All the planned stages were implemented, although curiously the regulations for medicinal use were not made, which was the way most of the countries that raised the issue began to address it. The North American scenario has also changed a lot, thirty-four states have already authorized medicinal use, and ten of them also include social use. Canada began regulating the medicinal use of cannabis in 2001, and in October 2018 it began regulating social use. In Latin America, there is the following scenario; in Brazil and Venezuela it is possible to import extracts and oils, in Chile there is cultivation in associations for medicinal use, Argentina and Colombia are preparing for the cultivation and national sale of medicinal products, Paraguay is authorizing the importation of seeds for cultivation.

What would have happened to this anti-magnet climate review? It seems possible to say that the rediscovery that the plant has several therapeutic properties and possibilities of safe use in the medical clinic has led to a resumption of research with cannabis, this would be a relevant factor in the new scenario. It also seems necessary to point out that there is a great popular pressure, mainly coming from family members and patients with serious disorders, mostly refractory to conventional treatments, which has required doctors to use marijuana products. The demand of patients on physicians has induced the medical class to review concepts and update

A. N. Matos (✉)
Conselho Regional de Psicologia de Minas Gerais, Divinópolis, MG, Brazil

D. De Micheli et al. (eds.), *Drugs and Human Behavior*,
https://doi.org/10.1007/978-3-030-62855-0_36

itself in relation to the subject. The medicinal marijuana industry has produced the unusual situation of having patients teaching their doctors about cannabis treatments. These situations have occurred in several countries in the world, the best known case is probably the girl Charlotte Figi, with the diagnosis of Dravet syndrome, about 50 daily convulsions debilitated the child more and more, taking her to the limit of what reached traditional allopathic medicine. The girl's parents became aware of reports on cannabis use in these cases and were able to medicate her with extracts rich in cannabidiol (CBD) that completely changed the child's clinical picture. The oil from the strain that was used on the girl received her name, *Charlotte's Web*, and her producers "have created a non-profit organisation in Colorado to facilitate access by people with severe epileptic syndromes to quality controlled cannabis with high amounts of Cannabidiol" (Ribeiro 2014).

Another illustrative situation would be the one set by Porter and Jacobson (2013) when the authors used parents belonging to a Facebook group dedicated to share information about the use of cannabis enriched with cannabidiol to treat seizures in children who were diagnosed with Dravet syndrome, Doose syndrome, and Lennox–Gastaut syndrome as a control group for the research. The media coverage of these cases has led to renewed scientific interest in cannabis. But certainly, the cherry on the cake is not the so controversial marijuana, but the endocannabinoid system was discovered only in the 1990s. In any case it is possible to say: marijuana, the 5000-year-old novelty returns to the scene with full force.

Historical Overview

Reports of medicinal use of cannabis are millenary, dating back to 2700 years before Christ, in Pen-ts'ao ching, a pharmacopoeia attributed to Emperor Shen-Nung there are indications for cannabis in rheumatic pain, intestinal constipation, disorders of the female reproductive system, malaria, and others. In India the records date from over 1000 AC., with reports of both religious and medical use analgesic, anticonvulsant, hypnotic, tranquilizer, anesthetic, anti-inflammatory, antibiotic, antiparasitic, antispasmodic, digestive, diuretic, aphrodisiac or anaphrodisiac, antitussive, and expectorant (Zuardi 2008). For the Assyrians, since the ninth century B.C., there was the use for edema, hematomas, depression, impotence, arthritis, renal lithiasis. Avicenas, a famous Arab doctor mentions the use of cannabis since 1000 A.D., and Muslim texts highlight the use of the plant as diuretic, digestive, antiflatulent, etc. There is a report made in 1464 by Ibn al-Badri which describes a treatment made with marijuana resin for a case of epilepsy, revealing the cure of the condition and highlighting the need to maintain the use of the plant continuously for the remission of symptoms (Zuardi 2008).

The Western world became familiar with these reports of medicinal marijuana in the nineteenth century through doctors who had experiences outside their home country and who found clinical applications and forms of treatment with the use of cannabis hitherto unknown both in Europe and the USA. William Brooke

O'Shaughnessy, an Irish doctor serving of England in Calcutta, published in 1839 "On the preparations of the Indian hemp, or Gunjah," on the occasion he reviewed the literature on the plant, tested the effect on different pathologies, described experiments where he carried out evaluating the toxicity in animals, and found therapeutic effects in humans for rheumatism, convulsions, muscle spasms of tetanus and rabies. Another report that gained prominence was the work done by the psychiatrist Jacques-Joseph Moreau, better known as Moreau du Tours. Accompanying patients on trips to exotic countries, a common practice at the time, Moreau observes the use of hashish by Arabs and decides to experiment on himself and later on his students. Moreau's expectation with the drug was to investigate the genesis of mental illness. He intended to produce an "experimental psychosis" with the use of hashish. The experiments led to the publication of the book "Du Hachisch et de l'Alienation Mental: Études Psychologiques," published in 1845. These publications impacted Western medicine, mainly due to the few therapeutic options of the time for disorders such as epilepsy, spasms, tetanus, and anger.

Soon Europe and the USA experienced the spread of cannabis products, and more than a hundred scientific papers on therapeutic cannabis were published in the second half of the nineteenth century. Several laboratories began marketing cannabis extracts or dyes, for example: Merck, Burroughs-Wellcome, Bristol-Meyers Squibb, Parke-Davis, and Eli Lilly (Zuardi 2008). In 1924 Sajou's Cyclopedia of Practical Medicine produced a summary of areas where there were clinical indications for cannabis, highlighting its use as a sedative, hypnotic, or analgesic for a substantial group of diseases (Zuardi 2008).

This would have been the "boom" in medical use of cannabis in the West, it lasted until other products or technologies emerged in both pharmacy and medicine that achieved greater efficiency or safety in handling. This would have been the case, for example, with the development of vaccines for infectious diseases such as tetanus, the emergence of aspirin, or hypodermic syringes for the injectable use of more powerful analgesics such as morphine (Zuardi 2008). But there would be other details that would influence the discontinuity of medicinal use of cannabis, such as the "active ingredient" of cannabis had not been identified, the biochemical bases of its pharmacology were unknown, the extracts from the nineteenth century were not standardized in terms of composition or dosage. There were still wide variations between products without adequate quality control and inconveniences in smoked use, and oral administration was problematic, so safety for modern standards was not clearly established (Russo 2010). Thus, although there were reports of the therapeutic effects of cannabis, and it had earned a place in the conventional pharmacopoeia for some decades, ignorance of some of its properties meant that it ended up being removed from the Western medical framework, leaving the American pharmacopoeia in 1941.

But other factors also influenced the scenario, as marijuana had already entered the scope of prohibitionism, which would become increasingly upward in the twentieth century. An international agenda had already been created since the Opium Conferences in the expectation of controlling the production, trade, and sale of some products, initially cocaine, opium, and its derivatives. At the 1924 conference in Geneva, marijuana was included in the discussions, Egyptian delegate El Guindy reported the existence of a cannabis epidemic in his country, and that the drug posed a social risk, and that it should be included in the list of substances to be proscribed. The plea received support from several delegations and led to the creation of a sub-committee to discuss the issue, composed of Britain, India, Greece, Egypt, and Brazil (França 2015). From then on, on the world stage, a climate antipathetic to marijuana arises that will gradually transform it into a drug proscribed for medicinal use and prohibited for social use.

But, the fact is, that, even receiving contraindications, the twentieth century would not see the plant disappear. The prohibition, even if it had the pretension of global reach, did not succeed, because ancestral uses, rituals, or those derived from popular practices resisted and even expanded. The counter-culture movement would make marijuana a symbol of resistance, and in the 1960s its recreational use "spread rapidly to the younger sections of the population, throughout the western world" (Zuardi 2008, p. 13). The prohibitionist climate gave more weight to the prohibition of the plant, with the Single Convention on Narcotic Drugs, promoted by the UN in 1961, and implemented in the USA by the "Controlled Substances Act" in 1970, which "gave the Drug Enforcement Administration (DEA) and the Food and Drug Administration (FDA) the responsibility to identify which substances were authorized or proscribed, according to classification in schedules I, II and III" (Pamplona 2014). Cannabis has been included in Schedule I, which characterizes drugs with no therapeutic potential and a high risk of producing addiction.

To maintain control over the plant and its prohibition, publications began to appear, and these were mainly aimed at reflecting the stance that was being built on the world stage regarding cannabis, which was the "pure and simple condemnation of marijuana as if it were an evil drug" (Carlini 2010). In an incomplete survey by the Brazilian Center for Information on Psychotropic Drugs (CEBRID) between the twentieth and twenty-first centuries, there were 470 articles made by Brazilians, 39 of them until 1955, the first being written in 1934, when the prohibitionist climate was intensifying (Carlini 2010).

The kind of focus given to marijuana will only change in the 1960s, with the pioneering work of José Ribeiro do Valle, a professor at the Escola Paulista de Medicina da Universidade Federal de São Paulo, who, through animal studies, is once again investigating the effects of cannabis extracts with the collaboration of researchers from Switzerland (Carlini 2010). But who consistently advances this research is Professor Elisaldo Carlini, who for 30 years has published no less than 57 papers, most of them in international journals (Carlini 2010).

A great leap was made in 1964 when Gaoni and Mechoulam succeeded in identifying, isolating, and synthesizing the chemical structure of Δ9 Tetrahydrocannabinol, the main psychoactive component of marijuana (Zuardi 2008). With the advancement of the studies we arrived at the discovery of cannabinoid receptors in 1988, and the endocannabinoid, anandamide, in 1992. From the moment a scientific basis was discovered it was possible to resume the use of cannabis in modern medicine (Russo 2010). Phytocannabinoids and an endogenous cannabinoid system reveals a NEW HORIZONT

Current Surveys

The discovery of the endocannabinoid system revealed the existence of natural chemical substances, it is as if the brain produced a kind of "natural marijuana." The endocannabinoid system is a neuromodulatory system consisting of two receptors coupled to protein G: cannabinoid 1 (CB1) and cannabinoid 2 receptors (CB2). CB1 receptors are located mainly in the central nervous system, in particular they are found in the cerebral cortex, cerebellum, hippocampus, and seem to play an important role in cognition, memory, learning, emotion, mood, motor activity, and motivation. In contrast, CB2 receptors are found primarily in organs and function predominantly within the immune system where they modulate cytokine release (Katzman et al. 2016).

From the cellular point of view, endocannabinoids and phytocannabinoids act on cannabinoid type 1 (CB1) receptors abundantly expressed in the brain, causing a reduction in the release of neurotransmitters and decreasing neuronal excitation. However, depending on the brain region in which the endocannabinoids are produced, they generate very different physiological effects. Some of the known functions are, for example, regulation of body temperature, regulation of appetite, reduction of pain threshold, and modulation of cognitive processes (Pamplona 2014, p. 29).

One issue that has been addressed is that the CBD is considered a beneficial molecule and THC is considered more conservative by the medical class, through the psychoactive effects known to be attributed to it, but new discoveries indicate that this may not be exactly the case:

> The CBD was initially considered non-psychoactive, i.e. devoid of brain effects. Although today it is known that this is not true […], it is true that isolated CBD does not induce the euphoric effects of THC, and still balances some adverse effects that isolated THC presents, for example, in relation to memory impairment […]. For this reason, more modern pharmacological strategies have focused on the use of a blend of THC and CBD in different proportions, to the detriment of the use of pure THC as previously thought. Pure oral THC can produce tachycardia, dysphoria, psychotic symptoms, physical and mental sedation in healthy individuals. (Pamplona 2014, p. 20).

Under the view that THC would be the "bad molecule" responsible for unwanted effects, a line of thought has focused on the idea that only CBD would be of therapeutic use, and that the absence of THC in medicinal products would be desirable. It is an idea that seems mistaken, researchers realize that the entourage effect, that is found when using the ingredients of the plant *in natura*, and not synthetic compounds, produces more beneficial effects than only the pure molecules alone, as Pamplona (2014) pointed out, reporting several adverse effects by ingesting pure THC, orally, in healthy patients.

A point that deserves attention in relation to the use of cannabis, refers to the proclaimed relationship between the use of the plant and the appearance of symptoms, psychotic symptoms, or even schizophrenia itself. Perhaps Moreau du Tours' accounts have created the basis for this hypothesis when he reports the use of hashish as an experimental psychotomimetic (Hallak et al. 2008).

Moreau located several psychological changes that could be observed under the effect of hashish; feeling of happiness, excitement and dissociation of ideas, changes in the perception of time and space, enhancement of the sense of hearing, fluctuations of emotions, irresistible impulses, delusions, and hallucinations. For Moreau some of his volunteers experienced "occurrences of delirium or real madness," which lead him to conclude that: "there is not a single elementary manifestation of mental illness that cannot be found in the mental changes caused by hashish" (Mechoulam and Parker 2013, p. 22). For Raphael Mechoulan, the discoverer of THC, this diversity of effects, contributed to confusing research on cannabis, at that time nothing was known about the molecules of the plant.

The idea that there would be a relationship between marijuana and psychosis was strongly reinforced by the first authors who talked about the plant and led researchers to try to advance more in this aspect. Professionals accompanying patients with psychotic symptoms should be concerned with making a differential diagnosis between a psychotic condition itself and an acute/transitory drug-induced psychosis. Psychotic symptoms produced by drug abuse or abstinence tend to present remission as soon as the drug is metabolized and excreted, unlike psychosis itself, which is usually longer. When psychotic symptoms occur after the use of cannabis, they usually occur acutely and soon after the use of the drug, there may be persecutory delusions and/or jealousy, anxiety, emotional lability, depersonalization, and amnesia, hallucinations are uncommon, and the pictures are usually remixed on 1 day (Hallak et al. 2008), so although it may be possible for specific psychotic symptoms to occur, it does not seem possible to say that they settle permanently. Studies that attempt to establish a causal relationship between psychosis and marijuana remain inconclusive; other studies have presented "inconsistent results in terms of differentiating or identifying a specific type of cannabis-induced psychosis" (Hallak et al. 2008).

Among attempts to explain whether there is a relationship between cannabis use and psychosis, there is the hypothesis that schizophrenic patients abuse this substance because "the occurrence of one disorder would facilitate the development of another. That is, schizophrenia could lead to substance abuse, or substance abuse could develop chronic psychosis" (Hallak et al. 2008). Another common hypothesis is that schizophrenic patients use drugs as a kind of "self-medication," also this hypothesis is controversial because it is known that "drugs such as cannabis and cocaine can exacerbate existing psychotic symptoms, precipitate the recurrence of an acute episode and cancel the effects of antipsychotic medications" (Hallak et al. 2008). However, other findings reveal that *post-mortem* studies in schizophrenic patients present a change in the cannabinoid system that occurs in schizophrenia and that is independent of recent cannabis use, that there would be a dysfunction of the endocannabinoid system, probably in a state of hyperactivity, and concluded that "the results reinforce the idea of a cannabinoid dysfunction in schizophrenia and that this anomaly would be associated with the acute phase of the disease" (Hallak et al. 2008). That is, if there appears to be some relationship between psychosis and marijuana, it appears to be more associated with a dysfunction of the endocannabinoid system itself.

Unlike the idea that cannabis could produce psychosis, it has been tested as a drug. GW Pharmaceuticals developed a study using cannabidiol in schizophrenic patients, phase II was done with 88 schizophrenic patients, who responded only partially to standard antipsychotic treatment, patients received cannabidiol or placebo in addition to their antipsychotic medication for 6 weeks. Cannabidiol was consistently superior to placebo in attenuating symptoms of schizophrenia and also in not inducing serious adverse events. Among the drugs that act on the endocannabinoid system, pre-clinical studies and subsequent data point to cannabidiol as the promising compound for the treatment of schizophrenia symptoms without inducing significant side effects (Peres et al. 2016).

It is not yet clear enough whether the cannabis–psychosis relationship is primarily beneficial or harmful. Only the progress of studies can make this field clearer, apparently the conclusion that seems most plausible is the one that points out:

> The existence of a causal relationship between substance use and long-lasting psychotic disorder remains questionable. For example, if drug use was responsible for the precipitation of schizophrenia, it would be expected that there would be a large increase in cases of people with this diagnosis, since consumption has become more common in the last 30 years. However, recent detailed epidemiological reviews have shown that this is not the case (Hallak et al. 2008, p. 167).

Another field on which several hypotheses hovered would be that of the harmful effects of marijuana on the production of "brain damage." A Mexican study (Aguirre-Velázquez 2017) addressed the relationship between the plant, its components and cases of childhood epilepsy. Epilepsy is a chronic neurological disorder that usually requires the use of several associated drugs (polypharmacy). It has been estimated that more than 50 million people worldwide suffer from epilepsy, with 85% of these patients in developing countries like Mexico. About 30–35% of patients have refractory epilepsy, which is defined as a failure to respond to two or more antiepileptic drugs. There are an estimated 1.5 million patients with epilepsy in Mexico, 30% of whom are diagnosed with refractory epilepsy. Some studies conducted in that country have reported a prevalence between 1.2% and 3% of cases of Lennox–Gastaut syndrome, a syndrome that presents in 3% of childhood epilepsy cases. Infantile epilepsy begins in the first years of life and is often characterized by frequent, severe, and resistant seizures, generating delayed neurological development and deterioration of the child's quality of life, many of these cases do not respond to conventional treatments that include antiepileptic drugs, ketogenic diet, high doses of steroids, and even neurosurgery. Realizing that the indicated treatments have failed to control their children's seizures, some parents resort to alternative treatments, one of these alternative treatments is cannabis enriched with cannabidiol. In the last decade, interest in using Cannabis sativa in household products to treat various types of childhood epilepsy has emerged and evidence of its success has spread through digital media according to Gupta (Aguirre-Velázquez 2017).

Gloss and Vickrey (2014) conducted a systematic review of four articles reporting the use of cannabis and concluded that animal studies provided sufficient justification for testing in humans. However, there is still no consistent evidence on its effectiveness and safety. Porter and Jacobson (2013) conducted an observational study of 19 children with refractory epilepsies between 2 and 16 years at Stanford University. The results of this study showed that 16 out of 19 patients (84%) had a reduced frequency of seizures with the use of cannabis sativa, other effects reported were: improved mood (79%), increased alertness (74%), improved sleep (68%), the only adverse effects reported were drowsiness (37%) and fatigue (16%). In another survey of 117 parents of children with refractory epilepsy, with a primary diagnosis of Lennox–Gastaut syndrome, with the presence of many spasms, Hussain et al. (2015) reported similar improvements over an average treatment time of 6.8 months using a mean dose of 4.3 mg/kg/day of cannabidiol (CBD). Devinsky et al. (2018) recently published the results of an FDA-approved open-center prospective clinical trial using a pharmaceutical product (Epidiolex) that is 99% CBD and reported a mean reduction in motor crises of 36.5% in the 162 children studied and an adequate safety profile for CBD was observed (Aguirre-Velázquez 2017).

Topics of Interest

In this work we highlight aspects related to psychiatric or neurological conditions. The choice was made because of the importance of this information, unknown to the majority of the public not affectionate to the subject, and which point to the possibility of questioning widely disseminated information on cannabis, such as that marijuana would cause schizophrenia, or that the use of cannabis would be particularly harmful to brain tissue. There are works that go in another direction, as some authors we have found point to the use of CBD as an antipsychotic:

> After some individual treatment attempts, the first randomized, double-blind, controlled clinical trial demonstrated that in acute schizophrenia cannabidiol exerts antipsychotic properties comparable to the antipsychotic drug amisulpiride and is accompanied by a placebo-like superior side effect profile. Since clinical improvement by cannabidiol has been significantly associated with high levels of anandamide, it seems likely that its antipsychotic action is based on mechanisms associated with increased anandamide concentrations (Rohleder et al. 2016, p. 1).

Regarding the possible damage to the brain, it is also possible to find divergent information, because some studies locate the possibility of neurogenesis from the use of cannabinoids.

> In recent years, considerable data have indicated that the endocannabinoid system plays a central role in neurogenesis […] activation of CB1 is necessary for axonal growth response […], the endocannabinoid system drives proliferation of neural progenitor cells […], cannabinoids actually promote neurogenesis. (Mechoulam and Parker 2013 p. 29.)

A large number of possibilities of using the plant in other pathologies must be considered, escaping the scope of this work to reach them on this occasion. As mentioned above, we have chosen to highlight only two types of disorders, belonging to the field of neurology and psychiatry, environments in which a number of controversies have reigned, with all sorts of captious information guiding for a long time the debate on the therapeutic or medicinal use of marijuana. Thus, it seemed appropriate to point out how wide and still unknown this universe is.

Final Considerations

The current Brazilian scenario, at the time of this work, is refractory, not very sensitive to these new findings in relation to marijuana, the debates, the legal norm, or even the access of patients to these therapies continue to be conducted by a conservative view, not very sensitive to reality. However, in spite of the internal environment, which is unfriendly to the signs that global reality reverberates over the plant, in countries where the climate is more pragmatic, companies are searching for millionaire figures from the regulated cannabis market, be it for adult or medicinal use.

At some point it seemed possible to think that advances in cannabis medicine would meet with great resistance from Big Pharma, which dominates the allopathic market. The conventional market would apparently have good reason to reject the presence of cannabis for several reasons, namely being a herbal medicine product, presenting wide therapeutic coverage without the important presence of undesirable side effects, the low toxicity, the possibility of making a very specific fine adjustment in the use of dosages, etc. But, the scenario has shown that what really happened was the emergence of cannabis pharmaceutical laboratories. Companies based in countries such as the USA, Canada, Israel, Holland already offer a wide range of products, with different delivery routes for the active ingredients, serving patients in the most diverse age groups, covering increasingly larger groups of disorders. These companies already export products, serving markets that do not yet have regulations that allow local production of cannabis or derivatives, as is the case in Brazil. In fact, these companies are already starting to set up commercial representation in these countries to remedy local demands. A report produced by The Green Hub highlights that: "With a population of more than 200 million people, the market for medicinal cannabis in Brazil may become substantial even in the context of relatively restrictive regulation" (The Green Hub 2019). Complementing the scenario immediately below:

> According to the 2016 Global Health Disease Study, one in five adults in Brazil suffer from back and neck pain, meaning that the decision to include or not include chronic pain as a clinical condition in a future medicinal cannabis program could have an influence as a determinant of patient size and population increase (The Green Hub 2019, p. 2).

And a little further on, the following projections emerge:

> If Brazil passes legislation favorable to medicinal cannabis, the number of patients could reach 959,000 in the first 36 months of legal cannabis sales in the case of a more restrictive list of approved diseases (i.e. a list that does not include chronic pain), and approximately 3.4 million in the case of a broader list of diseases and clinical symptoms that includes chronic pain. The program in which chronic pain is accepted as a condition for treatment, with the number of patients able to reach 3.4 million, could mean approximately R$4.4 billion (or US$1.4 billion) in annual revenues (The Green Hub 2019, p. 3).

Thus, the current scenario is slipping. Cannabis pharmaceutical groups are already emerging, foreseeing billionaire collections for the sector. Countries that have already made their laws and regulated markets more flexible have access to yet another therapeutic option for doctors and patients, improving with palliative care the quality of life of these patients and their families, in addition to the possibility of carrying out research with increasingly better parameters, and using products with safety and effectiveness, among other advantages. This reality is already a path without a return, cannabis is able to improve the quality of life of children in complex epileptic or autism, young and adults who have suffering of the type; anxiety, depression, psychotic symptoms, or even allergic or inflammatory symptoms that affect all ages, a very large number of elderly will reap benefits in degenerative diseases.

References

Aguirre-Velázquez, C. G. (2017). Report from a survey of parents regarding the use of cannabidiol (medicinal cannabis) in Mexican children with refractory epilepsy. *Neurology Research International., 2017*, 2985729. https://doi.org/10.1155/2017/2985729.

Carlini, E. A. (2010). A História da Cannabis Sativa L. (maconha, liamba, diamba, fumo de Angola, etc.) no Brasil. In *Centro Brasileiro de Informações sobre Drogas Psicotrópicas, Simpósio Internacional: Por uma agência brasileira da cannabis medicinal?* Retrieved from https://www.cebrid.com.br/wp-content/uploads/2012/10/Simpósio-Internacional-Por-uma-Agência-Brasileira-da-Cannabis-Medicinal.pdf

Devinsky, O., Verducci, C., Thiele, E. A., Laux, L. C., Patel, A. D., Filloux, F., et al. (2018). Open-label use of highly purified CBD (Epidiolex®) in patients with CDKL5 deficiency disorder and Aicardi, Dup15q, and Doose syndromes. *Epilepsy & Behavior, 86*, 131–137. https://doi.org/10.1016/j.yebeh.2018.05.013.

França, J. M. C. (2015). *A história da maconha no Brasil*. São Paulo, Brazil: Três Estrelas.

Gloss, D., & Vickrey, B. (2014). Cannabinoids for epilepsy. Cochrane database of systematic reviews, Wiley, Hoboken, NJ (3). doi:https://doi.org/10.1002/14651858.cd009270.pub2.

Hallak, J. E. C., Bressan, R. A., Crippa, J. A. S., & Zuardi, A. W. (2008). Cannabis e Psicose. In A. W. Zuardi, J. A. S. Crippa, & F. S. Guimarães (Eds.), *Cannabis e saúde mental: Uma revisão sobre a droga de abuso e o medicamento*. Ribeirão Preto, Brazil: FUNPEC-Editora.

Hussain, S. A., Zhou, R., Jacobson, C., Weng, J., Cheng, E., Lay, J., et al. (2015). Perceived efficacy of cannabidiol-enriched cannabis extracts for treatment of pediatric epilepsy: A potential role for infantile spasms and Lennox–Gastaut syndrome. *Epilepsy & Behavior, 47*, 138–141. https://doi.org/10.1016/j.yebeh.2015.04.009.

Katzman, M. A., Furtado, M., & Anand, L. (2016). Targeting the endocannabinoid system in psychiatric illness. *Journal of Clinical Psychopharmacology, 36*(6), 691–703. https://doi.org/10.1097/JCP.0000000000000581.

Mechoulam, R., & Parker, L. A. (2013). The endocannabinoid system and the brain. *Annual Review of Psychology, 64*, 21–47. https://doi.org/10.1146/annurev-psych-113011-143739.

Pamplona, F. A. (2014). Quais são e para que servem os medicamentos à base de Cannabis? *Revista de Biologia, 13*(1), 28–35. https://doi.org/10.7594/revbio.13.01.05.

Peres, F. F., Levin, R., Almeida, V., Zuardi, A. W., Hallak, J. E., Crippa, J. A., & Abilio, V. C. (2016). Cannabidiol, among other cannabinoid drugs, modulates prepulse inhibition of startle in the SHR animal model: Implications for schizophrenia pharmacotherapy. *Frontiers in Pharmacology, 7*, 303. https://doi.org/10.3389/fphar.2016.00303.

Porter, B. E., & Jacobson, C. (2013). Report of a parent survey of cannabidiol-enriched cannabis use in pediatric treatment-resistant epilepsy. *Epilepsy & Behavior, 29*(3), 574–577. https://doi.org/10.1016/j.yebeh.2013.08.037.

Ribeiro, F. T. (2014). Cannabis sativa: o que a neurociência tem a dizer. *Scientific American Mente e Cérebro, 259*, 28–37.

Rohleder, C., Müller, J. K., Lange, B., & Leweke, F. M. (2016). Cannabidiol as a potential new type of an antipsychotic. A critical review of the evidence. *Frontiers in Pharmacology, 7*, 422. https://doi.org/10.3389/fphar.2016.00422.

Russo, E. (2010). Therapeutic uses of cannabis: Lessons of the past, design for the future. In *Centro Brasileiro de Informações sobre Drogas Psicotrópicas, Simpósio Internacional: Por uma agência brasileira da cannabis medicinal?* Retrieved from https://www.cebrid.com.br/wp-content/uploads/2012/10/Simpósio-Internacional-Por-uma-Agência-Brasileira-da-Cannabis-Medicinal.pdf

The Green Hub. (2019). *Cannabis medicinal no Brasil: Visão geral 2018 – Resumo executivo.* Retrieved from https://cdn2.hubspot.net/hubfs/3324860/NFD-MedicalCannabisInBrazil-Port-ES-1.pdf

Zuardi, A. W. (2008). Aspectos históricos da cannabis na medicina e em saúde mental. In A. W. Zuardi, J. A. S. Crippa, & F. S. Guimarães (Eds.), *Cannabis e saúde mental: Uma revisão sobre a droga de abuso e o medicamento.* Ribeirão Preto, Brazil: FUNPEC-Editora.

Chapter 37
Drug Use and Suicidal Behavior at Work

Karina Borgonovi Silva Barbi, João Carlos Caselli Messias, and Liliana Andolpho Magalhães Guimarães

Introduction

The use of psychoactive substances is a behavioral phenomenon present all over the world, regardless of culture, social class, educational level, age, or gender, constituting one of the public health problems that still generates intense government demand for its combat. The consequences for the individual's life, in the personal, social, and work spheres, depend on the intensity of their consumption and the type of drug used. The World Health Organization (WHO) and the American Psychiatric Association (APA) define the type of consumption according to two main standards, classifying it as harmful use or abuse the pattern in which the harmful consequences may occur in the validity of the use, but without the occurrence of physical disorders (abstinence and tolerance) or behavioral related to the search for the drug, which are present in the pattern defined as dependence.

Epidemiological data on substance use indicate that alcohol is the most widely consumed legal substance in the world. According to the WHO, in 2016 the global average annual consumption of pure alcohol per person over 15 years of age was 6.4 liters (World Health Organization [WHO] 2016). In relation to illicit drugs, according to the most recent world report on drugs by the United Nations Office on Drugs and Crime (2019), *cannabis* is the most widely used substance, with an estimated use by 188 million people in the world in 2017, which is equivalent to about 3.8% of the world population between 15 and 64 years old, followed by opioids (53.4 million), amphetamines (28.9 million), and cocaine (18.1 million). In Brazil, a study on the main data regarding the use of alcohol and other drugs showed that, in

K. B. S. Barbi (✉) · J. C. Caselli Messias
Pontifícia Universidade Católica de Campinas, Campinas, SP, Brazil

L. A. M. Guimarães
Universidade Católica Dom Bosco, Campo Grande, MS, Brazil

D. De Micheli et al. (eds.), *Drugs and Human Behavior*,
https://doi.org/10.1007/978-3-030-62855-0_37

2005, 86.7% of the individuals interviewed reported having used alcohol at least once in their lives. Of these, 2.7% had an ingestion of up to twice a week, and 4.9% three or more times a week. The use of drugs other than alcohol and tobacco was reported by 8.9% of individuals (Bastos et al. 2008).

It is not uncommon to observe that many users of psychoactive substances exhibit risky behaviors, such as putting themselves in danger, having impulsive attitudes, and manifesting aggressiveness towards others or themselves. Such behaviors are mainly explained by the deficiency in self-control and increased impulsiveness, actions mediated by regulatory mechanisms located in the frontal lobe of the brain (Bari and Robbins 2013). The relationship between impulsivity, aggressiveness, and self-injurious behavior, such as suicidal behavior, is well known and scientifically based, but it is not yet possible to predict when and how the development of suicidal behavior may occur as a result of this relationship (Gvion and Apter 2011).

This chapter aims to better understand the association between drug use and suicidal behavior, specifically at work. Suicidal behavior is another complex and multifactorial behavioral phenomenon that, like drug use, cannot be delimited according to individual, collective, ethnic, socioeconomic or cultural characteristics. Thus, it is also part of the most worrisome picture for public health, since consensual and effective measures for its prevention have not yet been established, configuring one of the main causes of mortality worldwide. The concept of suicidal behavior refers to a variety of behavioral manifestations that range from suicide ideation and planning, followed by suicide attempts, to suicide effectiveness. The presence of a history of prior suicidal behavior is one of the most important risk factors for committing suicide, increasing in severity the more serious, frequent, and recent this behavior is (U.S. Department of Health and Human Services 2012).

In a 9-week prospective study, Mundt et al. (2013) reported a risk of suicide four to nine times higher in individuals who had previously shown some manifestation of suicidal behavior, compared to those without such a history. One of the existing hypotheses for the understanding of suicidal behavior is that suicide is a final occurrence of an evolutionary process of manifestation of death wish, in which suicidal ideation and planning appear as the starting point of this path. Millner et al. (2015), when evaluating 30 cases of recent suicide attempts, observed that most of them reported the presence of suicidal ideation years before the attempt. In the multicenter study on suicidal behavior SUPRE-MISS[1] carried out by the WHO in partnership with ten countries, the rates of suicide ideation varied from 2.6% to 25.4% among the countries involved, with the sample of the Brazilian population presenting an index of 17% (Bertolote et al. 2005). Together with the ideation, the presence of planning for the act of attempting suicide is quite common. This planning can be limited to the scope of the ideas or, in many cases, manifest itself in the form of

[1]The composition of acronyms SUPRE-MISS that name the study refers to the junction of SUICIDE PREvention (SUPRE), a global initiative of WHO for the prevention of suicide, which aims to reduce morbidity and mortality due to suicidal behavior; with the method of the study, *Multisite Intervention Study on Suicidal Behaviors* (MISS).

preparatory behaviors characterized by attitudes regarding how to commit the act of attempted suicide, such as storing medications, ropes, and weapons, with the intention of later use for this purpose.

Millner et al. (2015), in a study involving 1500 participants to evaluate scales of suicidal behavior, found that among those individuals who had suicidal ideation, 48.8% reported life-long preparatory behaviors, and among those with a history of suicide attempts, the preparatory behaviors were related to the presence of prior planning. In another study, when Arias et al. (2016) tracked 782 patients admitted to emergency services for 52 weeks due to ideation or attempted suicide in the last week, they observed the presence of preparatory behaviors during the entire follow-up period (Arias et al. 2016).

The suicide attempt is the manifestation of suicidal behavior that comes closest in terms of the seriousness of the risk for suicide. According to existing population data, the prevalence of attempted suicide in individuals over the age of 18 is 4 per 1000 inhabitants. Considering that the death rate from suicide for this age group is 15 per 100,000 inhabitants, it can be assumed that for each adult who dies from suicide, another 20 attempt suicide (WHO 2014).

The SUPRE-MISS study, cited previously, also evaluated the rates of attempted suicide in the participating countries, observing a variation for this scenario of 0.4–4.2%. The Brazilian study belonging to this project found a rate of 2.8% (Botega et al. 2009). A relevant difference in this behavior is found in the comparison between genders, with women committing suicide attempts up to two times more than men (Muheim et al. 2013).

The impact caused by death by suicide, in addition to repercussions on family and close friends, extends to society as a whole, generating government investment to create forms of identification and methods of prevention. According to WHO data, in 2012 there were about 804,000 deaths from suicide worldwide, equivalent to an average of 11.4 deaths per 100,000 inhabitants and representing 1.4% of all causes of death (WHO 2014).

It is observed that, although there is a reduction in the number of suicides, with the total decreasing to 788 thousand suicides and the average to 10.7 deaths per 100 thousand inhabitants in 2015, there is a great variation in the rates of these deaths according to the region, from 4.34 thousand suicides in the Mediterranean to 12.84 thousand per 100 thousand inhabitants in Africa (Vijayakumar and Phillips 2016). In Brazil, in 2015, suicide deaths reached a total number of 11,178 cases, corresponding to a rate of six deaths per 100,000 inhabitants. Of the Brazilian regions, the Southeast has the highest occurrence and the North the lowest. Contrary to what was observed for suicide attempts, men commit much more suicide than women. In Brazil, these rates correspond to 9.6 and 2.7 deaths per 100,000 inhabitants for men and women, respectively, in 2015. However, it is observed that, over the years, the rates show a progressive increase in women, but not in men (WHO 2015).

The etiology of suicide is heterogeneous, contributing to this behavior several factors that act on the individual. These factors can be of individual origin, related to particular individual aspects, or of social/environmental origin, referring to specific epidemiological aspects, such as culture, ethnicity, gender, among others.

Individual risk factors can be divided into three interrelated dimensions: (1) predisposing factors, related to family psychopathological inheritance and neurobiological aspects; (2) modulating factors, related to personality traits and behavior; and (3) precipitating factors, which act temporally, serving as precipitators of suicidal behavior, such as mental disorders and stressful personal experiences (Turecki and Brent 2016).

As a precipitating causal factor, the presence of some type of mental disorder is known to be the main risk factor evidenced. A review of studies carried out from 1959 to 2001 showed that, of the suicide deaths evaluated, about 98% were associated with some type of diagnosable mental disorder (Bertolote and Fleischmann 2002). Among the mentally caused disorders, mood disorders, especially depression, is one of the most widely studied diagnoses strongly associated with suicidal behavior. In suicide attempts in Urgency and Emergency Services, depressive disorder is among the main observed diagnoses (Santos et al. 2009). Besides mood disorders, other psychiatric diagnoses are strongly associated with suicidal behavior, and among the most observed are personality disorders, mainly called Cluster B, including, specifically, histrionic and borderline personality disorders (Tyrer et al. 2015). The diagnosis of substance dependence along with depression is observed in two thirds of suicide deaths (Hoven et al. 2010).

The Relationship Between Work and Use of Substances

The most relevant work elements in the production of both workers psychic wear and tear and motivation and well-being can be understood from the Job Demand–Resources (JD-R) model which has been widely employed in studies around the world (Bakker and Demerouti 2007). According to this model, the demands of work correspond to individual, group, and organizational aspects that require physical and psychological efforts to be met, while the resources encompass everything that, in these same dimensions, can be functional in achieving objectives, reducing wear and tear and promote professional growth.

Depending on how these factors combine, deleterious effects can arise to the psychic health of workers. When demands are high (such as pressure for productivity or complexity of the task) and resources are low (such as organizational support or clarity of procedures), high stress and wear are expected. The JD-R model evolved from the Karasek (1979) model known as Demand–Control (DCM) and also from the Siegrist (1996) model known as Effort-Reward Balance Imbalance (ERI), maintaining the general principles of these two pillars, but with a broader scope.

According to Bakker and Demorouti (2007), in the Demand–Control model the emphasis is placed on the latitude of autonomy that a person could have in their work. Thus, the less flexibility and the possibility of making decisions, the more vulnerable the worker would be to stress. In the ERI model, the emphasis is placed on the balance between how much one invests and what one earns from work, whether in material terms (salary and assets) or immaterial (prestige and recognition, for example). Psychic suffering would be proportional to the perception of an unsatisfactory return, which may constitute a risk factor for alcohol and drug consumption.

Nunes and Jólluskin (2007), when conducting a brief historical and social analysis of drug use concluded that, due to cultural characteristics, more and more problematic behaviors escape self-control and are expressed in the form of various types of addictions, not only by drugs, but also by exacerbated consumption, gambling, internet access, and even work. According to this view one can bring to light an issue that is often discussed today, which is the increasing demands and requirements on the recognition of a well-performed job function.

For Lima (2010) the use of drugs as a "tool for integration" not only to society, but especially to work, for its often excessive demands, must be seen as a problem that transcends the basic issue of dependency, since it refers to another problem: that of alienation and its inevitable relationship with the processes of health-disease. In this study, the author describes and discusses both the "functional" use of drugs in the context of work, when used as a source of greater productivity and performance, and its evolution towards "dysfunctionality," when used as a source of desire, to the detriment of the work functions themselves, causing various problems to the worker, such as punishments, transfers, downgrading of function, prejudice from other colleagues, and, consequently, isolation. In a descriptive and quantitative work on the use of alcohol and other drugs, carried out with 315 employees from different positions in a petrochemical company, Carrillo and Mauro (2004) highlighted the consumption of alcohol by 7.1% of the interviewees and highlighted the stress related to the organization of work, as well as the rivalries generated among colleagues resulting from this organization, as vulnerability factors possibly related to this problem.

Drug Use, Labor, and Suicidal Behavior

As described previosly, drug use is among the most related factors of suicidal behavior. The second Brazilian Survey on Alcohol and Drugs conducted in 2012 with more than 4000 individuals aged 14 years and older, demonstrated the existence of an association between the presence of ideation and attempted suicide and the use of substances (Abdalla et al. 2019). In the sample, 9.9% reported suicidal ideation and 5.4% attempted suicide during their lifetime. In the prevalence observed for each type of substance, alcohol dependents presented rates of 20.8% and 12.4%; cannabis users 31.5% and 16.5%; and cocaine users 40.0% and 20.8% for suicide ideation and attempted suicide during life, respectively. In all cases significant associations were found between substance use and the presence of suicidal behavior (Abdalla et al. 2019). In a meta-analysis conducted with 31 observational studies that evaluated the relationship between alcohol dependence and suicidal behavior, Darvishi et al. (2015) reached the conclusion that the presence of this condition should be considered an important factor in increasing the risk of any suicidal manifestation, and should be taken into consideration in the investigation of early death in individuals with this problem.

Taking up the issue of drug use in the workplace as a consequence of the emotional wear and tear caused by various factors faced by workers, it is necessary to discuss how these work stressors can also act as a primary cause for suicidal behavior. For this, besides substance addiction, mood disorders such as depression, which may or may not occur concomitantly, must be strongly considered. In a literature review that addresses aspects of the work environment involved in the development of mood disorders and suicide, Woo and Postolache (2008) concluded that mood disorders are closely related to the occupational environment and lead to harmful consequences ranging from impairment of the work function to suicide. For these reasons, it is important to emphasize that the approach of this picture in organizations should be done in a preventive way, with investments in education and guidance, as well as in the investigation of the presence of depressive symptoms and, in some way, of suicidal behavior in the periodic evaluations of workers.

Another important condition that may be associated with the relationship between drug use, work and suicidal behavior is Burnout Syndrome. The concept of burnout was first described by psychologist Herbert J. Freudenberger in 1974, when he observed a condition composed of feelings of failure and exhaustion, resulting from the labor attrition of professionals who worked with chemical dependents. Such professionals reported feelings of uselessness and incapacity in face of the few positive results obtained (Murofuse et al. 2005).

With the development of this concept, currently characterized as a multidimensional psychic syndrome, composed by three independent components, which may be interrelated: emotional exhaustion, characterized by the feeling of no longer having physical and/or psychic energy to meet the interpersonal demand of its work function; depersonalization, characterized by the feeling of "objectification" of the other, generating a reduction in affectivity and increased insensitivity; and lack of personal fulfillment, characterized by a negative self-judgment about its work capacity (Maslach et al. 1986; Murofuse et al. 2005).

Several studies were conducted in order to identify and analyze interrelated characteristics between this syndrome and the work. Aronsson et al. (2017) published a meta-analysis study analyzing a wide variety of work and burnout factors in a survey of different types of studies conducted between 1990 and 2013. In this work, the authors identified that high demands, little control and reward, high workloads and insecurity in the work environment are risk factors for the development of emotional exhaustion.

As an important consequence, the association between Burnout and the development of psychiatric disorders has been investigated and evidenced for more than 10 years, such as described in the literature review by Trigo et al. (2007), in which the authors collected data from studies that addressed several psychopathologies, such as depression, anxiety disorders, dissociative disorders, psychosomatic disorders, and suicidal behavior. Specifically on the relationship between burnout and the use of alcohol and other drugs, a meta-analysis work with 12 studies that had 27,936 individuals evaluated, Kempeman (2019) found a significant association between alcohol consumption and the presence of Burnout Syndrome, considering the hypothesis that the use of alcohol plays a role in relieving stress caused by work for some people, who presented a greater frequency of this association.

Trigo et al. (2007) also address substance dependence as one of the burnout disorders, finding data mainly related to the medical subpopulation. As a risk for suicidal behavior, the presence of burnout has been evidenced, mainly when associated with depressive conditions, besides other factors, such as negative work environment, quality of work, and propensity to suicide. When evaluating the prevalence of burnout in a sample of 92 individuals treated in an Emergency Unit for attempted suicide, Perju and Gallois (2016) found that 8.7% of those evaluated had this condition, of which 88% were women, 25% worked in a work context of many responsibilities, 75% had no history of psychiatric disorders and/or previous psychiatric treatment, and 88% had attempted suicide for the first time in their lives, concluding that the burnout presents an initial picture of psychic stress, but can evolve into self-aggressive behaviors such as suicide attempts.

Final Considerations

There is extensive information on the epidemiological data related to suicide and attempts to commit this act. WHO studies, with special emphasis on SUPRE-MISS, indicate important and elucidative aspects regarding such a serious issue.

This chapter sought to highlight a complex point of confluence that cannot be understood only in function of the individual, as if he were extraneous to the context in which he lives. In fact, personal elements linked to biology and personality are very important, however, one cannot ignore those relevant to the environment. In the specific case of this chapter, the environment corresponds to the daily tasks, demands, and immediate relationships, policies, culture and organizational values, labor laws, and the macroeconomic scenario of a globalized world. Such issues cannot be disregarded when seeking to understand the suffering of workers, the meaning of substance use and the plan to put an end to one's own life.

The care must be preventive, prior to psychological and psychiatric attention in an individual clinical setting. Thus, two dimensions need to be observed: the first, at the macro level, refers to public health and work policies. At the intermediate (meso) level, organizational policies, job design, interpersonal relationships, and the extent of autonomy can be important risk factors or factors that protect workers' psychic health. In the former case, changes depend on large-scale social, economic, and political movements. In the second, people management can intervene in a direct and effective way, provided that it is well directed and imbued with a genuine desire to promote the quality of life at work.

References

Abdalla, R. R., Miguel, A. C., Brietzke, E., Caetano, R., Laranjeira, R., & Madruga, C. S. (2019). Suicidal behavior among substance users: Data from the second Brazilian national alcohol and drug survey (II BNADS). *Brazilian Journal of Psychiatry, 41*(5), 437–440. https://doi.org/10.1590/1516-4446-2018-0054.

Arias, S. A., Miller, I., Camargo, C. A., Jr., Sullivan, A. F., Goldstein, A. B., Allen, M. H., et al. (2016). Factors associated with suicide outcomes 12 months after screening positive for suicide risk in the emergency department. *Psychiatric Services, 67*(2), 206–213. https://doi.org/10.1176/appi.ps.201400513.

Aronsson, G., Theorell, T., Grape, T., Hammarström, A., Hogstedt, C., Marteinsdottir, I., et al. (2017). A systematic review including meta-analysis of work environment and burnout symptoms. *BMC Public Health, 17*(1), 264. https://doi.org/10.1186/s12889-017-4153-7.

Bakker, A. B., & Demerouti, E. (2007). The job demands-resources model: State of the art. *Journal of Managerial Psychology, 22*(3), 309–328. https://doi.org/10.1108/02683940710733115.

Bari, A., & Robbins, T. W. (2013). Inhibition and impulsivity: Behavioral and neural basis of response control. *Progress in Neurobiology, 108*, 44–79. https://doi.org/10.1016/j.pneurobio.2013.06.005.

Bastos, F. I., Bertoni, N., Hacker, M. A., Berquó, E., França, I., Barbosa, R., et al. (2008). Consumo de álcool e drogas: Principais achados de pesquisa de âmbito nacional, Brasil 2005. *Revista de Saúde Pública, 42*, 109–117. https://doi.org/10.1590/S0034-89102008000800013.

Bertolote, J. M., & Fleischmann, A. (2002). Suicide and psychiatric diagnosis: A worldwide perspective. *World Psychiatry, 1*(3), 181–185.

Bertolote, J. M., Fleischmann, A., De Leo, D., Bolhari, J., Botega, N., De Silva, D., et al. (2005). Suicide attempts, plans, and ideation in culturally diverse sites: The WHO SUPRE-MISS community survey. *Psychological Medicine, 35*, 1457–1465. https://doi.org/10.1017/S0033291705005404.

Botega, N. J., Marín-León, L., Oliveira, H. B., Barros, M. B. D. A., Silva, V. F., & Dalgalarrondo, P. (2009). Prevalências de ideação, plano e tentativa de suicídio: Um inquérito de base populacional em Campinas, São Paulo, Brasil. *Cadernos de Saúde Pública, 25*(12), 2632–2638. https://doi.org/10.1590/S0102-311X2009001200010.

Carillo, P. L. L., & Mauro, M. Y. C. (2004). O trabalho como fator de risco ou fator de proteção para o consumo de álcool e outras drogas. *Texto e Contexto Enfermagem, 13*(2), 217–225.

Darvishi, N., Farhadi, M., Haghtalab, T., & Poorolajal, J. (2015). Alcohol-related risk of suicidal ideation, suicide attempt, and completed suicide: A meta-analysis. *PLoS One, 10*(5), e0126870. https://doi.org/10.1371/journal.pone.0126870.

Gvion, Y., & Apter, A. (2011). Aggression, impulsivity, and suicide behavior: A review of the literature. *Archives of Suicide Research, 15*(2), 93–112. https://doi.org/10.1080/13811118.2011.565265.

Hoven, C. W., Mandell, D. J., & Bertolote, J. M. (2010). Prevention of mental ill-health and suicide: Public health perspectives. *European Psychiatry, 25*(5), 252–256. https://doi.org/10.1016/j.eurpsy.2010.01.011.

Karasek, R. A., Jr. (1979). Job demands, job decision latitude, and mental strain: Implications for job redesign. *Administrative Science Quarterly, 24*(2), 285–308. https://doi.org/10.2307/2392498.

Kempeman, R. L. (2019). *Burnout and alcohol consumption: A meta-analysis.* (*Master's thesis*). Leiden University.

Lima, M. E. A. (2010). Dependência química e trabalho: uso funcional e disfuncional de drogas nos contextos laborais. *Revista Brasileira de Saúde Ocupacional, 35*(122), 260–268. https://doi.org/10.1590/S0303-76572010000200008.

Maslach, C., Jackson, S. E., & Leiter, M. P. (1986). *Maslach burnout inventory* (Vol. 21, pp. 191–217). Palo Alto, CA: Consulting Psychologists Press.

Millner, A. J., Lee, M. D., & Nock, M. K. (2015). Single-item measurement of suicidal behaviors: Validity and consequences of misclassification. *PLoS One, 10*(10), 1–17. https://doi.org/10.1371/journal.pone.0141606.

Muheim, F., Eichhorn, M., Berger, P., Czernin, S., Stoppe, G., Keck, M., & Riecher-Rössler, A. (2013). Suicide attempts in the county of Basel: Results from the WHO/EURO multicentre study on suicidal behaviour. *Swiss Medical Weekly, 143*, w13759. https://doi.org/10.4414/smw.2013.13759.

Mundt, J. C., Greist, J. H., Jefferson, J. W., Federico, M., Mann, J. J., & Posner, K. (2013). Prediction of suicidal behavior in clinical research by lifetime suicidal ideation and behavior ascertained by the electronic Columbia-suicide severity rating scale. *Journal of Clinical Psychiatry, 74*(9), 887–893. https://doi.org/10.4088/JCP.13m08398.

Murofuse, N. T., Abranches, S. S., & Napoleão, A. A. (2005). Reflexões sobre estresse e burnout e a relação com a enfermagem. *Revista Latino-Americana Enfermagem, 13*(2), 255–261. https://doi.org/10.1590/S0104-11692005000200019.

Nunes, L. M., & Jólluskin, G. (2007). O uso de drogas: breve análise histórica e social. *Revista Da Faculdade de Ciências Humanas e Sociais, 4*, 230–237.

Perju, E., & Gallois, E. (2016). The prevalence of the burnout syndrome among population examined at the psychiatric emergency department for attempted suicide. *European Psychiatry, 33*(S1), S443–S443. https://doi.org/10.1016/j.eurpsy.2016.01.1613.

Santos, S. A., Lovisi, G., Legay, L., & Abelha, L. (2009). Prevalência de transtornos mentais nas tentativas de suicídio em um hospital de emergência no Rio de Janeiro, Brasil. *Cadernos de Saúde Pública, 25*(9), 2064–2074. https://doi.org/10.1590/S0102-311X2009000900020.

Siegrist, J. (1996). Adverse health effects of high-effort/low-reward conditions. *Journal of Occupational Health Psychology, 1*(1), 27–41. https://doi.org/10.1037/1076-8998.1.1.27.

Trigo, T. R., Teng, C. T., & Hallak, J. E. C. (2007). Síndrome de burnout ou estafa profissional e os transtornos psiquiátricos. *Archives of Clinical Psychiatry, 34*(5), 223–233. https://doi.org/10.1590/S0101-60832007000500004.

Turecki, G., & Brent, D. A. (2016). Suicide and suicidal behaviour. *The Lancet, 387*, 1227–1239. https://doi.org/10.1016/S0140-6736(15)00234-2.

Tyrer, P., Geoffrey, M. R., & Crawford, M. J. (2015). Classification, assessment, prevalence, and effect of personality disorder. *The Lancet, 385*, 717–726. https://doi.org/10.1016/S0140-6736(14)61995-4.

U. S. Department of Health and Human Services. (2012). *2012 National Strategy for suicide prevention: Goals and objectives for action*. Retrieved from www.samhsa.gov/nssp

United Nations Office on Drugs and Crime. (2019). *World drug report 2019*. Retrieved from https://wdr.unodc.org/wdr2019/

Vijayakumar, L., & Phillips, M. (2016). Suicide prevention in low- and middle-income countries. In R. C. O'Connor & J. Pirkis (Eds.), *The International Handbook of Suicide Prevention* (2nd ed.). Hoboken, NJ: Wiley. https://doi.org/10.1002/9781118903223.ch29.

Woo, J. M., & Postolache, T. T. (2008). The impact of work environment on mood disorders and suicide: Evidence and implications. *International Journal on Disability and Human Development, 7*(2), 185–200. https://doi.org/10.1515/IJDHD.2008.7.2.185.

World Health Organization. (2014). *Preventing suicide: A global imperative*. Retrieved from https://apps.who.int/iris/bitstream/handle/10665/131056/9789241564779_eng.pdf?sequence=1

World Health Organization. (2015). *Age-standardized suicide rates (per 100 000 population)*. Retrieved from https://www.who.int/data/gho/data/indicators/indicator-details/GHO/age-standardized-suicide-rates-(per-100-000-population)

World Health Organization. (2016). *Harmful use of alcohol*. Retrieved from https://apps.who.int/iris/bitstream/handle/10665/274603/9789241565639-eng.pdf?ua=1

Chapter 38
Grief Experience and Substance Misuse: An Integrative Review

Caroline Matilde da Silva Ribeiro, Fernanda Beatriz Hodar Lobato, Beatriz Cortese Barbugli, Gabriella Di Girolamo Martins, Veronica Vidotto Caricati, Renata Thurler Lessa, Adriana Scatena, Denise De Micheli, Gabrielle Fernandes Fronza, Richard Alecsander Reichert, and André Luiz Monezi Andrade

Introduction

Psychoactive substances permeate human history and have been widely used since ancient times for medicinal, ritualistic, and recreational use. Over the centuries, they have exceeded religious and mystical bonds by meeting demands for immediate pleasures and relief from pain and suffering, which are inherent to all individuals (Medeiros et al. 2013). In this context, some drugs became popular in the decades that followed, since the factors correlated to the motivation for their use reach all social classes (Almeida et al. 2018; Santana 1999).

In the face of malaise and sacrifices, individuals seek measures to confront them (Silva et al. 2019). This reality, to which individuals are exposed daily, sets a precedent for resources such as substances of abuse to be used in order to alleviate possible displeasure (Ribeiro 2009).

In the same sense, the Polish sociologist Bauman (1998) characterized contemporary society as a liquid, in which relations are established in a fluid and quick way. Thus, post-modernity contemplates individualistic and hedonistic characteristics, awakening in individuals' feelings of dissatisfaction and inconstancy that make them insecure, anxious, stressed, and distressed. Through this panorama, the use of psychoactive substances is inserted as a symptom of contemporaneity.

C. M. da Silva Ribeiro · F. B. H. Lobato · B. C. Barbugli · G. D. G. Martins · V. V. Caricati · R. T. Lessa · G. F. Fronza · A. L. M. Andrade (✉)
Pontifícia Universidade Católica de Campinas, Campinas, SP, Brazil

A. Scatena · D. De Micheli
Universidade Federal de São Paulo, São Paulo, SP, Brazil

R. A. Reichert
Universidade do Vale do Itajaí, Itajaí, SC, Brazil

D. De Micheli et al. (eds.), *Drugs and Human Behavior*,
https://doi.org/10.1007/978-3-030-62855-0_38

Drug Use in the World and Brazil

The abusive use of psychoactive substances encompasses a significant population contingent, establishing itself as a severe public health problem. Data from the United Nations World Drug Report (United Nations Office on Drugs and Crime [UNODC] 2019) show that approximately 271 million people between 15 and 64 years of age have used some type of drug throughout their lives, of which one in 20 has used some illicit substance. Among the most commonly used illicit substances, *cannabis* is the most consumed in the world. The opioids, meanwhile, stood out as the ones responsible for two-thirds of the 585,000 deaths recorded for indiscriminate drug use in 2017, and include some 53 million users.

Another report indicated that approximately 3 million premature deaths occur due to excessive alcohol use (World Health Organization [WHO] 2018). In this sense, it is estimated that 27 million people have problems related to drug use, comprising 0.6% of the world population. Besides this aspect, it is valid to point out that only one out of seven people with some level of substance dependence receives the appropriate treatment (UNODC 2012).

Faced with this panorama, we observe the decrease in potential years of the life of the population in situations of vulnerability, violence, or accidental events facilitated by drug abuse (Barbosa et al. 2018). This scenario is intensified by the speed with which new substances are presented and their growing demands (Abreu et al. 2016).

In Brazil, epidemiological data from the Center for Information on Psychotropic Drugs ([CEBRID] 2012) indicate that 74.6% of the population has consumed alcohol at least once in their lives, followed by tobacco with 44% and 22.8% some illicit drug, among them marijuana is the most used. The average age for initial consumption of tobacco and alcohol is 16 and 17 years old, respectively, which proves its premature use (Queiroz et al. 2015). Also, 3.6% of the country's total population from the age of 18 years presents some difficulty due to drug use (Ronzani et al. 2019). Other studies also reported excessive use both among colleges (Bedendo et al. 2019; Bedendo et al. 2018; Bedendo et al. 2017) and adolescents in different socioeconomic conditions (Yamauchi et al. 2019; Silva et al. 2018a; Almeida et al. 2017; Oliveira et al. 2016; Bedendo et al. 2015). Substance abuse is also associated with various risk behaviors in these populations.

Diagnostic Criteria and Types of Addiction

Psychoactive substances are characterized by altering brain activity, generating changes in perception, cognition, mood, and behavior of an individual (Andrade et al. 2018; Fernandes et al. 2017; De Micheli et al. 2016, 2020). The periodic use of these substances increases the probability of dependence, as described as a set of physiological, cognitive and behavioral symptoms according to the International

Classification of Diseases (ICD-10) and is established as a biopsychosocial issue (Faria et al. 2015).

It should be noted that addiction differs from abuse and circumstantial use of substances. Abuse is characterized by a higher frequency and greater quantity on a single occasion, while occasional use represents a sporadic episode of substance consumption. (Silva et al. 2018b).

The diagnostic criteria described for addiction tables in the fifth edition of the Diagnostic and Statistical Manual of Mental Disorders (DSM-5; American Psychiatric Association [APA] 2013) include use of substances in larger quantities or for a longer time than planned; persistent desire; substantial time spent in obtaining them; fissure; abandonment of activities due to use; maintenance of consumption despite social adversities and/or physical damage; use in risky situations; tolerance; abstinence. From them, mental health professionals make diagnoses that correspond to the number of criteria presented by the individual during the minimum period of 1 year. Thus, the mild dependence is determined from two or three criteria, the average from four or five, and the severe one from six or more of the 11 criteria above.

Risk Factors of Substance Use

By altering neurological, cognitive, and behavioral functions, psychoactive substances can act to relieve symptoms triggered by stressful events and sometimes accompany mental comorbidities such as anxiety and depression (Andretta et al. 2018; Andrade et al. 2017)(Frade et al., 2013). Thus, there is a strong association between depressive disorders and attempts to ease them through drug use (Hunt et al. 2020). In addition to depression, the anxiety disorder, defined by DSM-V (APA 2013) as a set of maladjusted and frequent reactions to anticipate threats that are not always real, may also be associated with the misuse of psychoactive drugs for similar reasons as before (Galvão et al. 2017).

Comprising one of the categories of anxiety disorders, post-traumatic stress disorder (PTSD) is characterized by the intense manifestation of feelings related to impotence, horror or fear after a traumatic episode. In this sense, some studies have already identified the relationship between PTSD and substance abuse (Quitete et al. 2012). In addition to the greater vulnerability to substance addiction for individuals with a history of PTSD, a more complex clinical picture stands out among them (Tractenberg et al. 2012).

In PTSD scenario, avoidance behaviors are observed in situations that refer to trauma, as well as constant discomfort about the subject's memories. These reactions can act as triggers for the consumption of drugs, pointing to an inadequate attempt to relieve the sensations previously described (Pulcherio et al. 2008).

Studies show that 30–60% of users of psychoactive substances are diagnosed with PTSD, and, concomitantly, the intensity of symptom manifestation is associated with the number of traumatic events witnessed and individual factors before the episodes. Besides, a study conducted by Pulcherio et al. (2008) reveals that alcohol users are the majority among those classified with the disorder. However, the nature of the relationship between the abuse of this substance and PTSD remains controversial, considering that users may present other aspects in their prior history, in addition to other comorbidities that justify their abuse (Dantas and Andrade 2008).

Studies suggest that complicated mourning, i.e., the mourning in which the individual experiences significant mental disorganization that makes it impossible for him to carry out his daily activities, or even stops going through some phase, is more likely to facilitate the misuse of substances, which evidences the complicated Grief as a possible risk factor for the use of substances.

The Grieving Process: Revisiting the Concept

Reactions to significant losses have been transformed over the centuries by different beliefs and cultures. In ancient times, death was naturalized and accompanied by rituals that encouraged participants to expose their feelings for the loss suffered. During the Middle Ages, people welcomed their finitude with tranquility, supported by the personal religiosity of the time (Basso and Wainer 2011). Contemporary times began to deny this human condition (Ariès 2012).

Technological, medicinal, and pharmaceutical advances have made possible a significant increase in life expectancy and quality of life, which may give death the idea of the failure of new resources. Thus, a false sense of control over finitude was established, and this was now denied, censored, and restricted to hospitals (Machado et al. 2016). Currently, death is considered a taboo, which can make the mourning process more delicate and complex (Basso and Wainer 2011).

Grief is the concept used to refer to the feelings resulting from the loss of loved ones and is a phenomenon accompanied by pain and suffering. Although death is a certainty, according to Franco (2010), mourning is an expected process in the face of the breaking of a significant bond. The individual begins to understand, accept, and adapt to the conditions resulting from the loss suffered.

In this sense, there is the implication of personal issues that trigger behaviors and understand the ability to express and manage the pain of this disruption (Fukumitsu 2012). The grieving process can increase levels of anxiety and threaten the physical and psychological integrity of individuals, affecting their quality of life (Parkes 2001). As a result of the prolonged difficulty in adjusting to the broken bond, which can compromise social functions in a significant amount of time, what is conceptualized as complicated Grief is established. To this may be allied aspects related to denial, anger, or the repression of feelings of pain and loss, which prevent the individual from carrying out his activities with the same quality as they did before (Braz and Franco 2017).

Parkes (1998) points to the importance of care in the first classification of complicated grieving processes. This is due to the different reactions caused by loss and the particular way in which people react to crises. Symptoms linked to depression, insomnia, and increased use of psychoactive substances can be triggered by Grief, but do not necessarily make it complicated, revealing the need for a biopsychosocial look at this context raised by loss. In this same sense, the stress arising from this process is also considered a natural response, keeping its due proportions (Kovács 2008).

Faced with the complexity of the subject, the Swiss psychiatrist (Kübler-Ross 1985), proposed phases of reaction to loss, that is, stages that integrate the confrontation of the breaking of a bond. The first of these comprises the denial of loss and isolation, followed by the exteriorization of anger. The third involves bargaining; the fourth refers to reactive depression and, finally, the fifth, acceptance.

However, the steps for the mourning process raise controversy in the literature. Although they understand remarkable didactic importance and have made possible concrete studies on the subject, they can be transitory, and the duration of the phases can vary according to each individual. The aspects related to culture, the type of death (traumatic or not), the need to standardize the process, and the eagerness to maintain the routine activities, directly influence the way each person experiences his/her grieving process (Kovács 2008). In this sense, the progressive and individual nature of mourning is reaffirmed, which can transit between the stages in order to adequately reorganize mental issues (Braz and Franco 2017).

Mourning and Use of Substances

Research points to the relationship between the mourning process and the use of psychoactive substances. In this case, drug use is established as a defense strategy for the difficulties of elaboration in breaking meaningful bonds (Lobb et al. 2010). The substances act as an *escape valve* and an adaptive alternative to a moment of pain and suffering by altering neurological functions and assisting in the relief of displeasure (Ribeiro 2009).

Table 38.1 presents five several studies associating the use of substances and the mourning process, highlighting the possible correlated factors. The studies vary in methodology, including exploratory, qualitative, and review studies. Despite the methodological differences, the results obtained corroborate each other and are supported by the logic that places the harmful use of substances as a risk factor for a complicated bereavement.

Drabwell et al. (2020), Hamdan et al. (2013), and Kendler et al. (2002) point out in their studies the male predisposition to substance abuse resulting from the mourning process. This aspect is related to the possible difficulty of men to express emotions, especially in situations of vulnerability, when compared to women (Drabwell et al. 2020). Thus, some authors have identified an increase in the use of psychoactive substances during bereavement, especially among those who had previously used drugs (Parisi et al. 2019).

Another relevant aspect is related to the concomitance between the preparation of the bereavement and the treatment of substance abuse. Thus, when the individual

Table 38.1 Aspects associated with substance use and grief

Author	Publication date	Methodological design	Main results
Drabwell et al.	2020	Qualitative design	It points to the misuse of substances as a form of rebellion of bereaved children and presents a gender delineation by indicating consumption as a facilitator for the expression of emotions in men
Eng et al.	2019	Qualitative design	It indicates the relationship between increased substance use and coping strategies for grief triggered by suicide
Kendler et al.	2002	Exploratory design	There is an association between the loss of parents, alcoholic dependency (AD), and gender. The same is not perceived concerning the loss of parents and major depression (DM)
Hamdan et al.	2013	Longitudinal design	Young bereaved people, especially males, present a higher risk for alcohol dependence than those who are not going through a bereavement process
Parisi et al.	2019	Systematic review	It indicates the existence of a relationship between substance misuse and complicated grief. It points to greater use of alcohol and tobacco and a higher predisposition of individuals who had already misused them before bereavement

reorganizes psychically after a loss, influence on the intensity of drug use is expected to occur. However, some mourning processes may be more complex, directly implying in the possible dependence (Parisi et al. 2019).

Final Considerations

Contemporary life, characterized by unstable social relations driven by the growing capitalist system, demands from individual's dynamism and productivity that favor the fluidity of relations. In this sense, post-modernity gives individuals feelings of repression and anxiety. As a result, psychoactive substances act to alleviate the symptoms of discomfort, making harmful use a public health problem. Therefore, stressful events, such as the loss of a loved one, can drive the use of psychoactive drugs as a maladaptive and suffering form of Grief.

In this context, questions are discussed regarding the risk and protection factors available to the bereaved, as well as the culture in which they are inserted and the support network at their disposal. These aspects directly influence the consumption of psychoactive substances, both in an adaptive and maladaptive way. It is clear that, although it is established as a taboo, death is inherent to human beings. In this sense, the studies on finitude and the consequences triggered by it must be increasingly discussed and explored, especially concerning the association between the harmful use of substances and the difficulties of confronting the various contexts involved in the mourning processes.

References

Abreu, A. M. M., Parreira, P. M. S. D., Souza, M. H. N., & Barroso, T. M. M. A. (2016). Perfil do consumo de substâncias psicoativas e sua relação com as características sociodemográficas: Uma contribuição para intervenção breve na atenção primária à saúde. *Texto & Contexto - Enfermagem, 25*(4), e1450015. https://doi.org/10.1590/0104-07072016001450015.

Almeida, D. E. R. G., Andrade, A. L. M., Cruz, F. D., & Micheli, D. D. (2018). Perception of freedom in leisure among substance users and nonusers. *Psico-USF, 23*(1), 13–24. https://doi.org/10.1590/1413-82712018230102.

Almeida, D. E. R. G., De Micheli, D., & Andrade, A. L. M. (2017). Leisure and substance use among adolescents: A systematic review. *Estudos e Pesquisas em Psicologia, 17*(3), 970–988. https://doi.org/10.1590/1413-82712018230102.

American Psychiatric Association. (2013). *Diagnostic and statistical manual of mental disorders, fifth edition*. Arlington, TX: Author.

Andrade, A. L. M., Bedendo, A., Enumo, S. R. F., & Micheli, D. (2018). Brain development in adolescence: general aspects and update. *Adolescência e Saude, 15*(Supl. 1), 62–67.

Andrade, A. L. M., Teixeira, L. R. D. S., Zoner, C. C., Niro, N. N., Scatena, A., & Amaral, R. A. D. (2017). Factors associated with postpartum depression in social vulnerability women. *SMAD. Revista eletrônica saúde mental álcool e drogas, 13*(4), 196–204. https://doi.org/10.11606/issn.1806-6976.v13i4p196-204.

Andretta, I., Limberger, J., Schneider, J. A., & Mello, L. T. N. (2018). Sintomas de depressão, ansiedade e estresse em usuários de drogas em tratamento em comunidades terapêuticas. *Psico-USF, 23*(2), 361–373. https://doi.org/10.1590/1413-82712018230214.

Ariès, P. (2012). *História da morte no ocidente: Da idade média aos nossos dias*. Rio de Janeiro, Brazil: Nova fronteira.

Barbosa, L. A., Andrade, A. L. M., Oliveira, L. G., & De Micheli, D. (2018). Prevalence of psychotropic substance use by urban bus drivers: A systematic review. *SMAD. Revista eletrônica saúde mental álcool e drogas, 14*(4), 234–244. https://doi.org/10.11606/issn.1806-6976.smad.2018.000400.

Basso, L. A., & Wainer, R. (2011). Luto e perdas repentinas: Contribuições da Terapia Cognitivo-Comportamental. *Revista Brasileira de Terapias Cognitivas, 7*(1), 35–43.

Bauman, Z. (1998). *O mal-estar da pós-modernidade*. Rio de Janeiro, Brazil: Jorge Zahar.

Bedendo, A., Andrade, A. L. M., & Noto, A. R. (2015). Sports and substance use in high school students different perspectives of this relationship. *SMAD Revista Eletrônica Saúde Mental Álcool e Drogas, 11*(2), 85–96. https://doi.org/10.11606/issn.1806-6976.v11i2p85-96.

Bedendo, A., Andrade, A. L. M., & Noto, A. R. (2018). Internet-based alcohol interventions for college students: Systematic review. *Revista Panamericana de Salud Pública, 42*, e54. https://doi.org/10.26633/RPSP.2018.54.

Bedendo, A., Andrade, A. L. M., Opaleye, E. S., & Noto, A. R. (2017). Binge drinking: A pattern associated with a risk of problems of alcohol use among university students. *Revista Latino-Americana de Enfermagem, 25*, e2925–e2933. https://doi.org/10.1590/1518-8345.1891.2925.

Bedendo, A., Ferri, C. P., Souza, A. A. L., Andrade, A. L. M., & Noto, A. R. (2019). Pragmatic randomized controlled trial of a web-based intervention for alcohol use among Brazilian college students: Motivation as a moderating effect. *Drug and Alcohol Dependence, 199*, 92–100. https://doi.org/10.1016/j.drugalcdep.2019.02.021.

Braz, M., & Franco, M. H. P. (2017). Profissionais paliativistas e suas contribuições na prevenção de luto complicado. *Psicologia: Ciência a Profissão [online]., 37*(1), 90–105. https://doi.org/10.1590/1982-3703001702016.

Centro Brasileiro de Informações sobre Drogas Psicotrópicas. (2012). *VI levantamento nacional sobre o consumo de drogas psicotrópicas entre estudantes do ensino fundamental e médio das redes pública e privada de ensino nas 27 capitais brasileiras*. Retrieved from https://www.cebrid.com.br/wp-content/uploads/2012/10/VI-Levantamento-Nacional-sobre-o-Consumo-de-Drogas-Psicotr%C3%B3picas-entre-Estudantes-do-Ensino-Fundamental-e-M%C3%A9dio-das-Redes-P%C3%BAblica-e-Privada-de-Ensino-nas-27-Capitais-Brasileiras.pdf

Dantas, H. S., & Andrade, A. G. (2008). Comorbidade entre transtorno de estresse pós-traumático e abuso e dependência de álcool e drogas: Uma revisão da literatura. *Archives of Clinical Psychiatry, 35*(Suppl. 1), 55–60. https://doi.org/10.1590/S0101-60832008000700012.

De Micheli, D., Andrade, A. L. M., Silva, E. A., & Souza-Formigoni, M. L. O. (2016). *Drug abuse in adolescence* (1st ed.). New York: Springer. https://doi.org/10.1007/978-3-319-17795-3.

De Micheli, D., Andrade, A., & Galduróz, J. C. (2020). Limitations of DSM-5 diagnostic criteria for substance use disorder in adolescents: what have we learned after using these criteria for several years? *Brazilian Journal of Psychiatry*, in press. https://doi.org/10.1590/1516-4446-2020-1151.

Drabwell, L., Eng, J., Stevenson, F., King, M., Osborn, D., & Pitman, A. (2020). Perceptions of the use of alcohol and drugs after sudden bereavement by unnatural causes: Analysis of online qualitative data. *International Journal of Environmental Research and Public Health, 17*(3), 677. https://doi.org/10.3390/ijerph17030677.

Eng, J., Drabwell, L., Stevenson, F., King, M., Osborn, D., & Pitman, A. (2019). Use of alcohol and unprescribed drugs after suicide bereavement: Qualitative study. *International Journal of Environmental Research and Public Health, 16*(21), 4093. https://doi.org/10.3390/ijerph16214093.

Faria, E. A. F., Queiros, P. S., Medeiros, M., Rosso, C. F. W., & Souza, M. M. (2015). Concepções sobre drogas por adolescentes escolares. *Revista Brasileira de Enfermagem, 68*(3), 517–523. https://doi.org/10.1590/0034-7167.2015680320i.

Fernandes, T. F., Monteiro, B. M. M., Silva, J. B. M., Oliveira, K. M., Viana, N. A. O., Gama, C. A. P., & Guimarães, D. A. (2017). Uso de substâncias psicoativas entre universitários brasileiros: perfil epidemiológico, contextos de uso e limitações metodológicas dos estudos. *Cadernos Saúde Coletiva, 25*(4), 498–507. https://doi.org/10.1590/1414-462x201700040181.

Franco, M. H. P. (2010). Por que estudar o luto na atualidade? In M. H. P. Franco (Ed.), *Formação e rompimento de vínculos* (pp. 17–42). São Paulo, Brazil: Summus.

Fukumitsu, K. O. (2012). *Perdas no desenvolvimento humano: Um estudo fenomenológico*. São Paulo, Barzil: Digital Publish & Print Editora.

Frade, I. F., De Micheli, D., Andrade, A. L. M., & de Souza-Formigoni, M. L. O. (2013). Relationship between stress symptoms and drug use among secondary students. The Spanish journal of psychology, 16, e4. https://doi.org/10.1017/sjp.2013.5

Galvão, A., Pinheiro, M., Gomes, M. J., & Ala, S. (2017). Ansiedade, stress e depressão relacionados com perturbações do sono-vigília e consumo de álcool. *Revista Portuguesa de Enfermagem de Saúde Mental*, (spe5), 8–12. https://doi.org/10.19131/rpesm.0160.

Hamdan, S., Melhem, N. M., Porta, G., Song, M. S., & Brent, D. A. (2013). Alcohol and substance abuse in parentally bereaved youth. *The Journal of Clinical Psychiatry, 74*(8), 828–833. https://doi.org/10.4088/JCP.13m08391.

Hunt, G. E., Malhil, G. S., Lai, H., & Cleary, M. (2020). Prevalence of comorbid substance use in major depressive disorder in community and clinical settings, 1990–2019: Systematic review and meta-analysis. *Journal of Affective Disorder., 266*, 288–304. https://doi.org/10.1016/j.jad.2020.01.141.

Kendler, K. S., Sheth, K., Gardner, C. O., & Prescott, C. A. (2002). Childhood parental loss and risk for first-onset of major depression and alcohol dependence: The time-decay of risk and sex differences. *Psychological Medicine, 32*(7), 1187–1194. https://doi.org/10.1017/S0033291702006219.

Kovács, M. J. (2008). Desenvolvimento da tanatologia: estudos sobre a morte e o morrer. *Paidéia, 18*(41), 457–468. https://doi.org/10.1590/S0103-863X2008000300004.

Kübler-Ross, E. (1985). *Sobre a morte e o morrer: o que os doentes terminais têm para ensinar a médicos, enfermeiras, religiosos e aos seus próprios parentes*. São Paulo, Brazil: Martins Fontes.

Lobb, E. A., Kristjanson, L. J., Aoun, S. M., Monterosso, L., Halkett, G. K. B., & Davies, A. (2010). Predictors of complicated grief: A systematic review of empirical studies. *Death Studies, 34*(8), 673–698. https://doi.org/10.1080/07481187.2010.496686.

Machado, R. S., Lima, A. A., Silva, G. R. F., Monteiro, C. F. S., & Rocha, S. S. (2016). Finitude e morte na sociedade ocidental: uma reflexão com foco nos profissionais de saúde. *Cultura de los Cuidados, 20*(45), 91–97. https://doi.org/10.14198/cuid.2016.45.10.

Medeiros, K. T., Maciel, S. C., Sousa, P. F., Tenório-Souza, F. M., & Dias, C. C. V. (2013). Representações sociais do uso e abuso de drogas entre familiares de usuários. *Psicologia em Estudo, 18*(2), 269–279. https://doi.org/10.1590/S1413-73722013000200008.

Oliveira, B. P., Andrade, A. L. M., & De Micheli, D. (2016). Relationship between levels of physical activity and quality of life in drug use in teenagers. *SMAD. Revista eletrônica saúde mental álcool e drogas, 12*(3), 178–187. https://doi.org/10.11606/issn.1806-6976.v12i3p178-187.

Parisi, A., Sharma, A., Howard, M. O., & Wilson, A. B. (2019). The relationship between substance misuse and complicated grief: A systematic review. *Journal of Substance Abuse Treatment, 103*, 43–57. https://doi.org/10.1016/j.jsat.2019.05.012.

Parkes, C. M. (1998). *Luto: Estudos sobre a perda na vida adulta*. São Paulo, Brazil: Summus.

Parkes, C. M. (2001). A historical overview of the scientific study of bereavement. In M. Strobe, R. H. Hansson, W. Stroebe, & H. Schut (Eds.), *Handbook of bereavement research. Consequences, coping and care*. Washington, DC: American Psychological Association.

Pulcherio, G., Vernetti, C., Strey, M. N., & Faller, S. (2008). Transtorno de estresse pós-traumático em dependente do álcool. *Archives of Clinical Psychiatry, 35*(4), 154–158. https://doi.org/10.1590/S0101-60832008000400005.

Queiroz, N. R., Portela, L. F., & Abreu, A. M. M. (2015). Associação entre o consumo de bebidas alcoólicas e tabaco e a religiosidade. *Acta Paulista de Enfermagem, 28*(6), 546–552. https://doi.org/10.1590/1982-0194201500091.

Quitete, B., Paulino, B., Hauck, F., Aguiar-Nemer, A. S., & Silva-Fonseca, V. A. (2012). Transtorno de estresse pós-traumático e uso de drogas ilícitas em mulheres encarceradas no Rio de Janeiro. *Archives of Clinical Psychiatry, 39*(2), 43–47. https://doi.org/10.1590/S0101-60832012000200001.

Ribeiro, C. T. (2009). Que lugar para as drogas no sujeito? Que lugar para o sujeito nas drogas? Uma leitura psicanalítica do fenômeno do uso de drogas na contemporaneidade: A psychoanalytical view on the phenomenon of drug use nowadays. *Ágora: Estudos em Teoria Psicanalítica, 12*(2), 333–346. https://doi.org/10.1590/S1516-14982009000200012.

Ronzani, T. M., Fuentes-Mejía, C., Mota, D. C. B., Gomide, H. P., Ferreira, M. L., & Cruvinel, E. (2019). Intervenciones breves para el abuso de sustancias en América Latina: Una revisión sistemática. *Psicologia em Estudo, 24, e44393*. https://doi.org/10.4025/psicolestud.v24i0.44393.

Santana, A. (1999). A globalização do narcotráfico. *Revista Brasileira de Política Internacional, 42*(2), 99–116. https://doi.org/10.1590/S0034-73291999000200006.

Silva, M. A. A., Andrade, A. L. M., & De Micheli, D. (2018a). Evaluation of the implementation of brief interventions to substance abuse in a Socieducative context. *Revista Psicologia em Pesquisa, 12*(1). https://doi.org/10.24879/2018001200100125.

Silva, M. L., Hatanaka, Y. F., Rondina, R. C., & Silva, N. R. (2018b). Evaluation of the repertory of social skills of users of psychoactive substances under treatment. *Cadernos Brasileiros de Terapia Ocupacional, 26*(4), 849–858. https://doi.org/10.4322/2526-8910.ctoao1633.

Silva, R. A., Messias, J. C. C., Andrade, A. L. M., Souza, J. C. R. P., & Guimarães, L. A. M. (2019). The perception of truck drivers on the use of psychoactive substances at work: An ethnographic study. *SMAD. Revista eletrônica saúde mental álcool e drogas, 15*, 1–8. https://doi.org/10.11606/issn.1806-6976.smad.2019.150461.

Tractenberg, S. G., Viola, T. W., Rosa, C. S. d. O., Donati, J. M., Francke, I. D., Pezzi, J. C., & Grassi-Oliveira, R. (2012). Exposição a trauma e transtorno de estresse pós-traumático em usuárias de crack. *Jornal Brasileiro de Psiquiatria, 61*(4), 206–213. https://doi.org/10.1590/S0047-20852012000400003.

United Nations Office on Drugs and Crime. (2012). *World drug report 2012*. Retrieved from https://www.unodc.org/documents/data-and-analysis/WDR2012/WDR_2012_web_small.pdf

United Nations Office on Drugs and Crime. (2019). *World drug report 2019*. Retrieved from https://wdr.unodc.org/wdr2019/

World Health Organization. (2018). *Global status report on alcohol and health 2018*. Retrieved from https://apps.who.int/iris/bitstream/handle/10665/274603/9789241565639-eng.pdf?ua=1

Yamauchi, L. M., Andrade, A. L. M., Pinheiro, B. O., Enumo, S. R. F., & De Micheli, D. (2019). Evaluation of the social representation of the use of alcoholic beverages by adolescents. *Estudos de Psicologia, 36*, e180098. https://doi.org/10.1590/1982-0275201936e180098.

Index

D. De Micheli et al. (eds.), *Drugs and Human Behavior*,
https://doi.org/10.1007/978-3-030-62855-0

O

Q

R

Printed by Printforce, the Netherlands